THE ENCYCLOPEDIA OF

INFECTIOUS DISEASES
THIRD EDITION

THE ENCYCLOPEDIA OF

INFECTIOUS DISEASES

THIRD EDITION

Carol Turkington

Bonnie Lee Ashby, M.D.

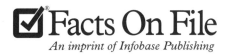

☑ Facts On File

An imprint of Infobase Publishing

The Encyclopedia of Infectious Diseases, Third Edition

Copyright © 2007, 2003, 1998 by Carol Turkington

Facts On File, Inc.
An imprint of Infobase Publishing
132 West 31st Street
New York NY 10001

ISBN-10: 0-8160-6397-4
ISBN-13: 978-0-8160-6397-0

Library of Congress Cataloging-in-Publication Data

Turkington, Carol.
The encyclopedia of infectious diseases / Carol Turkington, Bonnie Lee Ashby.—3rd ed.
p.; cm.
Includes bibliographical references and index.
ISBN 0-8160-6397-4 (hc.: alk. paper)
1. Communicable diseases—Encyclopedias. I. Ashby, Bonnie. II. Title. III. Title: Infectious diseases.
[DNLM: 1. Communicable Diseases—Encyclopedias—English.
WC 13 T939e 2007]
RC112.T87 2007
616.903—dc22   2006013795

Text and cover design by Cathy Rincon

Printed in the United States of America

VB Hermitage 10 9 8 7 6 5 4 3 2 1

This book is printed on acid-free paper.

Far better it is to dare mighty things, to win glorious triumphs
even though checkered by failure, than to take rank with
those poor spirits who neither enjoy much nor suffer much
because they live in the grey twilight that
knows not victory nor defeat.

—Theodore Roosevelt

For
William M. Roulston
(1948–1997)
In loving memory

CONTENTS

FOREWORD

In 1969, U.S. Surgeon General William H. Stew_ard told Congress that "the time has come to close the book on infectious diseases." Unfortunately, his optimism was unfounded. Today the health of the world's population continues to be threatened by infections ranging from such new entities as the avian influenza virus to mad cow disease. Humans face ever more insidious risks from potential bioterrorism, such as with anthrax. At the same time, many kinds of recognizable bacteria continue to mutate, such as the deadly versions of streptococcal and staphylococcal bacteria that have become completely resistant to most antibiotics.

As more awareness of health conditions throughout the world is gained, more is also learned about the shifting face of the microbial population that exists within and around us. The diseases caused by these invisible foes pose an ever-growing threat that requires improvement of the public health infrastructure at the local, state, and federal levels. The health of the American people is linked to the health of people in other nations. Infectious diseases can and do spread rapidly around the globe, and global surveillance for emerging infections is vital to public health.

In the field of microbiology there can be no patriotism and no isolationism. The entire human race is at equal risk from the denizens of the invisible space. Humans are, in fact, a biochemical species, with a life force controlled by chemical reactions. Each of our cells functions at a molecular level with all other cellular and subcellular entities. The computer as a medical research tool is now indispensable in the study of the human interaction with the microbiological world, when one considers that a single gene description would be hundreds of pages long.

For all the historical discussions of the Black Plague, the devastation brought by measles, by smallpox, TB, malaria, and influenza, nothing has compared to the social and scientific impact of the AIDS virus. No other single entity has been more thoroughly researched or written about in human history. I was barely into my medical career as an infectious disease specialist when the AIDS epidemic struck, and, for the next 18 years, the disease I treated most, the patients for whom I spent the most time caring, my greatest output of emotional angst was directed toward acquired immune deficiency syndrome. I went to more funerals than I want to count and made countless house calls for dozens of young people who were dying from AIDS.

AIDS in an insidious and horrible disease, and yet even today, it is not the kind of medical condition patients feel they can freely discuss with most people. Unlike more commonplace and socially acceptable infections such as the flu, where you can complain, for example, that you caught a bug after a long airplane flight, AIDS is a disease that carries profound stigma. It is bad enough to be fatally ill, but to be shunned because of that illness is infinitely worse.

Despite the recent development of new antiviral medicines, AIDS continues to spread rapidly throughout all parts of the world. Estimated numbers of infected people are mind boggling. At the end of 2001, 40 million people around the world were infected with AIDS, with 4 million newly diagnosed each year. In sub-Saharan Africa alone, 28 million people struggle with the disease, which has had devastating effects on the culture.

The identification in the early nineties of the structure of the AIDS virus made it possible to construct the drugs we use to treat it today and to develop drugs for use against many other viral diseases. In fact, the struggle against the AIDS epidemic has indeed led to many advances in medicine in general. The new group of AIDS drugs will, in the long run, improve the ability to treat viral diseases and will benefit humanity's ongoing fight with these invisible, often deadly residents of the cellular and subcellular terrain.

Scientists understand the people must try to live symbiotically with their coinhabitants on this Earth. Yet, efforts to fight off infection have created a dilemma. Microbes will continue to survive despite antibiotics because they replicate rapidly and genetically mutate frequently. As a result of the use of antibiotics, ever-more deadly types of bacteria and new illnesses are unwittingly being created.

Such a national problem is a diarrheal disease caused by the toxin produced by a normal bacteria in the bowel after a dose of antibiotics is given. This disease, *C. diff colitis*, (*Clostridium difficile* colitis), can be mild or so severe that colonic perforation and death can occur. The body contains both beneficial bacteria necessary for good health and harmful bacteria such as *C. difficile*. In healthy people, millions of good bacteria keep the *C. diff* under control, but when an antibiotic is taken, bacteria of all types are killed—both good and bad. If the *C. diff* survives, it is possible that these germs will overpopulate the colon. When this occurs, one gets *C. diff* colitis. Although it is treated with specific antibiotics, in the end, the bacteria are likely to win.

Another such phenomenon is the spread across the country of staph USA300, which causes boils and abscesses all over the skin and is easily acquired from one person to another. This bacteria appears to have borrowed genetic characteristics from an otherwise rather harmless organism but became lethal. USA300 was first isolated in September 2000, and it has since been linked to outbreaks of skin and soft tissue infections in healthy individuals in at least 21 states, as well as in Canada and Europe. Very few antibiotics help, and treatment options are dwindling.

Humans can never be smug or complacent about their place on Earth. In the Far East there originated a flu virus in chickens that is sweeping the globe and that carries the potential to wipe out half the human race if it obtains the ability to be transmitted among people. I would like to think that scientists around the world will win the race against the mutation rate of the bird flu virus and develop a combative vaccine or a treatment in time.

—Bonnie Lee Ashby, M.D., F.A.C.P.

ACKNOWLEDGMENTS

This book would not have been possible without the cooperation of countless men and women whose generosity of spirit contributed to the massive task of keeping track of the ever-evolving global picture on infectious disease.

Thanks to everyone who gave time and effort at the National Institutes of Health, the medical libraries of the National Library of Medicine, the Hershey Medical Center, and the University of Pennsylvania Medical Center. Thanks to staffers at Pharmaceutical Research and Manufacturers of America, to Eli Lilly, Astra USA, Bristol-Myers, Ciba-Geigy, Hoffmann-LaRoche, Pfizer, Smith-Kline Beecham, and Solvay Pharmaceuticals. Thanks also to the staffs of the Centers for Disease Control and Prevention, the National Institute of Allergy and Infectious Diseases, the World Health Organization and its Collaborating Centers on AIDS, the Food Safety and Inspection Service, the American Public Health Association, the International Research Foundation for Helicobacter and Intestinal Immunology, Allan Brownstein at the American Liver Foundation, the American Leprosy Missions, the National AIDS Clearinghouse, the National Vaccine Compensation Program, the Emerging Infections Information Network, the WHO Division of Control of Tropical Diseases, the WHO Emergine and Other Communicable Diseases Surveillance and Control, the National Center for Infectious Disease, the folks at the Bug Bytes Web site, and the American Lyme Disease Foundation.

Finally, my thanks as ever to my agents Bert Holtje, Gene Brissie and Ed Claflin, to the very patient James Chambers, Vanessa Nittoli, and Sarah Fogarty at Facts On File, and to Michael and Kara.

INTRODUCTION

Humans survive amid a dizzying sea of pathogens, awash in more than 1,400 germs and parasites capable of causing disease. The sobering realization is that science is not winning the fight against infectious disease. In this pathogenic war, a stalemate is perhaps the best for which we can hope, for even as drug companies devise new antibiotics, stronger antivirals, and more effective vaccines, germs continue to mutate, become resistant to standard treatment, and threaten to overwhelm those among the population least able to withstand the onslaught.

In the past 25 years, 38 completely new human germs have emerged, and three-quarters of these—including AIDS, avian flu, SARS, and new-variant CJD (human mad cow disease)—have originated in animals. Experts say that at least one new disease is jumping the species barrier from animals to human beings every year, exposing people to emerging infections at an unprecedented rate. This ability of animal germs to infect humans is likely caused by a number of changes in human behavior and the environment, including intensive agriculture, bush hunting, extensive international travel, and global warming. As humans interact with their environment in new ways, they are becoming exposed to novel pathogens against which they have no natural immunity. The deadliest examples of these include HIV, thought to have started out as an African monkey or ape virus, the Ebola and Marburg hemorrhagic fevers, the SARS coronavirus, the West Nile virus now endemic in the United States, and most frightening of all—the H5N1 bird flu that could one day cause the next worldwide influenza pandemic.

As science faces these newest challenges, having the most up-to-date reference information about infectious disease becomes more vital than ever. This third edition of *The Encyclopedia of Infectious Disease* has been designed as a guide and reference to a wide range of terms related to infectious diseases and includes extensive appendixes with information and addresses for organizations that deal with infection. However, it is not a substitute for prompt assessment and treatment by experts trained in the diagnosis of infectious disease.

In this revised edition, we have tried to present the latest information in the field, based on the newest information research and current government approvals of new treatments. Readers will find a number of new topics, including entries on new vaccines, such as the new vaccine against genital warts, against rotavirus, and a new booster (Boostrix Tdap) for children aged 10 to 18, which adds protection against whooping cough to the traditional booster against tetanus and diphtheria.

New overview topics have been added, including entries on food safety and natural disasters, neonatal infections, lung and respiratory infections, chlamydial infections, parasitic infections, immunizations for influenza, and stomach and intestinal infections.

New and emerging diseases are always a concern in the field of infectious disease. This volume includes entries on new discoveries such as defensins, along with a variety of new and emerging viruses, including Marburg virus, Napa virus, norovirus, Nipah virus, nanobacteria, Powassan (POW) virus, *Mycobacterium nebraskanses,* methicillin resistant staph A, and the newest information on the bird flu virus spreading throughout the world.

Other new entries discuss conditions and diseases, such as

- post-Lyme syndrome
- subacute sclerosing panencephalitis (SSPE)
- bronchiolitis obliterans with organizing pneumonia (BOOP)
- fungal pneumonia
- hemolytic uremic syndrome
- gram-negative bacterial pneumonia
- mycoplasma pneumonia
- *Clostridium perfringens* food poisoning
- gram-negative pneumonia
- SARS (severe acute respiratory syndrome)
- streptococcal toxic shock syndrome
- West Nile virus poliomyelitis

There are updates on terrorist-related infectious disease information in the entries about smallpox, bubonic plague, dioxin, and anthrax. At the same time, vaccines are always being developed, discarded, or improved upon—either due to fears of terrorist attacks or approaching pandemics. This revision includes the latest information on a variety of new vaccines, including new shingles prevention vaccines related to the chicken-pox shot and new or improved vaccines for rotavirus and papillomavirus (a precursor to cervical cancer).

Many entries have been almost totally revised, including new information on the disease, vaccines, or treatments for anthrax, avian flu, mad cow disease (including the new cases diagnosed in U.S. cows), chicken pox, cryptosporidium, Cyclospora, cholera, *Clostridium difficile,* Congo fever, Coxsackie virus, cryptosporidiosis, guinea worm disease, ECHOvirus, hemolytic uremic syndrome, hepatitis A, B, and C, mad cow, Marburg virus, bacterial meningitis, polio, POW virus, prion diseases, smallpox, chikungunya fever, and vancomycin-resistant enterovirus.

In addition, the majority of entries have been updated with the newest statistics and information on treatment for AIDS, anthrax, amebiasis, aspergillosis, bacillary angiomatosis, chancroid, B. cereus, ciguatera, clostridium, genital herpes, hospital-acquired infections, Lassa fever, Legionnaires' disease, Lyme disease, malaria, measles, pelvic inflammatory disease, penicillin, pinworms, pyelonephritis, rabies, syphilis, Norwalk virus, yellow fever, and tuberculosis.

All appendixes have been completely updated; new organizations have been added and the latest addresses, phone numbers, and Web sites added and checked for accuracy. New antibiotics have been added to the antibiotics page.

Information in this book comes from the most up-to-date sources available and includes some of the most recent research in new and emerging infectious diseases. Readers should keep in mind, however, that changes occur very rapidly in this field. References have been provided for readers who seek additional sources of information. All entries are cross-referenced, and appendixes provide additional information.

—Carol Turkington
Cumru, Pennsylvania

ENTRIES A to Z

abscess An inflammatory pus-containing nodule that is usually caused by a bacterial infection. The pus is made up of dead and live microorganisms and dead tissue from white blood cells carried to the area to fight the infection.

An abscess may either grow larger or smaller depending on whether the white blood cells or the bacteria win the fight.

While bacteria are the most common cause of abscesses, fungal infections sometimes cause abscesses as well.

Symptoms and Diagnostic Path

Abscesses are often found in the soft tissue beneath the skin (such as the armpit or groin), where a large number of lymph glands are located, or deep in the brain.

Abscesses can usually be diagnosed by sight, although a CAT or MRI scan may be used to confirm the diagnosis.

Treatment Options and Outlook

Antibiotics are usually prescribed to treat a bacterial infection, and antifungal agents can treat fungal infections. However, the lining of the abscess cavity tends to cut down on the amount of the drug that can pass from the blood into the source of the infection. Therefore, the cavity itself needs to be drained by cutting through the lining. This allows the pus to escape through a drainage tube, or by leaving the cavity open to the skin. Many abscesses heal after simple drainage; others require both drainage and drug treatment.

Acanthamoeba infection *Acanthamoeba* are microscopic amoeba commonly found in the environment, which can cause a serious infection in brain, lungs, or eyes. *Acanthamoeba* can enter the skin through a cut, wound, or through the nostrils. Once inside the body, the amoeba can travel to the lungs and through the bloodstream to other parts of the body, especially the brain and spinal cord.

Through improper storage, handling, and disinfection of contact lenses, the amoeba can enter the eye and cause a serious infection. The risk of infection is higher for those who make their own contact lens cleaning solution. Acanthamoeba enter the eye via contact lenses or through a corneal cut or sore, triggering infection or a corneal ulcer.

The species of *Acanthamoeba* that infect humans include *A. culbertsoni, A. polyphaga, A. castellanii, A. healyi (A. astronyxis), A. hatchetti,* and *A. rhysodes.*

Acanthamoeba are found worldwide in the soil and dust, in freshwater sources such as lakes, rivers, and hot springs and in hot tubs, or in brackish water and seawater. Amoeba also can be found in heating, venting, and air conditioner units, humidifiers, dialysis units, and contact lens equipment. The microbes have been found in the nose and throat of healthy people as well as those with compromised immune systems.

Symptoms and Diagnostic Path

Species of *Acanthamoeba* can cause skin lesions or a body-wide infection, and can lead to a serious, often deadly infection called granulomatous amebic ENCEPHALITIS (GAE). GAE causes headaches, stiff neck, nausea and vomiting, tiredness, confusion, lack of attention to people and surroundings, loss of balance and bodily control, seizures, and hallucinations. This condition is usually fatal.

Treatment Options and Outlook

Eye and skin infections are generally treatable with antibiotics. Although most cases of brain infection with *Acanthamoeba* have been fatal, a few patients have recovered from the infection with proper treatment.

Risk Factors and Preventive Measures

Eye infections may be prevented by using commercially prepared contact lens cleaning solution rather than making homemade solutions. There is little that can be done to prevent skin and body infection.

Acinetobacter A genus of aerobic bacteria, of the family Neisseriaceae. The genus do not produce spores or move of their own accord. Found everywhere in nature, some members of the family can cause illness in humans.

Although many species of *Acinetobacter* can cause infection, *A. baumannii* is one of the most common and can be linked to many hospital acquired infections including skin and wound infections, PNEUMONIA, and MENINGITIS. *A. lwoffi*, in particular, is responsible for most cases of meningitis caused by *Acinetobacter*. Because most species are resistant to older antibiotics, a combination of aminoglycoside and ticarcillin is usually recommended for treatment.

acquired immunodeficiency syndrome (AIDS) A fatal viral disease of the immune system for which there is no immunization and no cure. The disease has a crippling effect on the human immune defense system, rendering the patient unable to fight off many types of other infections, and prone to certain cancers. Eventually, these infections and cancers in themselves may be fatal. First identified in 1980, AIDS was soon recognized as epidemic throughout the world. Although initially AIDS cases occurred primarily in homosexual males in the United States, more recently the majority of new cases are being diagnosed in the heterosexual population. Caused by HIV (HUMAN IMMUNODEFICIENCY VIRUS), infection has now spread to every country in the world and affected more than 40 million people worldwide by the end of 2003. The disease has been particularly devastating in sub-Saharan Africa. At the same time, the proportion of adult women among those infected with HIV is increasing.

More than 1.1 million people in the United States have been infected with HIV, with about 25 percent unaware of their condition. U.S. government statistics indicate that the rate of HIV diagnosis decreased among African Americans from 2001 to 2004; however, the rate of HIV diagnosis among African Americans remained disproportionately high. In 2004, the rate among African Americans was still 8.4 times higher than among Caucasians.

The cumulative estimated number of diagnoses of AIDS through 2003 in the United States is 929,985, according to the CDC. In 2003, the estimated number of deaths of persons with AIDS was 18,017, including 17,934 adults and adolescents and 83 children under age 13.

The 10 states reporting the most number of cases (from most to least) are New York, California, Florida, Texas, Georgia, Pennsylvania, Illinois, Maryland, New Jersey, and North Carolina.

No one knows where the human virus originated. One theory is that the virus existed undetected for centuries in isolated African villages. Since a person can harbor the virus for years before developing AIDS, and because rural Africans often contract many diseases that kill them at an early age, it is possible that the virus could have been infecting people for a very long time without being identified. Other scientists believe the virus somehow "jumped" from infected African monkeys to humans fairly recently, since viruses in monkeys are genetically similar to the HIV. However, trying to place the origin of HIV infection in Africa angers some, who feel this is blaming Africa for the AIDS problem.

The earliest documented case of HIV infection was found in a 1959 blood sample from central Africa. Epidemiologists believe the virus may have traveled from Africa to the United States during the mid-1970s, where it was first transmitted via anal intercourse among gay men in New York and San Francisco. The Rwanda capital of Kigali and the capital of Zaire both reported epidemics in 1980, and by 1982 Uganda and Zambia reported similar epidemics.

Within 10 years, U.S. scientists began to notice among young gay men an outbreak of formerly rare diseases such as PNEUMOCYSTIS CARINII pneumonia and Kaposi's sarcoma that had previously been found only in those with damaged immune systems. Next, IV drug users began to come down with the disease, together with hemophiliacs and others who received blood transfusions or blood products.

By 1991, the cumulative number of cases from 52 African countries was almost 93,000, increasing to an estimated 7.5 million people infected with HIV in sub-Saharan Africa by 1993. By 1994, scientists reported as many as 30 different strains of HIV that often escape conventional tests to detect their presence in blood. (The new strains, first isolated in Cameroon, have not yet been detected in the United States.)

HIV (also called the AIDS virus) is found in all body fluids of infected people. However, only blood, semen, vaginal discharge, and breast milk have enough of the virus to spread it readily to others. The virus progressively destroys the body's ability to fight germs and malignant cells. It attaches to and attacks the helper T cells in the white blood cells. White blood cells are a part of the immune system and help fight infection and disease. When the immune system is damaged, it cannot keep the body healthy. In AIDS, T cells die slowly as the HIV invades and destroys them.

HIV is the third of five human RETROVIRUSES identified since 1980, although scientists believe there are more retroviruses in existence. (A retrovirus contains an enzyme—reverse transcriptase—that converts viral RNA into a DNA copy that becomes part of the host cell's DNA.) HIV is part of a class of retroviruses known as lentiviruses, ordinarily associated with arthritis and anemia. (Lentiviruses are retroviruses that cause slowly progressive, usually fatal diseases.)

In the case of the HIV, the virus attaches itself to the cells that control the immune system (the T lymphocytes). Once inside this T cell, the virus releases its RNA with a chemical that allows it to join the cell's own DNA. All offspring of this altered T cell therefore contains the virus's genetic code. The T cell produces new HIVs, which destroy the host cell as they are created.

HIV is spread by sexual contact with an infected person, by needle-sharing among injecting drug users, or (now rarely) through blood or blood-prod-uct transfusions. An infected mother may spread the virus to her unborn baby before or during birth or during breast-feeding. In the health care setting, workers have been infected with HIV after being stuck with a needle containing HIV-infected blood, or (rarely) when infected blood enters an open cut or splashes into a mucous membrane. There has been only one demonstrated case of patients being infected by a health care worker, which involved transmission from an infected dentist to six of his patients.

A person cannot get AIDS from someone else by touching, sneezing or coughing, sharing eating or drinking utensils, or from a swimming pool or other public place. AIDS is not spread from tears, urine, sweat, or saliva. In thousands of households where families have cared for AIDS patients, AIDS has not been transmitted via sharing laundry, kitchen or bathroom facilities, meals, eating utensils, drinking cups or glasses.

There has been no known risk of HIV transmission to coworkers, clients, or consumers. Food service workers known to be HIV infected need not be restricted from work, unless they have other infections such as diarrhea or HEPATITIS A, which are readily contagious.

HIV has not been transmitted through closed-mouthed kissing, although open-mouthed kissing is not recommended because of the slight risk of contact with blood. No case of AIDS has ever been reported that occurred from any kind of kissing.

While many people have been concerned about the possibility of transmission via insect bites, studies have shown no evidence that insects can transmit HIV, even in areas where there are many cases of AIDS and large populations of insects. This could be because when an insect bites a person, it does not inject blood into the victim; instead, it injects its own saliva. Some diseases (such as MALARIA or YELLOW FEVER) are transmitted by saliva, but HIV lives for only a short time within an insect. Even if a mosquito carried the virus, it does not become infected and cannot transmit the virus to the next person it bites.

Symptoms and Diagnostic Path

A person who has been infected with the AIDS virus may not have any symptoms for months or even years. Many patients remain relatively healthy from eight to 11 years after being infected. However, although there are no symptoms during this period, the virus is multiplying, infecting, and killing cells of the immune system, especially those cells that are the primary infection fighters (the CD4+ or T4 cells).

Once the immune system becomes weakened and vulnerable, a person infected with HIV can develop a number of symptoms, including lack of energy; weight loss; fevers and sweats; frequent yeast infections; skin rashes or flaky skin; short-term memory loss; and mouth, genital, or anal sores from herpes infections.

Eventually, the immune system is so debilitated during the advanced stage of HIV infection that a diagnosis of AIDS is appropriate. A person is diagnosed with AIDS when he or she has less than 200 CD4+ cells per microliter of blood. The definition also includes 26 conditions that are common in advanced HIV disease but that rarely occur in healthy people, most of which are caused by bacteria, viruses, fungi, parasites, and other organisms. Some of these conditions include TUBERCULOSIS, CYTOMEGALOVIRUS, *Pneumocystis carinii*, TOXOPLASMOSIS, and MYCOBACTE-RIUM AVIUM COMPLEX. Opportunistic infections are common in people with AIDS.

Some of the common symptoms of full-blown AIDS include cough and shortness of breath; seizures and lack of coordination; difficult or painful swallowing; confusion and forgetfulness; severe and persistent diarrhea; fever; vision loss; nausea, abdominal cramps, and vomiting; weight loss; extreme fatigue; severe headaches with neck stiffness; and coma.

In addition, people with AIDS are vulnerable to a number of cancers, such as Kaposi's sarcoma, cervical cancer, and lymphoma (cancers of the immune system). Kaposi's sarcoma is characterized by round, brown, reddish or purple spots in the skin or in the mouth.

HIV infection is diagnosed by detecting the presence of disease-fighting proteins, called antibodies, in the blood. These HIV antibodies are usually not apparent until between one and three months after infection. Early testing is important for anyone who has been exposed to the HIV virus, because experts believe the earlier treatment is begun, the better the person's chances of survival.

Two different types of antibody tests are available: a screening test called the enzyme-linked immunoassay (ELISA) and a confirming test called the Western blot. *Both of these tests can be negative for up to three months after exposure to HIV, even if the person has been infected.* If there is significant reason to believe that a person may have been infected during these first months, another more accurate test can be performed that directly looks for the actual HIV particles in the blood.

A diagnostic blood test was developed in 1985. The presence of HIV is determined by this blood test, which shows antibodies to HIV. The disease is defined as a positive AIDS test and a T-cell count less than 200. (A healthy person's T-cell count should be more than 440.) There are a number of different HIV home collection test systems and kits that have appeared on the market, available through the Internet and through magazine or newspaper promotions. However, only one HIV-1 home collection test system is currently approved by the U.S. Food and Drug Administration (FDA): Home Access Express HIV-1 Test System manufactured by Home Access Health Corporation.

This approved system uses a simple finger prick process for home blood collection which results in dried blood spots on special paper. The dried blood spots are mailed to a laboratory with a confidential and anonymous personal identification number (PIN), and analyzed by trained clinicians in a certified medical laboratory using the same procedures that are used for samples taken in a doctor's office. The results are obtained by the purchaser through a toll-free telephone number using the PIN, and post-test counseling is provided by telephone when results are obtained.

Other HIV-1 home test kits have not been approved by the FDA for use and marketing in the United States. These unapproved HIV home test kits claim to detect antibodies to HIV-1 (the virus that causes AIDS) in blood or saliva, providing results in the home in 15 minutes or less. The advertisers of the unapproved HIV home test kits claim that the presence of a visual indicator (such as a red dot) within five to 15 minutes shows a positive result for HIV infection. These unapproved test kits use a simple finger prick process for home blood collection or a special sponge for saliva collection; the sample is then added to a plastic testing device containing a special type of paper. A developing solution is added to determine if the sample is positive for HIV. The samples are not sent to a laboratory for professional analysis. Although this approach may seem faster and simpler, it may provide a less accurate result than can be achieved using an approved test, which is analyzed under more controlled conditions than is possible in the home.

Treatment Options and Outlook

While at present there is no cure for AIDS, intensive research has produced new medications that can prolong life. A number of medicines are used to treat AIDS: antiviral drugs, prophylactic medicines to protect against certain infections, and other drugs to fight infections and cancer.

Still, after a diagnosis of AIDS, the average survival time is two to three years. Over the past 10 years, several drugs to fight both the HIV infection and its associated infections and cancers have become available.

Atripla This brand-new once-a-day pill combines three drugs in a cocktail therapy. Approved in 2006, the medicine will cost more than $1,000 a month but will make it easier for patients to stick to a treatment regimen.

Reverse transcriptase inhibitors These drugs interrupt the virus from making copies of itself. These drugs are AZT (zidovudine, brand name Retrovir), ddC (zalcitabine, brand name Hivid; dideoxyinosine), d4T (stavudine, brand name Zerit), and 3TC (lamivudine, brand name Epivir). These drugs may slow the spread of HIV in the body and delay the onset of opportunistic infections.

Nonnucleoside reverse transcriptase inhibitors (NNRTIS) These medications are combined with other drugs to help keep the virus from multiplying. They include delavirdine (Rescriptor) and nevirapine (Viramune).

Protease inhibitors These medications interrupt virus replication at a later step in its life cycle. These include ritonavir (Norvir), a lopinavir and ritonavir combination (Kaletra), saquinavir (Invirase), indinavir sulphate (Crixivan), amprenavir (Agenerase), and nelfinavir (Viracept). Using both types of drugs reduces the chances of developing resistance in the virus.

Fusion inhibitors This is the newest class of anti-HIV drugs. The first drug of this class (enfuvirtide [Fuzeon]) has recently been approved in the United States. Fusion inhibitors block HIV from entering the human immune cell.

Currently available antiretroviral drugs cannot cure HIV infection or AIDS, and all these drugs have severe side effects. Some of the nucleoside RT inhibitors may deplete red or white blood cells, especially when taken in the later stages of the disease; some may also cause pancreatic inflammation and painful nerve damage. There have been reports of other severe reactions, including liver failure and death, to some of the antiretroviral nucleoside drugs when used alone or in combination.

The most common side effects associated with protease inhibitors include nausea, diarrhea, and other gastrointestinal symptoms. In addition, protease inhibitors can interact with other drugs and cause serious side effects. They also cause changes in body fat and serum lipids.

A major factor in reducing the number of deaths from AIDS in this country by 47 percent has been highly active antiretroviral therapy (HAART). HAART is a treatment regimen that combines reverse transcriptase inhibitors and protease inhibitors to treat patients who are newly infected with HIV as well as AIDS patients.

While HAART is not a cure for AIDS, it has greatly improved the health of many people with AIDS, reducing the amount of virus circulating in the blood to nearly undetectable levels. However, researchers have shown that HAART cannot eradicate HIV entirely from the body; it still lives in the lymph glands, for example.

A number of drugs are available to help treat opportunistic infections to which people with HIV are especially prone. These drugs include foscarnet (Foscavir) and ganciclovir (Vitrasert, Cytovene) to treat cytomegalovirus eye infections, fluconazole (Diflucan) to treat yeast and other fungal infections, and trimethoprim/sulfamethoxazole (Bactrim, Septra) to treat *Pneumocystis carinii* pneumonia (PCP).

Therefore, in addition to antiretroviral therapy, it is possible to treat adults infected with HIV whose CD4+ T-cell counts drop below 200 and become prone to other infections. Drugs can prevent the occurrence of PCP, one of the most common and deadly infections associated with HIV. Children also can receive PCP preventive therapy when their CD4+ T-cell counts drop to levels considered below normal for their age group. Regardless of their CD4+ T-cell counts, HIV-infected children and adults who have survived an episode of PCP take drugs for the rest of their lives to prevent a recurrence of the pneumonia.

HIV-infected individuals who develop Kaposi's sarcoma or other cancers can be treated with radiation, chemotherapy, or injections of alpha interferon, a genetically engineered naturally occurring protein.

Researchers are currently working on 28 new HIV vaccines, and many drugs for HIV- or AIDS-associated infections are being developed or tested. Researchers are also studying how the HIV virus damages the immune system and are trying to understand how the disease progresses in different people.

In addition, scientists are testing chemical barriers that can be used during sex to prevent HIV transmission.

Risk Factors and Preventive Measures

Abstinence from sexual contact and not sharing needles is the only sure way to prevent AIDS. Other than that, using a latex (rubber) condom during sexual intercourse is the best protection against the sexual transmission of HIV. Latex condoms should always be used for oral, anal, and vaginal sex in any relationship or if there is a chance that either partner is infected. Condom manufacturers in the United States electronically test all condoms for holes and weak spots. In addition, the FDA requires that manufacturers use a water test to examine samples from each batch for leakage. Only water-based lubricants should be used with latex condoms because oil-based lubricants, such as petroleum jelly, weaken natural rubber.

For people allergic to latex, the FDA has approved several polyurethane condoms, which are comparable to latex as a barrier to sperm and HIV virus.

In the United States, blood and blood products have been tested since 1985 for the AIDS virus and are considered safe. In addition, the FDA inspects the more than 3,000 donor centers where blood and blood components are collected and processed. The risk of HIV infection from transfusions has dropped from one in 2,500 units of blood in 1985 to one in 440,000 to 640,000 units by the end of 1995.

Outside the body, the HIV is easily killed by common disinfectants such as alcohol or peroxide.

actinomycosis A bacterial infection caused by *Actinomyces israelii* or *Arachnia propionica*, bacteria normally present in the mouth and tonsils that can cause infection when introduced into broken tissue. It is possible to transmit the bacteria via a human bite.

Abdominal actinomycosis usually follows an acute inflammatory process in the stomach or intestines, such as APPENDICITIS. Generalized actinomycosis may involve the skin, brain, liver, and urogenital system. A pelvic form of abdominal actinomycosis may occur with the use of an intrauterine contraceptive device.

Symptoms and Diagnostic Path

The most common form of the disease affects the mouth and jaw, causing a painful swelling. Small openings later develop on the skin of the face, discharging pus and characteristic yellow granules. Poor oral hygiene may contribute to this particular manifestation.

A diagnosis is usually confirmed by the presence of the microorganism.

Treatment Options and Outlook

All forms of the disease can be treated with PENICILLIN, which is usually successful, although treatment may be needed for several months in severe infections. Penicillin is the drug of choice, but other antibiotics are also effective. Adequate surgical drainage is important, together with bed rest and proper diet.

adenovirus A family of 49 DNA-containing viruses identified by sequential letters and numbers that cause infections of the eyes, upper respiratory tract, and gastrointestinal system. Whereas some adenoviruses attack only animals, the ones that inhabit humans account for 10 percent of all respiratory illness from mild flu to PNEUMONIA.

After the illness fades away, the virus persists in the tonsils, adenoids, and other lymph tissue. Adenoviruses do not become latent (like the HERPES viruses) but instead reproduce constantly and slowly. It is possible to be infected more than once with adenoviruses, because there are many different types.

The virus was first isolated in adenoids in the 1950s, but the virus probably was causing respiratory illnesses long before that. Respiratory disease caused by adenoviruses has been a problem since the Civil War and was known as acute respiratory disease (ARD) during World War II. There is no vaccine against this virus family. Adenoviral infections affect infants and young children much more often than adults; widespread respiratory infections and diarrhea caused by adenovirus often sweep through child-care centers and schools. Although these infections can occur at any time of the year, respiratory tract disease caused by adenovirus is more common in late winter, spring, and early summer. However, CONJUNCTIVITIS and pharyngo-conjunctival fever caused by adenovirus tend to affect older children mostly in the summer, when they are swimming in pools and lakes.

Although characteristics of the adenoviruses vary, they are all transmitted by direct contact, fecal-oral transmission, and sometimes via water. Some types are capable of establishing persistent infections in tonsils, adenoids, and intestines of infected hosts without exhibiting any symptoms; shedding can occur for months or years. Epidemics of febrile disease with conjunctivitis are associated with waterborne transmission of some adenovirus types, usually involving swimming pools and small lakes.

Although outbreaks of adenovirus-associated respiratory disease have been more common in the late winter, spring, and early summer; these infections can occur throughout the year.

Symptoms and Diagnostic Path

Symptoms may vary depending on which part of the body is affected by the particular adenovirus.

Respiratory disease If the virus infects the respiratory tract, the most common symptom is a fever. Other flu-like symptoms may include sore throat; a congested, runny nose; cough; swollen lymph glands; and possibly a middle EAR INFECTION (otitis media). Adenovirus also can infect the lower respiratory tract, causing BRONCHIOLITIS, CROUP, or viral PNEUMONIA.

Stomach Pain Adenovirus can inflame the stomach and the small and large intestines, causing watery diarrhea, vomiting, headache, fever, and abdominal cramps.

Eye Infections Adenovirus can cause pinkeye (conjunctivitis), a mild inflammation of the membranes covering the eye and inner surfaces of the eyelids. Symptoms include red eyes, discharge, tearing, and the feeling that there is something in the eye. Keratoconjunctivitis is a more severe infection that involves both the membrane covering the eye and the cornea (the transparent front part of the eye). This type of adenoviral infection is extremely contagious and occurs most often in older children and young adults, with symptoms of red eyes, photophobia, sensitivity to light, tearing, and pain.

Treatment Options and Outlook

Most infections are mild. Because there is no treatment specifically tailored to this virus, serious adenovirus illness can be managed only by treating symptoms and complications.

Risk Factors and Preventive Measures

There are vaccines for adenovirus serotypes 4 and 7, but these are available only to prevent ARD among military recruits. Strict attention to good infection-control practices is effective for stopping outbreaks of adenovirus-associated disease in hospitals. Adequately chlorinating pools can prevent swimming pool-associated outbreaks of adenovirus conjunctivitis.

Aedes A genus of mosquito found widely in tropical and subtropical areas. Several species are capable of transmitting to humans disease-causing organisms that cause a variety of illnesses, including DENGUE FEVER, EASTERN EQUINE ENCEPHALITIS, St. Louis encephalitis (see ENCEPHALITIS, ST. LOUIS), and YELLOW FEVER.

Aedes mosquitoes are painful and persistent biters when searching for a blood meal early in the morning, at dusk, and into the evening. Some, however, will bite during the day, especially on overcast days and in the shade. *Aedes* mosquitoes are strong fliers and are known to fly many miles from their breeding sources.

Aedes albopictus mosquito   Also called the Asian tiger, this type of mosquito can transmit the dengue and YELLOW FEVER viruses. This mosquito entered Houston, Texas, after hitching a ride with a used tire shipment from Japan in 1985. It is now established in 26 states and in 866 countries worldwide.

Although this mosquito has not yet caused any known cases of DENGUE FEVER in the United States, it was found to carry another dangerous arbovirus—EASTERN EQUINE ENCEPHALITIS.

It is found as far north in the United States as Chicago, and an infestation was found in Minnesota in 1997. It has been reported in the northeast as far as York County, Pennsylvania and in 1995, it was found in three counties in New Jersey. It has appeared as far south as Cameron County, Texas, and Monroe County, Florida. In the west, it has occurred in Lubbock, Texas, and Omaha, Nebraska.

Limited infestations in at least three northern states (Indiana, Minnesota, and Ohio) apparently have been eliminated through persistent control efforts by state and local agencies together with severe winter temperatures. Nonetheless, other areas in Indiana and Ohio continue to be infested.

During 1994, Georgia became the first state to document *A. albopictus* in all counties of the state and has since been joined by Florida, South Carolina, and Tennessee.

Aedes japonicus   An Asian mosquito that may transmit WEST NILE VIRUS and Japanese ENCEPHALITIS that was first detected in the United States in New York and New Jersey in 1998. Since that time, *Aedes japonicus* has been found in six other states: Ohio, Maryland, Connecticut, Massachusetts, Pennsylvania, and Virginia. Elsewhere, the mosquito can be found in Japan, Korea, Okinawa, Taiwan, South China, and Hong Kong.

Larvae are found in a wide variety locations, such as used tires, and especially at sites that are shaded and contain water. Eggs can survive several months under dry conditions.

The adult female of *A. japonicus* is a medium-sized dark- to black-brown mosquito, with white scales on body and legs. Adults rest in wooded areas and prefer to bite during the day.

AIDS   See ACQUIRED IMMUNODEFICIENCY SYNDROME.

alveolar hydatid disease   See ECHINOCOCCOSIS.

amebiasis (amoebiasis)   Also known as amebic dysentery, this infection of the liver or intestine is caused by the parasite *Entamoeba histolytica*, normally found in the human intestinal tract and feces. It is most serious in infants, the elderly, and those with impaired immune systems.

In the United States, amebiasis most often occurs among immigrants from developing countries or in people who have traveled to developing countries. It also may occur among institutionalized people who live in poor sanitary conditions. Men who have sex with men can become infected and can get sick from the infection, but they often do not have symptoms. Some people carry the parasite for weeks to years, often without symptoms.

Food can be tainted with the protozoa through fecal contamination, such as when infected food handlers do not wash their hands after using the bathroom. A person contracts the disease by swallowing the cyst stage of the parasite in contaminated food or water. The disease can also be spread by person-to-person contact, especially during anal intercourse.

Symptoms and Diagnostic Path

If there are symptoms, they may include tenderness over the abdomen and liver, abdominal pain, jaundice, loose morning stools, diarrhea, nervousness, loss of appetite, weight loss, and fatigue. Symptoms usually occur from a few days to a few months after exposure, but usually within two to four weeks. Most people exposed to the disease do not become seriously ill.

Rarely, the parasite will invade the body beyond the intestines, causing a more serious infection.

The disease is diagnosed by examining stools under a microscope; multiple samples of fresh feces may have to be studied because the number of parasites changes from day to day and they are hard to see.

However, diagnosis of amebiasis can be very difficult because other parasites can look like *E. histolytica* under a microscope. In particular, *E. histolytica* and another amoeba, *Entamoeba dispar,* look the same under a microscope; however, *E. dispar* is about 10 times more common. Unlike *E. histolytica* infection, which sometimes makes people sick, infection with *E. dispar* never causes disease and therefore does not need to be treated. Therefore, patients who have been diagnosed with *E. histolytica* infection but who feel fine might be infected with *E. dispar* instead.

Most labs do not yet have the tests that can differentiate between *E. histolytica* and *E. dispar.* Until these more sensitive tests become more widely available, physicians usually assume that the parasite is *E. histolytica.*

A blood test is available, but this is recommended only when it is suspected that the infection has invaded the wall of the intestine or some other organ. One drawback of the blood test is that it cannot differentiate between a past and current infection.

Treatment Options and Outlook
Metronidazole is often effective in curing the infection. It is not usually necessary to isolate an infected person, since casual contact at work or school is not likely to transmit the disease. Special precautions may be needed by food handlers or children enrolled in day care.

Risk Factors and Preventive Measures
Careful handwashing after toileting and proper disposal of sewage can help prevent the disease. Infected patients should refrain from intimate contact until effectively treated.

amebic abscess A collection of pus in the liver caused by the protozoan parasite *Entamoeba histolytica.* When the organism's cysts are ingested in contaminated food or water, they pass into the intestine and, from there, into the intestinal walls.

Symptoms and Diagnostic Path
Nausea and vomiting, abdominal pain, and severe diarrhea.

Treatment Options and Outlook
Oral metronidazole and chloroquine.

amebic carrier state A condition in which a patient may carry amebic organisms without showing symptoms of infection. A carrier appears to be healthy, but subsequently may develop the amebic infection. The carrier is always contagious if feces are not disposed of carefully.

aminoglycosides A family of antibiotics used to treat serious infections caused by Gram-negative bacteria. They work by killing bacteria or stopping their growth. They include gentamicin, amikacin, kanamycin, neomycin, netilmicin streptomycin, and tobramycin. These drugs have a narrow margin of safety; they may be toxic to the nerve involved in balance or hearing and can damage kidney function.

amoeba A microscopic single-celled parasite (a type of protozoan) that takes different shapes as it moves through its watery world. When an amoeba senses food (such as bacteria), it heads in that direction by stretching out a "pseudopod" (false foot) until it is right beside the food. Then the pseudopod stretches out and wraps around the food, trapping it.

Amoeba reproduce by cell division at an extremely fast rate—thousands of generations in one day. However, most of the cells die almost as quickly as they reproduce.

Several species prey on humans, including *Entamoeba coli* and *E. histolytica.*

anaerobic bacterial infections A bacterial infection that flourishes in complete or almost complete absence of oxygen, such as CLOSTRIDIUM BOTULINUM. These bacteria (called anaerobes) are found throughout nature and in the body. Infections are usually found in deep puncture wounds that are not exposed to air, or in damaged tissue as the result of trauma, tissue death, or an overgrowth of bacteria. Growth of anaerobic organisms can lead to GANGRENE, TETANUS, or BOTULISM.

ancylostomiasis See HOOKWORMS.

angiostrongyliasis Infection with one of two nematodes (roundworms), *Angiostrongylus (Parastrongylus) costaricensis* or *A cantonensis*. *A. cantonensis* is the most common cause of human eosinophilic MENINGITIS (inflammation of the lining of the brain, with eosinophils in the cerebrospinal fluid). Meningitis is caused by the *A. cantonensis* larvae in the brain and the patient's local reactions to them. *A. costaricensis* causes abdominal or intestinal angiostrongyliasis.

Symptoms and Diagnostic Path
Abdominal angiostrongyliasis mimics APPENDICITIS.

Meningitis symptoms include high fever, stiff neck, vomiting, sensitivity to light, and nausea.

Treatment Options and Outlook
There is no effective treatment.

anisakiasis A type of food poisoning caused by the parasitic worm *Anisakis simplex,* or related worms that are found in sushi, the Japanese dish made of raw fish.

Fewer than 10 cases are diagnosed in the United States every year; however, it is suspected that many cases go undiagnosed. Japan has the highest number of cases because of the large amounts of raw fish eaten there.

Anisakiasis can be misdiagnosed as acute APPENDICITIS, Crohn's disease, peptic ulcer, or cancer of the intestine.

The parasitic worm *Anisakis simplex* infests small crustaceans eaten by many kinds of fish, dolphins, and whales. Fertilized eggs from the female parasite are eliminated by the host fish, which develop into larvae that hatch in salt water.

The disease is transmitted by raw, undercooked, or insufficiently frozen fish and shellfish. Its incidence is expected to increase with the increasing popularity of sushi and sashimi bars. In addition to sushi, sashimi, and ceviche, the larvae can be found in raw herring and Pacific salmon and in cod, haddock, fluke, flounder, and monkfish.

Symptoms and Diagnostic Path
Symptoms may appear from an hour to two weeks after consuming raw or uncooked seafood, but usually begins within six hours.

If the worm is not coughed up or passed into the bowels, it can penetrate the stomach and cause severe pain, nausea, and vomiting. Removing the worms surgically is the only known method of reducing the pain and eliminating the infestation. If the larvae pass into the bowel one to two weeks following infection, a severe eosinophilic granulomatous response may also occur, causing symptoms mimicking Crohn's disease.

In North America, the disease is usually diagnosed when the patient begins to feel a tingling or tickling sensation in the throat, and coughs up a worm. In more severe cases, the pain is akin to acute appendicitis.

In cases where the patient coughs up the worm, the diagnosis may be made by examining the worm itself. Otherwise, the physician may need to examine the inside of the stomach and the small intestine.

Treatment Options and Outlook
Most patients improve spontaneously without specific therapy. If necessary, the worm can be removed surgically. Prescribed medications can be effective if surgery is not needed.

Risk Factors and Preventive Measures
The worm is killed by cooking or freezing the fish. Fish should be cooked at 140°F for at least 10 minutes. Fish should be frozen for more than five days at or below 5°F to ensure killing the worm. Marinating raw fish in lemon or vinegar does *not* kill all the harmful bacteria or parasites that the fish could contain. Visual inspection of the raw fish, even by the most experienced Japanese chef, will not guarantee the absence of worms.

***Anopheles* mosquito** A genus of mosquito, many species of which transmit the MALARIA parasites to humans. This genus is the most important of all the vectors for parasitic disease.

Anopheles mosquitoes breed in permanent bodies of fresh water that have plenty of aquatic plants to provide protection from fish and other predators. Eggs are laid singly on the water's surface. Of the 400 species of *Anopheles,* about 30 to 40 species (females only) are vectors for malaria (*Plasmodium* spp.) in humans. Mosquitoes also transmit canine heartworm (*Dirofilaria immitis*).

Once ingested by a mosquito, malaria parasites must develop within the mosquito for up to three weeks before they can infect humans. If a mosquito does not survive longer than the incubation period, then she will not be able to transmit any malaria parasites.

anthrax A bacterial infection primarily affects livestock, but it is occasionally spread to humans, causing a skin or lung infection.

Because anthrax is considered to be a potential biological warfare agent, all military personnel on active duty who might be involved in combat must be vaccinated.

Bible experts believe the "very severe plague" on the Pharaoh's cattle described in Exodus 9 was almost certainly anthrax. Anthrax is one of the zoonotic diseases, which means that it resides mainly in animals, not in people.

In the 1800s, anthrax was known as "woolsorter's disease" in England and "ragpicker's disease" in Germany because workers caught it from spores in hides and fibers (respectively). By 1876, bacteriologist Robert Koch developed a way to grow pure anthrax cultures in a lab. Within a year, as anthrax raced through French sheep herds, Louis Pasteur began work on developing a vaccine. He was successful in 1881.

In the 1920s, the United States enacted laws to require testing of horsehair or pig bristle shaving brushes. A large outbreak in this country occurred in 1957, when nine employees of a goat hair processing plant got sick after touching a contaminated shipment from Pakistan; four of the five patients with the pulmonary form of the disease died. Other cases appeared in the 1970s when contaminated goatskin drumheads from Haiti were brought into the country as souvenirs.

On October 4, 2001, the first confirmed outbreak associated with intentional anthrax release occurred in Florida, killing a journalist who came in contact with anthrax-contaminated mail. Since then, four more people died of anthrax, including two Washington postal workers; more than a dozen people were infected in New York, New Jersey, Florida, and Washington. None of them were the intended recipients of the letters, but were citizens, government workers, and postal workers who somehow inhaled anthrax spores expelled from the tainted envelopes as they moved along their delivery routes. Before October 2001, the last case of inhalation anthrax in the United States had occurred in 1976.

Epidemiologic investigation indicated that the outbreak, in the District of Columbia, Florida, New Jersey, and New York, resulted from intentional delivery of BACILLUS ANTHRACIS spores through mailed letters or packages. Anthrax contamination temporarily closed several postal facilities and kept a Senate office building shut for three months.

In the wake of the anthrax-contaminated mail, doctors injected four dozen workers with the anthrax vaccine as thousands weighed the government's printed list of the pros and cons of the experimental inoculations. The vaccine does cause side effects, and because it has never been used after exposure to anthrax, there is no guarantee the vaccine will help prevent disease after exposure. One health department in the nation's capital advised against the vaccinations, saying two months of antibiotic treatment already prescribed to people exposed to anthrax during the mail attacks in fall 2001 was enough.

The U.S. Centers for Disease Control and Prevention (CDC) offered voluntary vaccinations or 40 more days of antibiotics to thousands of workers because animal studies suggest that in rare cases, anthrax can lurk in the body for more than 60 days, erupting after people finish their antibiotics.

Side effects of the vaccine include burning at the injection site and soreness, redness, itching, and swelling of that arm for up to a week. Up to 35 percent of recipients have muscle and joint aches, malaise, rashes, chills, a low fever or nausea for up to a week. Serious allergic reactions occur less than once in every 100,000 doses. Studies of more than

500,000 vaccinated people suggest that reports of more severe reactions, such as muscle diseases, are not caused by the vaccine. It is not possible to get anthrax from the vaccine.

Since the first cases of anthrax were identified in October 2001, more than 15,000 anthrax hoaxes and threats have been reported to the postal service and more than 540 post offices have been closed as a result. The originator of the anthrax mailings has never been identified.

In the second half of the 20th century, anthrax was developed as part of a larger biological weapons program by several countries, including the Soviet Union and the United States. The number of nations believed to have biological weapons programs has steadily risen from 10 in 1989 to 17 in 1995, but how many are working with anthrax is uncertain.

Anthrax bacteria is a leading choice for use as a biological weapon because it can produce spores that can be processed to become easily airborne. Mail-sorting machinery can easily aerosolize anthrax in envelopes sent via regular methods through the U.S. Postal Service. Anthrax spores can be spread in the air by missiles, rockets, artillery, and aerial bombs and sprayers, and it can travel downwind for hundreds of miles.

It is dangerous because spores remain potent for decades. During World War II, the British experimented with anthrax on Gruinard Island, and 40 years later, the island was still uninhabitable and had to be decontaminated. Naturally occurring anthrax spores remain dormant in the soil for decades. Grazing animals can ingest them and become infected with the disease.

Anthrax can be produced in large quantities with relatively basic technology. All of the technology needed to produce anthrax also has legitimate uses in the biological and pharmaceutical industries. Therefore, the technology is available on the open market with few controls to its purchase. Any country with basic health care or a basic pharmaceutical industry has the expertise to produce anthrax. The Japanese cult Aum Shinrikyo spent millions of dollars on the development of biological weapons and actually attempted to release anthrax in Tokyo.

In a terrorist attack, 50 percent of those who inhale between 8,000 and 10,000 spores would die,

according to the U.S. Defense Department. Indeed, the largest documented outbreak ever of human inhalation anthrax occurred in Russia in 1979. While officials at the time claimed that the 77 victims got anthrax after eating contaminated meat, in 1992 Russian president Boris Yeltsin said the KGB had admitted a military cause. Two years later, an independent team of American and Russian experts found that a windborne aerosol of anthrax spores from a military lab on April 2, 1979, produced the epidemic that killed 69 of the 77 victims. Why the release occurred has never been explained.

Anthrax is caused by the bacterium *Bacillus anthracis,* which produces spores that can remain dormant for years in soil and animal products such as hides, wool, hair, or bones. *B. anthracis* can live in pastures for a long time, multiplying rapidly during damp, warm weather. It is especially hardy in the alluvial soil of the Nile valley and the Mississippi River valley (the first North American cases were found among animals in Louisiana in the early 1700s). The disease is often fatal to cattle, sheep, and goats, and their hides, wool, and bones are often heavily contaminated. However, the bacillus is not highly infectious in humans and does not depend on multiplication within humans to survive.

If the bacteria are breathed in, they can cause a type of rare and fatal anthrax known as pulmonary anthrax, which attacks the lungs. Intestinal anthrax is a very rare, fatal form of the disease caused by eating the flesh of animals who have died of anthrax. Cutaneous anthrax is the milder form, caused when spores enter the body via a cut.

Symptoms and Diagnostic Path

Cutaneous anthrax causes a raised, itchy area at the site, which progresses to a large blister. This is followed by a black scab surrounded by swollen tissue (in fact, the disease gets its name from the Greek word for "coal" because of this characteristic coal-black sore). Patients also experience shivering and chills, but few other symptoms.

In more than 90 percent of humans cases, the bacteria remain within the sore. Occasionally, the bacteria may spread to the nearest lymph node, or in rare cases it may escape into the bloodstream, causing rapidly fatal blood poisoning, internal bleeding, or anthrax meningitis.

Intestinal anthrax causes stomach and intestinal inflammation and ulcers, with nausea, vomiting, and fever. This may be followed by vomiting blood and severe diarrhea.

Pulmonary anthrax patients experience a suffocating bronchitis.

Anthrax is diagnosed by isolating *B. anthracis* from the blood, skin lesions, or respiratory secretions, or by measuring specific antibodies in the blood.

Treatment Options and Outlook

Anthrax is curable in the early stages with high doses of antibiotics, but it can be fatal in advanced stages.

One or two out of 10 patients will die from anthrax of the skin if it is not properly treated; 100 percent of patients will die of inhalation anthrax if untreated. The abdominal form is fatal in 25 percent to 60 percent of cases. Pulmonary anthrax is usually fatal.

Risk Factors and Preventive Measures

The anthrax vaccine is reported to be 93 percent effective in protecting against anthrax. The immunization consists of three subcutaneous injections given two weeks apart, followed by three more injections given at six, 12, and 18 months. Annual booster injections of the vaccine are recommended thereafter.

About 30 percent of recipients experience mild local reactions that consist of slight tenderness and redness at the injection site. Severe local reactions are infrequent and consist of extensive swelling of the forearm in addition to the local reaction. Systemic reactions occur in fewer than 0.2 percent of recipients.

antibacterial drugs A group of drugs used to treat infections caused by bacteria. These drugs share the same actions as antibiotics but (unlike the antibiotics) have always been produced synthetically. The largest group of antibacterial agents are the sulfonamides. Medically, physicians do not differentiate antibacterials from antibiotics.

antibiotic drugs A group of drugs used to treat infections caused by bacteria. Originally prepared from molds and fungi, antibiotic drugs are today produced synthetically. Antibiotics fight infection when the body has been invaded by harmful bacteria, or when the bacteria in the body begin to multiply uncontrollably.

Some drugs, known as broad-spectrum antibiotics, are effective against a wide range of bacteria, whereas others are useful only in treating a specific bacterium. Some of the best-known antibiotics include the macrolides (erythromycin and clarithromycin); the penicillins (amoxicillin, penicillin V, and oxacillin); the aminoglycosides (gentamicin and streptomycin); the cephalosporins (cefaclor and cephalexin); the quinolones (ciprofloxacin and ofloxacin); and the tetracyclines (doxycycline and oxytetracycline).

These drugs can cause some side effects. Antibiotics kill bacteria, but they can also reduce the "good" bacteria naturally present in the body. When this happens, different bacteria or fungi can grow in their place, causing oral, intestinal, or vaginal candidiasis (THRUSH).

Some patients are allergic to antibiotics and can develop swelling, itching, or breathing problems if they take these drugs. A severe allergic reaction to antibiotics (especially PENICILLIN) can be fatal.

When penicillin was first introduced in the 1940s, doctors finally had a good way to treat infections that had previously claimed thousands of lives. Penicillin and its cousin, ampicillin, were called "wonder drugs" and were soon among the most widely prescribed drugs in the world. Unfortunately, even the best of these drugs cannot kill every single bacterium. When an antibiotic was used against a bacterial infection, it destroyed only those bacteria that were susceptible to the drug; resistant strains were left behind, to survive and spread. Over time, this occurred often enough so that today there are many bacteria resistant to the most-prescribed antibiotics. Resistance occurs when a bacterium is able to evolve so that it is no longer harmed by the specific antibiotic.

The problem is worse in other parts of the world (Europe, the Far East, and South America), where antibiotics are widely available without a prescription. This has led even more quickly to drug-resistant strains in other parts of the world, which are now circulating the globe. See also ANTIBACTERIAL DRUGS.

Resistance

Resistance is likely to develop if a person does not take antibiotics long enough; this leaves a few super-strong germs behind. Drugs kill the vulnerable strains of germs, but the tough survive and flourish. Indeed, half of all antibiotics prescribed in the United States today are either misused or unneeded, according to medical experts.

Resistance also occurs when doctors overprescribe antibiotics instead of saving them for specific infections that really require such a drug. Too often, doctors prescribe antibiotics for viral infections which antibiotics cannot treat. Some doctors defend this practice by saying the cost of a culture to identify the source of the infection is more expensive than the antibiotic. Patients also pressure physicians to prescribe antibiotics. For this reason, the U.S. Centers for Disease Control and Prevention (CDC) has issued guidelines urging hospitals and doctors to use antibiotics more sparingly to slow the development of drug-resistant strains of germs.

Among bacteria that have concerned public health officials are certain types of "flesh eating" strep, and bacteria that cause EAR INFECTION, TUBERCULOSIS, PNEUMONIA, MENINGITIS, and sepsis (an often-fatal blood infection). Some hospitals cannot treat enterococci that can infect kidneys, bladders, wounds, and blood because they have become resistant even to vancomycin, the drug of last resort. Every year, 60,000 to 70,000 patients die from hospital-acquired infections, half of which are caused by drug resistant superbugs. Scientists believe that antibiotic resistance is a major threat to the nation's health, since many diseases are no longer treatable by antibiotics that were effective against them even a few years ago.

Bacteria and other microorganisms that have developed resistance to antimicrobial drugs include

- Methicillin/oxacillin-resistant *Staphylococcus aureus*
- Vancomycin-resistant enterococci
- Penicillin-resistant *Streptococcus pneumoniae*

Scientists are racing against time to develop new types of drugs that will be effective against some of the most deadly infections. Because scientists had

---

WHO'S AT RISK FOR RESISTANT BACTERIA?

Certain groups of people are considered more vulnerable to drug-resistant infections. They include the following:

- anyone who takes small amounts of antibiotics to ward off frequent infections
- health-care workers
- child-care workers
- anyone with impaired immune function
- patients during prolonged hospital stays

---

mistakenly thought the world had enough antibiotics, drug companies began moving away from antibiotic research in the 1980s. Drug development is also expensive: it costs about $237 million to bring one new drug to the market. For every drug that does make it that far, many others are abandoned along the way.

Among the newest antibiotics in development include self-assembling antibiotics—small rings of amino acids that can assemble themselves into tubes that punch holes in bacteria. Other research is focusing on tiny viruses that target and infect bacteria, which could someday be the source of a new class of antibiotics. Some of these viruses, which are known as bacteriophages, produce a protein that wreaks havoc with a bacterium's ability to construct its cell wall. The viruses infect a bacterium, replicate and fill the bacterial cell with new copies of the virus, and then break through the bacterium's cell wall, causing it to burst.

See also VANCOMYCIN-RESISTANT ENTEROCOCCI.

ANTIBIOTIC CAUTIONS

It is possible to cut down on resistant bacterial infections if patients change the way they use antibiotics. Patients should

- not self-medicate with antibiotics
- not pressure a physician to prescribe antibiotics
- not use antibiotics for minor infections
- complete the full course of medicine, as prescribed
- never share antibiotics
- never save leftover pills for future use

FDA SAFE ANTIBIOTIC INGREDIENTS FOR TOPICAL USAGE

The FDA has listed the following antibiotic active ingredients as safe and effective:

- bacitracin
- bacitracin zinc
- chlortetracycline hydrochloride
- tetracycline hydrochloride
- neomycin sulfate
- oxytetracycline hydrochloride (only in combination products)
- polymyxin B sulfate (only in combination products

antidiarrheal drugs A type of medicine used to relieve the symptoms of diarrhea. These drugs work by several means: absorbing water from the digestive tract, changing the action of the intestines, altering electrolyte transport, or adsorbing toxins or microorganisms.

The drug loperamide (Imodium A-D) slows the passage of stools through the intestines. Adsorbents such as attapulgite (Kaopectate) pull diarrhea-causing substances from the digestive tract. Bismuth subsalicylate (Pepto-Bismol) decreases the secretion of fluid into the intestine and inhibits the activity of bacteria. It not only controls diarrhea, but relieves the cramps that often accompany diarrhea.

Patients should not use antidiarrheal drugs for more than two days unless told to do so by a doctor. Elderly people should not use attapulgite (Kaopectate, Donnagel, Parepectolin), but may use other kinds of antidiarrheal drugs. People in this age group may be more likely to have side effects, such as severe constipation, from bismuth subsalicylate.

Bismuth subsalicylate may cause the tongue or the stool to temporarily become pitch black; this is harmless. Children with flu or CHICKEN POX should not be given bismuth subsalicylate because the salicylate it contains can lead to Reye's syndrome, a life-threatening condition that affects the liver and central nervous system. Children may have unpredictable reactions to other antidiarrheal drugs; loperamide should not be given to children under six years and attapulgite should not be given to children under three years unless directed by a physician.

Anyone who has a history of liver disease or who has been taking antibiotics should check with a doctor before taking the antidiarrheal drug loperamide. Loperamide should not be used by people whose diarrhea is caused by certain bacterial infections, such as SALMONELLA or SHIGELLA, because it tends to prolong the illness.

Side Effects

The most common side effects of attapulgite are constipation, bloating, and fullness. Bismuth subsalicylate may cause ringing in the ears, but that side effect is rare. Possible side effects from loperamide include skin rash, constipation, drowsiness, dizziness, tiredness, dry mouth, nausea, vomiting, and swelling, pain, and discomfort in the abdomen. Some of these symptoms are the same as those that occur with diarrhea, so it may be difficult to tell if the medicine is causing the problems. Children may be more sensitive than adults to certain side effects of loperamide, such as drowsiness and dizziness. Other rare side effects may occur with any antidiarrheal medicine.

See also TRAVELER'S DIARRHEA.

antifungal/antiyeast drugs A group of drugs prescribed to treat infections caused by either fungi or yeasts (and sometimes both) and that can be administered directly to the skin, taken orally, or by injection. They are commonly used to treat different types of TINEA, including ATHLETE'S FOOT, JOCK ITCH, and scalp ringworm. They are also used to treat THRUSH and fungal infections such as CRYPTOCOCCUS.

Side Effects

Agents applied to the skin, scalp, mouth, or vagina may sometimes increase irritation. Systemic antifungal agents that are given by mouth or injection may cause more serious side effects, damaging the kidney or liver.

Types

Antifungal agents are available as creams, injections, tablets, lozenges, suspensions, and vaginal suppositories. The most commonly used antifungals include terbinafine, amphotericin B, ciclopirox, clotrimazole, econazole, griseofulvin (by mouth only), itraconazole (by mouth and IV only), fluconazole (by mouth and IV only), ketoconazole, miconazole, and tolnaftate. While amphotericin B is the standard drug for treating serious systemic fungal infections, it is usually given in the hospital because of the danger of side effects. Itraconazole and fluconazole are two more recently approved drugs. These two cause fewer side effects and can be taken orally on an outpatient basis.

Nonprescription creams may help treat typical vaginal yeast infections. They are of no use in treating candidal infections affecting the brain, kidney, or other organs, which tend to occur in immuno-compromised patients.

Antiyeast agents such as mycostatin do not kill most fungi, although most antifungals inhibit yeasts as well (except for griseofulvin). Drugs that are used for both systemic fungal and yeast infections include fluconazole, ketoconazole, amphotericin B, and itraconazole.

Most yeast infections are superficial. Systemic, life-threatening yeast infections do not occur in healthy people.

antihelmintic drugs A group of drugs used to treat worm infestations. A large proportion of the world's adult population harbor many worms in their intestines. The amount of parasites is described as their "worm burden."

Because the body's immune system does not fight worms well, persistent infestations are not uncommon. The antihelmintic drugs eliminate the worms from the body, preventing potential complications.

Different types of antihelmintic drugs—including niclosamide, niridazole, piperazine, praziquantel, thiabendazole, albendazole, and mebendazole—are used to treat infestation by different types of worms. For intestinal worms, drugs work by either killing or paralyzing the worms, thus preventing them from gripping onto the intestinal walls. They are then eliminated from the body in the feces. To speed up this process, laxatives may be used at the same time. When worms are present in other tissues, antihelmintics kill worms by boosting their vulnerability to the immune system; once these worms have died, they may need to be surgically removed along with any cysts that they have caused.

Adverse effects of antihelmintics include nausea and vomiting, stomach pain, headache, dizziness, and rash.

antimalarial drugs A type of medicine used to destroy or prevent the development of plasmodia (protozoa that cause MALARIA). Chloroquine hydrochloride and hydroxychloroquine sulfate are effective against *Plasmodium vivax, P. malariae,* and certain strains of *P. falciparum.* Anyone with drug-resistant strains of *P. falciparum* may be treated with a combination of different antimalarial drugs. Resistance by the malarial organism to usual forms of therapy is becoming a worldwide problem.

antimicrobial drugs Drugs that destroy or inhibit the growth of microorganisms.

See also ANTIBACTERIAL DRUGS and ANTIBIOTIC DRUGS.

antipyretic drugs A type of medicine designed to lower fever by reducing body temperature. Most popular types of antipyretics include acetaminophen, aspirin, and other nonsteroidal anti-inflammatory drugs (NSAIDs), such as ibuprofen.

antiseptic A germicide that slows down the growth and reproduction of germs on human skin or tissue (not inanimate objects). They weaken microbes but do not usually kill them. Health-care antiseptics in soaps or other products help prevent the spread of infection in medical facilities. Antiseptics include alcohol (ethanol or isopropanol), iodine (iodophor), povidone-iodine (Betadine), hydrogen peroxide, chlorhexidine, or hexachlorophene (pHisoHex).

Experts advise against using hydrogen peroxide as an antiseptic in open wounds, since it does not kill bacteria and interferes with capillary blood flow and wound healing. Other experts note that ethyl alcohol is not a good wound antiseptic because it irritates already damaged tissue and causes a scab to form, which may protect bacteria.

FDA LISTS SAFE ACTIVE INGREDIENTS IN ANTISEPTICS
• ethyl alcohol (48 to 95 percent)
• isopropyl alcohol
• benzalkonium chloride
• benzethonium chloride
• camphorated metacresol
• camphorated phenol
• phenol
• hexylresorcinol
• hydrogen peroxide solution
• iodine tincture
• iodine topical solution
• povidone-iodine
• methylbenzethonium

The U.S. Food and Drug Administration advisory review panel has found some antiseptics not generally recognized as safe and effective. These include cloflucarban, fluorosalan, and tribromsalan.

Over-the-counter antiseptics applied to the skin can help prevent infection in minor cuts, scrapes, or burns. They can be kept in the first-aid kit to pour on a dirty cut after cleaning it with soap and water. If an injury is extensive, it should be taken care of by a doctor. Antiseptics should not be used for cuts that are deep, that keep bleeding, or that require stitches. Antiseptics should not be used for scrapes with imbedded particles that cannot be flushed away, large wounds, or serious burns.

Over-the-counter antiseptics should not be used for more than one week on an injury; if it persists or gets worse, consumers should seek medical care.

antiserum A preparation containing antibodies to a specific germ that combine with specific foreign invaders (antigens). Antiserum usually includes components of living things such as viruses or bacteria, and is usually used as an emergency treatment when an unvaccinated person has been exposed to a dangerous infection. Treatment includes immunization as well.

Antiserum is prepared from the blood of animals or humans who have already been immunized against the organism.

The antiserum helps to provide some immediate protection against the microorganisms while full immunity develops. However, these measures are not as effective in preventing disease as is immunization before exposure.

antitoxin An antibody produced by the body to fight off a toxin formed by invading bacteria or a biological poison such as BOTULISM or snakebite. Antitoxins are also produced commercially to contain an antibody that can neutralize the effect of a specific toxin released into the blood by bacteria (such as those that cause TETANUS or DIPHTHERIA). They are often life saving, especially in the case of food poisoning (see FOOD-BORNE INFECTIONS) from botulism.

Antitoxins are prepared by injecting animals (usually horses) with specific toxins that provoke the animal's immune system into producing antibodies that neutralize the toxin. The extracts are taken from the animal's blood to be used as an antitoxin.

Antitoxins are usually injected into the muscle of the patient. Once in a while, the antitoxin may cause an allergic reaction or, more rarely, anaphylactic shock.

Antivenin is an antitoxin specifically made to combat snakebite poison. Antivenins are specific for each poisonous snake.

antitussive drugs A type of medicine used to suppress coughing, possibly by reducing the activity of the cough center of the brain and by depressing breathing. These drugs include both narcotics and nonnarcotics that act on the central and peripheral nervous systems to suppress the cough reflex. Because the cough reflex is important in clearing the upper respiratory tract of secretions, antitussives should not be used with a productive cough (one that produces mucus). Codeine and hydrocodone are strong narcotic antitussives. Dextromethorphan is equally effective but does not carry the danger of inducing patient dependence. Antitussives are given by mouth (usually in a syrup with an expectorant and alcohol). They may also be given as a capsule with an antihistamine and mild painkiller.

antiviral agents A group of drugs used to treat viral infections. To date, there is no drug that completely eradicates viruses and cures the illnesses they cause. This is because viruses live only within cells; a drug capable of killing a virus would also kill its healthy host cell. Antiviral drugs are one type of antimicrobial medication, a larger groups of drugs that also includes ANTIBIOTICS, antifungal and antiparasitic drugs.

However, scientists are making exciting discoveries in the race to discover a drug that will fight viruses. Antiviral agents that interfere with viral replication or that otherwise disrupt chemical processes of viral metabolism have been developed. Some of these agents prevent viruses from penetrating into healthy cells.

Researchers are studying how to create antiviral medications that attack viruses at every stage in their life cycles. Although viruses are not alike, they all share similar replication patterns. Scientists have discovered that the best time to attack a virus is early in its life cycle. Vaccines that target viruses usually are made of a weakened or killed version of a virus, which stimulates the immune system without injuring the host. Then, when the real virus attacks the vaccinated person, the immune system quickly recognizes the invader and responds to it quickly. While vaccines work very well, they are not much help for someone already infected.

Antiviral drugs are devised to do just that. One of the ways that scientists are trying to target viruses is to interfere with their ability to enter a person's cells. For example, several "entry-blocking" drugs are being developed to fight HIV. Two entry-blocking drugs (amantadine and rimantadine) have been developed to fight influenza; scientists are trying to develop other entry-inhibiting drugs to fight HEPATITIS B and C.

Scientists are also working on a new entry-blocker named pleconaril, the first antiviral drug that targets the RHINOVIRUSES that cause the common cold. The drug also appears to work against ENTEROVIRUSES, which can cause diarrhea, MENINGITIS, CONJUNCTIVITIS, and ENCEPHALITIS.

Scientists are also targeting the processes that produce virus components after a virus invades a cell. One way to do this is to develop substances that look like the building blocks of RNA or DNA (called nucleotide or nucleoside analogues) but interfere with the enzymes that produce the RNA or DNA. The first successful antiviral drug—ACYCLOVIR—is a nucleoside analog that is effective against herpesvirus infections. Zidovudine (AZT), the first antiviral drug approved to treat HIV, is another nucleoside analogue. Nucleoside analogues that treat HIV infections include lamivudine, which also has been approved to treat hepatitis B.

Antiviral drug developers have also targeted the final stage in the life cycle of a virus, when completed viruses are released from the host cell. Two drugs named zanamivir and oseltamivir have been recently introduced to treat influenza by preventing the release of viral particles.

Another way to fight viruses is to encourage the body's immune system to attack the germs, rather than attacking them directly. Some of these antivirals do not focus on a specific pathogen; instead, they prompt the immune system to attack many different pathogens. One of the best-known of this class of drugs are INTERFERONS, which interfere with the production of viruses in infected cells. Interferon alpha is used to treat hepatitis B and C, and other interferons are being studied as treatments for a variety of diseases.

A more specific approach is to produce proteins called antibodies that can attach to a virus and mark it for attack by the immune system.

All drugs designed to fight viruses and bacteria eventually become less effective because the germs acquire resistance to the drugs. Therefore, no antiviral drug will ever result in a permanent cure.

The antivirals are not without problems, however; some useful antivirals have a wide variety of side effects and patients receiving these drugs must be monitored carefully. Some resistant virus strains have developed in patients receiving initially effective therapy.

Some of the better-known antivirals include acyclovir, amantadine, rimantadine, ribavirin, idoxuridine, vidarabine, trifluridine (trifluorothymidine), valcyclovir, ganciclovir, zidovudine (ZDU, formerly called AZT, or azidothymidine), foscarnet, interferon, protease inhibitors, and combinations of these.

appendicitis   Infection of the appendix, a small tube of tissue that connects to the beginning of the large intestine, usually at the lower right side of the abdomen. Appendicitis is the most common reason for emergency abdominal surgery. Young people between the ages of 11 and 20 are most often affected, and most cases of appendicitis occur in the winter between October and May. A family history of appendicitis may increase risk for the illness, especially in boys. People with cystic fibrosis are also at increased risk.

The inside of the appendix usually opens into the large intestine. When the inside of the appendix is blocked by a piece of stool or something that has been swallowed, the appendix becomes swollen and easily infected by bacteria. If the infected appendix is not removed, an abscess may form and eventually burst or perforate. This may happen as soon as 48 to 72 hours after symptoms begin.

Symptoms and Diagnostic Path

In older children and young adults, the classic symptoms of appendicitis are abdominal pain, fever, and vomiting. Abdominal pain usually begins in the center of the abdomen near the navel; often, the pain then moves down and to the right, roughly where the appendix is located in the lower right part of the abdomen. After the abdominal pain begins, patients with appendicitis usually develop a slight fever, lose their appetite, and may vomit. The fact that abdominal pain begins before nausea and vomiting instead of after is one clue to suspect appendicitis.

Other symptoms that may be seen in older children with appendicitis include diarrhea (small stools with mucus), urinating often or having an uncomfortably strong urge to urinate, constipation, and occasionally breathing problems.

In children younger than age two, the most common symptoms are vomiting and a bloated or swollen abdomen. There may be abdominal pain, but children may be too young to describe this pain. Because appendicitis is rare in infants, and their symptoms are not "classic," the diagnosis of appendicitis is more difficult.

Correctly diagnosing appendicitis in anyone can be difficult, since symptoms may mimic many other more common conditions, such as gastrointestinal infections. Even the most experienced physicians and surgeons are not able to diagnose appendicitis 100 percent of the time. Children between ages five and nine with appendicitis are often misdiagnosed with either gastroenteritis or a respiratory infection, which are much more common illnesses in this age group.

A diagnosis of appendicitis is made based on a physical examination, together with tests of blood and urine. To help support or eliminate the diagnosis, a doctor may also order X-rays of the abdomen and chest. No laboratory test is specifically designed to identify appendicitis. Instead, surgeons are beginning to rely on CT scans of the appendix to confirm appendicitis when the diagnosis is not clear.

Treatment Options and Outlook

Appendicitis is a medical emergency that must be treated surgically; it cannot be treated at home. Anyone with a suspected case of appendicitis should see a doctor immediately. Since the doctor will need to examine the abdomen for signs of pain and tenderness, no pain medication should be given without a doctor's permission. If there is a suspicion of appendicitis, no food or liquids should be given in case surgery is required.

The decision whether to operate or not is most often based on the patient's history and a physical exam. Surgeons have the option of removing the appendix either through the traditional abdominal incision, or by using a small surgical device called a laparoscope to create a smaller opening in the abdomen. However, if the appendix has perforated, surgery becomes more complex and the risk of complications increases.

If the appendix is removed surgically before it perforates, complications are rare. Even if the appendix has not perforated, the doctor may prescribe antibiotics to decrease the risk for wound infection after surgery.

However, if appendicitis is not treated, the infected appendix may break open and spread the infection inside the abdomen. If perforation does occur, the abdominal pain may spread out to involve the whole abdomen, and fever may spike. Once symptoms of appendicitis begin, it takes as little as 24 hours for an infected appendix to perforate. Perforation with appendicitis is more common with younger children. It may be life-threatening if bacteria enter the bloodstream.

Risk Factors and Preventive Measures

There is no way to prevent appendicitis. Although appendicitis is rare in countries where people eat a high-fiber diet, experts have not yet proven that a high-fiber diet prevents appendicitis.

arboviral infections Arboviral (short for *arthro-pod-bo*rne) infections are caused by any of a number of viruses transmitted by arthropods such as mosquitoes and ticks. The infections, which include ENCEPHALITIS, EASTERN EQUINE ENCEPHALITIS, WEST NILE VIRUS, RIFT VALLEY FEVER, hemorrhagic fever, St. Louis encephalitis, and California encephalitis, usually occur during warm weather months when insects are active. There are more than 520 known arboviruses; about 100 of these can cause human disease.

Anyone can get an arboviral infection, although youngsters and the elderly are most susceptible. Most of these type of infections are spread by infected mosquitoes, but only a few types of mosquitoes are capable of transmitting disease—and only a few of these actually carry a virus. Infection with one arbovirus can provide immunity to reinfection by that specific virus and may also protect against other related viruses.

Symptoms and Diagnostic Path

Symptoms of the different types of arboviruses are usually similar, although they differ in severity. Most infections do not cause any symptoms at all; mild cases may involve a slight fever or headache. Severe infections quickly cause an intense headache, high fever, disorientation, coma, tremor, convulsions, paralysis, or death. Symptoms usually occur between five and 15 days after exposure.

Treatment Options and Outlook

There are no specific treatments for these kinds of infections. Treatment is typically aimed at relieving symptoms.

Risk Factors and Preventive Measures

The arboviral diseases can be prevented by using insect repellents, screening, and community control programs. Epidemics are not likely to occur when insects that carry the diseases are kept under control. See also ENCEPHALITIS, CALIFORNIA; ENCEPHALITIS, ST. LOUIS.

Arctic Investigations Program A program of the Centers for Disease Control and Prevention (CDC) that is designed to prevent infectious diseases in people of the Arctic and Subarctic, with special emphasis on diseases of concern among Alaska natives and American Indians. Priority activities include prevention of diseases caused by STREPTOCOCCUS PNEUMONIAE, HAEMOPHILUS INFLUENZAE TYPE B, HELICOBACTER PYLORI, and RESPIRATORY SYNCYTIAL VIRUS (RSV), as well as control of viral HEPATITIS and BOTULISM.

The AIP conducts infectious diseases surveillance, provides and evaluates prevention services, and conducts applied research in collaboration with other programs within CDC and with the Alaska State Division of Public Health, Native Health Corporations, Indian Health Service, foreign ministries of health, industry, and universities. Approximately 35 epidemiologists, research nurses, statisticians, and support staff are based at the AIP facility on the Alaska Native Health Campus in Anchorage, Alaska.

arenavirus A family of viruses named for the Latin word for "sand," a reference to the virus's granular outer appearance. The arenaviruses were first identified during a 1933 ENCEPHALITIS outbreak in St. Louis. The various viruses include Ampari, Junin, Lassa, Latino, Machupo, Parana, Pichinde, Tacaribe, Tamiami (Guanarito, and Sabia); they may cause MENINGITIS or hemorrhagic fevers when humans encounter these viruses in excrement from bats, rats, or mice. The arenaviruses are divided into two groups: the New World or Tacaribe complex and the Old World or LCM/Lassa complex, according to the Centers for Disease Control and Prevention. Viruses in these groups that cause illness in humans include Lassa virus (LASSA FEVER), Junin virus (Argentine hemorrhagic fever), Machupo virus (Bolivian hemorrhagic fever), Guanarito virus (Venezuelan hemorrhagic fever), and Sabia virus (Brazilian hemorrhagic fever).

These unusual viruses can be deadly. Argentinian hemorrhagic fever, which is caused by the Junin virus, was identified in 1953 near the Junin River; the disease kills 20 percent of those infected by causing fatal hemorrhaging. The mortality rate for the Bolivian variety (Machupo, named for another river) is 30 percent; this disease was first called the black typhus. Lassa fever may kill as many as 60 percent of its victims.

Most of these viruses have been limited to certain geographic areas, and since direct person to person contagion is unusual, worldwide pandemics are not expected to occur.

arthritis, septic   Also known as infective arthritis or pyogenic arthritis, this joint disease is caused by the invasion of bacteria into the joint from a nearby infected wound or from a blood infection.

In addition to a nearby infection, septic arthritis also may occur as a complication of an infection elsewhere in the body, such as with GONORRHEA or STAPHYLOCOCCAL INFECTION.

Symptoms and Diagnostic Path

The infected joint usually becomes hot, painful, and swollen.

Diagnosis is made from the appearance of the joint and the joint fluid, which may be withdrawn through a needle from the affected joint and examined for the presence of microorganisms; a culture may be made from this fluid as well.

Treatment Options and Outlook

Antibiotic drugs are used to treat septic arthritis. Occasionally, surgical cleansing of the joint space is necessary.

ascariasis   See ROUNDWORMS.

Asian flu   See INFLUENZA.

Asian tiger mosquito   See *AEDES ALBOPICTUS* MOSQUITO.

aspergillosis   An infection in which the fungus *Aspergillus fumigatus* (found in old buildings or decaying plants) affects the lungs or other organs.

Symptoms and Diagnostic Path

The fungus can cause illness in one of three ways. It can trigger an allergic reaction in people with asthma (a condition called pulmonary aspergillosis—allergic bronchopulmonary type). In patients with a healed lung wound from previous disease, such as TUBERCULOSIS, the fungus can produce a fungus ball called an aspergilloma.

Third, it can lead to an invasive infection followed by pneumonia, which spreads to other parts of the body via the bloodstream (a condition called pulmonary aspergillosis—invasive type). This invasive infection can lead to blindness or attack any other organ of the body, such as the heart, lungs, brain, or kidneys. This form is found almost exclusively in people with an impaired immune system due to cancer, AIDS, leukemia, organ transplants, high doses of corticosteroid drugs, or other diseases that lower the white blood cell count.

Treatment Options and Outlook

Amphotericin B is used to treat systemic aspergillosis (especially if it has spread to the lungs). Oral prednisone is used to treat acute allergic reactions to *ASPERGILLUS.*

A fungus ball in the lung usually does not require treatment unless the infection is accompanied by bleeding into the lung tissue; in this case, the ball must be surgically removed.

Endocarditis (inflammation of heart valves) caused by *Aspergillus* is treated by surgically removing the infected heart valves, along with administration of amphotericin B.

Patients with allergic aspergillosis will slowly improve over time.

Invasive aspergillosis may not respond to medication and can be fatal. With invasive aspergillosis, the patient's underlying disease and immune system strength will affect the overall prognosis.

Aspergillus   A genus of fungi (including many common molds), some of which cause respiratory infections in humans. It is a common contaminant in the laboratory and is a rare cause of hospital-acquired infection. The fungus is found everywhere in soil and proliferates rapidly. The species *A. fumigatus* causes ASPERGILLOSIS. *A. niger* is commonly found in the external ear. Inhalation of *A. fumigatus* and *A. flatus* is common, but infection is rare. More commonly, an allergic reaction ensues.

athlete's foot A common fungal condition causing the skin between the toes (usually the fourth and fifth toes) to itch, peel, and crack. Associated with wearing shoes and sweating, the condition is rare in young children and in places of the world where people do not wear shoes. It is primarily found in adolescents and men, especially those who wear sneakers without socks. A person with athlete's foot is infectious for as long as the lesions exist.

Itchy skin on the foot is probably not athlete's foot if it occurs on the top of the toes. If the foot is red, swollen, sore, blistered, and oozing, it is more likely some form of contact dermatitis, although inflammatory fungal infections can sometimes look like this. Secondary bacterial infections of the eroded skin can also resemble athlete's foot.

The fungi that are responsible for athlete's foot are called DERMATOPHYTES; they live only on dead body tissue (hair, the outer layer of skin, and nails). The two main dermatophytes responsible for athlete's foot are TRICHOPHYTON *rubrum* and *T. mentagrophytes*. The condition occurs both by direct and indirect contact; it can be passed in locker rooms, showers, or shared towels and shoes.

Symptoms and Diagnostic Path

Symptoms may include scaling and cracking of the skin between the toes and the sides of the feet; the skin may itch and peel. There may be small water blisters between the toes; it can spread to the instep or the hands. There is often an odor.

Scrapings from the affected area will be examined under a microscope for certain fungal characteristics.

Treatment Options and Outlook

The condition may clear up without any attention, but it usually requires treatment. An untreated fungal infection can lead to bacterial invasion in cracks in the skin. The affected area should be kept dry, clad in dry cotton socks or in sandals, or kept uncovered.

A number of nonprescription fungicide sprays will cure athlete's foot, including clotrimazole, ketoconazole, miconazole-nitrate, sulconazole, or tolnaftate. Before applying, the feet should be bathed well with soap and water, then well dried (especially between the toes). The sprays should be applied to all sides of the feet twice a day for up to four weeks. After the spray has been applied, the feet should be covered in clean, white cotton socks. For cases that do not respond to the sprays, a physician may prescribe one of several oral medicines.

When the acute phase of the infection passes, the dead skin should be removed with a bristle brush in order to remove the living fungi. All bits of the dead skin should be washed away. In addition, the skin underneath toenails should be scraped every two or three days with an orange stick or toothpick.

Risk Factors and Preventive Measures

Good hygiene is the best way to prevent athlete's foot. Disinfecting the floors of showers and locker rooms can help control the spread of infection.

Once an infection has cleared up, the patient should continue using antifungal cream now and then—especially during warm weather. Plastic or too-tight shoes should be avoided. Natural materials (cotton and leather) and sandals are the best choices, whereas wool and rubber can make a fungal problem worse by trapping moisture.

Shoes should be aired out regularly in the sun and wiped inside with a disinfectant-treated cloth to remove fungi-carrying dead skin. The insides of shoes should then be dusted with antifungal powder or spray. Those individuals who perspire heavily should change socks three or four times daily. Only natural white cotton socks should be worn, and they should be rinsed thoroughly during washing.

Feet should be air dried after bathing and then powdered. To reduce the risk of infection, it is important to wear sandals or flip-flops in public bathing areas.

avian flu (bird flu) A deadly type of influenza normally affecting chickens that abruptly jumped to humans in Hong Kong in 1997, infecting 18 people and killing six. To date, there have been 135 cases of humans with bird flu, and 69 deaths around the world.

As of June 2005, 103 people have been infected with bird flu in Vietnam, Thailand, and Cambodia, according to the World Health Organization, and more than half of the cases have been fatal, suggesting an unprecedented level of harm for a modern flu. It also led to the slaughter of millions of poultry across the region.

Bird flu is an infection caused by avian influenza viruses that occur naturally among birds. Wild birds worldwide harmlessly carry the viruses in their intestines, but because avian influenza is very contagious among all birds, the virus can make some domesticated birds (including chickens, ducks, and turkeys) fatally ill.

Infected birds shed the virus in their saliva, nasal secretions, and feces; other birds become infected from contaminated secretions or excretions. Domesticated birds may become infected with avian influenza virus through direct contact with infected waterfowl or other infected poultry, or through contact with contaminated surfaces.

Infected domestic poultry may contract one of two main forms of the disease, one of which is not very virulent, but the other is quite deadly. The "low pathogenic" form may cause only mild symptoms, such as ruffled feathers and a drop in egg production. The deadly form spreads faster through flocks, causing disease that affects all of the internal organs and kills almost every bird within 48 hours.

Avian flu, popularly known as "bird flu," is caused by the avian flu virus, a Type A rod-shaped virus that can cut through protective mucus and attach to cells that line the nose and throat. For reasons that are not clear, it travels more efficiently from chickens to humans than from humans to humans. Unlike the more traditional flu viruses that cause little more than chills, fever, and aches, this viral version attacks not just the respiratory system but every tissue in the body including the brain, leading to severe hemorrhaging throughout the body.

Type A flu viruses are subtyped according to proteins on their surfaces. There are 16 different H proteins and nine different N proteins; all H and N proteins occur in birds. Human disease has traditionally been caused by three H subtypes—H1, H2, and H3—but recently humans have gotten sick after catching new H subtypes (H5, H7, and H9) from birds. Experts fear that one of these subtypes will emerge as the next flu pandemic—particularly the H5N1 virus that is causing an unprecedented global epidemic among domestic and wild birds.

Bird flu viruses come in two varieties, depending on how efficiently they kill birds. Low pathogenicity avian influenza (LPAI) is not as deadly, but high pathogenicity avian influenza (HPAI)—apparently limited to the H5 and H7 viruses—kills up to 100 percent of infected birds. The current H5N1 bird flu virus is an HPAI virus.

In May 2001, Hong Kong authorities ordered the slaughter of virtually all poultry in the territory to prevent the further spread of an outbreak of bird flu. Imports of poultry from the rest of China were also suspended, and as many as 1.2 million birds were slaughtered. However, this virus does not affect people and was different from the 1997 strain, which killed six people. However, the latest infection was a new and highly virulent strain of avian flu that killed almost 800 chickens in cages in three separate markets during the first 24 hours. After that, all the chickens, ducks, geese, and quail in the territory's markets, along with all mature poultry on its farms, were slaughtered.

The appearance of the H5N1 virus in Hong Kong in humans in 1997 prompted fears of a worldwide epidemic. A 1998 study showed similarities between the virus and Spanish flu, an outbreak of which killed between 20 and 40 million people in 1918. A less serious strain infected two children in 1999, and there were unconfirmed reports of further cases in China's southern provinces. Fortunately, most bird flu viruses do not replicate efficiently in humans.

Outbreaks of avian influenza H5N1 occurred among poultry in eight countries in Asia (Cambodia, China, Indonesia, Japan, Laos, South Korea, Thailand, and Vietnam) during late 2003 and early 2004. At that time, more than 100 million birds in the affected countries either died from the disease or were killed in order to try to control the outbreaks. By March 2004, the outbreak was reported to be under control. After late June 2004, however, new outbreaks of influenza H5N1 among poultry were reported by several countries in Asia (Cambodia, China [Tibet], Indonesia, Kazakhstan, Malaysia, Mongolia, Russia [Siberia], Thailand, and Vietnam). Experts suspect that these outbreaks are ongoing. Influenza H5N1 infection also has been reported among poultry in Turkey and Romania and among wild migratory birds in Croatia. Human cases of influenza A (H5N1) infection have been reported in Cambodia, China, Indonesia, Thailand, and Vietnam.

The World Health Organization's conservative estimate of the number of deaths that an epidemic would cause is 7 million worldwide. Experts calculate that a pandemic on the scale of the devastating global influenza epidemic of 1918 would kill at least 180 million people today.

There is no vaccine, but, even if one could be produced to fight the constantly evolving strains of the virus, it would be impossible to meet the overwhelming demand.

Virologists consider the emergence of this new virus to be one of the most troubling medical events of the century. The danger with this purely avian virus is that unlike the common flu, humans would have no immunity against it. High-speed travel linking countries around the world means that a pandemic of this unusually deadly influenza virus could circle the globe in a matter of months.

The virus is termed *H5 flu*, because it carries the H5 variation of the H gene, a variation that is notoriously lethal in chickens. In the Hong Kong epidemic, the many outdoor markets held the key to why the confirmed cases of H5 avian flu were sprinkled throughout the city. Some people had had direct contact with poultry, and then others appeared to have caught the disease from contact so casual that the people were not aware of it.

It is believed that the epidemic was temporarily halted when the city government decided to kill every chicken in Hong Kong. The decision, which was widely ridiculed at the time, apparently prevented a more widespread disaster.

Scientists fear that the virus could exchange genetic material with the common flu virus. If someone were to be infected with both viruses at once, the RNA from one virus could combine with the RNA from the other, producing a new virus that is both highly contagious and deadly. This is exactly what happened in the deadly flu epidemic of 1918 that killed more than 20 million people, many of them young and healthy. Warnings have grown much more stark as officials warn of a catastrophic economic shutdown and a global political crisis if bird flu strikes an unprepared world.

The H5N1 virus that has caused human illness and death in Asia is resistant to amantadine and rimantadine, two antiviral medications commonly used for influenza. Two other antiviral medications (oseltamivir and zanamavir) would probably be effective against influenza caused by H5N1 virus, but additional studies still need to be done to demonstrate their effectiveness.

There currently is no commercially available vaccine to protect humans against the H5N1 in Asia and Europe. However, research studies testing a human vaccine against H5N1 virus began in April 2005, and a series of clinical trials is under way. However, even if a vaccine is effective, manufacturers could not quickly make enough to protect the U.S. population.

babesiosis (babesiasis) A rare, occasionally fatal disease caused by a tick-borne microorganism that is similar to both LYME DISEASE and human granulocytic ehrlichiosis (HGE). Also known as Nantucket fever, it is most often seen in the elderly and those with impaired immune systems. Severe cases have been diagnosed in those who have had their spleen removed prior to exposure.

Most cases of babesiosis have been reported in summer and fall in the northeastern United States, especially Nantucket, Shelter Island in New York, and other offshore islands in New England. However, cases have recently been identified in the upper Midwest, the Pacific Coast states, and Europe. A related species has caused a babesiosis-like illness in Washington and California.

Babesiosis is caused by protozoa similar to those that cause MALARIA (the species *Babesia microti*). It is passed via the bite of ticks; the most common is the species *Ixodes scapularis* which prey on meadow voles, mice, and deer. The disease can also be transmitted via contaminated blood transfusions. The protozoa causing babesiosis was first identified by Roman bacteriologist Victor Babes, for whom the organism and the disease was named.

Symptoms and Diagnostic Path

Babesiosis typically causes mild illness in otherwise healthy people, but it can be overwhelming to those with impaired immune systems. Symptoms appear within a week after a tick bite and include fever, fatigue, and hemolytic anemia lasting from several days to several months. A person may also have the disease with no symptoms at all. It is not known if a past infection renders a patient immune.

The disease is diagnosed by identifying the parasite in blood samples.

Treatment Options and Outlook

Seven days of oral quinine plus clindamycin are the drugs of choice. Fatigue, malaise and low fever may linger for weeks or months after treatment.

Risk Factors and Preventive Measures

The spread of babesiosis can be curtailed by controlling rodents around houses and using tick repellents. No vaccine is available.

bacillary angiomatosis A life-threatening but curable infection characterized by purple lesions on or under the skin, found almost exclusively in patients with AIDS. It causes blood vessels to grow out of control in bone, liver, and skin, forming tumor-like masses that look like Kaposi's sarcoma lesions.

Bacillary angiomatosis is a reemerging bacterial infection caused by two versions of the same bacteria. It is found among homeless AIDS patients and those afflicted with CAT-SCRATCH DISEASE. The infection is rarely seen today in patients who do not have HIV. According to the U.S. Centers for Disease Control and Prevention (CDC), an HIV patient diagnosed with bacillary angiomatosis is considered to have progressed to full-blown AIDS.

Two varieties of the BARTONELLA bacteria cause bacillary angiomatosis: *B. quintana* (formerly *Rochalimaea quintana*) and *B. henselae* (cause of cat-scratch disease). *B. quintana* infection (known as trench fever), was associated with body lice that sickened European troops during World War I. Lice carry the bacteria, and can transmit the infection to humans. The incidence of trench fever had disappeared after World War I and was not diagnosed in the United States until 10 cases were reported among homeless men in 1992.

The related bacteria *B. henselae* was first identified several years ago as the cause of cat-scratch fever, and was transmitted to AIDS patients from cat fleas. It also can lead to bacillary angiomatosis in AIDS patients.

Symptoms and Diagnostic Path

The disease is characterized by blood vessels that form firm, tumor-like masses in the skin and organs. The masses can occur anywhere on the body in large or small groups they are rarely found on palms of the hands, soles of the feet, or in the mouth.

As the number of masses increase, the patient may develop a high fever, sweats, chills, poor appetite, vomiting, and weight loss.

In addition to the basic disease process, the two different types of bacteria cause slightly different symptoms. Patients infected with *B. henselae* also experience blood-filled cysts in the liver and abnormal liver function; *B. quintana* patients may develop tumors in the bone.

This life-threatening but curable infection is often misdiagnosed, and mistaken for other conditions such as Kaposi's sarcoma. A blood test can detect antibodies to the bacteria. Biopsy of a small sample of the lymph node is unnecessary unless cancer is suspected.

Treatment Options and Outlook

Antibiotics used to treat HIV opportunistic infections can prevent and treat bacillary angiomatosis. Treatment is usually given for three or four weeks. A severely affected lymph node or blister may have to be drained. Acetaminophen may relieve pain, aches, and fever over 101°F.

Early diagnosis is crucial to a cure. If untreated, the patient may die.

Risk Factors and Preventive Measures

Antibiotics may prevent the disease. Patients also should treat cats for fleas.

bacillary dysentery   See SHIGELLOSIS.

Bacillus   A large genus of gram-positive, spore-bearing bacteria (in the family Bacillaceae) that includes 33 species, three of which cause disease. Bacilli are found in soil and air and are responsible for many diseases, including ANTHRAX and food poisoning (see FOOD-BORNE INFECTIONS). Most feed on dead matter and are responsible for food spoilage. The genus includes BACILLUS ANTHRACIS, BACILLUS POLYMYXA, and BACILLUS SUBTILIS.

Bacillus anthracis   A species of gram-positive bacteria that causes ANTHRAX, a disease mostly affecting cattle and sheep. If inhaled, the spores of this organism can cause a pulmonary form of anthrax. Spores live for many years in hides and wool.

Bacillus pestis   See YERSINIA (PASTEURELLA) PESTIS.

Bacillus polymyxa   A species of *Bacillus* that is commonly found in soil and is the source of the polymyxin group of antibiotics.

Bacillus subtilis   A species of BACILLUS that may cause CONJUNCTIVITIS in humans; it is also used to produce the antibiotic bacitracin.

bacteremia   An invasion of bacteria into the bloodstream. This is an uncommon complication of STREP THROAT, TONSILLITIS, or streptococcal skin infection; it may also occur a few hours after minor surgery or dental cleaning. Infection can spread via the bloodstream to other parts of the body, producing ABSCESSES, peritonitis (inflammation of the abdomen), inflammation of the heart, or MENINGITIS. Bacteremia may also lead to shock, causing a generalized illness with high fever, circulatory collapse, and eventually, organ failure.

Those at greatest risk include patients with an impaired immune system, children with CHICKEN POX, burn victims, elderly patients with CELLULITIS, diabetes, blood vessel disease, cancer, or anyone taking steroids or chemotherapy. IV drug users are also at risk.

Bacteremia may occur as well in healthy young adults with no known risk factors.

bacteria Bacteria are microbes whose genetic material is not organized into a cell nucleus, like plants or animals. Some bacteria feed on other organisms, some make their own food (like plants do) and some bacteria do both. Some need air to survive, and others exist without air (anaerobic). Some move by themselves, and others cannot move at all. Bacteria also come in a variety of shapes, colors, and sizes.

It is important to remember that not all bacteria are harmful; most are helpful, such as those that break down dead plant and animal matter in the soil. Some (like the actinomycetes) produce antibiotics such as streptomycin. Plants cannot grow without nitrogen, and bacteria help nitrogen to form in the soil. Bacteria are also used to make cheese out of milk and leather out of animal hide. Grazing animals use bacteria to digest the grass they eat.

Bacteria can be found in the air, the water, food, and everything we touch. Since few of these are harmful, humans are seldom bothered by them. When harmful bacteria do enter the body, the immune system usually can kill the invading microbes.

Bacteria are of incredible importance because of their extreme flexibility, capacity for rapid growth and reproduction, and their great age—the oldest known fossils are those of bacteria-like organisms that lived nearly 3.5 billion years ago.

Bacteria in humans are essential to digestion. More than 400 different kinds help digest food and fill niches in the intestine that might otherwise be colonized by harmful bacteria. At least one type of bacteria (*Bacteroides thetaiotaomicron*) interacts with cells lining the intestine, benefitting both the human host and the bacteria. Without this type of bacteria, cells in the intestines may fail to produce a sugar found in human milk that is used as food by the bacteria and other beneficial intestinal organisms. When these naturally occurring bacteria are killed (because of ANTIBIOTIC use or other illnesses) harmful bacteria can take over. Diarrhea is one result.

As scientists understand more about the interaction between helpful bacteria and intestines, they may be able to use these bacteria to protect a patient with an impaired immune system or who is taking antibiotics.

Unfortunately, some disease-causing bacteria are beginning to become resistant to many of the antibiotics doctors use to treat the infections. Drug-resistant strains of microbes causing TUBERCULOSIS, PNEUMONIA, CHOLERA, and traveler's diarrhea are on the rise. Certain drug-resistant microbes in the United States cause up to 60 percent of hospital-acquired infections.

See also ANTIDIARRHEAL DRUGS; DIARRHEA AND INFECTIOUS DISEASE; TRAVELER'S DIARRHEA.

bacterial infections One of the most important types of infectious disease. Bacterial infections include GONORRHEA, bacterial MENINGITIS, WHOOPING COUGH, bacterial PNEUMONIA, TUBERCULOSIS, TYPHOID FEVER, and many others.

bacterial names Bacteria are named and are classified into families according to shared properties. Names are always italicized. Because bacterial names are usually derived from Latin or Greek, their meaning may not be obvious to the non-Latin scholar. The naming of organisms is left to the discoverer. Sometimes a species or genus is named after a person, a place, an element of metabolism, or the shape of the organism.

The family name or genus is used first and is followed by a species name, as in *Eschericia coli* ("Eschericia" is the genus, and "coli" is the species name). Both names may indicate some special property or identifying feature of the organism.

A species can be further broken down to identify individual strains within the species, such as *ESCHERICHIA COLI* O157:H7. Strains share the major properties that identify a species but differ in secondary properties such as antibiotic sensitivity, transmissibility, and virulence. The human equivalent would be individual members of the same family belonging to the same sex but having different eye color.

bacterial pneumonia See PNEUMONIA, BACTERIAL.

bactericide Any substance that kills bacteria.

Bang's disease The common name for BRUCEL-LOSIS.

Bartonella A genus of small, Gram-negative type of bacteria that infect red blood cells and cells of the lymph nodes, liver, and spleen. Named for the 18th-century Peruvian bacteriologist who discovered them (Alberto Barton), they are transmitted at night by the bite of a sandfly of the genus *Phlebotomus*. The only known species of *Bartonella* is *B. bacilliformis*, the organism that causes BARTONELLOSIS.

bartonellosis An acute or chronic bacterial infection transmitted to humans by the bite of the sandfly. The risk of this disease is greatest in the mountain valleys of southwest Colombia, Ecuador, and Peru, at altitudes between 2,500 and 8,000 feet.

The *Phlebotomus* sandfly carries the disease-producing bacterium *Bartonella bacilliformis*. Transmission occurs between dusk and dawn (which is sandfly feeding time).

Symptoms and Diagnostic Path

Bartonellosis has two distinct types: Oroya fever and Veruga peruana. Symptoms of Oroya fever begin between two to three weeks after being bitten, with fever, weakness, headache, and bone or joint pain followed by severe anemia and swollen lymph nodes. The disease lasts between two and six weeks and then subsides, but it is occasionally fatal.

Veruga peruana is characterized by the appearance of nodules on the face and limbs that bleed easily and last for up to a year. They finally heal without scarring.

Treatment Options and Outlook

Chloramphenicol or ampicillin is the preferred treatment, although tetracycline, PENICILLIN, or streptomycin also are effective. More recently, doctors may combine two or more antibiotics because of the frequent presence of *Salmonella*. Death from Oroya fever is usually associated with secondary and overwhelming *Salmonella* infection.

Risk Factors and Preventive Measures

This disease can be prevented by avoiding high-risk areas between sundown and sunup, together with the use of insect repellents.

basidiobolomycosis, fungal A chronic, subcutaneous, fungal infection that usually affects humans, horses, and dogs. Subcutaneous disease is found most commonly among adolescent males in East and West Africa and Southeast Asia.

It is caused by a fungus (*Basidiobolus ranarum*) found mainly in the soil and on decaying vegetation. It also has been isolated from the river banks of tropical rivers in West Africa, and has also been found in association with some insects. The fungus is known to be present in the gastrointestinal tracts of reptiles, amphibians, and some bat species.

Symptoms and Diagnostic Path

The disease usually starts as a painless, slow-growing lump underneath the skin that can eventually become large and disfiguring. The nodules may block the lymphatic drainage, causing swelling or ELEPHANTIASIS in an arm or leg.

Treatment Options and Outlook

Several medicines have been successfully used to treat basidiobolomycosis, including itraconazole, ketoconazole, co-trimoxazole, or potassium chloride. All of these oral medications require many months of treatment.

See also BASIDIOBOLOMYCOSIS, GASTROINTESTINAL.

basidiobolomycosis, gastrointestinal A rare emerging infection of the gastrointestinal tract that is often misdiagnosed as cancer or inflammatory bowel disease. Only six cases have been described in the world's medical literature, three in Brazil, one in Kuwait, and two in the United States. Half of the patients died despite medical therapy.

Symptoms and Diagnostic Path

Basidiobolomycosis of the gastrointestinal tract usually begins with pain. Sometimes, a mass can be felt in the abdomen.

Treatment Options and Outlook

There is no standardized treatment, but itraconazole or ketoconazole may be used together with surgical removal of the mass.

See also BASIDIOBOLOMYCOSIS, FUNGAL.

BDV   See BORNA DISEASE VIRUS.

bilharziasis   See SCHISTOMOMIASIS

bird flu   See AVIAN FLU.

black death   See PLAGUE.

bladder infection   See URINARY TRACT INFECTION.

blastomycosis   A mild, often self-limiting yeast infection that usually begins in the lungs and spreads to other sites in the body, especially skin and bone. The disease is found most often in children and in men between the ages of 40 and 60.

The disease is also known as Chicago disease, Gilchrist's disease, or North American blastomycosis.

The disease is caused by the yeast *Blastomyces dermatitidis*; it can be confused with *Coccidioides immitis* or *Cryptococcus neoformans*.

Symptoms and Diagnostic Path

The amount and type of inflammation may vary from one site on the body to another and from one patient to another. There is usually widespread inflammation in the lungs, with small areas of ABSCESSES.

Treatment Options and Outlook

Amphotericin B is the drug of choice; hydroxystilbamidine has been successful in treating the form of the disease that affects the skin, but it is less helpful with other types. Both ketaconazole and itraconazole have been used successfully.

blepharitis   A chronic or long-term inflammation of the eyelids and eyelashes affecting people of all ages. It is characterized by red, irritated scaly skin at the edges of the lids.

Among the most common causes are poor eyelid hygiene, excess oil produced by the glands in the eyelids, a bacterial infection, or an allergic reaction. Seborrheic blepharitis is the most common form. It is often associated with dandruff of the scalp or skin conditions such as acne.

Symptoms and Diagnostic Path

Blepharitis usually appears as greasy flakes or scales around the base of the eyelashes and as a mild redness of the eyelid. Sometimes, seborrheic blepharitis may cause a roughness of the tissue that lines the inside of the eyelids or in nodules on the eyelids. Styes also can result from an acute infection of the eyelids.

A less common form of blepharitis is ulcerative blepharitis. It is characterized by matted, hard crusts around the eyelashes which, when removed, leave small sores that may bleed or ooze.

Treatment Options and Outlook

Blepharitis is usually not serious. In many cases, good eyelid hygiene and a regular cleaning routine can control it. Scales can be removed with cotton moistened with warm water. The inflammation often recurs, which requires more treatment. Ulcerated eyelids must be treated by a physician, since severe cases can lead to problems with the cornea.

bloodborne infectious disease   See INFECTIOUS DISEASES.

blood fluke   See FLUKE.

blood poisoning   See SEPTICEMIA.

boil   An inflamed, pus-filled section of skin (usually an infected hair follicle) found often on the back of the neck or moist areas such as the armpits and groin. A very large boil is called a CARBUNCLE.

Boils are usually caused by infection with the bacterium *Staphylococcus aureus*. After invading the body through a break in the skin, it infects a blocked oil gland or hair follicle. When the body's immune system sends in white blood cells to kill the germs, the resulting inflammation produces pus.

Symptoms and Diagnostic Path

A boil begins with a red, painful lump that swells as it fills with pus, until it becomes rounded with a yellowish tip. It may continue to grow until it erupts, drains, and fades away. Recurrent boils may occur in people with known or unrecognized diabetes mellitus or other diseases involving lowered immune resistance.

Treatment Options and Outlook

Putting pressure on a boil may spread the infection into surrounding tissue. Instead, a hot compress should be applied for 20 minutes every two hours to relieve discomfort and hasten drainage and healing. After treating a boil, hands should be washed thoroughly before cooking to guard against staph infection getting into food.

It may take up to a week for the boil to break on its own. To further reduce chance of infection, the patient should shower, not bathe. If the boil is large and painful, a physician may prescribe an antibiotic or open the boil with a sterile needle to drain the pus. Occasionally, large boils must be lanced with a surgical knife; this is usually done using a local anesthetic.

More seriously, bacteria from a boil may find its way into the blood, causing blood poisoning; for this reason, doctors advise against squeezing boils that appear around the lips or nose, since the infection can be carried to the brain. (Other danger areas include the groin, the armpit, and the breast of a nursing woman.) Signs of a spreading infection include generalized symptoms of fever and chills, swelling lymph nodes, or red lines radiating from the boil.

Risk Factors and Preventive Measures

Some experts note that boils are usually infected cysts and recommend leaving cysts untouched or having them lanced by a physician. For patients prone to boils, some experts recommend washing the skin with an antiseptic soap.

Skin around a boil should be kept clean while drainage is occurring.

Boostrix The first combination booster vaccine approved to prevent WHOOPING COUGH, TETANUS, and DIPHTHERIA for young adults. The booster vaccine (produced by GlaxoSmithKline) is intended for youths aged 10 to 18 years.

Currently, vaccinations against whooping cough, diphtheria, and tetanus are given in early childhood, but protection from these vaccines begins to wear off after five to 10 years. The drug company says it expects Boostrix will replace diphtheria-tetanus boosters that are routinely given to children at about ages 11 or 12 years, since those current boosters do not include whooping cough.

Boostrix has the same components (but in smaller quantities) as Infanrix, a diphtheria-tetanus-whooping cough vaccine for infants and young children. Testing showed that teens' response to Boostrix was considered adequate, according to the U.S. Food and Drug Administration, but it is not known how long whooping cough immunity will last.

It is important to realize that Boostrix is a booster and is not intended as a replacement for the primary whooping cough vaccine normally given during childhood. It has not yet been studied in people who did not complete recommended childhood vaccinations.

The original whooping cough vaccine was developed for infants and young children. However, since the late 1980s, whooping cough infection rates have been rising in very young infants who have not received all their immunizations and in adolescents and adults, according to the FDA. According to GlaxoSmithKline, almost 40 percent of the nearly 20,000 whooping cough cases reported to the CDC in 2004 were diagnosed in teens aged 10 to 19. Still, even with the increase in reports among teens and very young infants, the number of reported cases is more than 97 percent lower than in the pre-vaccine ara, according to the CDC.

Side Effects

Boostrix caused pain, redness, and swelling at the injection site, but these temporary problems were the same as those that occur with a tetanus-diphtheria vaccine. However, pain at the injection site was more common with adolescents who received Boostrix. Other side effects included brief headaches, fever, and fatigue.

Bordetella   A genus of gram-negative bacteria discovered by Belgium bacteriologist Jules J. B. V. Bordet. Some species cause respiratory disease in humans involving the bacteria *Bordetella bronchiseptica*, *B. parapertussis*, and *B. pertussis*.
   See WHOOPING COUGH; *BORDETELLA PERTUSSIS*.

Bordetella pertussis   A species of tiny gram-negative anaerobic bacterium (in the genus *Bordetella*) that causes WHOOPING COUGH, one of the most common infections on earth. All the other species of the *Bordetella* genus cause diseases that resemble whooping cough.

It is extremely virulent, infecting more than 90 percent of susceptible victims after close contact. It usually strikes during childhood; before the advent of modern medicine it was a major cause of infant death around the world. It is still a significant health problem in underdeveloped areas, causing about 40 million cases worldwide and about 400,000 deaths. A vaccine against the bacteria was developed in the mid-1940s, although local outbreaks still occur among unvaccinated individuals.

The disease was named *pertussis* (from the Latin word for "intense cough") and was known popularly as "whooping cough" in the 17th century; earlier, it was called "chin cough." French physicians called it *quinta* because of the five-hour respites between coughing spasms, or "coqueluche."

Since 1940, the vaccine against *Bordetella pertussis* (a combination of DIPHTHERIA, TETANUS, and pertussis), or "DTP," has cut the incidence of whooping cough by 99 percent, but the shot has been linked to rare but serious side effects, including high fever, convulsions, and rarely, brain damage and death. In 1988, the United States established an $80 million fund to compensate children who were injured by the vaccine, which initiated 4,700 claims. Since then, the National Institutes of Health spent $16 million to develop a safer vaccine—the acellular

vaccine (DTaP), so named because it was derived from only part of a *B. pertussis* cell.

Borna disease virus (BDV)   A type of virus known to cause behavior disruptions and neurological disease in several animal species, and recently found in humans as well. Infection with this virus may trigger depressive episodes in humans who are already vulnerable to major depression or manic depression.

Borna disease virus is a single-stranded RNA virus that establishes a persistent infection without directly damaging host cells. BDV infection may contribute to depressive illness by altering neurol cells in the limbic system. The leading hypothesis is that BDV, as it inserts itself into neurons, may disrupt the function of those cells.

Symptoms and Diagnostic Path

BDV causes neurological symptoms in domestic animals, which is where it gets its nickname, "crazy virus." The neurological symptoms resemble those seen in humans with manic depression. This virus is entirely separate from MAD COW DISEASE, although the neurological symptoms are what led researchers to study BDV more closely.

The virus infects cells of the limbic system implicated in many psychiatric disorders, including bipolar depression and schizophrenia. BDV infects cells in the nervous system just as its distant viral relative rabies, causing brain damage in animals and humans. Previous studies have shown that a large proportion of psychiatric patients with certain affective disorders, such as depression and manic depressive disorder, have antibodies specific to proteins of BDV. Since Borna viral material tends to appear during episodes of depression, scientists suspect that the virus brings on depressive episodes in people predisposed to mood disorders by their genes or other factors (perhaps by disrupting communication between brain cells). In most people, however, the infection appears to cause no problems.

Doctors do not know how big a factor Borna virus might be in mental disorders and it is not clear whether Borna virus can jump from animals to people, nor how it might spread among people. However, scientists do know that humans cannot get Borna virus from eating meat or other products of infected animals.

BDV was first reported more than a century ago as a cause of neurological disease in horses in Borna, Germany. Since then, outbreaks of the virus have been documented in cattle, sheep, and cats. Rats injected with BDV exhibit damage to brain cells in the limbic system, the part of the brain that governs mood and emotions. Interestingly, the virus affects various animal species differently. While rats' brains are destroyed, the virus causes only subtle abnormal social patterns in tree shrews. Further animal studies as well as larger studies of psychiatric patients may help scientists better understand how the virus causes disease and how to develop a way to diagnose and treat it.

The cause of most of the common psychiatric disorders, including depression, manic depression, anxiety, and schizophrenia, remains a mystery. In some cases, symptoms appear suddenly and the disease follows a catastrophic course, while in other cases the disease may be intermittent. Despite a large amount of research, and a lot of familial association evidence, the search for causative genes has produced mixed results. This has helped fuel the search for other factors, such as viral infection.

One group of investigators at the National Institute of Mental Health is pursuing the hypothesis that schizophrenia might be caused by viruses transmitted from household pets to pregnant women or young children. Another group of researchers at the University of Southern California is looking for a link between chronic fatigue syndrome and "stealth viruses" (viruses that have been incorporated into the host DNA and are no longer recognized by the immune system). These viruses cannot be detected by standard immunological methods or standard culture techniques. However, they can be detected with techniques that match DNA sequences with known viral DNA.

borrelia See LYME DISEASE; RELAPSING FEVER.

Borrelia burgdorferi A species of large parasitic spirochete bacteria (in the genus _Borrelia_) that cause

LYME DISEASE. The species _B. duttonii, B. persica,_ and _B. recurrentis_ cause RELAPSING FEVER.

botulism The most common type of the infectious disease known as botulism is a food-borne illness involving the toxin produced by the bacteria _Clostridium botulinum,_ which is both rare and very deadly (two-thirds of those afflicted die). Another type is known as "infant botulism," an uncommon illness that strikes infants under the age of one. Because botulism is technically a poisoning, not an infection, the patient cannot infect others even though the bacteria will be excreted in feces for months after the illness.

Botulism is more common in the United States than anywhere else in the world owing to the popularity of home canning; there are about 154 cases of food-borne botulism poisoning each year. Botulism got its name during the 1800s from _botulus,_ the Latin word for "sausage," because of a wave of poisoning from contaminated sausages at that time.

Botulism toxins are a type of neurotoxin that attaches to the nerves, blocking the messages that are sent to the muscles. The _C. botulinum_ spores (latent form of the bacteria) are found in air, water, and food; they are harmless until deprived of oxygen, such as inside a sealed can or jar. If conditions are favorable, the spores will start to generate and multiply, producing one of the most deadly toxins known—7 million times more deadly than cobra venom.

Cases of botulism from commercially canned food are rare because of strict health standards enforced by the U.S. Food and Drug Administration, although some people have gotten botulism from eating improperly handled commercial pot pies. In Canada, cases have been reported from seal meat, smoked salmon, and fermented salmon eggs. However, most cases occur during home canning.

Canned foods that are highly susceptible to contamination include green beans, beets, peppers, corn, and meat. Although the spores can survive boiling, the ideal temperature for their growth is between 78°F and 96°F. They can also survive freezing.

Botulism can also occur if the _C. botulinum_ bacteria in the soil enters the body through an open wound, although this is extremely rare.

Symptoms and Diagnostic Path

Onset of symptoms may be as soon as three hours or as late as 14 days after ingestion, although most symptoms usually appear between 12 and 26 hours. The first sign is usually muscle weakness beginning with the head, often leading to double vision. This is followed by problems in swallowing or speaking, followed by the paralysis of the muscles needed to breathe. Other symptoms can include nausea, vomiting, diarrhea, and stomach cramps. The earlier the onset of symptoms, the more severe the reaction. Symptoms generally last between three to six days; death occurs in about 70 percent of untreated cases, usually from suffocation as a result of respiratory muscle paralysis. In infants, symptoms may go unrecognized by parents for some time until the poisoning has reached a critical stage.

Large commercial labs or state health labs can test for the toxin in food, blood, or stool; it is also possible to grow the bacteria from food or stool in a special culture. The diagnosis is most often made by an astute health care practitioner who recognizes the signs and symptoms. In an outbreak, the first victim to become sick usually dies because the condition was not immediately diagnosed.

Treatment Options and Outlook

Prompt administration of the antitoxin (type ABE botulinus) lowers the risk of death to 10 percent. Most untreated victims will die. The Centers for Disease Control and Prevention is the only agency with the antitoxin, and it makes the decision to treat. Local health departments should be called first for this information. While induced vomiting may help following ingestion of food known to contain botulism toxin, it may not be complete. Because the disease can occur with only a small amount of toxin, botulism may still develop. Patients are usually put on a respirator to ease breathing.

In infant botulism, if symptoms are present it may be too late to administer antitoxin, since the damage has probably already been done.

Risk Factors and Preventive Measures

It is easy to prevent, since botulism is killed when canned food is boiled at 212°F for one minute, or if the food is first sterilized by pressure cooking at 250°F for 30 minutes.

While the tightly fitted lids of home-canned food will provide the anaerobic environment necessary for the growth of botulism toxins, the spores will not grow if the food is very acidic, sweet, or salty (such as canned fruit juice, jams and jellies, sauerkraut, tomatoes, and heavily salted hams).

Even though botulism spores are invisible, it is possible to tell if food is spoiled by noticing if jars have lost their vacuum seal; when the spores grow, they give off gas that makes cans and jars lose the seal. Jars will burst or cans will swell. Any food that is spoiled or whose color or odor does not seem right inside a home-canned jar or can should be thrown away without tasting or even sniffing, since botulism can be fatal in extremely small amounts.

botulism, infant Unlike BOTULISM in adults, which occurs after eating contaminated food, infant botulism occurs in babies under six months of age and is less serious. There are about 92 cases of infant botulism in the United States each year.

While all botulism is caused by toxins given off by *Clostridium botulinum* bacteria, in infant botulism the baby does not ingest the toxin. Instead, the spores from botulism bacteria reproduce the toxin in the baby's digestive tract, which then travels to the baby's nerve cells.

Fortunately, most babies will recover with prompt hospital treatment. The illness is found in all races in North and South America, Asia, and Europe.

This rare disease may be difficult to trace, since the spores may survive for a long time in the environment. It is clear that about 10 percent of commercial honey contains botulism spores and occasionally, light and dark corn syrup also harbors the bacteria. For this reason, parents are advised not to feed either food to infants under a year of age.

Although an infected baby will excrete toxin for weeks in feces, the baby cannot pass on the infection to others.

Symptoms and Diagnostic Path

Infant botulism symptoms include constipation, facial muscle flaccidity, sucking problems, irritability, lethargy, and floppy arms and legs.

Treatment Options and Outlook

The antitoxin used to treat adults with botulism is not safe for infants. Antibiotics may be used to treat secondary infections. In severe cases, the baby may need breathing assistance; while recovery may be slow, most usually completely recover.

Some experts believe that infant botulism may be responsible for up to 5 percent of all cases of sudden infant death syndrome.

Risk Factors and Preventive Measures

Babies under age one should not be fed honey or corn syrup. They should be kept away from dust (both from vacuum cleaners and from the outdoors), especially around construction sites.

bouba   See YAWS.

bovine spongiform encephalopathy   The medical name for MAD COW DISEASE, a chronic, degenerative disease affecting the central nervous system of cattle. It is one of a group of fatal brain diseases called transmissible spongiform encephalopathies (TSEs). These infectious diseases, which are always fatal, create holes in the brain, making it look like a sponge. The first known TSE appeared in sheep, but now humans, cows, elk, deer, mink, rats, mice, hamsters, and possibly monkeys all get various types of the disease.

BSE was first identified in Britain in 1986, and was thought to be transmitted to humans via contaminated meat and bone meal. The human version of BSE is called new variant CREUTZFELDT-JAKOB DISEASE.

As of November, 2000, more than 177,500 cases of mad cow disease in cattle were confirmed in the United Kingdom in more than 35,000 herds; it peaked in January, 1993 at almost 1,000 new cases a week. The outbreak may have resulted from the feeding of tainted sheep meat and bone meal to cattle, amplified by feeding rendered cow meat-and-bone meal to young calves. Since the feeding of bovine offal to cows was stopped in Britain, the incidence of the disease has declined significantly.

Worldwide there have been more than 180,000 cases in cattle since the disease was first diagnosed

in 1986. While there is a decline in the number of cases of BSE in the United Kingdom, confirmed cases of BSE have risen in other European countries, including Belgium, Czech Republic, Denmark, France, Germany, Greece, Ireland, Italy, Luxembourg, Liechtenstein, the Netherlands, Northern Ireland, Portugal, Spain, and Switzerland. More than 90 percent of all BSE cases have occurred in the United Kingdom.

In the United States, officials restricted imports of live cattle and meat from countries with BSE in 1989.

The first case of mad cow disease in the United States was reported on December 23, 2003, when an infected cow from a Washington farm had been slaughtered two weeks earlier. The edible parts went to meat processors for making into hamburgers and steaks, while the inedible parts went to renderers to grind into meal for animal feed and fat for soap. The brain went to a U.S. Department of Agriculture (USDA) laboratory in Ames, Iowa, for BSE testing. Informed that the tissue revealed mad cow disease, the FDA and the USDA had to try to destroy as many parts of the infected cow as possible. FDA investigators traced potentially contaminated products to renderers, grocery stores, meat suppliers, and even a hide recycler. Officials wanted to make sure that no parts of the hide from the cow, not even any flesh scrapings, could have been diverted to animal feed or other use.

A second infection was identified in June 2005 in a cow that was first identified in November 2004. Results from this test were inconclusive in screening, but negative in further tests. However, when the USDA recently conducted an additional test, the results were positive for BSE. The USDA sent the samples to Britain, where BSE was confirmed. The cow had been born before the United States banned the use of most mammalian protein in feed for ruminant animals, which is believed to be the most critical way to prevent the spread of BSE among cattle. The cow was presented at slaughter as a "downer" cow, which means that government's mad cow regulations kept it out of the human food supply.

The cause of BSE has been linked to three main theories: an unconventional virus, an abnormal PRION, or a virino ("incomplete" virus) composed of naked nucleic acid protected by host proteins. What scientists do know is that the BSE agent is smaller than most viral particles and is highly resistant to heat, ultraviolet light, ionizing radiation, and common disinfectants that normally inactivate viruses or bacteria. They also know that it causes no detectable immune or inflammatory response and has not been observed microscopically. At present, most scientists blame prions as the most likely cause.

There is no test to detect the disease in a live animal, but two lab methods can confirm a diagnosis of BSE on autopsy: microscopic examination of the brain tissue to identify characteristic changes or techniques to detect the infectious agent.

brain abscess A pocket of infection, most commonly found in the frontal and temporal lobes, usually caused by the spread of infection from another part of the body, such as the sinuses. A brain abscess also may result from spread of an infection in the bones, the nervous system outside the brain, or the heart. These abscesses cause symptoms due to increased pressure and local brain injury.

About 10 percent of cases are fatal; the remaining patients often have some brain function impairment. A seizure disorder is a common complication.

Brain abscesses are almost always caused by infection spreading from somewhere else in the body. About 40 percent of abscesses are from middle ear or sinus infections. Blood-borne infections may also cause multiple brain abscesses. Fluid, dead tissue cells, white blood cells, and live and dead microorganisms collect and form a mass that usually becomes enclosed by a membrane that forms at the edges of the fluid collection. The brain swells in response to the inflammation, and the mass may put pressure on the structures of the brain. Infected material can block the vessels of the brain, further damaging brain tissues. As a result, pressure within the brain rises, causing more extensive damage and dysfunction.

Symptoms and Diagnostic Path

The most common symptoms are headache, sleepiness, and vomiting. There may be visual problems, with fever and seizures. There may be evidence of local brain damage as well, including partial paralysis or speech problems.

Brain scans (CT scans or magnetic resonance imaging) of the brain can diagnose a brain abscess.

Treatment Options and Outlook

High doses of antibiotics and usually surgery; the abscess may be accessible via a small hole in the skull.

Brainerd diarrhea A syndrome of watery diarrhea lasting for a month or longer that can occur in outbreaks or as sporadic cases. The disease is named after Brainerd, Minnesota, the town where the first outbreak occurred in 1983.

Symptoms and Diagnostic Path

Patients typically experience 10 to 20 episodes per day of explosive watery diarrhea, characterized by urgency and often by incontinence. Accompanying symptoms include gas, mild abdominal cramping, and fatigue. Nausea, vomiting, and systemic symptoms such as fever are rare, although many patients experience slight weight loss.

Symptoms may last a year or more, and typically have a waxing and waning course. Long-term follow-up studies have shown virtually all patients are completely cured by the end of three years. There have been no known cases of complications or relapse once the illness has completely healed.

Despite extensive clinical and laboratory investigations, the cause of Brainerd diarrhea has not yet been identified. Although scientists think it must be an infectious agent, intensive searches for bacterial, parasitic, and viral causes have not yet been successful. The possibility remains that Brainerd diarrhea is caused by a chemical toxin, but no such toxin has yet been found.

Seven outbreaks of Brainerd diarrhea have been reported since 1983, six in the United States; five of these were in rural settings. One outbreak occurred on a South American cruise ship based in the Galápagos Islands. The original Brainerd outbreak was the largest, involving 122 people. An outbreak in Henderson County, Illinois, involved 72 people; the Galápagos Islands outbreak involved 58. However, many patients who are not associated with a recognized outbreak seek treatment for illness compatible with Brainerd diarrhea.

In the original Brainerd outbreak, unpasteurized milk was implicated as the cause of the disease transmission. Contaminated and inadequately chlorinated or unboiled water has been identified as a source of Brainerd diarrhea in several other outbreaks. For example, illness was strongly associated with drinking untreated well water in the Henderson County outbreak. People who drank the same water after it was boiled did not get sick. Contaminated water was also implicated in the Galápagos Islands outbreak. The diarrheal illness does not spread contagiously from one person to the next.

Because the cause is unknown, there is no lab test that can confirm the diagnosis. Brainerd diarrhea should be suspected in any patient who experiences sudden nonbloody diarrhea lasting for more than a month, and for whom stool cultures and examinations do not reveal any eggs or parasites. Other causes of chronic infectious and noninfectious diarrhea must be ruled out in order to diagnose Brainerd diarrhea, which is not characterized by any specific laboratory abnormalities.

Treatment Options and Outlook

There is no known treatment for Brainerd diarrhea. Approximately half of patients report their symptoms improve with high doses of opioid antimotility drugs, such as loperamide, diphenoxylate, and paregoric.

Risk Factors and Preventive Measures

Avoiding drinking unpasteurized milk and water that has not been properly chlorinated or boiled will help reduce the risk for Brainerd diarrhea and many other diseases. Once the cause of Brainerd diarrhea is identified, more specific prevention measures can be formulated.

Brazilian purpuric fever A serious systemic illness that may be caused by bacterial infection, which was first recognized in 1984 in Brazil. Since then there have been occasional outbreaks in a number of towns in the surrounding area, and cases with similar symptoms have also been reported in

Australia. Little is actually known about the bacteria that cause the disease or its mode of spread, but it almost always affects children under 10.

Cases being treated for presumed meningococcemia may in actuality be cases of BPF. In many areas a blood culture may not have been drawn to determine the diagnosis.

Brazilian purpuric fever appears to be related to *Haemophilus aegyptius* (*H. influenzae,* biotype III). If untreated, the infection spreads and can lead to fatal purpura (bleeding into the skin), release of toxins, and overwhelming shock.

Symptoms and Diagnostic Path

The illness typically begins with eye infection caused by *H. influenzae* III; in a small number of patients, the bacteria spread throughout the body, causing fever and bleeding into the skin. If untreated, this bleeding continues; the bacteria release a toxin that overwhelms the body's defenses and ends in death. Symptoms resemble meningococcemia.

Treatment Options and Outlook

Systemic antibiotics to treat BPF (usually ampicillin with or without chloramphenicol) before the skin bleeding begins may prevent progression of the disease.

breast cancer and virus For many years controversial claims suggesting some cases of breast cancer may be linked in some form to a virus have been debated.

Cancerous breast cells often contain genetic sequences similar to an infectious virus that triggers mammary tumors in mice, which is why some researchers continue to question whether a virus plays a role in at least some types of breast cancer.

Over the last few decades, investigators have linked a number of viruses (specifically retroviruses) to cancer in animals and people. A retrovirus can transform a normal cell into a cancer cell by inserting its genetic material into the cell, disrupting the function of crucial genes. For example, mouse mammary tumor virus (MMTV) produces cancer in about 95 percent of the mice it infects.

The idea that viruses may cause some types of breast cancer dates to the 1930s, when scientists identified virus-like particles in mothers' milk. While mice can transmit MMTV to their babies through milk, no evidence was found that children who were breast-fed by mothers with breast cancer had a higher chance of developing the disease themselves.

Still, over the decades since then, research groups have reported some genetic evidence that an MMTV-like virus is associated with breast cancer. The problem with those reports was that in those days, scientists could not tell the difference between MMTV-like viruses and human endogenous retrovirus (HER), an ancient virus whose genetic code is integrated into everyone's genome.

In recent years, however, scientific procedure has become more sophisticated. Scientists have sequenced many of MMTV's genes and found regions of various genes that differ quite a bit from those of HER. The new research looked at samples of human breast tissue for MMTV-specific gene fragments. In 1995, the group reported that in almost 40 percent of breast cancer tissue tested, they found sequences similar to those in one of the MMTV's genes. Less than 2 percent of normal breast samples yielded this so-called env gene. This env gene encodes a protein that helps form the outer surface of the virus.

In 1996, the group reported that they found a different sequence of the env gene in 13 of 19 breast cancer samples, and in none of the normal breast tissue samples. Interestingly, hormones such as estrogen stimulate the activity of an MMTV-like env gene in a cell line derived from breast cancer cells.

bronchiolitis An acute viral infection of the small airways in the lungs that primarily affects infants and young children. Winter epidemics tend to occur every two or three years, affecting thousands of children in the United States. A virus that may induce only a mild head or chest infection in an adult can cause a severe bronchiolitis in an infant. With prompt treatment, even the sickest infants usually recover completely within a few days.

The smaller airways that branch off the bronchial tubes become inflamed, usually because of the RESPIRATORY SYNCYTIAL VIRUS (RSV) infection, although

other viruses associated with the flu or ADENOVIRUS may be responsible. Adult attacks may follow BRONCHITIS brought on by INFLUENZA. The viruses may be transmitted from person to person through airborne drops and are highly contagious. Hospitalized patients will be placed in respiratory isolation.

Symptoms and Diagnostic Path
The first symptoms of bronchiolitis are usually the same as those of a COMMON COLD and include a stuffy, runny nose and a mild cough. After a few days, symptoms get worse, and the patient begins to wheeze when breathing out. More severe respiratory difficulties may gradually develop, including rapid, shallow breathing; rapid heartbeat; sucking in of the neck and chest with each breath; flaring nostrils; irritability; sleeping problems; fatigue. Other symptoms may include fever, poor appetite, and vomiting after coughing.

A few infants (especially premature babies) may experience apnea, when they briefly stop breathing, before developing other symptoms.

In severe cases, symptoms get worse very quickly, and the child may become very tired from struggling to breathe. In this case, the lips and fingernails may turn blue (cyanosis). The child also may become dehydrated as a result of fever, vomiting, and not drinking enough.

Treatment Options and Outlook
In mild cases no treatment is needed, but in severe cases the child may need to be hospitalized for oxygen and respiratory therapy to clear the mucus. Antibiotics and CORTICOSTEROID DRUGS would not work against this viral infection, although antibiotics may be prescribed to prevent a secondary bacterial infection. Sometimes a child may need to be placed on artificial ventilation until normal breathing returns. Although bronchiolitis is often mild, some vulnerable infants are at risk for a more severe disease that can require hospitalization. Conditions in infancy that increase the risk of severe infection include prematurity, chronic heart or lung disease, and a weakened immune system as a result of disease or medications.

Children who have had bronchiolitis may be more likely to develop asthma when they are older, although it is not clear whether bronchiolitis directly triggers asthma or whether children who eventually go on to develop asthma were at higher risk to develop bronchiolitis in infancy.

Risk Factors and Preventive Measures

Frequent hand washing is the best way to prevent the spread of viruses that can cause bronchiolitis; avoiding people who are sick also may help. It is also a good idea to keep infants away from cigarette smoke, since research suggests that babies exposed to cigarette smoke are more likely to develop more severe bronchiolitis.

There is as yet no vaccine for bronchiolitis. Infants at high risk of severe disease (such as those who were born prematurely or who have chronic lung disease) may be given antibodies to the virus that are injected monthly during peak RSV season.

bronchiolitis obliterans with organizing pneumonia (BOOP)

Inflammation that partially obliterates the small airways (bronchioles) and nearby lung tissue. It may affect either a small area or the entire lung but is not linked to infection, smoking, or lung cancer. The condition is not infectious or caused by a germ; instead, it is due to inflammation of lung tissue around the inflamed bronchioles.

In many cases, the cause cannot be identified, but the condition has been linked to certain medications, connective tissue disorders such as lupus, organ and tissue transplantation (especially bone marrow transplants), and radiation therapy (especially for breast cancer).

Symptoms and Diagnostic Path

There may be no symptoms at all. If symptoms do appear, they may develop slowly over several weeks and include shortness of breath and fever.

This condition is difficult to diagnose. BOOP may be found during a chest X-ray performed for another reason. Otherwise, a diagnosis may be based on medical history, lung scans, or lung tissue biopsy.

Treatment Options and Outlook

Treatment depends on the underlying cause but typically may include prednisone.

bronchitis   Inflammation of the airways that connect the windpipe (trachea) to the lungs, resulting in persistent cough with quantities of phlegm or sputum. Attacks usually occur in the winter among smokers, babies, the elderly, and those with lung disease, although anyone can get bronchitis.

Bronchitis presents in one of two forms: acute (of sudden onset and short duration) and chronic (persistent over a long period, and recurring several years).

Acute bronchitis is usually a complication of a viral infection (such as a cold or the flu), although it can also be caused by air pollution. A bacterial infection also may lead to acute bronchitis. Attacks occur most often in winter.

Cigarette smoking is the primary cause of *chronic bronchitis*, because it stimulates the production of mucus in the lining of the bronchi and thickens the bronchi's muscular walls and those of smaller airways in the lungs, narrowing those passages. The passages then become more susceptible to infection, which cause further damage. Air pollution can have the same effect. The disease is most prevalent in industrial cities and in smokers, and more common in manual and unskilled workers.

Symptoms and Diagnostic Path

The symptoms of both chronic and acute bronchitis are the same. As the bronchial tubes swell and become congested, symptoms appear: wheezing, breathlessness, and a persistent cough that produces yellow or green phlegm. There also may be pain behind the breastbone. Acute bronchitis is also characterized by fever.

In chronic bronchitis, symptoms do not quickly clear up, and there is usually no fever. The persistence of symptoms also differentiates this disease from chronic asthma, in which wheezing and breathlessness vary in severity from day to day.

As the disease progresses, emphysema may develop. The lungs become more resistant to the flow of blood, leading to pulmonary hypertension. Those with chronic bronchitis usually have two or more episodes of acute viral or bacterial infection of the lungs every winter. Occasionally, blood may be coughed up.

Treatment Options and Outlook

Humidifying the lungs either with a humidifier or by inhaling steam will ease symptoms. Drinking plenty of fluids also helps bring up phlegm. Most acute bronchitis clears up on its own without further treatment. If there is a suspicion of an underlying bacterial infection, antibiotics will be prescribed.

In chronic bronchitis, an inhaler containing a bronchodilator may relieve breathlessness. In specific cases, the patient may improve by inhaling oxygen from a cylinder. Antibiotics may treat or prevent any bacterial lung infection. Chronic bronchitis often leads inexorably to increased shortness of breath.

Pleurisy or PNEUMONIA may rarely occur in cases of acute bronchitis. A physician should be consulted if any of the following symptoms appear:

- severe breathlessness
- audible wheezing
- no improvement after three days
- blood in sputum
- fever over 101°F

Brucella A genus of Gram-negative spherical or rodlike parasitic bacteria that cause BRUCELLOSIS (undulant fever) in humans, and contagious abortion in animals. The principal species include *B. abortus* and *B. melitensis.* The genus was named after David Bruce, a surgeon who first identified the bacteria in 1887.

brucellosis A chronic bacterial disease carried by farm animals that may be transmitted to humans, affecting various organs of the body. It is also known as undulant fever, Malta fever, Gibraltar fever, Bang's disease, or Mediterranean fever.

Anyone is susceptible to the bacteria and may get the disease if exposed, but it is more likely to be found among those who work with livestock. Up to 200 cases of brucellosis are diagnosed in the United States each year. In areas where milk pasteurization is not widely practiced (such as in Latin America and in the Mediterranean) the disease is contracted from eating unpasteurized dairy products. Untreated, the disease may persist for years.

The disease is caused by several different species of bacteria of the genus *BRUCELLA. B. abortus* is found in cattle. *B. suis* is most often isolated in hogs and is more deadly when contracted by humans than the version found in cattle. *B. melitensis* is found in goats and sheep and causes the most severe illness in humans. *B. rangiferi* occurs in reindeer and caribou, and *B. canis* in dogs.

The bacteria are transmitted to humans by contact with an infected animal (through a cut or breathing in bacteria) or by consuming nonpasteurized contaminated milk or fresh goat cheese. It is also found in the afterbirth from infected cattle or goats that have aborted a fetus. It is not likely that the disease spreads from person to person or that a person will be reinfected after recovery. In the United States the disease is primarily confined to workers at slaughterhouses. The late President Richard Nixon suffered from brucellosis as a child.

Symptoms and Diagnostic Path

The disease is not usually fatal, but the intermittent fevers (a source of the name, "undulant fever"), can be debilitating. Symptoms usually appear within five to 30 days after exposure. The acute form of the disease involves a single bout of high fever, shivering, aching, and drenching sweats that last for a few days. Other symptoms include headache, poor appetite, backache, weakness, and depression. Mental depression can be so severe that the patient may be suicidal. In rare, untreated cases, an acute attack is so serious it can cause fatal complications such as PNEUMONIA or bacterial MENINGITIS. *B. melitensis* can cause abortions in women, especially during the first three months of pregnancy.

Chronic brucellosis is characterized by symptoms that recur over a period of months or years.

Blood tests can diagnose the disease.

Treatment Options and Outlook

Prolonged treatment with antibiotics (including tetracyclines plus streptomycin) and sulfonamides is effective. Bed rest is imperative. After an apparent recovery, the disease sometimes recurs a few months later, requiring another course of treatment.

Risk Factors and Preventive Measures

Human disease can be prevented by immunizing livestock that have first been checked to make sure they are not already infected. Infected animals are usually destroyed.

bubonic plague   See PLAGUE.

Bunyaviridae   One of the largest viral families that includes more than 300 viruses, BUNYAVIRUS have presented a significant challenge to scientists trying to define them. This viral family contains five genera: bunyavirus, PHLEBOVIRUS, NAIROVIRUS, HANTAVIRUS, and tospovirus, all with similar features.

bunyavirus   A group of mosquito-borne viruses that can infect humans. Named after the Bunyamwera virus found in Uganda, almost all of the more than 161 viruses in this family are transmitted by mosquitoes but have a wide variety of vertebrate hosts. Within this genus, the California serogroup viruses are those that most commonly affect humans. The bunyaviruses cause a feverish illness that can include California encephalitis, RIFT VALLEY FEVER, La Crosse encephalitis, SANDFLY FEVER, and others.

See also BUNYAVIRIDAE; ENCEPHALITIS, CALIFORNIA; ENCEPHALITIS, La CROSSE.

Burkholderia cepacia   A bacterium formerly known as *Pseudomonas cepacia* whose natural habitats are river sediments and the moist areas of soil around the roots of plants. In the past, it was best known as the cause of a type of onion rot (the Latin name for "onion" is *cepia*).

B. cepacia is one of the most adaptable of all bacteria and has an uncanny ability to survive in hostile environments. Soil contains many natural antibiotics to which *B. cepacia* has become resistant—so much so that it can even use PENICILLIN as a nutrient.

Although the bacteria rarely infect healthy people, serious infections can threaten immunocompromised patients and those with serious lung diseases such as cystic fibrosis (CF).

While *B. cepacia* can spread from one person to the next, it is unclear exactly how it is transmitted from person to person.

Although originally identified as a plant organism, it is now recognized as a useful organism for plant protection and plant-growth promotion, while at the same time becoming notorious as a resistant and life-threatening pathogen in the immune suppressed such as patients with chronic granulomatous disease.

Before the early 1980s, reports of human infections caused by *B. cepacia* were rare and generally restricted to hospitalized patients exposed to contaminated disinfectant and anesthetics.

By the early 1980s, however, more cases began to appear, particularly in patients with CF. Infection with the bacteria cuts survival in half, and about a third to a half die of "cepacia syndrome," a rapidly fatal necrotizing pneumonia. During the 1980s and 1990s, several major outbreaks of *B. cepacia* infections caused many deaths in CF populations worldwide. Each of the nine species of the *B. cepacia* complex has been given a formal species name. Two species (*B. cenocepacia* and *B. multivorans*) account for most *B. cepacia* complex infection in patients with cystic fibrosis. Research suggests that specific *B. cepacia* complex strains infect many cystic fibrosis patients, which implies that the bacteria may spread quickly among patients. Studies suggest that at least some of these epidemic strains are also more deadly in a person with cystic fibrosis.

California encephalitis   See ENCEPHALITIS, CALIFORNIA.

camp fever   See TYPHUS.

Campylobacter   A genus of bacteria that infects the gastrointestinal tract and is the most common cause of diarrhea in the world. The bacteria are usually transmitted via contaminated water or food. For many years, scientists had thought the bacteria were related to the VIBRIO germs that cause intestinal illnesses and CHOLERA. In fact, the bacteria are much less dangerous, but much more common.

The bacteria were first identified in 1909 by two English veterinarians who were studying aborted cattle fetuses and who named the bacterium *Vibrio fetus*. The same bacteria were then isolated in 1947 in a woman's blood, but it was not until 1972 that researchers identified it as a new genus and named it *Campylobacter* for its characteristic shape from the Greek for "curved rod."

The *Campylobacter* organism is actually a large group of spiral-shaped bacteria. Almost all human illness is caused by one species, called CAMPYLOBACTER JEJUNI, but 1 percent of human *Campylobacter* cases are caused by other species such as *C. fetus*, which looks like *C. jejuni* but usually attacks newborn babies or people with weakened immune systems. Although much more rare than *C. jejuni*, *C. fetus* also causes a more severe illness, which typically requires prolonged treatment with antibiotics. *C. jejuni* is carried by birds without them becoming ill.

The bacterium is fragile; it cannot tolerate dryness and can be killed by oxygen. Freezing can reduce the number of *Campylobacter* bacteria in food.

The bacteria survive best at body temperatures of humans and cattle, poultry, horses, and pets. They are one of the four most important types of disease-causing organisms that infect the intestines; the others are SHIGELLA, SALMONELLA, and GIARDIA LAMBLIA. All are ingested in much the same way, via tainted food and water in places where proper sanitation, hygiene, or cooking methods are not strictly observed.

See also ANTIDIARRHEAL DRUGS; CAMPYLOBACTERIOSIS; DIARRHEA AND INFECTIOUS DISEASE; TRAVELER'S DIARRHEA.

campylobacteriosis   A form of food-borne illness, first recognized in the 1970s, that causes gastroenteritis—one of the many types of so-called TRAVELER'S DIARRHEA. Much more common than diseases caused by either SALMONELLA or SHIGELLA, campylobacteriosis is responsible for between 5 to 14 percent of all diarrheal infections in the world. It may affect between 2 and 4 million Americans each year. Although anyone can get an infection, children under age five and young adults aged 15 to 29 are more frequently afflicted.

In the 1970s, more than 3,000 residents in Bennington, Vermont, became ill with diarrhea when their town's water supply was contaminated by a dead dog, which produced the rod-shaped bacterium CAMPYLOBACTER JEJUNI. It has subsequently spread everywhere.

Without treatment, the stool is infectious for several weeks, but three days of antibiotics will eliminate the bacteria from the stool. While the illness can be uncomfortable and even disabling, deaths among otherwise healthy patients are rare. Still, it is estimated that 500 people die from CAMPYLOBACTER each year.

While there are several different forms of *Campylobacter*, the most common is *Campylobacter jejuni*, which accounts for 99 percent of all *Campylobacter* infections. Campylobacteriosis is caused by eating or drinking food or water contaminated with the bacteria; only a small amount is necessary to cause illness. It can survive in undercooked food such as chicken, lamb, beef, or pork, in water, and in raw milk. The disease may also spread throughout a child care center or from the diarrhea of affected young dogs or cats.

The most common source of *Campylobacter* infection is in contaminated poultry (between 20 percent and 100 percent of all raw chicken on the market is contaminated). This is not surprising considering that many healthy chickens carry the bacteria in their intestines. Raw milk is also a source of infection. Consumers get sick when they eat undercooked chicken or when the organisms are transferred from the raw meat or raw meat drippings to the mouth. The bacteria are common among healthy chickens on chicken farms, where they may spread undetected among the flocks (perhaps through drinking water supplies). When the birds are slaughtered, the bacteria are transferred from the intestines to the meat.

Other forms of *Campylobacter* are harder to diagnose and appear to be much more rare than *C. jejuni*; it is not yet clear what the source of those infections are.

Symptoms and Diagnostic Path

Symptoms begin between two to 10 days after tainted food or water is consumed and may last up to 10 days. Primary symptoms are fever, nausea and vomiting and abdominal pain followed by watery or bloody diarrhea. Other symptoms may include headaches, fatigue, and body aches. Diarrhea can lead to dehydration.

The infection is diagnosed by culturing stool using special lab techniques.

Treatment Options and Outlook

Antibiotics taken at the very beginning of the illness can shorten the duration of symptoms. For mild cases, rest and fluids should be sufficient. Young children are usually given antibiotics (usually erythromycin) as a way of reducing the risk of passing the infection on to other children via infected stool.

Most people recover completely within two to five days, although recovery may take up to 10 days. About 20 percent of the time, diarrhea may last as long as three to four weeks or recur after a period of improvement. Rarely, some long-term complications may include either arthritis or Guillain-Barré syndrome, a rare disease that affects the nerves of the body several weeks after the diarrheal illness. Guillain-Barré syndrome occurs when a person's immune system attacks the body's own nerves, and can lead to paralysis that lasts several weeks. Experts estimate that about one in every 1,000 reported campylobacteriosis cases leads to Guillain-Barré syndrome. As many as 40 percent of Guillain-Barré syndrome cases in this country may be triggered by campylobacteriosis.

Risk Factors and Preventive Measures

Hands should be washed after using the toilet. Anyone with diarrhea should use a separate towel and washcloth and should not prepare food (especially uncooked food). Properly cooking chicken, pasteurizing milk, and chlorinating drinking water will kill the bacteria.

See also ANTIDIARRHEAL DRUGS; DIARRHEA AND INFECTIOUS DISEASE.

Campylobacter jejuni   A slender type of bacteria of the genus CAMPYLOBACTER, now recognized as the leading cause of bacterial diarrheal illness (called CAMPYLOBACTERIOSIS) in the United States, causing more disease than *SHIGELLA* and *SALMONELLA* combined. Estimates suggest there may be 2 to 4 million cases annually.

Although this bacterium is not carried by healthy individuals, it is often isolated from healthy cattle, chickens, birds, and flies. It may be found in nonchlorinated water (such as in ponds and streams). Not all strains of *C. jejuni* cause disease, but so far it is not possible to differentiate among them.

Complications are relatively rare, but infections have been associated with reactive arthritis, hemolytic uremic syndrome, and infections of nearly any organ. The death rate is estimated at one per 1,000 cases; fatalities are rare in healthy people. Meningitis, recurrent colitis, acute cholecystitis, and Guillain-Barré syndrome are very rare complications. Reactive arthritis is a rare complication of these infections.

Although anyone can have a *C. jejuni* infection, children under five and young adults aged 15 to 29 are more often affected.

Campylobacter pylorii The former name for HELICOBACTER PYLORII.

Candida albicans The yeast that causes the infection called candidiasis (THRUSH), often found within the vagina or on other mucous membranes (such as the inside of the mouth). The infection is also known as moniliasis.

Because this yeast is so commonly found in the body, it is a problem only when it grows too abundant due to changes in the mucous membranes. It is also the cause of diaper rash, which has nothing to do with a baby's immune system but is simply a result of the perfect yeast environment.

Thrush, which causes patches that look like cottage cheese in the mouth, may be a sign of AIDS in young adults, but it is also common among healthy children or among those who take inhaled steroids in the treatment of asthma.

C. albicans, while it is a yeast, has nothing to do with the food-grade yeast used to bake bread (*Saccharomyces cerevisiae*).

See also CANDIDA LUSITANIAE INFECTION.

Candida lusitaniae infection A rare but emerging human pathogen that can cause fungal infection in the lining of the brain, lungs, lower urinary tract, kidney, gastrointestinal tract, bone, skin, and soft tissue. It appears to resist antifungal drugs, including amphotericin B.

C. lusitaniae was first isolated in 1959 from the gastrointestinal tract of mammals, but it was not recognized as a cause of human disease until 1979. While this infection is very rare, there is evidence that it is becoming more of a problem, especially as a hospital-acquired infection. Because of its growing drug resistance scientists expect this fun-

gal infection to be an increasing problem, especially among those patients with impaired immune function.

The infection can affect people of all ages; as with other *Candida* species, the main risk factors seem to be the use of antibacterial drugs, having an intravascular catheter, and having an impaired immune function.

The *C. lusitaniae* infection usually begins in the throat or gastrointestinal tract.

The presence of the fungus can be determined via blood tests.

Treatment Options and Outlook
Since the fungus is resistant to amphotericin B, flucytosine is often combined with other antifungal drugs. Even with this treatment, however, 30 percent of patients with this disease die.

See also CANDIDA ALBICANS.

candidiasis See THRUSH.

canker sore A small painful ulcer on the inside of the mouth, lip, or underside of the tongue that heals without treatment. About 20 percent of Americans at any one time are experiencing a canker sore, which occurs most commonly between ages 10 and 40. The most severely affected people have almost continuous sores, while others have just one or two per year.

Because hemolytic STREPTOCOCCUS bacteria have so often been isolated from canker sores, experts believe the lesions may be caused by a hypersensitive reaction to the bacteria. Other factors often associated with a flareup include trauma (such as biting the inside of the cheek), acute stress allergies, or chemical irritants in toothpaste or mouthwash. More women than men experience canker sores, which are more likely to occur during the premenstrual period. They are also more likely to occur if other members of the family suffer from them. Interestingly, the older a person gets, the less likely a canker sore will occur. Some experts believe the lesions may be caused by an underlying immune system defect similar to an allergy.

Symptoms and Diagnostic Path

A canker sore is usually a small oval ulcer with a gray center surrounded by a red, inflamed halo, which usually lasts for one or two weeks. They are similar but not identical to COLD SORES (or "fever blisters"), which also appear on the mouth. Both usually cause small sores that heal within two weeks. However, canker sores are not usually preceded by a blister. Canker sores are usually larger than fever blisters, but they do not usually merge to form one large sore as fever blisters do. Finally, canker sores usually erupt on movable parts of the mouth (such as the tongue and the cheek or lip linings) whereas cold sores usually appear on the gums, roof of the mouth, lips, or nostrils.

Treatment Options and Outlook

While the ulcers will heal themselves, topical painkillers may ease the pain; healing may be speeded up by using a corticosteroid ointment or a tetracycline mouthwash. Patients also may cover the sore with a waterproof ointment to protect it.

Over-the-counter medications containing carbamide peroxide (Cankaid, Glyoxide, and Amosan) may be effective in treating the sore. Other treatment possibilities include medications in liquid or gel form of benzocaine, menthol, camphor, eucalyptol, and/or alcohol or pastes (such as Orabase) that form a protective "bandage" over the sore. For short-term pain relief, a prescription mouthwash rinse containing the anesthetic lidocaine, may help. A canker sore should heal within two weeks; if not, or if the sufferer cannot eat, speak, or sleep, medical help should be sought.

Risk Factors and Preventive Measures

Patients should avoid coffee, spices, citrus fruits, walnuts, strawberries, and chocolates if prone to canker sores. Eating, at least four tablespoons daily of plain yogurt containing *Lactobacillus acidophilus* will introduce helpful bacteria into the mouth to fight canker sore bacteria.

Also, patients should avoid commercial toothpastes and mouthwashes; instead teeth should be brushed with baking soda followed by warm salt water for a month or two. Toothpaste with the detergent sodium lauryl sulfate has been linked to canker sores in susceptible people.

carbuncle A cluster of BOILS (pus-filled inflamed hair roots) infected with bacteria, commonly found on the back of the neck and the buttocks.

Carbuncles are usually caused by the bacterium *Staphylococcus aureus*.

Symptoms and Diagnostic Path

Carbuncles usually begin as single lesion that spreads; they are less common than single boils. They primarily affect patients with lowered resistance to infection, or irritation of an area of skin.

Treatment Options and Outlook

Carbuncles are treated with oral and topical antibiotics and hot compresses. These may relieve the pain by causing the pus-filled heads to burst; if this occurs, the carbuncle should be covered with a dressing until it has healed completely. However, the lesion must often be cut and drained; the cavity may then need to be packed to improve drainage.

In some rare cases, draining is not necessary. Antibiotics given by mouth may prevent spread of bacteria from the pus pockets into the bloodstream or surrounding tissues.

Risk Factors and Preventive Measures

Recurrent carbuncles usually mean that patients are constantly reinfecting themselves. Regular washing with antibacterial soap (especially around rashes, irritations, shaving, or areas of heavy sweating) can help get rid of the infection. Hands and bedding also should be washed often.

carditis Inflammation of the heart muscles usually caused by viral infection. Most of the time, more than one layer of the heart is involved. Types of carditis include endocarditis (inflammation of the internal lining of the heart chambers and valves, usually caused by bacteria); myocarditis (inflammation of the heart muscle, usually caused by a virus); and pericarditis (inflammation of the outer lining of the heart, caused by a virus or bacteria).

Endocarditis is caused by a direct infection of the endocardium or indirectly as a result of rheumatic fever. Direct infection is called "infective endocarditis." Almost all bacteria and many fungi, if they manage to invade the bloodstream, can cause infective endocarditis. However, up to 80 percent are caused by streptococci or staphylococci.

Many species of viruses, bacteria, chlamydiae, rickettsias, fungi, and protozoa can cause myocarditis, but viruses (especially the enteroviruses) are the most common. The virus is typically ingested via water or food contaminated with fecal material, which may first infect the skin and then eventually reach the heart. The virus invades the heart muscle cells and causes necrosis of the cells and clinical effects.

Pericarditis is an inflammation of the sac enclosing the heart that may appear as one of three types depending on whether it is caused by viruses, bacteria, or fungi.

Symptoms and Diagnostic Path
Symptoms include chest pain, circulatory failure, heartbeat irregularities, and damage to the structure of the heart.

Treatment Options and Outlook
Endocarditis is treated with antibiotic therapy for at least two weeks, even if symptoms disappear before the end of the 14 days. A combination of antibiotics should be used. If antibiotic therapy is not successful, the infected endocardium may need to be surgically removed, especially in the case of fungal infections.

Viral myocarditis is typically a mild disease and responds well to bed rest. Bacterial, fungal, and protozoan myocarditis can be treated with the appropriate antibiotics, but glucosteroids and other drugs that suppress the immune system should not be administered.

The treatment for pericarditis includes bed rest, control of pain with nonsteroidal anti-inflammatory agents, and antimicrobial therapy, depending on the type of virus or bacteria.

cats and infectious disease   Cats may spread multi-drug-resistant bacteria that can cause serious illness. Researchers suspect the cats pick up infection from their food (either by eating scraps of contaminated human food or from eating raw or undercooked meat). Therefore, cats should not be given free access to unprotected food and cooking areas, and people who touch cats should wash their hands before eating or preparing food.

See also CAT-SCRATCH DISEASE; PETS AND INFECTIOUS DISEASE.

cat-scratch disease (CSD)   A mild bacterial infection following the lick, scratch, or bite of a kitten or cat, caused by *Bartonella henselae*. Three-quarters of cases occur in children, more often in fall and winter.

While the disease causes few problems in healthy individuals, in those with a weakened immune system the infection can become life threatening. There are about 22,000 cases of CSD in the United States each year.

The disease was first recognized in the 1950s, but the organism that causes it has only been recently discovered.

The bacteria are transmitted among cats by the common cat flea. About 90 percent of cases are caused by kittens; the rest result from grown cats, dogs, and other animals.

Researchers still do not understand how the bacteria can live in the bloodstream, since blood is normally sterile and bacteria are usually killed by the immune system. While cats with the disease are not ill and have no symptoms, many have large numbers of organisms in their blood.

The disease cannot be transmitted from one person to another, and it is not clear if one infection confers immunity.

Symptoms and Diagnostic Path
The symptoms of CSD resemble the early stages of other infectious diseases, such as TUBERCULOSIS. About two weeks after a bite or scratch, the patient reports a red round lump at the site of infection and one or more swollen lymph nodes near the scratch, which may become painful and tender, with an occasional discharge. Other symptoms may include mild fever, rash, malaise, sore throat, appetite loss, and headache. In most cases, symptoms disappear on their own.

Rarely, more severe infections occur, involving the liver, spleen, bones, or lungs. Some individuals may develop a lingering high fever as the only symptom. Some have an eye infection known as

Parinaud oculoglandular syndrome, characterized by a small sore on the membrane lining the eye or inner eyelid, redness, and swollen lymph nodes in front of the ear. Even more rare symptoms may involve brain inflammation or seizures. Even these serious complications usually resolve without any lasting illness.

CSD can be diagnosed by symptoms, history, and negative tests for other diseases that cause swollen lymph glands. A blood test developed by the CENTERS FOR DISEASE CONTROL AND PREVENTION, detects antibodies to the bacteria. The test is available free to doctors and state health departments. Biopsy of a small sample of the swollen lymph node is not necessary unless there is question of cancer of the lymph node or some other disease.

Treatment Options and Outlook

Antibiotics are occasionally prescribed. A severely affected lymph node or blister may have to be drained, and a heating pad may help swollen, tender lymph glands. Acetaminophen may relieve pain, aches, and fever over 101°F. In most cases, the illness fades after one or two months.

Risk Factors and Preventive Measures

Other than avoiding cats, there is no way to prevent the disease. However, cats only carry the infecting organism for a few weeks during their lives, so the likelihood of being reinfected, or infected by just one pet in the home, is minimal.

Patients with weakened immune systems do not need to get rid of their cats, but they should inform their physicians that they own cats and avoid getting scratched. If a scratch does occur, it should be washed thoroughly with soap and water. It is also important to control fleas.

See also CATS AND INFECTIOUS DISEASE; PETS AND INFECTIOUS DISEASE.

cellulitis A bacterial infection of the skin and the tissues underneath it. Untreated, the disease may lead to BACTEREMIA and SEPTIC SHOCK; facial cellulitis may spread to the eye and the brain. Before the advent of antibiotics, the disease was sometimes fatal. Today, any form of cellulitis is likely to be more serious in those with impaired immune systems. Cellulitis begins when bacteria enters a cut or scratch, leading to inflammation, pain, swelling, warmth, and redness. Children with skin conditions such as ECZEMA or severe acne, which create broken skin, are at higher risk for developing cellulitis. Children who scratch the lesions from insect bites or CHICKEN POX are also at risk.

However, cellulitis also may develop in people who do not have broken skin, if they have conditions such as diabetes or a weakened immune system.

Many different types of bacteria can lead to cellulitis, but the most common are STREPTOCOCCUS GROUP-A and STAPHYLOCOCCUS AUREUS. PASTEURELLA MULTOCIDA bacteria introduced by a cat or dog bite, or Pseudomonas infection after nail-puncture wounds, also may lead to cellulitis.

Symptoms and Diagnostic Path

The affected area (usually the skin of the face, neck, or legs) is usually hot, tender, and red; other symptoms include fever and chills, with swollen lymph glands. Perianal cellulitis may occur with itchy, painful bowel movements. A rash may appear on face, arms, or legs, with raised borders. Infection may recur, causing chronic swelling of arms or legs.

The organism is hard to culture from skin lesions, but it may be identified in blood. Antibodies can be found in blood.

Treatment Options and Outlook

Cold compresses and aspirin may bring relief. Antibiotics effective against the organism causing the infection must be taken for up to two weeks. At the beginning of antibiotic treatment, symptoms may temporarily get worse because of the abrupt death of many organisms. Often, antibiotics must be given intravenously for a period of time, especially if the infection is spreading quickly or is located on the face.

Periorbital cellulitis (infection of the eyelid and tissues surrounding the eye) more often occurs in children as a result of a scratch or insect bite around the eye, or by the spread of infection from another part of the body, such as the sinus. Untreated cases can go on to infect the entire eye socket (orbital cellulitis)—a much more severe infection causing a bulging eyeball, eye pain, restricted eye movements, or visual disturbances. Orbital cellulitis is an emergency that requires hospitalization and intravenous antibiotics.

Centers for Disease Control and Prevention (CDC) The federal organization responsible for preventing and controlling infectious diseases. Established as the Communicable Disease Center in 1946 in Atlanta, its mission was to protect Americans from germs, including TYPHUS, dengue, PLAGUE, malaria, and other infectious diseases. Since then, CDC has led efforts to prevent MALARIA, polio, SMALLPOX, TOXIC SHOCK SYNDROME, LEGIONNAIRES' DISEASE, LYME DISEASE, hospital infections, and more recently, HIV/AIDS.

The center's responsibilities have expanded over the years and continue to evolve as the agency addresses other threats to health such as injuries and environmental and occupational hazards. CDC supports surveillance, research, prevention efforts, and training in the area of infectious diseases through its NATIONAL CENTER FOR INFECTIOUS DISEASES.

Today, the public mission of the CDC ranges far beyond the U.S. border. Fighting disease today is a global effort, requiring the talents of public health officials in every county, state, city, and country in the world.

CDC epidemiologists continue to study microbes, from EBOLA in Africa to CRYPTOSPORIDIUM in Milwaukee, but the agency also combats health threats such as gun violence, poverty, and poor nutrition. In so doing, it has been criticized by those who believe the agency should stick to bugs and keep out of social policy.

The CDC maintains centers, institutes, and offices, including the National Center for Infectious Diseases; the National Center for Chronic Disease Prevention and Health Promotion; the National Center for Environmental Health; the National Center for Health Statistics; the National Center for HIV, STD, and TB Prevention; the National Center for Injury Prevention and Control; the National Center for Occupational Safety and Health; the Epidemiology Program Office; the International Program Office; the Public Health Practice Program Office; and the National Immunization Program. It maintains offices in Anchorage; Atlanta; Cincinnati; Fort Collins, Colorado; Morgantown, West Virginia;

Pittsburgh; Research Triangle Park, North Carolina; San Juan; Spokane; and Washington, D.C.

The infectious disease center houses the maximum containment lab, which can handle the most deadly organisms. High-tech filters keep the microbes inside from getting outside, and scientists at the lab wear spacesuits to protect themselves from microbes. The lab is locked, guarded, and under constant video surveillance.

cephalosporins A class of antibiotics used to treat infections that occur in a variety of places in the body. They are used to treat most common URINARY TRACT INFECTIONS (UTIs) and upper respiratory infections such as PHARYNGITIS or TONSILLITIS. The cephalosporins include cefadroxil, cefixime, cefuroxime axetil, cefaclor, and cephalexin. As with other antibiotics, some cephalosporins can treat certain bacterial infections better than others.

They can be taken either with food or on an empty stomach; in case of nausea, they should be taken with food or milk. Liquid suspensions should be refrigerated (except for cefixime suspension). Any unused suspension should be thrown away after 14 days.

These drugs should always be taken at the same time of day and for the exact amount of time prescribed, *even if the patient feels better*. The infection may return if the drug is not taken for the full amount of time. Heart or kidney complications can result if a STREPTOCOCCUS infection is not completely treated.

If the infection is caused by a type of bacteria that responds to cephalosporins, the symptoms should improve within a few days, although sometimes it may take longer to get relief. If the symptoms remain after all the drug is taken or gets worse during the medication period, a physician should be contacted.

Cephalosporins appear to be relatively safe to use during pregnancy. They do pass into breast milk in small amounts. The drugs also may cause diabetics to get a false-positive reading for glucose in the urine if copper sulfate urine test tablets are used.

Side Effects

Common side effects include mild temporary stomach cramps, nausea, vomiting, and diarrhea. As other antibiotics, cephalosporins may encourage the growth of fungus normally found in the body, causing a sore tongue, mouth sores, or a vaginal yeast infection.

More serious (but rarer) side effects include allergic reactions ranging from itchy, red, or swollen skin rash to severe breathing problems and shock. A patient allergic to PENICILLIN also may be allergic to a cephalosporin.

Specific allergic reactions to cephalosporin can include skin rash, joint pain, irritability, and fever.

A rare side effect is serious colitis, with severe watery diarrhea, stomach cramps, fever, weakness, and fatigue.

cerebrospinal fluid analysis   See SPINAL TAP.

cereus   A type of food poisoning caused by the *Bacillus cereus* bacteria, which multiplies in raw foods at room temperature. The *B. cereus* bacteria produces toxins most often found in steamed or fried rice. It is believed that poisoning with *B. cereus* is underreported because its symptoms are so similar to other types of food poisoning (especially staphylococcal and *CLOSTRIDIUM PERFRINGENS* poisoning).

Symptoms and Diagnostic Path

This bacterium produces two distinct types of food poisoning: The first begins after a short incubation period (usually less than six hours), causing cramps and vomiting, and occasionally a short bout with diarrhea. Almost 80 percent of patients with these symptoms who test positive for *B. cereus* poisoning have eaten steamed or fried rice at Chinese restaurants.

The second type of *B. cereus* poisoning is very similar to *C. perfringens* poisoning; it appears within eight to 24 hours after eating tainted food and causes abdominal cramps and diarrhea with very little vomiting.

A wide variety of foods including meats, milk, vegetables, and fish have been associated with the diarrheal type of cereus food poisoning. The vomiting-type outbreaks have generally been associated with rice products, but other starchy foods such as potatoes, pasta, and cheese products have also been

implicated. Food mixtures such as sauces, puddings, soups, casseroles, pastries, and salads have often been linked to food poisoning outbreaks.

Many outbreaks go unreported or are misdiagnosed because symptoms are so similar to STAPHYLOCOCCUS AUREUS intoxication (*B. cereus* vomiting-type) or *C. perfringens* food poisoning (*B. cereus* diarrheal type).

Between 1972 and 1986, 52 outbreaks of foodborne disease associated with *B. cereus* were reported to the CENTERS FOR DISEASE CONTROL AND PREVENTION, but experts suspect this only represents about 2 percent of the total cases that have occurred during that time.

In 1993, 14 cases related to fried rice at two day-care centers in Virginia were reported.

Treatment Options and Outlook

Treatment of both types of the disease is aimed only at making the patient comfortable. There are no medications that will shorten the course of the disease.

cestode   See TAPEWORM.

Chagas disease   A parasitic disease found only in Latin America also known as American TRYPANOSOMIASIS transmitted by the bite of blood-sucking insects, and occasionally by blood transfusions. Named for 19th-century Brazilian physician Carlos Chagas, the disease is endemic in Central and South America, where it is recognized as a serious public health problem. Officials there rank their need to control this disease third, behind MALARIA and SCHISTOSOMIASIS.

More than a quarter of the total population in Central and South America are at risk, with more than a million new cases diagnosed each year. Of these, 50,000 people will die, and up to 18 million people may be currently infected. Of these, 3 million may have already developed chronic complications, and more than 3 million are still in the incubation period. The disease is also known as Brazilian trypanosomiasis, Chagas-Cruz disease, Cruz trypanosomiasis, and South American trypanosomiasis.

The disease is caused by the single-celled parasite *Trypanosoma cruzi*, very similar to those that cause sleeping sickness in Africa. The parasite infects bugs commonly known as "assassin bugs" or "cone-nosed bugs" (reduviid); when the bugs defecate, the excrement includes the parasite, which can then enter a human through a break in the skin or through a mucous membrane. The parasites live in the bloodstream and also can affect a person's heart, intestines, or nervous system.

Symptoms and Diagnostic Path

The disease may occur in an acute or chronic form. The acute form (common in children, rare in adults) is marked by a lesion at the site of infection, together with fever, weakness, enlarged spleen and lymph nodes, facial and leg swelling, and rapid heartbeat. This form disappears on its own in about four months, unless complications (such as ENCEPHALITIS) set in.

About 10 to 20 years after the initial acute phase, incurable lesions of the disease develop. In addition, 27 percent of those infected develop a chronic heart disease problem. Six percent have chronic lesions in the digestive tract, and about 3 percent may have neurological problems. Patients with chronic disease become progressively sick and ultimately die, usually as a result of heart failure.

Treatment Options and Outlook

Benznidazole and nifurtimox can treat the early stages of Chagas disease. There is no accepted antiparasitic treatment for chronic illness.

Risk Factors and Preventive Measures

The best prevention is to avoid potential reduviid habitats (mud, adobe, and thatch buildings, especially those with cracks or crevices). If this is not feasible, infection may be prevented by spraying infested areas with insecticide, using fumigant canisters and insecticidal paints, and using bed nets. Housing improvements also help. In addition, screening blood donors at blood banks helps to control the spread of the disease via blood transfusions.

In 1991, the health ministers of Argentina, Bolivia, Brazil, Chile, Paraguay, and Uruguay began a program to eliminate Chagas disease. By 2001, disease transmission had been stopped in Chile, Uruguay, and Brazil, according to the World Health Organization.

Chagres fever   An arbovirus infection transmitted to humans through the bite of the sandfly. The disease, which is rarely fatal, is most common in Central America. It was named after the Chagres River in Panama and is also known as Panama fever.

Symptoms and Diagnostic Path

This disease is characterized by fever, headache, and muscle pain of the chest or abdomen, with nausea and vomiting, giddiness, weakness, sensitivity to light, and pain on moving the eyes. It usually passes within a week.

Treatment Options and Outlook

Bed rest, fluids, and painkillers.

chancroid   A sexually transmitted disease (STD) no longer common in industrialized nations, it is a frequent cause of genital ulcer disease in developing countries. Chancroid cases peaked in the United States in 1987, when 5,035 cases were reported to the CENTERS FOR DISEASE CONTROL AND PREVENTION (CDC). The number of cases has declined steadily since then, with 773 cases reported in 1994 and just 140 in 1999.

However, because of a lack of accurate diagnostic tests, the worldwide incidence of the disease is unknown, but estimates suggest as many as 6 million people may contract chancroid each year. It is common in the world's poorest areas in Africa, Asia, and the Caribbean, which also have some of the highest rates of HIV infection in the world.

Those most at risk are men under age 24, men and women with multiple sex partners, those with other STDs (especially SYPHILIS), prostitutes and their customers, and those in tropical areas. However, any sexually active person can be infected with chancroid. It is more commonly seen in men than women, especially in uncircumcised males.

Chancroid is caused by *Hemophilus ducreyi*, a rod-shaped bacterium that grows only in the absence of oxygen (much like GONORRHEA bacteria). The bacteria are transmitted from the draining sores of an infected person during sex. It is more likely to be transmitted to another person with a small cut or scratch in the genital area. The chances of transmission are greater if a person is very active sexually and does not practice good personal hygiene.

Symptoms and Diagnostic Path

Symptoms usually appear within a week of infection. In some women, there may be a small pimple with a reddish base that will gradually fill with pus, opening and hollowing. Eventually, several ulcers usually appear that are very painful and soft. About a week later, the pelvic lymph gland on one side of the groin may become enlarged and painful. Other women do not notice sores, but have pain during sex or while urinating. Still others never notice any symptoms, especially if ulcers are on the vaginal walls or cervix.

Men experience painful sores under the foreskin or on the underside of the penis that fill with pus and turn into ulcers. About 50 percent of infected men will go on to develop painful, enlarged lymph glands in the groin.

Both men and women are infectious until the lesions are completely healed, which may take up to two weeks. It is not possible to become immune.

The disease is diagnosed by symptoms and negative test results for other more common causes of genital ulcers (such as syphilis or HERPES). About half the time, microscopic examination of the fluid from a draining ulcer will correctly diagnose the infection; a culture of the drainage or biopsy of the ulcer will provide a correct diagnosis.

Treatment Options and Outlook

Antibiotics for both partners, such as azithromycin or erythromycin, or a shot of ceftriaxone, will cure the disease in about a week. Chancroid is now resistant to PENICILLIN and tetracycline. Lesions and ulcers will heal in about two weeks.

Untreated chancroid often causes ulcers on the genitals that may persist for weeks or months. The infection does not harm the fetus of a pregnant woman. However, the lesion does increase the chances of contracting HIV if a person has sex with an HIV-infected partner.

chicken pox   A common childhood infectious disease characterized by a rash and slight fever that affects about 4 million children each year in the United States. About 90 percent of cases occur in children under age 10, primarily in winter and spring. Chicken pox is also known as varicella, after the virus that causes the disease (varicella-zoster, or VZV). The name *varicella* dates to the 1700s and derives from the Latin term for "little pox."

Most people throughout the world have had the disease by age 10, and chicken pox is rare in adults. When it does occur after childhood, it is a far more serious illness.

There were 120,624 reported cases in 1995, which dropped to 40,016 by 1999.

VZV is a member of the family of herpesviruses, which includes more than 100 types, such as the herpes simplex virus (causing cold sores and genital herpes), Epstein-Barr virus (causing infectious mononucleosis), and varicella-zoster virus (causing chicken pox and SHINGLES).

Once a person has chicken pox, the virus stays in the body in a latent stage, hiding in the nerves of the lower spinal cord for the rest of the person's life. When reactivated (in old age or during times of stress), it can lead to the painful skin rash known as shingles.

Symptoms and Diagnostic Path

The VZV virus, which is spread by airborne droplets, is extremely contagious. The incubation period ranges from 10 to 23 days. One to three weeks after exposure, a rash appears on the torso, face, armpits, upper arms and legs, inside the mouth, and sometimes in the windpipe and bronchial tubes, causing a dry cough.

The rash is made up of small red itchy spots that turn into fluid-filled blisters within a few hours. After several days, the blisters dry out and form scabs. New spots usually continue to form over four to seven days. Children usually have only a slight fever, but an adult may experience fever with severe pneumonia and breathing problems. Adults also usually have higher fevers, more intense rash, and more complications than children.

The average child will have between 250 and 500 blisters over about five days; the more blisters the child has, the harder the body has to fight to make enough antibodies to destroy the virus. The fight between the virus and the immune system causes fevers, fatigue, and poor appetite. Those who catch the disease from a sibling instead of a classmate usually have a more severe illness, with from 300 to 5,000 blisters. This is because the close contact at home causes a much larger amount of virus to enter the system.

The patient is infectious from five days before the rash erupts until all the blisters are completely healed, dried, and scabbed over. This can take from six to 10 days after the rash appears.

Treatment Options and Outlook

In most cases, rest is all that is needed for children, who usually recover within 10 days. Adult patients take longer to recover. Acetaminophen may reduce the fever, and calamine lotion, baking soda baths, and oral antihistamines ease the itch. Compresses can dry weeping lesions. *Aspirin should never be given to a child who has flu-like symptoms or has been exposed to (or has recently recovered from) chicken pox.* In these cases, aspirin has been linked to Reye's syndrome.

The drug acyclovir may be prescribed for chicken pox patients over age 12 or any who have chronic skin or lung disorders, or a compromised immune system (such as AIDS). Unlike the herpes simplex viruses, VZV is relatively resistant to acyclovir, and doses required for treatment are much larger and must be administered intravenously. While the drug may shorten the length of the illness and lessen symptoms, its high cost and marginal effectiveness have prompted the American Academy of Pediatrics not to recommend it as a routine treatment. Acyclovir is not prescribed for children under age 12 because of possible side effects.

Scratching should be avoided, as it may lead to secondary bacterial infection and increase the chance of scarring.

If possible, a child with suspected chicken pox should not be brought into the doctor's office where others will be exposed to the disease; it can be very dangerous to newborns or those with suppressed immune systems. The virus can be spread both through the air and by direct contact with an infected individual. Instead, symptoms should be described on the phone if chicken pox is suspected.

In children, complications may include bacterial infection and, rarely, Reye's syndrome, or in even rarer cases, ENCEPHALITIS. Immunocompromised patients who are susceptible to VZV are at high risk for having severe varicella infections with widespread lesions.

Between 40 and 200 patients die every year in the United States; half are previously healthy people and the other half are those with impaired immune systems.

Risk Factors and Preventive Measures

Since 1995, a varicella vaccine has been given to children older than 12 months, as well as adults. The vaccine is about 70 to 85 percent effective at preventing mild infection, and more than 95 percent effective in preventing moderate or severe disease. People who do develop chicken pox after vaccination have much milder symptoms with fewer skin blisters and a fast recovery.

The vaccine stimulates the immune system to make protective antibodies to the virus, which last for life. The chicken pox vaccine is made from a live, weakened virus that works by creating a mild infection similar to natural chicken pox, but without the related problems. The mild infection spurs the body to develop an immune response to the disease. These defenses are then ready when the body encounters the natural virus.

The vaccine is recommended to be routinely given to children 12 to 18 months old. Older children, adolescents, and adults who have not had chicken pox also should be immunized. Children 12 months to 12 years receive a single vaccine dose, but teens and adults need two doses at least four weeks apart.

An infected child should not play with anyone at risk for serious disease from chicken pox, and should be kept away from infants younger than six weeks of age. They should also stay away from crowded public places where high-risk people might congregate.

Varicella-zoster immune globulin offers temporary protection for high-risk susceptible patients. This can abort or modify infection if administered within three days of exposure. Passive immunization is the administration of antibodies from donor's blood; since a person's blood is complete replaced every three months, the immunity lasts only that long. VZIG is given to newborns whose mothers had chicken pox during delivery, high-risk patients such as those with leukemia or a weakened immune system, and children taking drugs that suppress the immune system.

chikungunya fever An infectious disease whose name is Swahili for "that which bends up," in reference to the stooped posture of patients afflicted with the severe joint pain associated with this disease. The disease was first recognized in epidemic form in East Africa in 1952. Although it is not typically fatal, it is extremely painful.

The virus is found in eastern, southern, western, and central Africa and southeastern Asia, where it has caused illnesses in thousands of people. Epidemics have occurred in the Philippines, Thailand, Cambodia, Vietnam, India, Myanmar (Burma), and Sri Lanka.

In 2006, an epidemic in Mauritius ravaged the Indian Ocean region. Within the first two months of 2006, the virus affected more than 20 percent of the population (157,000 people) along the southeast island coast of Africa, including Reunion, Seychelles, and Mauritius. Athough the tropical virus is rarely fatal, it can weaken the immune system, allowing other deadly diseases to set in. During the Indian Ocean epidemic of 2005–06, 77 deaths were indirectly associated with the disease in Reunion Island, and the disease was linked to one death in Mauritius in February 2006.

The *Aedes aegypti* mosquitoes carry the chikungunya virus, which they pass on to humans when they bite. Epidemics are sustained by human-mosquito-human transmission, similar to the way that epidemics of DENGUE FEVER and urban YELLOW FEVER are maintained.

Symptoms and Diagnostic Path

The fever is characterized by sudden onset of severe arthritis like joint pain in many joints that can be debilitating. It also causes chills and fever, headache, nausea and vomiting, joint pain, and rash that lasts up to a week. While chikungunya is often confused with dengue fever, chikungunya has a shorter period of fever, persistent joint pain, and lack of fatalities. Joint stiffness can last for weeks or months.

Treatment Options and Outlook

There is no specific treatment; painkillers can lower fever and ease joint pain. The infection passes with time.

Risk Factors and Preventive Measures

There is no vaccine available for this mosquito-borne infection. Insecticides to kill mosquitos can be effective in limiting the spread of an epidemic.

child-care centers and infectious disease Since young children are often vulnerable targets for infectious disease due to their immature immune systems, it stands to reason that grouping many infants and preschoolers together in day-care centers would contribute to the spread of infectious disease. The problem is exacerbated by the fact that young children are not particularly concerned with good hygiene, and that many day-care centers include care for children who are not yet toilet trained.

Still, day care centers do not have to be breeding grounds for infectious diseases. In fact, recent research indicates that after the first year, children in child care get sick at about half the rate as do youngsters who are cared for at home. This is because youngsters at day care are simply exposed to germs sooner, and their immune systems learn to cope with the onslaught of exposure.

Many studies have shown that if the center staff understand, are supervised and educated about infection control, there is much less infectious illness spread among the youngsters. Simply by emphasizing hand washing, some centers have managed to cut diarrhea in half.

Before a child-care facility can be licensed, they must meet certain hygiene standards in a variety of areas, as set by local and state licensing authorities. Among other things, centers should clean all surfaces with a safe disinfectant. Surfaces should be dried with paper towels after being sprayed. Adequate ventilation and sanitation are necessary. Chemical air fresheners should not be used because many people are allergic to them.

Many infections in child-care centers are spread by fecal contamination. When diapers are changed, tiny amounts of feces on hands can be transferred to countertops, toys, and door handles, so that if one child is shedding an infection in the feces, it is not long before the infection spreads. Some infectious viruses will appear in feces before the diarrhea starts and remain in feces until more than a week after symptoms disappear.

To head off these problems, diapers should be checked every hour. Diaper-changing areas should not be located where food is prepared, stored, or served. The changing table should be cleaned after use. Soiled diapers should be disposed of in separate covered waste containers. Staffers should wash hands before and after changing diapers. If a child has diarrhea, staff should wear disposable gloves when changing the diaper.

Hands should be washed after using the toilet or handling diapers; after helping a child at the toilet; before preparing, handling, or serving food; before feeding an infant; before setting the table; after wiping or blowing noses; after touching blood, vomit, saliva, or eye secretions; after handling pets; and before and after eating.

chlamydial infections Infections caused by a unique type of bacteria that can live and reproduce inside human cells; three of the four known species can cause disease in humans. *Chlamydia trachomatis, Chlamydia pneumonia,* and *Chlamydia psittaci* all cause infections affecting many different organs, including the eyes, lungs, urinary tract, or genitals, depending on the species involved, the age of the person infected, and how the infection is transmitted.

The name "chlamydia" is derived from the Greek word *chlamys,* meaning "cloak," which refers to the fact that the bacteria infect a cell by draping themselves around its nucleus. When inside the cell, chlamydia can reproduce without damaging the cell, which can lead to prolonged infections with few if any symptoms—one of the major characteristics of this bacteria.

See also CHLAMYDIA PNEUMONIAE INFECTION; CHLAMYDIA PSITTACI INFECTION; CHLAMYDIA TRACHOMATIS INFECTION.

chlamydial pneumonia See PNEUMONIA, CHLAMYDIAL.

***Chlamydia pneumoniae* infection** A disease caused by infection with *Chlamydia pneumoniae,* one of the varieties of *chlamydia* organisms that has been linked to respiratory illness and coronary heart disease. Some experts think that because the germ can be killed by antibiotics, a link to heart disease could be of enormous importance for public health. Up to 10 percent of community-acquired PNEUMONIA may be caused by this bacteria.

Most people are first infected during childhood or early adolescence. Up to 60 percent of all adults around the world have antibodies to *C. pneumoniae,* and reinfection may be common. There is suspicion that this organism may also be related to the development of asthma.

TRANSMISSION OF INFECTIONS IN CHILDREN

Children catch infectious diseases in a variety of ways.

In the air:
- chicken pox
- colds
- fifth disease
- influenza
- meningitis
- TB

By direct contact:
- cold sores
- cytomegalovirus
- head lice
- scabies
- strep infections (strep throat, scarlet fever, and impetigo)

Fecal-oral route:
- diarrheal disease
- hepatitis A

By contact with infected blood:
- hepatitis B

This organism is spread from person to person by coughing or sneezing. Outbreaks of infection have been reported in families, schools, military barracks, and nursing homes. Often, there is a simultaneous infection with other bacteria or with a virus such as INFLUENZA or RESPIRATORY SYNCYTIAL VIRUS.

Symptoms and Diagnostic Path

Between seven to 21 days after exposure, symptoms of upper respiratory infection appear. Infection is usually mild, but it may be severe, especially among the elderly.

A variety of lab tests can reveal the infection.

Treatment Options and Outlook

Clarithromycin or azithromycin are used to treat this infection.

Chlamydia psittaci infection Infection with an organism that infects birds, and that causes a rare type of PNEUMONIA in humans known as psittacosis (ORNITHOSIS). *C. psittaci* is carried by infected birds, especially parrots.

Since 1996, fewer than 50 confirmed cases were reported in the United States each year, although many cases may not be correctly diagnosed or reported.

The infection is acquired through breathing in droplets of bacteria from infected birds and is an occupational hazard for employees of pet shops and poultry processing plants. Birds can be healthy carriers of the organism; increased shedding of bacteria and susceptibility to disease occur during stress, starvation, or egg laying. Person to person transmission is rare, but there have been instances where it has occurred.

In the *C. psittaci* pandemic of 1929–30, infected Argentine birds were shipped to different parts of the world, causing sporadic outbreaks with death rates of up to 40 percent. Since then, the bacterium has been isolated from more than 130 species of birds. All avian species should be considered potentially infectious.

Outbreaks of psittacosis in duck and turkey processing plants show that the infections continue to be a public health concern, despite diagnostic testing, medicated feed, and poultry screening.

Sources of human infection other than infected birds have been identified and may be more common than had previously been thought. *C. psittaci* has been identified in cats and breeding catteries, for example, which suggests that human infection from pets other than birds may occur.

Symptoms and Diagnostic Path

Within six to 19 days after exposure to the organism, the patient experiences a flu-like illness with fever, chills, headache and cough, facial pain, rash, joint pain, and swelling. In severe cases, there may be an atypical pneumonia.

Conditions associated with exposure to infected animals include spontaneous abortion, symptoms of kidney and liver disease, and heart inflammation. There also have been reports of eye infections and heart problems in people exposed to infected cats and pigeons. Blood tests can reveal the infection.

Treatment Options and Outlook

Recommended treatment is tetracycline for three weeks. The death rate is low, but many patients experience a lengthy recovery and relapse.

Chlamydia trachomatis infection The most common sexually transmitted disease (STD) in the United States, infecting more than 4.5 million people each year. *C. trachomatis* also is responsible for nonspecific urethritis (inflammation of the urethra), PELVIC INFLAMMATORY DISEASE, LYMPHOGRANULOMA VENEREUM (a sexually transmitted disease affecting the lymph nodes as well as the genitals), and TRACHOMA (a severe inflammatory eye infection).

Chlamydia is a serious but easily cured disease that is three times more common than GONORRHEA, six times more common than genital HERPES, and 30 times more common than SYPHILIS. Between 1988 and 1992, the rate of reported cases of chlamydia more than doubled. Sexually active teens have high rates of chlamydia infections.

The chlamydia organism is classified as a bacterium, even though it is similar to a virus and was once identified as such by scientists. A parasite that—like a virus—cannot reproduce outside living cells, it is enough like bacteria to be vulnerable to antibiotics. It is known as an "energy parasite," since it possesses all the biological features needed for independence except the ability to generate its own energy.

C. trachomatis was first described in China and in the Ebers papyrus in Egypt thousands of years ago; it continues to be a major cause of preventable blindness, with an estimated 500 million cases of active trachoma in the world.

Symptoms and Diagnostic Path

The organism *C. trachomatis* has two strains; one infects the eyes and/or genitals, the other causes swelling and ulceration of the lymph tissue near the groin, called lymphogranuloma venereum. The first strain attacks the eyes, causing a disease known as trachoma, now rare in the United States and Europe but one that remains the leading cause of blindness in the Third World.

The second strain has been steadily spreading since the 1960s, causing a range of symptoms from CONJUNCTIVITIS (inflammation of the rim of the eyes) to infertility. When transmitted sexually, it can cause a range of urinary tract infections in men and women, pelvic inflammatory disease, and ectopic pregnancy. The disease may be passed from an infected mother to a newborn, causing PNEUMONIA. Like other genital organisms, it is often found among young nonwhite, unmarried poor people. More than half of patients have no symptoms.

Treatment Options and Outlook

Antibiotics can kill this pathogen, but condoms are the best protection against spreading chlamydia.

cholera An infection of the small intestine characterized by profuse, painless, watery diarrhea. It has been one of the great social and political forces in history. If untreated, severe cases can cause rapid dehydration and death within a few hours. If patients are given enough fluids, most will recover. The death rate soars in pandemics where there is not enough clean water, or if so many people become ill that there are not enough healthy people to care for the sick. After one infection, resulting antibodies will protect the patient from reinfection with the same strain.

There has been a dramatic increase in cholera in the United States and its territories, and many cases may go undetected by physicians who are not familiar with the disease, according to the National Center for Infectious Diseases. The disease thrives in places without running water or treated sewage disposal. This is why in the United States and Canada, cholera does not spread from one person to the next; any cholera organisms in infected feces are killed by sewage treatment and chlorinated water.

Historically, the spread of cholera in the Western world was tied to the problems of 19th-century urbanization, with its lack of sewage control, public water supply, and burgeoning population. While tainted water supplies carry the bacillus, it is also passed in human feces. Therefore, preparing food with unwashed hands, contamination by roaches or flies, and the location of homes and buildings near raw sewage compounded the problem. During the industrialization of the 19th century, families crowded together in dirty tenements and those struggling in coal mining districts were especially at high risk, as were nurses and laundresses who handled soiled linen.

For centuries, cholera thrived only in northeast India, where outbreaks still occur regularly, because of the lack of clean water. In 1784, 20,000 pilgrims died from cholera at an Indian holy place known as Hurdwar. As the world trade routes opened in the 1800s, cholera spread throughout the world, killing millions of people in six distinct pandemics since 1817. The second pandemic reached England in the early 1800s, where London physician John Snow began his investigation of the Broad Street pump, a public source of water drawn from a well near a Soho cesspool. Snow, a general practitioner, was convinced that cholera was found in water and carried by the excretions of victims, and it was Snow who correctly identified sewage-contaminated drinking water as the source of the epidemic. In his research, he compared the incidence of cholera in a neighborhood with two different sources of water, one of which was contaminated with sewage. After he convinced authorities to remove the pump's handle (shutting off the water supply) the neighborhood's outbreak stopped.

In Paris, the pandemic of 1848–49 killed 18,000 people out of a population of 785,000. It was not until the fifth pandemic in 1881 that German and French scientific teams discovered the source of the disease. German microbiologist Robert Koch identified the "comma bacilli" (now called *VIBRIO CHOLERAE*) under the microscope as the actual cause of cholera.

All cases today are part of a pandemic that began in Indonesia in 1961 with a new strain, called *V. cholerae*, 01 biotype El Tor. Not a single case was reported anywhere in the entire Western Hemisphere between 1911 and 1973. Then between 1974 and 1988, a few cases appeared in U.S. states bordering the Gulf of Mexico (Florida, Louisiana, and Texas). In 1989, no cases were reported.

Unexpectedly, in 1991 this cholera epidemic spread to Peru when a ship arrived from the Far East dumped cholera-infected bilge water into the Lima harbor. The bacteria contaminated the fish and shellfish, which Peruvians ate raw; from there the bacteria got into the sewers and from there into the water supply. The disease then spread throughout South and Central America, where the epidemic continues to this day.

By September 1994, more than a million people in 20 countries had contracted the disease, and more than 9,000 had died.

Only a handful of cases have appeared in the United States, usually among people who have traveled to South America. Experts suggest the reported cases are probably only a fraction of the actual incidents of cholera, since as many as 90 percent of people with the disease have only mild diarrhea.

Cholera is caused by the comma-shaped bacterium *Vibrio cholerae*, which is acquired by swallowing food or water contaminated with human feces. A person may also contract cholera from eating fruits or vegetables that are washed in tainted water and eaten raw, by eating raw or undercooked shellfish harvested from contaminated water, or by eating food prepared by someone with contaminated hands. Sometimes, flies can carry the bacteria to food.

The rapid fluid loss that is the primary symptom of cholera occurs because of the action of a toxin produced by the bacterium. This boosts the passage of fluid from the blood into the large and small intestines.

Still, unless there is a huge source of germs (such as from contaminated water or the clothes of victims), the disease is fairly hard to acquire. Chlorina-tion can kill the bacteria, and acids in saliva and the stomach are a natural defense.

Symptoms and Diagnostic Path

Up to three fourths of all victims show no symptoms. But severe forms of the disease known for hundreds of years as "cholera morbus"—usually caused by drinking contaminated water—can be quickly fatal. Between a few hours and five days after infection, symptoms appear suddenly, beginning with incessant diarrhea and vomiting, severe muscular cramps, and prostration. Facial features and soft body tissues shrink because of the radical loss of fluid, and discoloration of the skin from ruptured capillaries turns the shriveled patient black and blue. More than a pint of fluid may be lost hourly, and if this is not replaced, death will occur within a few hours. Because the bacteria are inhibited by stomach acid, those with high levels of gastric acid will have only a mild infection. Those who are poorly nourished and have less gastric acid may have more severe diarrhea.

Many people (especially those living in areas where cholera is common) may have no symptoms, but they can still spread the disease to others. If the diarrhea is very bloody, the cause is probably not cholera but may be *SHIGELLA, E. COLI,* or *CAMPYLOBACTER.*

A positive stool culture will confirm the diagnosis. Stool specimens must be cultured on special culture media. A blood test taken a few weeks after the illness begins will show antibodies to cholera.

Treatment Options and Outlook

Cholera is treated by quickly replacing the lost fluids with water containing salts and sugar, together with intravenous fluids (if needed). Antibiotics (such as tetracycline) may shorten both the period of diarrhea and the infectiousness. While it is usually taken by mouth, IV tetracycline may be needed for very sick patients. Antidiarrheal medicine should not be taken.

As soon as vomiting stops, the patient should eat a bland diet rich in carbohydrates and low in protein and fats. Airlines are required to carry onboard packets of oral rehydration solution if they carry passengers to and from cholera-infected areas so that anyone developing severe diarrhea on a long flight will not get dehydrated. With proper treatment, most patients will recover with no permanent damage. Without prompt treatment, half the people with severe cholera will die within a few hours from profound dehydration.

Risk Factors and Preventive Measures

The manufacture and sale of the only licensed cholera vaccine in the United States (by Wyeth-Ayerst) has been discontinued; it was not recommended for travelers because of its brief and incomplete immunity. No cholera vaccination requirements exist for entry or exit in any country.

Two new vaccines for cholera are licensed and available in other countries, both of which seem to provide better immunity and fewer side effects than the vaccine that had been available in the United States. However, neither of these two vaccines is recommended for travelers nor are they available in the United States.

The bacteria can be killed by chlorine or boiling. Contaminated shellfish must be boiled or steamed for 10 minutes to kill all bacteria. The core temperatures of cooked food should be 158°F. Unless all the bacteria are killed by cooking, they will multiply rapidly at room temperature in cooked shellfish.

Cholera can be controlled by improved sanitation, especially by maintaining untainted water supplies. Travelers to high-risk areas in Latin America, Africa, and Asia must not:

- bring perishable seafood back to the United States
- consume unboiled or untreated water or ice
- eat food or beverages from street vendors
- eat raw or partially cooked fish or shellfish
- eat raw vegetables or salads

They should

- treat unbottled water with chlorine or iodine tablets
- drink carbonated bottled water or bottled soft drinks (the carbonation destroys the bacteria)
- drink tea and coffee made only with boiled water

- eat only fruits that the person peels
- eat only foods that are cooked and hot

See also ANTIDIARRHEAL DRUGS; DIARRHEA AND INFECTIOUS DISEASE; TRAVELER'S DIARRHEA.

chromomycosis An invasive, chronic fungal infection of the top two layers of the skin on the feet and legs. The infection almost always begins in the skin at the site of trauma, and is most common in the tropics. Called chromomycosis or verrucous dermatitis, the infection may remain localized, or become a generalized infection throughout the body.

This uncommon tropical infection is caused by a group of closely related molds found in the soil, affecting people involved in manual labor. While it is not clear why the infection occurs only in the tropics, it is believed that in colder climates, workers wear shoes, which protect the feet. Still, even in the tropics this disorder is not common.

Symptoms and Diagnostic Path

The disease begins with an itchy, watery, warty nodule on the leg or foot that develops in a cut or break in the skin. Appearing first as a small dull red lesion, it gradually develops into a large ulcer; over a period of weeks or months, more warty, foul-smelling growths appear in other parts of the skin along the path of lymphatic drainage of the foot, ankle, knee, elbow, or hand. As the ulcer spreads, the central area becomes scarred.

Treatment Options and Outlook

Bed rest, elevation of the affected part, and antibiotic therapy to control secondary infections are recommended. Many patients develop secondary bacterial infections. Surgical excision of the affected area, destruction of the affected tissue, or drug treatment (potassium iodide, flucytosine, thiabendazole, ketoconazole, and topical heat) may be successful.

This condition is chronic and may last for years or decades, leading to the necessity of amputation, the development of ELEPHANTIASIS, or to squamous cell cancer.

chronic fatigue syndrome A complex disorder characterized by severe fatigue, weakness, poor concentration and memory, once derisively dismissed as a new "yuppie flu." Contrary to popular notions, however, the disease is not new; clinical reports of the condition have appeared for more than 100 years. The modern stereotype of "yuppie flu" began because those who sought help in the early 1980s were primarily affluent, well-educated women in their 30s and 40s. Since then, however, physicians have realized the disease strikes those of all ages, races, and social classes in countries around the world, although it is still diagnosed two to four times more often in women than in men.

In the 1860s, it was called "neurasthenia," and considered to be a neurosis characterized by weakness and fatigue. In the 1960s it was called "Icelander's disease." Since then, physicians have blamed the symptoms variously on "iron-poor blood" (anemia), low blood sugar (hypoglycemia), allergies, or a body-wide yeast infection (CANDIDIASIS). In the mid-1980s, the disease was believed to be caused by the EPSTEIN-BARR VIRUS, after scientists found signs of the EBV antibodies in affected patients. Since then, scientists realized that the EBV is so common, it is actually found in the blood of many healthy Americans, while some people with no EBV antibodies have the symptoms of chronic fatigue syndrome.

The degree to which patients are disabled varies widely. Some can still function at home and work, but others become severely disabled and cannot perform many of the routine activities of daily living. The total number of affected people in the United States is unknown.

In other countries, CFS is known as myalgic encephalomyelitis, post-viral fatigue syndrome, chronic fatigue and immune dysfunction syndrome.

No one knows the cause of CFS, and no virus or antibody has been identified. This has made it more difficult to determine how many people actually have the illness. Based on the first three years of an ongoing surveillance study in four U.S. cities, the CENTERS FOR DISEASE CONTROL AND PREVENTION estimates the minimum rate of CFS in the United States to be four to 10 cases per 100,000 adults.

Scientists have studied a range of possible causes, including Epstein-Barr and other HERPES infections, the yeast organism *CANDIDA ALBICANS,* and immune system or hormone regulation problems. Many of these problems are found among CFS patients, but scientists have not yet been able to establish any of them as the source of CFS.

Symptoms and Diagnostic Path

To be diagnosed with chronic fatigue syndrome, a patient must have an unexplained persistent chronic fatigue for six months that is not caused by exertion or alleviated by rest; it must severely curtail activities. In addition, the patient must have any four of the following symptoms for at least six months that were not present before the fatigue:

- impaired memory or concentration
- sore throat
- tender lymph nodes in neck or under arms
- muscle pain
- multi-joint pain with no swelling
- headache (of new type or pattern)
- sleep that is not refreshing
- malaise after exercise lasting more than 24 hours

Many of these symptoms mimic the flu, but the flu goes away while CFS symptoms persist or recur frequently for more than six months. Many people first notice symptoms after an acute infection (cold, BRONCHITIS, HEPATITIS, MONONUCLEOSIS, or intestinal flu).

The course of the disease varies from one patient to the next. For most, the disease hits a plateau early on and ebbs and flows thereafter. Some get better, but are not completely well. Others spontaneously recover.

Treatment Options and Outlook

Although no specific treatment has been identified for CFS, there have been anecdotal reports of success with small numbers of patients using a range of treatment, including antiviral drugs, antidepressants, or drugs that boost the immune system. Many physicians prescribe tricyclic antidepressants, since these drugs help people with fibromyalgia (a disease much like CFS). Some patients improve with benzodiazepines (a class of drug used to treat anxiety and sleep problems) or antianxiety drugs.

Nonsteroidal anti-inflammatory drugs may help ease body aches and fever; nonsedating antihistamines may help relieve allergic symptoms.

ciguatera A common clinical syndrome caused by eating certain tropical marine reef fish (mostly barracuda, red snapper, amberjack, surgeonfish, sea bass, and grouper). The fish are toxic at certain times of the year when they ingest a certain type of dinoflagellate called *Gambierdiscus toxicus,* which contains "ciguatoxin," an odorless, tasteless poison that cannot be destroyed by either heating or freezing.

Ciguatera is the most frequently reported seafood-related illness in the world, affecting up to 500,000 people a year around the world. In the United States between 1977 and 1981, 37 percent of the seafood-borne illness reported to the CENTERS FOR DISEASE CONTROL AND PREVENTION were attributed to ciguatera.

Ciguatera fish poisoning is the most important type of seafood poisoning. Complex and hard to detect, it is impossible to predict outbreaks; contaminated fish look, taste, and smell normal. The toxins are not destroyed by cooking, and if enough are eaten, they can cause symptoms that last for years. With global warming and widespread bleaching and death of coral, the incidence of ciguatera is expected to increase.

Ciguatera occurs most often in the Caribbean Islands, Florida, Hawaii, and the Pacific Islands. Recent reports cited 129 cases over a two-year period in Dade County, Florida, alone.

Ciguatera occurs after eating any of more than 300 species of fish that may contain ciguatoxin, which is found in greatest concentration in internal organs, but cannot be detected by inspection, taste, or smell. The likelihood that ciguatoxin is present is greater with larger, more predatory coral reef fish.

Symptoms and Diagnostic Path

Eating a fish contaminated with ciguatoxin produces both stomach and neurologic symptoms within six hours. Patients often report a curious type of sensory reversal, so that picking up a cold glass would cause a burning hot sensation. Other symptoms include a tingling sensation in the lips and mouth followed by numbness, nausea, vomiting, abdominal cramps, weakness, headache, vertigo, paralysis, convulsions, skin rash, altered heart rate, arrhythmia, and low blood pressure; coma and death from respiratory paralysis occur in about 12 percent of cases. Subsequent episodes of ciguatera may be more severe.

Treatment Options and Outlook

Effective antidotes are available.

Ciguatera poisoning usually subsides on its own within several days. However, in severe cases the neurological symptoms can persist for months. In a few isolated cases neurological symptoms have persisted for several years. In other cases, recovered patients have experienced recurrence of neurological symptoms years after recovery. Such relapses are most often associated with changes in diet or with drinking alcohol.

clonorchiasis A parasitic infection caused by the trematode *Clonorchis sinensis* in raw or improperly cooked or pickled freshwater fish. Saltwater fish don't carry these parasites.

Endemic areas include Korea, China, Taiwan, and Vietnam. Clonorchiasis has been reported in nonendemic areas including the United States among Asian immigrants, or after ingestion of imported, undercooked, or pickled freshwater fish. The infection is rarely fatal, and most victims recover completely.

The infestation begins when the eggs are eliminated into water in human or animal feces and are eaten by certain snails. The eggs hatch inside the snail, where they develop into many free-swimming larval organisms that escape into the water and penetrate under the scales or in the flesh of freshwater fish. Humans become infected when they eat the fish raw or undercooked. Once inside a human host, the organisms migrate to the human bile ducts, where they mature and remain for their life span, shedding eggs into the bile.

Symptoms and Diagnostic Path

Most people are not infected with many parasites, and have no symptoms. If acute symptoms do occur, they include fatigue, fever, and abdominal pain. Chronic symptoms include weakness, lack of appetite, abdominal pain, diarrhea, prolonged low-grade fever, and jaundice.

Treatment Options and Outlook

Praziquantel or albendazole are the drugs of choice.

Risk Factors and Preventive Measures

Pickling, smoking, or drying fish may not destroy these infective organisms in freshwater fish.

Thorough cooking is the best way to prevent the infection.

clostridial myonecrosis See GANGRENE.

Clostridium A genus of spore-producing bacteria that contains more than 60 species, named for the Greek word meaning "spindle," found in earth throughout the world. Some forms of the bacteria are found in the intestines and stools of different mammals (including humans). Others produce toxins as they multiply. These germs, which cannot thrive in the presence of oxygen, can cause food poisoning and wound infection. Seven types (A, B, C, D, E, F, and G) of botulism have been identified based on the specific toxin produced by each strain. Types A, B, E, and F cause human BOTULISM; types C and D cause most cases of animal botulism. Although type G has been isolated from soil in Argentina, no outbreaks have been identified.

These bacteria are typically found in soil everywhere in the world; some species even live harmlessly in human intestines. When *Clostridium* bacteria cause human illness, it is usually because they produce a poisonous chemical called a toxin.

The genus includes the deadly CLOSTRIDIUM BOTULINUM, cause of botulism. CLOSTRIDIUM PERFRINGENS is a cause of gas GANGRENE, and also a more common and much less dangerous cause of food poisoning in the United States and is found most often in cooked beef and poultry. It is found widely in nature, and its spores can survive high cooking temperatures; if the food cools slowly, the spores germinate and the bacteria become activated. If the tainted food is served without reheating properly, live toxin-producing bacteria can be consumed, causing cramps and diarrhea in about 16 hours. Two separate outbreaks were traced to tainted corned beef served on a 1993 St. Patrick's Day.

CLOSTRIDIUM TETANI is a third deadly member of this bacterial family. The toxin produced by this bacteria causes TETANUS, not as often when eaten as when entering the body via a wound.

C. difficile is a recently identified cause of colitis linked to the administration of antibiotics. About 3 percent of healthy adults carry this bacterium in the intestines. When a patient takes antibiotics, the drugs can alter the balance of bacteria in the intestines and stomach, allowing *C. difficile* to reproduce to the point where its toxins cause diarrhea.

However, not all the types of bacteria in the genus are deadly. *C. pasteurianum* is a type of bacteria found in the soil that helps plants acquire nitrogen, a fundamental requirement in producing food.

See also ANTIDIARRHEAL DRUGS; CLOSTRIDIUM BOTULINUM; CLOSTRIDIUM DIFFICILE; CLOSTRIDIUM PERFRINGENS; CLOSTRIDIUM TETANI; DIARRHEA AND INFECTIOUS DISEASE.

Clostridium botulinum A species of spore-producing bacteria that cause BOTULISM in humans. Botulinus food poisoning is caused by the ingestion of food containing toxins produced by this species. The spore's resistance to heat makes them an important cause of poisoning in improperly cooked or canned foods. In addition, the bacteria are commonly found in soil, where the spores can survive for years.

Clostridium difficile A species of bacteria that has emerged as an increasing threat to hospital patients in Europe and North America, since it produces two toxins that lead to pseudomembraneous colitis among those taking antibiotics aimed at another infection.

One study estimates that as many as 2,000 people may have died in Quebec in 2003–04 because of *C. difficile* infection, according to the Canadian Medical Association. Recent cases in four U.S. states show it is appearing more often in healthy people who have not been admitted to health-care facilities or even taken antibiotics, according to the CENTERS FOR DISEASE CONTROL AND PREVENTION.

The bacteria are found in the colon, causing diarrhea and a more serious intestinal condition known as colitis. It is spread by spores in feces, which are difficult to kill with conventional household cleaners.

However, the bacteria have grown resistant to certain antibiotics that work against other colon bacteria, so that when patients take those antibiotics (especially clindamycin), competing bacteria die off, and *C. difficile* grows rapidly out of control.

Patients who are infected with this bacteria should be treated with vancomycin or metronidazole and stop taking any antibiotic that is causing the problem.

Clostridium perfringens A species of anaerobic Gram-positive bacteria (bacteria which grow in the absence of oxygen) capable of causing gas GANGRENE in humans, and a variety of digestive and urinary tract disease in livestock. The oval spores of this bacteria, also known as *Clostridium welchii*, are found mainly in soil and in human intestines.

Clostridium perfringens food poisoning A mild food-borne illness caused by *Clostridium perfringens* bacteria in human and animal feces and in soil and water. The bacteria may contaminate cooked meats or gravy that have been allowed to remain for too long at room temperature before being eaten. At room temperature, the bacteria grow in the contaminated food and produce a toxin that can kill cells along the inside lining of the intestines. These bacteria also are normally found in raw meat.

This type of food poisoning is among the most common in the United States, with an estimated 10,000 cases each year, according to the U.S. CENTERS FOR DISEASE CONTROL AND PREVENTION. Most cases go unreported.

The toxin-producing organism occurs in undercooked meat (such as rare beef; meat pies; burritos; tacos; enchiladas; reheated meats; or gravies made from beef, turkey, or chicken). The bacteria multiply quickly in reheated foods; once ingested, the bacteria produce illness in the digestive tract. A large amount of the bacteria must be ingested in order to cause illness. Outbreaks have been traced to restaurants, caterers, and cafeterias.

The bacteria have a spore form that is not killed by cooking; however, the spores cannot reproduce into bacteria at temperatures below 40°F or above 140°F.

Symptoms and Diagnostic Path

The illness appears suddenly (within six to 24 hours after eating), causing severe colic or cramps and abdominal gas pains followed by a 24-hour bout of watery diarrhea. There may be nausea and fever, but usually not vomiting. While typically a mild illness, it can be dangerous to infants and the elderly, who may become dehydrated. Having the disease does not confer immunity but patients are not infectious.

Following an injury, this type of bacteria proliferates in the injured tissues, causing the potentially fatal gas GANGRENE.

Treatment Options and Outlook

Because this is technically not an infection but an intoxication, no antibiotic will cure it. Patients should try to replace fluid losses by drinking clear liquids. If dehydration is suspected, medical care should be sought. If food poisoning is suspected, local health departments should be notified.

Clostridium tetani A bacterial member of the genus CLOSTRIDIUM that causes TETANUS. The bacteria are not dangerous by themselves, but because of the toxin they release. Spores of this bacteria are found in soil, which can enter the body via any type of wounds, from the classic deep puncture cuts to injuries as innocuous as a splinter.

As the bacteria are activated by decomposing tissue, the toxin travels though the nervous system into the spinal cord, triggering spasms, giving rise to the common name for this syndrome, "lockjaw." A terrible grin, called *RISUS SARDONICUS*, can transform the face of any untreated victim.

CMV See CYTOMEGALOVIRUS INFECTION.

Coccidioides immitis The infectious fungal spores that cause the acute or chronic illness COCCIDIOIDO-MYCOSIS.

coccidioidomycosis The medical name for valley fever, an infectious fungal disease caused by inhaling bacterial spores, which may be either acute or chronic. It is endemic in hot, dry areas of the Southwest—the Central and San Joaquin valleys and desert areas of California, as well as the arid areas of

Nevada, Utah, Arizona, West Texas, and New Mexico. A person who lives in one of these areas is quite likely to be affected by valley fever. For example, almost 60 percent of the residents of Bakersfield, California, have positive skin tests for this condition. (A positive skin test means the person has had an infection and has developed immunity to the fungus, and will never contract valley fever again.) The disease is also found in Mexico, Central America, and South America.

Animals also can develop the disease—especially horses, cattle, dogs, and llamas, but cats are not usually affected. Coccidioidomycosis is also known as desert fever, desert rheumatism, or San Joaquin fever.

The bacterial spore *Coccidioides immitis,* which is carried on wind-borne dust particles, is the cause of the disease. The cocci fungus lives in a sort of hibernation in alkaline soil, blooming when weather conditions are good. When it blooms, the tiny spores are stirred by wind or other movement and become airborne, floating in the air for many miles. When a person or animal who is not immune breathes them in, the spores enter the lungs and cause an infection. In general, the more spores that are inhaled, the more serious the infection.

Symptoms and Diagnostic Path

About 60 percent of infections cause no symptoms; in these cases, the condition is diagnosed only by a positive skin test. Symptoms range from mild to severe in the remaining 40 percent. Patients with an impaired immune system have more serious infections, and patients with AIDS are at higher risk for pulmonary coccidioidomycosis, as well as forms of the disease that affect the skin (cutaneous coccidioidomycosis) and that spread throughout the body (disseminated coccidioidomycosis).

Acute coccidioidomycosis is rare. Chronic pulmonary coccidioidomycosis can develop as long as 20 years after an initial infection. Rarely, lung infections can form and rupture, releasing pus between the lungs and ribs. Occasionally, the infection can spread to the bones, lungs, liver, meninges, brain, skin, heart, and sac around the heart.

Along with the flu-like symptoms, patients experience skin rash and joint aches (especially the knees). Dark-skinned patients appear to have more severe symptoms and to have the disease spread to other parts of the body. However, the most serious form that valley fever takes—when it infects the lining of the brain, called cocci meningitis—is most likely to occur in Caucasian males. Cocci meningitis is the form most likely to end in death.

The diagnosis can be confirmed if the patient has recently visited an endemic area, and if the fungus has been identified in sputum, body fluid, or tissue.

Treatment Options and Outlook

Most patients with valley fever do not need to be treated. However, those whose disease has spread to other parts of the body need medication. Ketoconazole, fluconazole, and itraconazole are all antifungal agents approved for the treatment of valley fever. The most effective medication for treating valley fever infections is amphotericin B.

ABSCESSES in soft tissue, bone, and joints may need to be drained, and bone infections may need to be removed.

cold, common An upper respiratory infection caused by one of at least 200 different types of viruses. Colds are most likely to occur during "cold season," which begins in the fall and continues throughout the spring; tropical areas tend to encourage cold viruses during the rainy months. While cold viruses are found throughout the world, they infect only humans with what are considered to be upper respiratory infections, which means they are limited to the nose and throat. After one bout with a particular virus, the victim will develop an immunity to that precise virus. This is why adults have fewer colds than young children, and why the oldest Americans have the fewest colds of all.

A person who smokes or lives in a polluted atmosphere has a higher chance of coming down with a cold. This is because air pollution and the nicotine and tars in tobacco smoke can irritate the lining of the nose and throat, making it easier for a cold virus to enter the cells and cause an infection. This irritation can also prolong the length of the infection. This is why people who live in heavily polluted areas or who smoke (or live with smokers) have more colds and have them longer than those who do not.

The common cold costs Americans millions of days of missed work and school every year and more than $2 billion for over-the-counter and prescription remedies, none of which will cure the infection.

Different types of viruses proliferate at different times; in the fall and late spring, a cold may be caused by one of the more than 100 types of rhinovirus. These are the most common villains, and appear to be related to crowding indoors, school openings, and seasonal variations. Between December and May, several types of coronaviruses are responsible for most cases. Besides these two types of viruses, colds may also be caused by PARAINFLUENZA, RSV, ADENOVIRUS, ENTEROVIRUS, and INFLUENZA. All of these viruses seem to be able to change their characteristics from one season to the next.

A cold is not transmitted by sitting in a draft, getting wet feet, or going outside without a jacket. Because the cold viruses are so specific, a person can only get a cold if the virus travels high up inside the nose, into the nasopharynx. A cold virus can only reach this area by touch, or (less often) through the air. One study found that while contact with saliva did not pass on germs, even a very brief contact with a nasal mucus-contaminated hand (as quick as a 10-second touch) led to transmission of virus in 20 of 28 cases.

While cooling the body does not seem to bring on a cold, fatigue, stress, and anything else that weakens the body's immune system *can* influence susceptibility. It is possible to catch a cold from other people who have colds or from the things they use or touch: faucets, phones, doorknobs, light switches, straps on buses or subways, office equipment. A virus can survive for many hours on these objects, unless it is washed off with alcohol, a household disinfectant, or hot, sudsy water. Everyone who touches one of these contaminated objects and then touches the nose, eyes, or mouth can get the virus. Once the virus is on the hands, others can be exposed by shaking hands or by touching other things that they touch.

Cold viruses are not carried very far through the air, however. If someone with a cold sneezes across the room, neighbors would not come down with the cold, too—but if someone should cough or sneeze right into a person's face, the person could get sick.

Healthy people have a film of mucus lining the nose and throat; tiny hairs called cilia move this mucus from sinuses and throat to the stomach. As the mucus is moved along, it traps harmful bacteria and viruses and carries them along to the stomach, where they are broken down by acids. A healthy mucous membrane can snag germs trapped in the nose and throat, so the person can then breathe, cough, or sneeze them back out. The mucus around the tonsils and adenoids can trap these germs, where they can be destroyed by the immune system.

If a person is not so healthy, the mucous membranes in the nose will be either too thick (causing a stuffy nose and congested throat) or too thin (runny nose). The germs would not be cleared away. Once the viruses enter the nose, they set up housekeeping in the mucous layer of the nose and throat, attaching themselves to cells found there. The viruses drill holes in the cell membranes, inserting their own genetic material to enter the cells. Soon, the virus takes over and forces the cells to pump out thousands of new little virus particles.

In response to this invasion, the body's immune system swings into action. Injured cells in the nose and throat release chemicals called prostaglandins, which trigger inflammation and attract infection-fighting white blood cells. (The throat will begin to feel scratchy and swollen.) Tiny blood vessels stretch, which allows spaces to open up and specialized white cells to enter. Body temperature rises and histamine is released (causing a fever), which steps up the production of mucus in the nose, trapping and removing viral particles. The nose starts to run. As the nose and throat stimulate the extra mucus production, it irritates the throat and triggers a cough. Cold viruses are also responsible for congestion in the sinuses.

All of this activity comes at a price, of course— the unpleasant symptoms experienced as a cold. Actually, by the time a person starts feeling sick, the body has already been fighting the invader for a day or two. When people are in the process of catching a cold, they probably feel fine. It is not until they are actually getting better that they feel ill.

In order to break through the body's defenses (hair, mucus, and other barriers in the human nose) viruses must attack in huge numbers in order to successfully cause a cold. Most of the time, a brief encounter with a sick stranger would not cause disease, even if a person sits in a doctor's office filled with sick patients for 10 or 20 minutes.

On the other hand, working all day in an office building filled with people who have colds could be a risk. Traveling on a plane carrying sick passengers is an even bigger risk for catching a cold, since the recirculated air in a pressurized cabin evenly distributes viruses to everybody, while drying out mucous membranes that would normally trap viruses and get rid of them.

Symptoms and Diagnostic Path

A stuffy congested nose, sneezing, sore scratchy throat, cough, headache, runny eyes, and (possibly) a low fever. Viruses that attack the lower respiratory tract—the windpipe, bronchial tubes, and lungs—are more serious but less common and are responsible for PNEUMONIA and BRONCHITIS, among others.

The symptoms of a cold (scratchy throat, runny nose, and congestion) are not caused by the virus itself but are the result of the immune system's fight to get rid of the invader.

Because the symptoms of a cold are actually caused by the body's attempt at healing itself, there are times when the patient should not interfere. It is best to let a fever below 101.5°F burn itself out, for example, since this type of fever will also help the body burn up viruses and toxins. And mucus from a runny nose is a good way of getting rid of germs.

Treatment Options and Outlook

There is no treatment that will cure a cold, which is caused by a virus. Symptoms may be treated by a wide variety of over-the-counter medications and many different home remedies. While the use of vitamin C to treat colds is still controversial, several well-controlled studies demonstrate that it can lessen a cold's symptoms and duration. Other studies have shown that zinc lozenges can shorten the duration of symptoms.

A cold usually lasts for about 10 days, although it can range from three days to several weeks. A doctor should be consulted if the patient still feels sick after 10 days. A person should call even sooner if the face starts to swell or teeth become

extremely sensitive, because these symptoms can signal a bacterial infection in the sinuses or middle ear.

When the sinuses become clogged with nasal secretions, they may become infected with bacteria. While antibiotics will not touch a cold, they *will* be effective in treating this secondary bacterial infection.

Colds may also trigger asthma attacks in those who suffer with this condition. In children, colds may also lead to middle-ear infections (the most common complication of colds).

Pneumonia may also set in at the end of a cold; a patient who suddenly develops a fever after the symptoms seem to be going away, should see a doctor.

Risk Factors and Preventive Measures

A person remains infectious from 24 hours before symptoms appear until five days *after* the cold starts. A person is most infectious for the first three days, from the time when the first symptoms show up. Young children are infectious for a longer period of time (up to three weeks), since it takes their immune systems longer to fight off the virus.

It may not seem practical, but a person with a cold should stay home. While most adults feel that they should force themselves to go to work if they have a cold, in fact it would be much better for everyone if they would isolate themselves to decrease the spread of the virus.

The most important factor in reducing the transmission of colds is to keep hands away from nose and eyes. By scratching the nose or rubbing the eyes with a contaminated hand, the virus can easily be inhaled higher up in the nose or enter the nasopharynx through the tear ducts of the eye. According to research, most people touch their nose or eyes about once every three hours.

Since most people find it difficult *not* to touch their face occasionally, washing hands often may help prevent colds. It is especially important for people who already have colds to wash their hands, since they are even more likely to be wiping, blowing, scratching, or touching the nose area. Washing the hands vigorously with soap and water for 20 seconds will remove the virus. Disposable towelettes are a good alternative.

Hands should be washed

- after sneezing or coughing
- before eating
- after wiping, blowing, or touching the nose
- after using the toilet
- before touching another person

Disposable tissues should be used instead of cloth handkerchiefs when coughing, sneezing, or blowing the nose and thrown away immediately afterward. A used tissue is filled with virus just waiting to be passed on to someone else.

In addition to not touching the face and washing the hands, it is also a good idea to disinfect areas likely to be contaminated with germs, such as door handles, telephones, light switches, and so on.

By being careful, it is really possible to stop the spread of colds, even in a household where others are sick.

Since plane travel brings a higher risk of catching someone else's cold, it is a good idea to drink at least eight ounces of water for each hour spent on a plane to rehydrate the nose.

Diet   There is some evidence that certain strains of rhinoviruses can be destroyed by high levels of vitamin C. Several German studies have suggested that the herb echinacea (*E. purpurea, E. angustifolia,* or *E. pallida*) appears to be mild stimulant of the immune system that may help fend off colds. Because its effect appears to fade when used on a daily basis for longer than eight weeks, it is best to use it intermittently.

Stress   There is a definite link between emotions and infections, according to studies reported in the *New England Journal of Medicine.* In one study by Sheldon Cohen, Ph.D., professor of psychology at Carnegie-Mellon University in Pittsburgh, it is reported that a high level of psychological stress lowers resistance to viral infections and nearly doubles the chance of getting a cold. Other studies have found that mental and emotional stress impairs the ability to fight off viruses and doubles the risk of catching a cold.

Studies found that about 25 percent of those who were infected with the rhinovirus *did not* develop cold symptoms; the reason, studies suggest, may be that some people have healthier immune systems than others.

Humor may also help. Levels of protective chemicals (such as IgA) jumped significantly when volunteers watched comics, according to research. Those who watched a documentary had no rise in IgA levels.

Humidity   Studies suggest that the relative humidity of the air may affect the risk of colds.

IS IT A COLD, THE FLU, OR AN ALLERGY?

A cold is *not* the same thing as the flu. Head colds are just what they say they are—limited to the head, whereas the flu will affect the entire system. A cold will come on gradually, beginning with a vague feeling of unease; the sore throat may be slight; chills or aches will not be severe, and fever will not usually rise above 100°F. The common cold causes

- scratchy throat
- runny nose
- itchy eyes

On the other hand, INFLUENZA strikes fast and hard, with symptoms that are much more severe than those characterized by a simple cold. The flu often causes

- nausea
- vomiting
- diarrhea
- high fever (from 101–104°F)
- body aches (especially in the back)
- chills
- cough
- eye pain
- light sensitivity
- headache

Allergies share a few symptoms with colds, but they have significant differences. If a cold seems to be hanging on for months, it could be an allergy. Winter allergies (known as perennial allergic rhinitis) cause

- itchy eyes
- itchy, runny, stuffy nose
- itchy throat
- postnasal drip
- coughing
- sneezing
- season-long symptoms

During the winter and the start of winter heating (with its lowered humidity), there is a sharp increase in the number of colds. This low humidity causes dry throats and nose, which increases the chance of infection.

The nose, throat, and lungs work best when the air has a relative humidity of about 45 percent. If the air during the winter falls below that level, moisture will be absorbed into the heated air from the mucous membranes. Since dried mucous membranes cannot clean themselves they become more vulnerable to invasion from cold viruses.

Air circulation   Good ventilation can also help disperse germs and hinder the spread of colds.

The closed circulation systems of airplanes are another potential danger for the transmission of colds. Airplane air usually has very low humidity.

WHEN TO CALL THE DOCTOR

A doctor should be contacted if there is

- fever of 101°F or above that stays up after fever medication has been given
- fever of 102°F in children
- any fever that lasts more than three days
- difficulty breathing, very rapid breathing, shortness of breath, wheezing or stridor (rattling or crackling noises in the chest or high-pitched sounds when inhaling)
- blue or dusky color around mouth, nail beds, or skin
- extreme pain (ears, headache, throat, sinuses, teeth)
- skin rash
- white or yellow spots on tonsils or throat
- coughing episode lasting longer than interval between coughs
- cough that produces thick yellow-green, gray, or bloody sputum or that lasts longer than 10 days
- shaking chills
- delirium
- enlarged, tender glands in neck
- symptoms that get worse instead of better
- extreme difficulty swallowing
- headache and stiff neck with no other symptoms (could be meningitis)
- headache and sore throat with no other symptoms (could be strep throat)

To combat this, passengers should drink lots of fluids on planes and avoid alcohol, which can dehydrate the body.

Personal hygiene   If there are cold germs circulating in a household, members should not share eating or drinking utensils with others (especially babies). The sick person should use a separate set of towels and washcloths and change the bedding more often. (Actually, bedding should be changed more often for *everyone*, healthy or sick, during the winter months to help cut down on virus transmission.)

It is not likely that rhinovirus (the most common cold virus) can cause illness by hitching a ride on a toothbrush—they must get into the nose to cause a cold. However, viruses such as the enteroviruses (found in the stomach/intestines) can occasionally cause a cold. To be safe, experts suggest replacing a toothbrush every three months. A toothbrush should not be shared with anyone else.

Rest/exercise   Plenty of exercise and sufficient rest will improve circulation, lymphatic system, organs, and emotions. In one study, volunteers who exercised regularly showed improved immune function, and only half as many days of cold symptoms. But too much of a good thing can be harmful—those who exercised too strenuously depressed their immune systems and actually increased their risk of getting colds. Any moderate noncompetitive exercise can work. Experts recommend exercise several times a week—not every day.

cold sore   A small skin blister, also known as a "fever blister," that appears on the mouth when a person has a cold. Cold sores are extremely common and are usually first transmitted during childhood. The term *fever blister* comes from the fact that such blisters often appear during fevers.

Cold sores are harmless in healthy children and adults, although they are painful to the touch and can be unattractive. They are similar, but not identical to, CANKER SORES, which also appear on the mouth. Both usually cause small sores to develop in the mouth that heal within two weeks. However, canker sores are not usually preceded by a blister, and they are usually larger than fever blisters, without merging to form one large sore as fever blisters do. Finally, canker sores usually erupt on movable parts of the mouth (such as the tongue and the cheek or lip linings) whereas cold sores usually appear on the gums, roof of the mouth, lips, or nostrils. Cold sores may occur on any part of the body.

People are most infectious when the sores first appear, but the virus is shed in the saliva for a long time (up to two months after the sores have healed). Cold sores can be spread to others during this entire time. Patients with an active cold sore should limit contact with newborns or anyone else with a weakened immune system.

Once a person has been infected, the virus remains in a latent stage in the body and may be reactivated when the immune system is stressed.

Cold sores are caused by the HERPES SIMPLEX virus. The viral strain usually responsible for cold sores is herpes simplex Type 1 (HSV1); up to 90 percent of all people around the world carry this virus. This strain usually appears on the mouth, lips, and face.

The virus is highly contagious when the blisters are present; it is often transmitted by kissing. The virus can also be spread by children who touch their blister and then touch other children. About 10 percent of oral herpes cases in adults are acquired by oral-genital sex with a person with active genital herpes.

Cold sores tend to appear when the victim is stressed, exposed to sunlight, a cold wind, another infection, or feels run down. Women tend to experience more cold sores around their menstrual periods, but some people are afflicted at regular intervals throughout the year. People with compromised immune systems may experience prolonged attacks.

One study suggests that the tendency for relapses might be inherited.

Symptoms and Diagnostic Path

Most people have their first infection before age 10, although most will not have symptoms. About 10 percent will go on to develop many fluid-filled blisters inside and outside the mouth about five days after exposure, together with fever, swollen neck, and aches. This is followed by a yellow crust that forms over the blister, healing without scars in about two weeks. Once the infection occurs, the virus remains in a nerve located near the cheek-

bone. There it may remain, forever inactive, or it may travel down the nerve to the surface of the skin to cause a new blister. Recurrent attacks tend to be less severe.

The first attack may not even be noticed; the first infection in childhood usually causes no symptoms. However, about 10 percent of newly infected children experience a mild to fairly severe illness with fever, tiredness, and several painful cold sores in the mouth and throat.

Subsequent outbreaks are often signaled by a tingling in the lips, followed by a small water-filled blister on a red base that soon grows, causing itching and soreness. Within a few days the blisters burst, encrust, and then disappear. The virus then retreats back along the nerve where it lies dormant in the nerve cell; in some patients, however, the virus is constantly reactivated.

Treatment Options and Outlook

There is no cure for recurrent fever blisters. For mild symptoms, the sore should be kept clean and dry and it will heal itself. For particularly virulent outbreaks, the antiviral drug acyclovir may relieve symptoms. Otherwise, there are a range of nonprescription drugs available containing some numbing agent (such as camphor or phenol) that also contain an emollient to reduce skin cracking.

Some studies have suggested that zinc may help prevent outbreaks because the zinc interferes with herpes viral replication. Studies found that both zinc gluconate and zinc sulfate helped speed up healing time, but zinc gluconate was less irritating to the skin. Both zinc products are available at health food stores.

Sores can be protected with a dab of petroleum jelly (applied with a clean cotton swab). Patients should avoid drinks with a high acid content (such as orange juice).

Anyone with an impaired immune system is at risk of complications; the virus may spread throughout the body, causing a severe illness.

Risk Factors and Preventive Measures

While there is no effective preventive treatment, some patients find applying a lip salve before going out in the sun prevents outbreaks. Research has shown that the virus can live up to seven days on a toothbrush, causing a reinfection after the sore heals. Once a sore develops, an infected toothbrush can also lead to multiple sores, so a new toothbrush should be used after the sore heals. It is also better to use small tubes of toothpaste, since the paste can transmit germs, too.

An infected individual should not touch sores, which could spread the virus to new sites (such as the eyes or the genitals). Kissing should be avoided during an outbreak if the blisters will come in contact with the lips.

coliform count   A method of determining the level of fecal coliform bacteria (such as *E. coli*) in water. While these bacteria are abundant in the lower intestines of warm-blooded animals (including humans), they are rare or absent in unpolluted waters. As a result, their presence serves as a reliable indication of sewage or fecal contamination in water.

Total coliform measurements include all types of coliform bacteria strains. Various methods are available for determining the presence and amount of coliform bacteria in water. Results are usually given as the number of bacteria per 100 mL of water, or by the "presence" or "absence" method. Because the bacteria are too small to count directly, a basic method is used to "magnify" their presence using a special broth that can detect acidity formed during lactose fermentation by the bacteria.

Commonly, ocean water along public beaches is regularly tested in the summer for coliform bacteria; contaminated water can result in beach closings, since the bacteria can cause disease.

communicable disease   Any disease that is transmitted from one person or animal to another, either directly—by contact with feces or urine or other bodily discharges—or indirectly, via objects or substances such as contaminated glasses, toys, or water. It also may be transmitted via fleas, flies, mosquitoes, ticks, or other insects.

Control of a communicable disease rests on properly identifying the organism that transmits it, preventing its spread to the environment, protecting others, and treating the infected patients.

By law, many communicable diseases must be reported to the local health department. Diseases that must be reported include bacterial MENINGITIS, AIDS, FOOD-BORNE INFECTIONS, MEASLES, HEPATITIS, RABIES, LYME DISEASE, SYPHILIS, MALARIA, and TUBERCULOSIS. However, not all communicable diseases must be reported, since they are not all considered to be a danger to society.

condylomata acuminata   See WARTS, GENITAL.

congenital infectious diseases   A wide variety of bacteria, viruses, and microorganisms can cross the placenta from the mother's blood into a fetus and cause disease. Organisms that cause particularly serious diseases include RUBELLA, SYPHILIS, TOXOPLASMOSIS, and CYTOMEGALOVIRUS. Often, the effect these microorganisms have on the fetus depends on the stage of pregnancy at which the infection was acquired. For example, a rubella infection at the ninth or 10th week of pregnancy may cause deafness, heart disease, and other damage. If the same infection occurs much later in pregnancy, no harm usually results.

The infant is also vulnerable to maternal infection while passing through the birth canal. At this time, any active infection in the mother's genital area can have serious repercussions to her child. Conditions acquired in this way include CONJUNCTIVITIS, genital HERPES, or chlamydial infection. Staph or strep infections, MENINGITIS, HEPATITIS B, or LISTERIOSIS may also be passed on.

Some of these diseases may be prevented by proper medical care. All girls should be immunized against rubella and pregnant women should have any sexually transmitted diseases treated immediately.

A baby who is born with an infectious disease is treated immediately, although some diseases that occurred in the uterus cannot be reversed at birth.

Congo fever   An infectious disease transmitted via tick bite that causes a fever and bleeding from mucous membranes and the skin. The disease, which was first observed in the Crimea by Russian scientists in 1944 and 1945, is fatal in about 30 percent of cases. The virus that causes this disease was isolated in Africa in the mid-1960s and named Crimean, but African researchers found the same organism and named it Congo; therefore, it is called either Congo fever or a combination of both names (Crimean-Congo hemorrhagic fever). The disease is endemic in many countries in Africa, Europe, and Asia, and during 2001 and 2002, outbreaks were recorded in Kosovo, Albania, Iran, Pakistan, and South Africa.

The viral infection is usually transmitted to humans by a tick in the genus *Hyalomma*. The virus has been classified as a *Nairovirus* in the genus *Bunyavirus*. (The *Nairovirus* group includes the Hazara virus isolated from ticks in Pakistan, and to Nairobi sheep disease virus.) In Africa, the virus has been isolated from a variety of animals, including cattle, sheep, goats, hares, and hedgehogs and from a number of ticks found on these animals. More and more cases have been reported among medical and nursing staffs caring for patients in hospitals and in lab personnel studying these patients. In these cases, the infection was apparently acquired by contact with the patient's blood or blood-contaminated specimens. Exposure to the blood of infected animals (especially cattle and sheep) has led to severe, often fatal, infections.

Antibodies to the disease have been widely found in farm workers, cattle, sheep, and small mammals in southern Africa without evidence of disease.

Symptoms and Diagnostic Path

Within two to seven days after exposure, the onset of illness begins suddenly with fever, chills, severe muscular pains, headache, and vomiting. Between the third and fifth day of the infection, a red rash or hemorrhages in the skin appear, and blood pours from all body orifices. At this stage, the face is flushed and the tongue is dry and often coated with dried blood. As blood loss continues, the pulse starts to race and blood pressure drops. This is followed by signs of shock and collapse, with massive hemorrhage and cardiac arrest. In fatal cases, death usually occurs between seven and nine days after onset.

The diagnosis may be confirmed in the lab by a variety of methods for testing the blood for presence of the virus and its antibodies.

Treatment Options and Outlook

There is no cure. The antiviral drug ribavirin seems to be effective.

Among patients who recover, the fever falls between 10 and 20 days after infection begins and bleeding stops. However, recovery may take more than a month in these cases.

Risk Factors and Preventive Measures

Although an inactivated vaccine has been developed and used on a small scale in eastern Europe, there is no safe and effective vaccine widely available for human use. People who live in endemic areas should avoid tick-infested areas and use repellents. Those who work with animals in endemic areas should use repellents on the skin (DEET) and clothing (permethrin) and protect skin from contacting infected tissue or blood. Hospitalized patients with suspected or confirmed CCHF should be isolated.

conjunctivitis The medical name for "pink eye," an inflammation of the transparent membrane covering the white of the eye and the lining of the eyelid. This common infection of childhood, also referred to as a "cold in the eye," causes redness, discomfort, and a discharge from the eye.

Most conjunctivitis is caused by bacteria (staphylococci) spread by hand-to-eye contact or by viruses associated with a cold, sore throat, or illness such as measles. Viral conjunctivitis can spread like wildfire through schools and other group settings.

Newborns sometimes contract a type of conjunctivitis called neonatal ophthalmia, caused by infection in the mother's cervix during birth from either GONORRHEA, genital HERPES, or chlamydia (see CHLAMYDIA TRACHOMATIS INFECTION). The infection may spread to the entire eye and cause blindness.

Symptoms and Diagnostic Path

All types of conjunctivitis lead to redness, itchy, scratchy, or painful feelings; discharge; and photophobia (discomfort from bright lights). There may be so much discharge that the eyelids stick together in the morning.

Treatment Options and Outlook

Antibiotic eye drops or ointments are given if a bacterial infection is suspected; however, this will not cure a viral infection. Warm water may wash away the discharge and remove crusts; in babies, the eye may be washed with sterile saline. In addition to eye drops, the discharge must be cleaned from the eyes (on an hourly basis for the first day).

A doctor should be called immediately if any of these symptoms appear: swollen red eyelids, blurry vision, severe headache, fever higher than 101°F, or a very painful eye. A doctor should be seen within 24 hours for any of the following symptoms: no improvement after drops or ointment, eye pain, decreased vision, or eyes that get more red or *itchy* after drops or ointment (which may be an allergic reaction).

Risk Factors and Preventive Measures

Careful hand washing may prevent conjunctivitis, since the disease is spread from hand-to-eye very easily. Anyone with the disease should have separate washcloths and towels. It is also important that swimming pools and hot tubs be properly chlorinated. Children with conjunctivitis should be kept at home until 24 hours after antibiotics have been taken or until the eye is better.

contagious disease   Any COMMUNICABLE DISEASE. (Previously, the term referred to any disease transmitted by direct physical contact.) The contagious diseases include ACTINOMYCOSIS, AMEBIASIS, CANDIDIASIS, CHICKEN POX, CHOLERA, COLDS, CONJUNCTIVITIS, DIPHTHERIA, GASTROENTERITIS, GIARDIASIS, HEPATITIS, HERPES, INFLUENZA, MENINGITIS, MONONUCLEOSIS, MUMPS, PARATYPHOID FEVER, PEDICULOSIS, PNEUMONIA, RINGWORM, ROUNDWORM infection, RUBELLA, SHIGELLOSIS, STREP THROAT, SYPHILIS, TUBERCULOSIS, TYPHOID FEVER, and WHOOPING COUGH.

coronavirus   Any one of a family of viruses that includes several types capable of causing respiratory illness and the common cold, especially during the winter and spring. Coronaviruses rarely cause fatal illness in humans. Named for their appearance, which includes a sort of thorny crown when visualized under an electron microscope, they are among the most common of the cold viruses.

It takes only about three days after exposure to these viruses for symptoms to appear, and they last up to about a week (a few days shorter than is typ-

ical for a cold caused by a RHINOVIRUS). However, the coronavirus tends to cause more nasal congestion and is capable of reinfecting the same person.

See also COLD, COMMON.

corticosteroid drugs   An extremely important group of drugs, commonly called steroids, that are similar to the natural corticosteroid hormones produced by the adrenal glands. These drugs, which are used to fight a variety of inflammatory conditions, include beclomethasone, betamethasone, cortisone, dexamethasone, hydrocortisone, prednisolone, and prednisone.

Side Effects

The severity of effects depends on the dose, the form of the drug, and the length of treatment. The effect of the steroids is to prepare the body for stress; they do this by increasing blood pressure, blocking histamine release, increasing sugar in the bloodstream, reducing the body's response to infection or inflammation, boosting appetite, and storing more fat. Short-term use of steroids, therefore, can produce beneficial "side effects," especially by decreasing inflammation (such as in the case of the asthmatic who stops wheezing).

Long-term treatment, which is often necessary in certain diseases, can cause high blood pressure, obesity, diabetes, and soft bones. High-dose steroid use can cause acute psychosis, which stops when the medication is discontinued.

Corynebacterium diphtheriae   A bacterium that causes DIPHTHERIA, found in the mouth, throat, and nose of an infected individual. The bacteria are easily transmitted to others during coughing or sneezing or through close contact with discharge from nose, throat, skin, eyes, and lesions.

Diphtheria is usually a disease of the throat that mimics STREP THROAT (although diphtheria may be more severe), characterized by a dense white membrane over the tonsils and the back of the throat.

In the United States, diphtheria is uncommon because of childhood immunizations. The immunity of adults is kept current by the practice of giving diphtheria vaccine whenever a tetanus booster is given.

cowpox   An infection that usually affects cows caused by the VACCINIA virus. In the past, an attack of cowpox in humans conferred immunity against SMALLPOX, since the two viruses were so similar. In fact, this was the basis for the smallpox vaccination. Vaccinia virus (for which the term *vaccine* was named) continued to be used as a smallpox vaccine until smallpox was eradicated in the 1970s.

See also MONKEYPOX.

Coxiella burnetti   Another name for *Rickettsia burnetti*, the organism that causes Q FEVER.

Coxsackie virus   Any of 30 different viruses associated with a variety of symptoms that primarily affect children during warm weather. The germ resembles the polio virus (especially in size). Named for the city in New York where it was discovered, the viruses are members of the digestive tract–dwelling enterovirus family, which includes ECHOVIRUSES, POLIOMYELITIS, and HEPATITIS A viruses. Coxsackie viruses can spread from person to person, usually via unwashed hands or feces, where they can live for several days.

Coxsackie viruses are separated into group A and group B viruses, with group B leading to more serious infections. These viruses infect primarily through the gastrointestinal tract, although they may also infect via the respiratory tract such as mucus droplets, especially when droplets come from people with TONSILLITIS, PHARYNGITIS, or PNEUMONIA.

There are many viral types or strains identified by antibody testing or viral cultures, neither of which are often performed. These different strains may cause all manner of different symptoms. The following types of Coxsackie virus are associated with specific clinical diseases:

- Coxsackie virus A16 and enterovirus 71 with HAND, FOOT, AND MOUTH DISEASE
- Coxsackie virus A24 and enterovirus 70 with eye infections
- Coxsackie viruses B1–B5 with heart infections

Because these viruses spread chiefly by contact with feces scrupulous handwashing is always the best defense against spread of these infections.

Symptoms and Diagnostic Path

About half of all patients experience no symptoms. Those who do may first notice an abrupt fever between 101 to 104°F, headache, muscle aches, mild sore throat, stomach pain, or nausea. Typically, the fever continues for about three days and then disappears; others experience a fever that waxes and wanes. In addition to the fever, coxsackie viruses can cause several different patterns of symptoms that affect different body parts.

It may cause hand, foot, and mouth disease, characterized by painful red blisters in the throat and on the tongue, gums, inside of the cheeks, and the palms of the hands and soles of the feet. The virus also may cause HERPANGINA, a throat infection with red blisters and ulcers on the tonsils, soft palate, and the roof of the mouth.

A related coxsackie virus is pleurodynia, which causes painful chest and upper abdomen spasms. Boys with pleurodynia may also have pain in the testicles about two weeks after the chest pain begins. A coxsackie virus infection in the whites of the eyes is called hemorrhagic conjunctivitis, which usually begins with pain suddenly followed by red, watery eyes, swelling, light sensitivity, and blurry vision.

Coxsackie viruses also cause an infection of the heart muscle (MYOCARDITIS) or MENINGITIS, an infection of the lining of the brain and spinal cord. Rarely, it may cause a more serious brain infection called ENCEPHALITIS.

Newborns (infected by their mothers during or shortly after birth) are at higher risk of a serious infection. These infants typically develop symptoms within two weeks of birth, experiencing fever, poor feeding, irritability, and lethargy. Infants with Coxsackie-related heart infections have trouble breathing and sometimes develop a bluish color of the skin, lips, and nails caused by too little oxygen in the blood.

Coxsackie virus is diagnosed from a physical exam and the appearance of telltale symptoms, such as rash or blisters. Stool or fluids from the back of the throat can be tested to detect the virus.

Treatment Options and Outlook

Treatment may differ depending on the type of infection and symptoms, but most children with a simple Coxsackie infection recover completely after a few days. Acetaminophen may ease any minor aches and pains. An antiviral medication may be given for Coxsackie meningitis. The rarest forms of Coxsackie virus infection (heart infection and encephalitis) can be fatal, especially in newborns.

crabs   The popular term for pediculosis pubis, or lice in the pubic hair. The pubic louse may also be found in eyebrows, beards, eyelashes, chest hairs, and armpits, but it is not found in hair on the head.

While the scientific name for the pubic louse is *Phthirius pubis,* it gets its common name from its crablike appearance; it even has tiny pincer claws that it uses to hang onto the hairs. The pubic louse is a cousin of the body louse and the head louse and infects only humans.

Pubic lice do not live more than a few days away from humans, which makes reinfestation less likely.

Crabs are caught through close body contact with an infected person (usually a sex partner) although it is possible to catch lice by sharing a bed, clothing, or towels with someone who has lice. Pubic lice are more common among those who live in crowded places with poor laundry facilities.

The pubic louse lays tiny round eggs (called nits) that hatch in about a week; eight to 10 days after that, the louse matures. Once it is attached to the hair, the louse hangs upside down and bores into the skin to feed on the blood vessels close to the skin's surface.

Symptoms and Diagnostic Path

Severe itching begins in the pubic area about a week after exposure to lice. Nits can be seen attached to the base of the pubic hairs; the lice leave a bluish stain on the skin on the upper thigh. In particularly bad infestations, there may be swelling of the lymph glands in the groin. The longer the infestation has been going on, the more lice there will be and the worse the itching.

Inspection of the pubic area will reveal nits. Tests are not necessary.

Treatment Options and Outlook

Pubic lice are eliminated the same way as other types of lice, using permethrin 1 percent or pyrethrins available without prescription; over-the-counter shampoos are available with RID. Lindane 1 percent is no longer considered to be the treatment of choice because of concerns about side effects.

After treatment, all visible nits should be removed with a nit comb. The patient should be checked daily for the first week after treatment to make sure all nits are gone. If itch remains after seven days, another treatment is needed. Close physical contact (including sex) should be avoided until the treatment is complete. Nits in eyebrows or eyelashes should not be treated (they are too close to the eyes); instead, nits in these areas should be removed with tweezers. All bedding, towels, and clothing should be washed in hot sudsy water, then dried in the dryer for 20 minutes on high. Anything that cannot be washed should be left isolated for three to four days, since lice can't survive long without a human host.

Risk Factors and Preventive Measures

All sex partners and roommates should be treated, since lice can be passed on to others as long as there are live, unhatched nits attached to the pubic hairs. Vigilant checks for nits should continue for one week.

Creutzfeldt-Jakob disease   A rare, fatal brain disease that causes memory impairment, behavior change and ultimately, dementia that strikes about 250 Americans each year. The three varieties of this brain-wasting disease (acquired, sporadic, and hereditary) are caused by a PRION: a misshapen protein that alters the shape of other proteins, causing cavities in the brain.

Acquired CJD includes variant CJD linked directly to eating meat from cattle infected with BOVINE SPONGIFORM ENCEPHALOPATHY (mad cow disease). At least 80 people in Europe have died of vCJD since the mid-1990s. Mad cow disease destroys an animal's brain, causing infected animals to act in bizarre ways. It was first diagnosed in Britain where about 177,000 cattle were infected.

Cases also have been reported in France, Italy, Germany, and Spain. It is estimated that about a million pounds of contaminated cattle may have entered the human food chain, and experts estimate this could result in up to 136,000 cases of vCJD in humans. Because of its long incubation period, it may be years before the toll of vCJD can be determined. VCJD is actually much rarer than classic CJD, and there have been no identified cases of vCJD in the United States.

Sporadic CJD accounts for at least 85 percent of all CJD, and occurs in the United States but is not linked to eating meat. This form of the disease occurs in patients who have no known risk for the disease.

Hereditary CJD occurs in people with a family history for the condition and who test positive for the genetic mutation in their prions. This version of the condition accounts for between 10 percent and 15 percent of all cases.

Symptoms and Diagnostic Path

All three forms of the disease are considered infectious but not contagious—it is not possible to get the condition in casual contact such as hugging, kissing, or sexual intercourse. The first symptoms involve a sudden, progressive memory loss, with insomnia, personality changes, bizarre behavior, visual distortions, hallucinations, and thinking problems. Patients soon lose the ability to communicate and lapse into a coma.

Doctors use a series of tests (including a very specific pattern on brain scans) to diagnose the condition, but the diagnosis cannot be confirmed beyond doubt until autopsy.

Treatment Options and Outlook

There is no cure for CJD. Current treatment alleviates symptoms and makes the patient as comfortable as possible. Painkillers can ease discomfort, and clonazepam and sodium valproate may help relieve involuntary muscle jerks.

About 90 percent of patients die within one year of diagnosis.

croup A group of conditions involving inflammation of the upper airway that causes a barking cough. Once very common in children up to age four, croup is a frightening but not terribly serious illness. In older children and adults, the air passages are too wide and the cartilage in the air passages too stiff for swelling or inflammation to cause the walls to collapse.

One bout of croup does not confer immunity, and some children get several attacks. However, most cases are mild and children recover uneventfully. Children outgrow the tendency toward croup.

Croup is caused by one of several different types of viral infections (often a cold) that affect the larynx, windpipe, and airways into the lungs. The most common is PARAINFLUENZA VIRUS (which usually occurs in late fall). RESPIRATORY SYNCYTIAL VIRUS (RSV) and INFLUENZA may appear in winter and early spring. ADENOVIRUSES, RHINOVIRUS, and sometimes MEASLES may lead to croup. While croup cannot be passed on to anyone else, it is possible to catch a virus that can cause croup.

Some babies appear to be more likely to get croup than others, possibly because of a sensitive larynx; premature infants may also be prone to croup. Twice as many boys get croup as girls; some infants never get it, and others get it every time they have a cold.

Symptoms and Diagnostic Path

Croup begins like a cold. About one to seven days later, fever, cough, and breathing problems often appear at night. The child may awaken with the characteristic barking cough, with shallow, fast, and noisy breathing. The high-pitched sounds occur during inhaling, not exhaling.

The child may feel better during the day but suffer the barking cough during the night for three or four nights.

A doctor can diagnose croup from the symptoms; tests are not needed, although a neck X-ray may be used to rule out foreign bodies or obstructions.

Treatment Options and Outlook

Cool mist vaporizers or cool night air help a child to breathe; the child should be kept upright while breathing in the cool air. Steam from a shower will work if no vaporizer is available.

A doctor should be called if the coughing does not get better or if the illness is severe (fever above

101°F or severe breathing problems). For serious cases, doctors may check oxygen levels in the blood and provide oxygen together with epinephrine or corticosteroids. A tube may be inserted down the throat or through the throat (tracheostomy). The infant may be placed in a croup or mist tent, but such a tent should not be constructed at home.

Croup that enters the windpipe and small airways leading into the lungs is called acute tracheobronchitis, a more serious condition that can interfere with breathing and may require hospitalization.

EPIGLOTTITIS is a rare (but dangerous) condition that may be confused with croup. Epiglottitis is caused by a sudden bacterial infection of the epiglottitis that causes so much swelling in the upper throat that the child's airway is blocked. A doctor should be called if there are any of these warning signs of epiglottitis:

- fever higher than 103°F
- drooling with open mouth
- agitation, restlessness, flaring nostrils
- bluish lips, skin, or nail beds
- muffled speech
- rapid, difficult breathing
- respiratory noise
- failure to breathe
- movement in and out in the areas between the ribs during breath
- severe sore throat
- refusal to swallow

Risk Factors and Preventive Measures

If the child has a tendency toward developing croup, to prevent the disease from occurring parents should:

- keep a cool-mist vaporizer in the room during sleep
- not smoke in the house
- give clear fluids to a baby with a cold

cryptococcosis A rare fungal infection caused by inhaling *Cryptococcus neoformans*, a type of fungus found throughout the world, especially in soil con-taminated with pigeon droppings. Untreated, this infection may be progressive and ultimately fatal. The disease is also known as Buschke's disease or European blastomycosis.

Although the infection usually affects adults, it can occur at any age. In North America, it is most likely to be found among those already ill with cancer (such as leukemia or lymphoma) or those with impaired immune systems, such as patients with AIDS. Infection with this fungus is unusual in patients who are otherwise healthy.

Symptoms and Diagnostic Path

Cryptococcosis is characterized by the development of fever and other symptoms depending on the specific organ involved. Because the lungs are the first site of infection, initial symptoms may include coughing. The fungus spreads from the lungs to the central nervous system, skin, skeletal system, and urinary tract. After the fungus spreads to the meninges, neurologic symptoms may develop, including headache, blurred vision, and difficulty in speaking.

While MENINGITIS is the more usual and serious form of the disease, it can also cause a range of granular lesions, including ULCERS, ABSCESSES, tumors, papules, nodules, and draining sinuses into the skin, lungs, and so on.

The diagnosis is made by isolating and identifying the fungus in specimens of sputum, pus, spinal fluid, or tissue biopsy.

Treatment Options and Outlook

Fluconazole freely passes into the central nervous system and is the drug of choice; intravenous amphotericin B and oral flucytosine also may be helpful.

Cryptococcus A genus of yeasty fungus that reproduce by budding instead of by producing spores. Many harmless types of this fungus are found in soil, on the skin, and in the mucous membranes of healthy humans. However, there are a few disease-causing species, including *C. neoformans*, the cause of CRYPTOCOCCOSIS.

cryptosporidiosis A diarrheal disease caused by a protozoan *CRYPTOSPORIDIUM*, which means "hidden spore" in Greek. The tiny invisible microbe infects cells lining the intestinal tract. First identified as a cause of human disease in 1976, it is a major threat to the water supply of the United States.

Since the 1980s, "Crypto" has become one of the most common waterborne diseases in the United States. It is found in every region of the United States.

This parasite lives its entire life within the intestinal cells; it produces worms (oocysts) that are excreted in feces. These infectious oocysts can survive outside the human body for long periods of time, passing into food and drinking water, onto objects, and spread from hand to mouth. Chlorine does not kill the protozoan; instead, drinking water must be filtered to eliminate it. Many municipal water supplies do not have the technology to provide this filter.

Because the parasite is transmitted by the fecal-oral route, the greatest risk occurs in those infected people who have diarrhea, those with poor personal hygiene, and diapered children.

Cryptosporidium is found in soil, food, water, or surfaces that have been contaminated with infected human or animal feces. A person becomes infected by sallowing something that has come in contact with these feces or by swallowing contaminated water in a lake, hot tub, river, pond, or pool. *Cryptosporidium* can survive for long periods of time, even in properly chlorinated swimming pools. A person also can be infected by eating uncooked food contaminated with *Cryptosporidium*.

It is not possible to become infected by contact with blood.

Symptoms and Diagnostic Path

Between one to 12 days after infection, the most common symptom is a watery diarrhea together with stomach cramps, nausea and vomiting, fever, headache, and loss of appetite. Some people with the infection do not experience any symptoms at all.

Healthy patients usually exhibit symptoms for about two weeks, but those with impaired immune systems may have a severe and lasting illness.

The infection is diagnosed by identifying the parasite during examination of the stool. If cryptosporidiosis is suspected, a specific lab test should be requested, since most labs do not yet routinely perform the necessary tests.

Treatment Options and Outlook

A new drug (nitazoxanide) has been approved for treatment of diarrhea caused by *Cryptosporidium* in otherwise healthy people. Most people who have a healthy immune system will recover without any treatment. Patients with diarrhea should drink plenty of fluids to prevent dehydration. Fluid replacement is especially important for infants, for whom rapid loss of fluids from diarrhea may be especially dangerous. Antidiarrheal medicine may ease diarrhea.

People who are in poor health or who have impaired immune systems are at higher risk for more severe illness. The effectiveness of nitazoxanide in patients with lowered immunity is unclear. Patients with AIDS may find that antiretroviral therapy designed to boost immunity also eases symptoms of Crypto. However, in these patients cryptosporidiosis is usually not curable, and the symptoms may return if the immune system weakens.

Risk Factors and Preventive Measures

Eradication of the organism from drinking water depends on adequate filtration, not chlorination. Scientists are studying new ways to protect water supplies, including reverse osmosis, membrane filtration, or radiation.

Because patients with Crypto are highly contagious, they must be careful to avoid spreading the disease to others. Patients should be careful to wash their hands with soap and water after using the toilet, changing diapers, and before eating or cooking. People with Crypto should not swim in pools, hot tubs, lakes or rivers, or the ocean for at least two weeks after their diarrhea ends. It is still possible to transmit *Cryptosporidium* in stool and contaminate water for several weeks after symptoms end.

Individuals can avoid becoming infected by not swallowing water in which people are swimming. They also should avoid drinking untreated water from shallow wells, lakes, rivers, springs, ponds, and streams; avoid drinking untreated municipal water during community-wide outbreaks of disease; avoid using untreated ice or drinking water when traveling in foreign countries.

Individuals who cannot avoid using potentially contaminated water can make the water safe to drink by either heating the water to a rolling boil for at least one minute or using a filter with an absolute pore size of at least one micron (or one that has been rated for cyst removal). Consumers should not rely on chemicals to disinfect water and kill *Cryptosporidium*. Its thick outer shell makes this parasite very resistant to disinfectants such as chlorine and iodine. Consumers also should avoid potentially contaminated food by washing or peeling all raw vegetables and fruits; using safe, uncontaminated water to wash all foods to be eaten raw; and avoiding uncooked foods when traveling in countries with poor sanitation.

See also ANTIDIARRHEAL DRUGS; DIARRHEA AND INFECTIOUS DISEASE; TRAVELER'S DIARRHEA.

Cryptosporidium A type of parasite that causes the waterborne infection CRYPTOSPORIDIOSIS. This organism is about 1/60 the size of an average dust particle and has been found in up to 87 percent of surface water samples across the United States.

The egg-like form of the organism, called an oocyst, is passed into the feces of infectious animals, eventually finding its way into water supplies, where it can then enter human intestines. Once in the intestine, an oocyst releases an infective spore that begins another reproductive cycle.

A healthy infected human will experience watery diarrhea and cramps that pass in about a week, but those with impaired immune systems may have a much more serious (or fatal) case.

Boiling water for one minute is the only way to kill this parasite, since it can live in chlorinated water. (Consumers who live above 6,562 feet should boil water for three minutes.)

cutaneous larva migrans Also known as creeping eruption, this disease is caused by HOOKWORM larvae that normally parasitize dogs, cats, or other animals. It occurs in southeastern and Gulf states.

Hookworm infestation occurs whenever human skin touches soil contaminated with cat or dog feces; shaded, moist, and sandy areas—such as beaches, children's sandboxes, and areas underneath houses—are the most likely spots to find larvae. Eggs passed in the feces hatch into infective larvae that can penetrate human skin (even through beach towels). The larvae penetrate the skin of the feet and move randomly, leaving intensely itchy red lines (sometimes accompanied by blisters).

Because several different parasites produce similar symptoms, there may be confusion about the diseases included under the umbrella of "cutaneous larva migrans." It usually refers to disorders caused by cat or dog hookworm larvae.

Symptoms and Diagnostic Path

Skin lesions usually appear in areas that often contact soil, such as feet, hands, and buttocks, appearing like a red papule a few hours after the larvae penetrates the skin. After a latency period of a few days to a few months, the larvae migrate, causing a red, raised, intensely itchy red line that may loop and meander all over the skin. Bacterial infection from scratching may occur. About half of the larvae die within three months even without treatment.

Treatment Options and Outlook

Thiabendazole can be administered on the skin over the tracks, and to normal-appearing skin around the lesions (because there may be larvae outside the visible lines).

Older methods of treatment, such as freezing the track with carbon dioxide or liquid nitrogen, is unreliable and painful.

Thiabendazole taken internally is effective but associated with a high probability of side effects such as dizziness, nausea, and vomiting.

Cyclospora cayetanensis A parasitic microbe that infects the intestine and causes intense diarrhea, weight loss, and fatigue. The United States is currently battling its fourth epidemic of cyclospora, which began in the spring of 1996.

The first outbreak in the United States was first identified in 1979. Before 1996 only three outbreaks in the U.S. were reported; by June 1997 there were 21 clusters of cases from eight states. This was followed by reports of outbreaks in Morocco, Peru, and New Guinea.

Cyclospora is spread by people swallowing water or food contaminated with infected stool. For example, outbreaks of cyclosporiasis have been linked to various types of fresh produce. Because

Cyclospora does not become infectious until days or weeks after being passed in a bowel movement, it is not likely that it can be passed directly from one person to another. Experts do not know whether animals can be infected and pass infection to humans.

The organism is a distant cousin of CRYPTOSPORIDIUM, the protozoan that infiltrated a Milwaukee water supply in 1993 and caused an epidemic of stomach problems and 40 deaths, but this new organism is twice as large. Because the organism is a parasite of the small bowel, patients continue to lose weight even after the diarrhea stops because they cannot absorb nutrients.

The organism does not appear to be halted by iodine or chlorine and can even elude filtration systems. The only thing that kills it is boiling the water in which it lives.

Symptoms and Diagnostic Path

About a week after ingestion, the disease begins with severe diarrhea, stomach cramps, nausea, and vomiting. It then progresses to weeks of mild fever, debilitating fatigue, and loss of appetite; patients can lose 15 to 20 pounds. While the disease is not normally fatal, some patients have been hospitalized because of dehydration.

Cyclospora is diagnosed by inspecting several stool specimens over several days. Identification of this parasite in stool requires special lab tests that are not routinely performed, so they must be specifically requested. Typically, stool also will be checked for other organisms that can cause similar symptoms.

Treatment Options and Outlook

The antibiotic combination of sulfa and trimethoprim (Bactrim, Septra, or Cotrim) can shorten the term of the illness, although most other diarrhea-causing organisms are now resistant to the drugs. Those with impaired immune systems require higher doses and longer therapy.

Risk Factors and Preventive Measures

Scientists advise those in epidemic areas not to eat strawberries or raspberries, especially for those with impaired immune systems. All fruit and vegetables should be thoroughly washed before eating.

cysticerosis   See TAPEWORM.

cytomegalovirus infection (CMV)   A disease caused by cytomegalovirus, one of the HERPES family of viruses. The CMV is the largest, most complex virus that infects humans. First discovered in 1956, this extremely common infection has affected almost all children, yet rarely produces symptoms. By adulthood, up to 85 percent of Americans have been infected.

While not usually a serious disease, those with impaired immunity may have more severe symptoms. Cytomegalovirus also may cause significant problems during pregnancy if a woman has an acute infection, which would be transmitted to her unborn child. This can lead to minor impairments affecting hearing, vision, or mental capacity; a few of these babies are born with severe brain damage, including mental retardation or severe hearing loss.

Once a person has been infected, the virus remains latent in the body like other herpes viruses and can be reactivated later on during periods of stress or weakened immunity.

CMV is present in almost all body fluids, including urine, saliva, semen, breast milk, and blood. It can be sexually transmitted, although most people don't get it this way. It is commonly found in day care centers, where it is passed around in children's saliva or urine-soaked diapers and transmitted from unwashed hands or shared toys.

Women with toddlers in day care are often infected, since CMV transmission occurs often in these institutions. While young children rarely have symptoms, they excrete the virus in their urine and saliva for months to years. Anyone who works with young children is exposed to CMV. It is also possible to acquire CMV from transfused blood or transplanted organs, since so many individuals have an infection without having symptoms.

A person having an organ transplant or chemotherapy for cancer takes drugs that suppress the immune system; if such a patient had been infected with CMV earlier in life, the dormant virus can reactivate, resulting in life-threatening illness. If a patient taking these drugs has a first exposure to the virus, the new infection can cause a serious illness. In AIDS patients, reactivation of a CMV infection can

lead to serious eye infections called retinitis, PNEU-
MONIA, HEPATITIS, ENCEPHALITIS, and colitis.

Symptoms and Diagnostic Path

Very few adults (including pregnant women) have
symptoms when infected; if they do, symptoms will
be mild, including achiness, low fever, and sore
throat. Young children may experience a mild cold
or flulike illness with fever.

However, if a woman is first exposed to this virus
early in pregnancy, the resulting infection can cause
serious fetal abnormalities. About 40,000 infants in
the United States are infected each year, but almost
all babies infected before birth are normal. About 10
percent of babies infected before birth are sick with
the symptoms listed above. Of these 10 percent, 20
to 30 percent have a "congenital CMV syndrome"
with serious symptoms that may be fatal. These
symptoms include problems of major organs, including the liver, brain, eyes, and lungs together with
convulsions, lethargy, and breathing problems. If
such a profoundly affected infant survives, there
may be permanent damage (mental retardation,
water on the brain, small brain, hearing loss, eye
inflammation, poor coordination, and liver disease).

Some studies suggest that a few apparently normal babies who were infected at birth may encounter health problems later in life. Babies infected
before birth excrete the virus intermittently for
years and are infectious when shedding the virus.

While CMV does not usually cause a problem for
healthy people, it can sometimes lead to an acute
illness resembling infectious MONONUCLEOSIS that is
almost identical to the infection associated with
EPSTEIN-BARR VIRUS, including a fever of two to
three weeks, inflamed liver, and sometimes a rash.
Healthy people with CMV mono have an excellent
prognosis.

Test results for CMV can be misleading. Blood
can be tested for the CMV antibody, but all the
presence of antibody indicates is that there was an
earlier infection. The test will not reveal whether
the virus is presently in blood, urine, or saliva. If a
patient has symptoms that imply a recently acquired
infection, sequential tests may reveal changes in
antibody levels that indicate an active infection.
However, since these changes can be hard to distinguish from normal fluctuations, researchers are trying to develop tests that are more specific.

The test for virus in these fluids is available in
most large hospital and commercial labs, but results
may take between two and six weeks.

Newborns with possible congenital CMV infection must have the virus cultured from their
urine, nose, eyes, or spinal fluid to confirm CMV.
This can be helpful in diagnosing potential future
problems such as hearing loss. Researchers are
now refining tests that would measure CMV in
saliva.

In patients with impaired immunity, tests can be
helpful to measure the effectiveness of therapy.

Treatment Options and Outlook

There is no cure for congenital CMV; babies with
the disease need to be hospitalized. In AIDS patients,
treatment includes two intravenous antiviral drugs,
ganciclovir or foscarnet. These drugs are not recommended for those with healthy immune systems
because the side effects from the drugs are more
severe than the risks of the illness.

Risk Factors and Preventive Measures

Good hygiene can reduce the risk of transmission at
day care centers, but intensive infection control is
not practical when dealing with a virus as common
as CMV. Scientists are presently researching a preventive vaccine.

People who need organ transplants are tested for
antibodies to CMV; those who do not have the antibodies will be matched to donors without antibodies as well. Because a match is not always possible,
the recipient faces a risk of serious CMV infection
from the transplanted organ later.

CMV-negative organ recipients who need blood
transfusions will be given special CMV-negative
blood, which is rare and saved for special cases.

There is no vaccine currently available for CMV.
Antibodies from those with high levels of immunity are available in the form of hyperimmune
globulins for certain high-risk patients, but use of
these products is expensive and of limited value.
Researchers studying the feasibility of a CMV vaccine believe that widespread vaccination of children with a safe, effective vaccine is justified to
protect unborn children from birth defects by
reducing the risk that mothers are exposed to
infected children. Researchers are studying a possible recombinant CMV vaccine.

dacryocystitis   Inflammation of the lacrimal sac or tear gland at the corner of the eye, caused by obstruction of the duct. This causes tearing and discharge from the eye.

Symptoms and Diagnostic Path
In the acute phase, the sac becomes inflamed and painful. The disorder almost always occurs only on one side and is usually seen in infants.

Treatment Options and Outlook
Systemic treatment with antibiotics will cure the problem. Occasionally surgery to insert a small plastic tube to hold the duct open is necessary.

deer tick   See TICKS AND DISEASE.

DEET (diethyltoluamide)   A type of insect repellent that can be sprayed on the skin to repel mosquitoes, gnats, and other insects that carry disease. In low concentrations, DEET is generally considered to be nontoxic, but it is not recommended for use on children. While poisoning with DEET is rare, there have been a few cases of toxicity.

Every year, about a third of the U.S. population uses DEET in a variety of liquids, lotions, sprays, and impregnated materials (such as wrist bands). DEET is available in formulations registered for direct application to human skin containing from 4 percent to 100 percent DEET. Except for a few veterinary uses, DEET can be used by consumers.

DEET is designed for direct application to human skin to repel insects. Developed by the U.S. Army in 1946, DEET was registered for use by the general public in 1957. More than 230 products containing DEET are currently registered with the Environmental Protection Agency (EPA).

In 1998, the EPA concluded that as long as consumers follow label directions and take proper precautions, insect repellents containing DEET do not present a health concern. Based on extensive toxicity testing, the EPA decided that normal use of DEET "does not present a health concern" to the general population.

DEET is approved for use on children over two months of age. There is no restriction on the percentage of DEET in any product for use on children, since research did not detect any difference in effects between young animals and adult animals.

defensins   Peptides naturally produced by the immune system to ward off viruses that were first identified more than 20 years ago at UCLA. However, it was unclear how defensins worked. Now UCLA and National Institutes of Health scientists have discovered that a specific defensin called retrocyclin-2 (RC2) binds to carbohydrate-containing proteins in cell membranes. This mechanism erects molecular barricades that block attacking viruses from entering and infecting the cell. RC2 stops the virus in its tracks, preventing it from replicating and spreading throughout the body.

dengue fever   An infectious viral disease with four distinct types, causing severe pain in the joints, fever, and rash. Infection with one of the four types does not provide immunity against the others, so a person living in a dengue-endemic area could have four separate dengue infections.

Dengue is primarily a disease of the tropics; it is endemic in 100 countries throughout the Americas, southeast Asia, the western Pacific islands, Africa, and eastern Mediterranean. The viruses that cause it are maintained in a cycle that involves humans and *AEDES aegypti,* a mosquito that prefers to feed on humans during the day. Infection with dengue viruses produces a spectrum of clinical illness ranging from a nonspecific viral syndrome to fatal DENGUE HEMORRHAGIC FEVER.

The first reported epidemics of dengue fever occurred in 1779–80 in Asia, Africa, and North America; the near-simultaneous occurrence of outbreaks on three continents indicates that these viruses and the mosquitoes that carry them have existed in the tropics for more than 200 years. During most of this time, dengue fever was considered a benign, nonfatal disease of visitors to the tropics. There were usually long intervals (between 10 and 40 years) between major epidemics, mainly because the viruses and the mosquitoes could only be transported between population centers by sailing vessels.

Its name may be a Spanish adaptation of the Swahili *Ki denga pepo* that describes cramps that seize victims like a spirit. Others believe the term is derived from the Spanish word meaning "affectation," referring to the mincing walk adopted by untreated victims suffering from severe joint pain. For the same reason, the English called it "Dandy fever."

Dengue fever is a rapidly spreading disease now found in most tropical areas of the world. After decades of being only a minor nuisance in Latin America, as mosquito control programs shut down over the past 20 years it has become the most widespread arbovirus disease of humans. There are now 2 billion people at risk and millions of new cases each year as epidemics caused by all four types of virus have become larger and progressively more frequent.

A global pandemic of dengue began in Southeast Asia after World War II and has intensified during the last 15 years. Epidemics caused by multiple types are more frequent, the geographic distribution of dengue viruses and their mosquito vectors has expanded. In Southeast Asia, epidemic dengue hemorrhagic fever first appeared in the 1950s, but by 1975 it had become a leading cause of hospitalization and death among children in many countries in that region.

In the 1980s, dengue began a second expansion into Asia when Sri Lanka, India, and the Maldive Islands had their first major epidemics; Pakistan first reported an epidemic of dengue fever in 1994. The recent epidemics in Sri Lanka and India were associated with multiple dengue virus types. After an absence of 35 years, epidemic dengue fever occurred in both Taiwan and the People's Republic of China in the 1980s. Singapore also had a resurgence of dengue from 1990 to 1994 after a successful control program had prevented significant transmission for more than 20 years. In other countries of Asia, the epidemics have become progressively larger in the last 15 years. Despite poor surveillance for dengue in Africa, epidemic dengue fever caused by all four types has increased dramatically since 1980. Most activity has occurred in East Africa, and major epidemics were reported for the first time in the Seychelles (1977), Kenya (1982), Mozambique (1985), Djibouti (1991–92), Somalia (1982, 1993), and Saudi Arabia (1994).

The emergence of dengue as a major public health problem has been most dramatic in the American region. In an effort to prevent urban yellow fever, which is also transmitted by *A. aegypti,* the Pan American Health Organization organized a campaign that eradicated the mosquito from most Central and South American countries in the 1950s and 1960s. As a result, epidemic dengue occurred only sporadically in some Caribbean islands during this period. However, the eradication program, which was officially discontinued in the United States in 1970, gradually eroded elsewhere, and this species began to reinfest countries from which it had been eradicated. In 1997, the geographic distribution of *A. aegypti* was wider than its distribution before the eradication program.

Although the United States has not had any major epidemics of dengue since the 1940s, health authorities fear the disease may appear here at any time. A small number of people have developed dengue from local mosquitoes in Texas in 1980, 1986, and 1995, and both species of mosquitoes that carry the dengue virus are firmly established in several southeastern states. In 1995, an outbreak infecting more than 200,000 people in Latin America and the Caribbean threatened thousands of Americans along the entire southern United States border. That year, Texas recorded almost 50 cases, the highest number in 10 years. Six of the patients got dengue without leaving the country. While scientists cannot predict the future incidence, it is anticipated that there will be increased dengue transmission in all tropical areas of the world during the next several years.

Dengue was called "break-bone fever" by 18th-century doctor Benjamin Rush during a Philadelphia epidemic in 1780, because of the severe bone pain; others called it "breakheart" fever because of the depression that often follows the illness. Through September, 1996, 140,000 cases of classic dengue have been reported in Latin America; dozens have died from hemorrhagic dengue.

During the mid-20th century, mosquito-eradication efforts almost wiped out dengue in much of the Americas. Population growth and urban sprawl, together with lax official policies, led to the return of the mosquito.

Dengue fever is transmitted by urban *Aedes* mosquitoes (usually *A. aegypti*), which can be found across the United States and which prefers to feed on humans during the daytime. The mosquito may bite at any time during the day (especially indoors), in shady areas or when it is overcast. Frost wipes it out in northern areas, but the mosquito survives in many parts of the south, especially along the Gulf of Mexico.

Symptoms and Diagnostic Path

Typically, the virus feels like a bad case of the flu, with sudden fever and severe frontal headaches and deep-muscle aches. There may be nausea and vomiting; the rash appears three to five days after onset of fever and may spread from torso to arms, legs, and face. The rash may be accompanied by itching and scaling. Most cases are mild, treated only with bed rest and fluids.

Health officials are concerned about dengue because people who have suffered a bout with one of the viruses face a potentially life-threatening complication if they later catch any other dengue virus. The danger is dengue hemorrhagic fever, accompanied by a red rash, bruises, and bleeding from gums, nose, and gastrointestinal tract. This bleeding can trigger a loss of blood pressure that can lead to shock; as many as one out of 10 patients who develop the hemorrhagic fever will die.

Treatment Options and Outlook

There is no specific treatment. Painkillers are given to relieve headache and other pain.

Risk Factors and Preventive Measures

The only way to control dengue and DHF is to eliminate the mosquitoes that carry the disease, by applying chemicals and altering the environment. Community-based clean-up campaigns remove tires, bottles, cans, and anything else that retains water to eliminate potential breeding sites. People traveling to dengue- and malaria-infested areas should use insect repellents containing DEET and stay in places with screened windows and mosquito nets for sleeping. Preventive drug therapy for malaria is also a good idea.

No dengue vaccine is available. Research is being conducted to develop dengue vaccine viruses. The CDC believes that an effective dengue vaccine for public use will not be available for five to 10 years.

dengue hemorrhagic fever (DHF) A grave form of DENGUE FEVER characterized by shock, collapse and hemorrhages. The incidence of dengue hemorrhagic fever has increased dramatically in southeast Asia in the past 20 years, with major epidemics occurring in most countries every three to four years. DHF first occurred in the Americas in 1981, with a major epidemic in Cuba. A second major DHF epidemic occurred in Venezuela in 1989–90; smaller outbreaks have occurred in Brazil, Colombia, French Guyana, and Nicaragua.

Although not completely understood, data suggest that the type of virus, together with the patient's age, immune status, and genetic background are the most important factors for developing DHF. In Asia, children under the age of 15 who are experiencing a second dengue infection appear to have the highest risk. Although adults can also develop DHF, most international travelers from the United States appear to be at low risk.

Symptoms and Diagnostic Path

Cold, clammy extremities; weak, thready pulse; respiratory distress; plus all the symptoms of dengue fever. Hemorrhage, bruises, and small red spots all indicate bleeding from skin capillaries; bloody vomitus, urine, and feces may occur and herald impending circulatory collapse.

Treatment Options and Outlook

Fluid and electrolyte replacement and fresh blood, plasma, or platelet transfusions. Oxygen and sedatives also may be given.

dermatophytes   Superficial fungi (also called tineal infections, including RINGWORM) that infect the skin, hair, and nails, usually caused by the fungi *Microsporum, Epidermophyton*, and *Trichophyton*. This type of fungi can be spread from person to person or from an animal to a person. The infections they cause usually have a Latin name using the term *tinea* with the part of the body affected (such as tinea pedis for ATHLETE'S FOOT). Although there are many different kinds of dermatophytes, seven species cause more than 90 percent of all infections.

dermatophytosis   See RINGWORM.

desert fever   A popular name for COCCIDIOIDO-MYCOSIS.

desert rheumatism   A popular name for COCCIDI-OIDOMYCOSIS.

diarrhea, viral   See GASTROENTERITIS, VIRAL.

diarrhea and infectious disease   Many infectious diseases cause diarrhea, with frequent passage of loose, watery stools that also may contain pus, mucus, blood, or fat. In addition to frequent trips to the bathroom, a patient with diarrhea may complain of abdominal cramps and weakness, nausea, and vomiting.

Acute diarrhea affects almost everyone at some time, usually from eating contaminated food or drinking contaminated water. Diarrhea is not a disease in itself, but a symptom. While it may not seem to be a serious problem, if it remains untreated severe diarrhea can lead to dehydration and electrolyte imbalance. This is a particular concern among the very young and the very old.

Symptoms and Diagnostic Path

Diarrhea usually starts suddenly and lasts between a few hours to two or three days. Diarrhea beginning within six hours of eating usually indicates that the food has been contaminated by bacteria such as *Staphylococcus,* CLOSTRIDIUM, or *E. coli.* If it takes longer (between 12 to 48 hours after eating), the diarrhea is probably from contamination of food or water by bacteria such as *CAMPYLOBACTER* or *SALMO-NELLA* or by a virus such as ROTAVIRUS or NORWALK VIRUS. Infective GASTROENTERITIS may be caused by inhaling droplets filled with ADENOVIRUS or ECHOVI-RUS. Less often, infectious diarrhea may be related to SHIGELLOSIS, TYPHOID, or amebic DYSENTERY.

Treatment Options and Outlook

During a severe attack, water and electrolytes must be replaced to prevent dehydration. Drinking water with sugar and salt added is one way to do this (one teaspoon salt and four teaspoons sugar dissolved in one quart of water). ANTIDIARRHEAL DRUGS should not be taken to treat diarrhea caused by infection, since they may in fact prolong the illness.

See also CHOLERA; CRYPTOSPORIDIOSIS; ENTEROVI-RUS; *ESCHERICHIA COLI; ESCHERICHIA COLI* O157:H7; MARBURG VIRUS.

diphtheria   A preventable bacterial disease that affects the tonsils, throat, nose, or skin, and that was once feared throughout the world. Through the 1920s, diphtheria killed 13,000 babies and children in the United States each year and sickened another 150,000. Today it is most common among the impoverished and in crowded conditions. Unimmunized children under age 15 are most likely to contract the disease.

The conquest of diphtheria is one of the greatest vaccination success stories in modern times. Only one case was reported in the United States in 1998 and 1999.

Although diphtheria is rare in the United States, the bacteria still circulate in parts of the country. In 1996, for example, 10 isolates of the bacteria were obtained in an American Indian community in South Dakota, although no one developed the disease. From 1980 through 2002, 54 cases of diphtheria were reported in the United States, averaging between two and three a year. No cases were reported in 1986, 1993, and 1995. Only one case was reported each year in 1984, 1998, 1999, 2000, and 2002. This does not mean that the disease has been eliminated, however.

Because so many Russian children did not get vaccines, a serious outbreak began in Moscow in 1990; by 1992, there were 4,000 cases in the Russian federation and 24 deaths in Moscow. The problem has gotten worse since then, spreading throughout Russia with 50,000 recorded cases and 1,100 deaths in 1994. Most of the patients are adults, but the outbreak has spread because many children had not been receiving their vaccines and adults who had been vaccinated were no longer immune. Today, the epidemic is most severe in cities on the Sea of Japan north of North Korea, where an immunization campaign has been going on at airports, hotels, and train stations.

Travelers to these areas must have completed a series of the vaccine and must have had a booster within the last five years. There is no risk if the traveler is fully immunized.

In the United States, confirmed cases of diphtheria must be reported to, and investigated by, the local and state health departments.

Since the time of Hippocrates, periodic outbreaks of diphtheria occurred around the world, becoming more common during the 16th century. Italian physicians began to perform tracheotomies during the Naples epidemic of 1610 in an attempt to help patients breathe despite the terrible swollen throat that is characteristic of the disease.

Some 50 years later, New England minister Cotton Mather described a disease he called "Malady of Bladders in the Windpipe," which was particularly deadly among Massachusetts children. A second epidemic began in New Hampshire in 1735, killing more than 1,000 citizens, most of them children. The Spanish called it *garrotillo*, after the executioner's garrotte, a string around the neck that could be tightened by twisting a stick.

The disease got its modern name during the French epidemic of 1826, when French physician Pierre-Fidèle Bretonneau called it after the Greek word for leather, *dipthera*, a reference to the tough gray membrane that often formed across the back of the throat.

As the disease spread during the 19th century, it appeared to grow stronger and more deadly; fatalities in New York skyrocketed to more than 2,300 in 1872. The bacterium that caused the disease was identified in 1883, and seven years later scientists determined that a poison produced by the bacterium (an exotoxin) could be used in weakened form to trigger an immune response in humans. This "antitoxin" was similar to tetanus, which scientists were beginning to understand at about the same time. Routine immunizations began in the 1920s.

Diphtheria is caused by a bacterium (*Corynebacterium diphtheriae*) named for the Greek word *koryne*, meaning "club-shaped." The bacteria thrive in dark, wet places such as the mouth, throat, and nose of an infected individual. They are easily transmitted to others during coughing or sneezing, or through close contact with discharge from nose, throat, skin, eyes, and lesions. Bacteria do not travel very far through the air, and they infect only humans. Crowded, unhealthy places help the germs spread from one person to another.

The infection also can be spread by carriers (those with the bacteria who have no symptoms). Untreated patients who are infected can be contagious for up to two weeks, but not usually more than a month. Recovery from the disease does not always confer immunity.

Symptoms and Diagnostic Path

Once established in the tonsils, *C. diphtheriae* produce symptoms faster than almost any other organisms, as a result of its powerful exotoxin. Symptoms usually appear within two to five days of being exposed.

There are two types of diphtheria; one type involves the nose and throat, and the other involves the skin. Diphtheria that develops in the throat causes fever, red sore throat, weakness, and headache. There may be swelling and a gray membrane that completely covers the throat. This membrane can interfere with swallowing and talking and causes an unpleasant, distinct odor; if the membrane covers the windpipe, it can block breathing and suffocate the patient. Other symptoms include slight fever and chills. The exotoxin produced by the bacteria can spread throughout the body and can damage tissue in the kidneys, heart, or nervous system. Death often comes as a result of an inflamed heart.

The skin variety causes skin lesions that may be painful, swollen, and red.

A sample of the nose or throat discharge must be cultured to diagnose the disease. Results are available within eight hours.

Treatment Options and Outlook

Diphtheria is a preventable and treatable disease, but if treatment is inadequate or not begun in time, the powerful toxin produced by the bacteria may spread throughout the body, causing serious complications.

Intensive hospital care and prompt treatment with diphtheria antitoxin offers the best hope for cure. The antitoxin neutralizes the toxin if it has not yet invaded cells but is still circulating in the blood. Antibiotics (PENICILLIN or erythromycin) can help destroy the bacteria and decrease infectiousness of the respiratory secretions. Patients should be kept isolated and in bed for 10 days to two weeks, and fed a liquid or soft diet. Secretions in nose and throat must be suctioned; tube feeding may be necessary if swallowing is impossible. A tracheotomy may be necessary if the breathing muscles are paralyzed.

A person is infectious from two to four weeks, or until two to four days of antibiotic treatment. Anyone with a confirmed case must be isolated until after completion of antibiotic treatment, when negative results are obtained from two cultures from the nose and throat taken 24 hours apart.

If the bacteria has time to produce the toxin, complications can include bronchial pneumonia, heart failure, or paralysis of the throat, eye, and breathing muscles. Severe paralysis of the breathing muscles or diaphragm can be fatal. The toxin can inflame the heart muscle, which can lead to heart failure and death. About one out of every 10 untreated patients with diphtheria will die.

Risk Factors and Preventive Measures

Diphtheria vaccine is almost always given to U.S. infants in a combination with pertussis and TETANUS (DTaP). Because the original DTP vaccine was believed to cause unwanted side effects in some children, the improved DTaP vaccine was introduced in 1997. This vaccine uses only the parts of the bacteria to help children develop immunity, leaving out the parts that may have been responsible for the harmful side effects of the old DTP vaccine. (The "a" in DTaP stands for "acellular," which means there are no whole bacteria in the vaccine.) The DTaP is about 10 times less likely to cause adverse reactions such as fever, vomiting, and seizures.

Further improvements were introduced on March 7, 2001, when the U.S. Food and Drug Administration (FDA) approved a new version of the DTaP vaccine—this one without preservatives and with only a trace amount of thimerosal. Although thimerosal is a very effective preservative, the Public Health Service recommended that thimerosal should be reduced or eliminated from vaccines as soon as possible to minimize the exposure of infants and young children to mercury.

The new vaccine now contains less than 0.5 micrograms of mercury per dose—more than a 95 percent reduction in the amount of thimerosal per dose compared to the original version.

The DTaP shots are given at a baby's two-, four-, six-, and 12- or 18-month checkups, and then again when the child is four to six years old. At 11 or 12 years of age and every 10 years after that, a child should get a booster shot to prevent diphtheria and tetanus.

If a child has had a severe reaction to either the DTP or the DTaP, including difficulty breathing, hives, fainting, high fever, or seizure, the child should not receive another dose of the DTaP vaccine. Children also should avoid the DTaP if they have had any swelling of the brain within seven days of any vaccination not known to be due to another cause.

Children who are moderately to severely ill at the time the vaccine is scheduled should probably wait until they recover before getting the shot.

All infants should be immunized; boosters throughout life will prevent resurgence. The vaccine is made of a toxoid (weakened form of the toxin) that stimulates the immune system to make antibodies (called antitoxin) against the toxin. However, this immunity wanes; a booster is required every 10 years.

The toxoid comes in two strengths; children under age seven need a higher concentration to develop immunity. Older patients should get the lower concentration, since it has fewer side effects yet will still boost immunity.

Anyone exposed to diphtheria must receive a vaccine booster (DTP, DT, or Td) if one has not been given within five years. Exposed people must have a throat culture and be under observation for one week; anyone with a positive culture (even without symptoms) needs seven days of antibiotics.

Anyone with a high fever or serious illness should not get a vaccination until recovered, but children with mild colds and low fevers may be vaccinated.

Common side effects of the vaccine and booster include slight fever and irritability in the first 24 hours, with redness, swelling, or pain at the injection spot. Giving acetaminophen at the time of the shot may prevent a fever. A fever more than one day after the shot requires a call to the physician.

diphtheria, skin A bacterial infection common in the tropics, but also found in Canada and the southern United States, that causes a rash similar to IMPETIGO. It is found in areas of poverty and crowded conditions.

Skin diphtheria is caused by the same organism that causes DIPHTHERIA (*Corynebacterium diphtheriae*), found in the mucous membranes of the nose and throat and probably on human skin. Rarely, it is caused by food contaminated with the bacteria. A person can contract skin diphtheria by touching the open sores of a patient.

Symptoms and Diagnostic Path

Skin diphtheria is characterized by superficial ulcers on the skin with a gray-yellow or brown-gray membrane in the early stages, which can be peeled off; later, a black or brown-black eschar appears, surrounded by a tender inflammatory area. Nasal discharge also may be present.

Treatment Options and Outlook

Antibiotics and specific antitoxin are recommended; oral penicillin V potassium is effective in mild cases. Whereas the antibiotics will inhibit the bacteria, diphtheria antitoxin is required to inactivate the toxin.

diphyllobothriasis A disease caused by broad fish tapeworms that occurs after eating infested fish. Rare in the United States, it was formerly common in the Great Lakes area. It was known as Jewish or Scandinavian housewife's disease because the preparers of gefilte fish or fish balls tended to taste their food as they prepared it, before the fish was fully cooked, and got the disease. The parasite is now supposedly absent from Great Lakes fish; however, cases are still sometimes reported on the West Coast.

Foods are not routinely analyzed for this parasite. In 1980, an outbreak involving four Los Angeles physicians occurred when they ate sushi made of tuna, red snapper, and salmon.

The disease is caused by the parasitic flatworm *Diphyllobothrium latum* and other members of this tapeworm genus. The larva is often found in the viscera of fresh and marine fishes. *D. latum*, a broad, long tapeworm, often grows to lengths between three and seven feet and is potentially capable of reaching 32 feet. It is sometimes found in the flesh of freshwater fish, or fish that migrate from salt water to freshwater for breeding. Bears and humans are the final hosts for this parasite. The closely related *D. pacificum* usually matures in seals or other marine mammals and grows to only half that length.

Symptoms and Diagnostic Path

Symptoms include distended abdomen, flatulence, cramping, and diarrhea about 10 days after eating raw or poorly cooked fish. Those who are susceptible (usually those of Scandinavian heritage) may experience a severe anemia as a result of this tapeworm infection, caused by the tapeworm's absorption of vitamin B_{12}.

The disease is identified by finding eggs in the patient's feces.

Treatment Options and Outlook

The drug niclosamide is used to treat the infestation.

Diphyllobothrium The genus of flat tapeworms that causes DIPHYLLOBOTHRIASIS.

disinfectant A chemical germicide used to disinfect surfaces; most should not be used on human skin. Any household product that is called a disinfectant contains either ethyl alcohol (ethanol), isopropyl alcohol (isopropanol), hydrogen peroxide, chlorine, ammonia, phosphoric acid, or pine oil.

- *Alcohol* Sold at drug stores or supermarkets and can be used to wipe off thermometers.
- *Ammonium* Found in many household disinfectants; quaternary ammonium compounds are used in hospitals to wipe down floors, walls, and furniture.
- *Chlorine* The ingredient in household bleach that kills germs, usually found as sodium hypochlorite. It will kill bacteria and viruses and can be used to wipe down bathrooms, diaper changing tables, diaper pails, toys, and cutting boards. Chlorine can be used in solution: ¼ cup (4 tablespoons) bleach in 1 gallon water, or 1 tablespoon bleach to 1 quart water. CHLORINE should NEVER BE USED WITH ANY ACID PRODUCT OR AMMONIA; the resultant chlorine gas will react with water to form hydrochloric acid, which can cause serious symptoms from eye irritation to lung damage and pneumonia.

disinfection The elimination of most germs on surfaces. Low-level disinfection is used in most hospitals for items that will only come in contact with intact skin; this is usually all that is required in the home. Alcohol, chlorine bleach, and other chemical DISINFECTANT products are used for low-level disinfection.

Household detergents or cleaners are not disinfectants or germicides; they usually contain phosphates and are good for general cleaning.

Division of Bacterial and Mycotic Diseases A division of the National Center for Infectious Diseases, part of the U.S. CENTERS FOR DISEASE CONTROL AND PREVENTION in Atlanta, Georgia.

The division is dedicated to preventing and controlling diseases caused by bacteria or fungi. These organisms are important causes of illness and death in the United States and abroad and are major causes of new and emerging diseases as well as drug-resistant diseases.

dracunculiasis (dracontiasis) A parasitic disease caused by infection with a guinea worm and which occurs just beneath the skin surface. Dracunculiasis, also known as guinea worm disease, is the only parasitic illness that may be totally eradicated in the very near future. At the beginning of the 20th century the disease was widely distributed; active pockets of the disease are now found only in certain parts of Africa south of the Sahara, on the Arabian peninsula, and in India.

In 1991 the World Health Assembly vowed to eradicate the disease by the end of the 1990s.

Many organizations, including the Global 2000 program of the Carter Center, UNICEF, CENTERS FOR DISEASE CONTROL AND PREVENTION, and the World Health Organization are helping the last 12 countries in the world (all in Africa) eradicate the disease. By 2003, only 32,193 cases of dracunculiasis were reported; most of those cases were from Sudan, whose civil war makes it impossible to eradicate the disease. All affected countries except Sudan are trying to eliminate this disease as soon as possible.

Humans are infected by swallowing contaminated drinking water from shallow tropical wells and ponds. Worm larvae penetrate the intestinal wall, develop and mature in the abdominal cavity, and finally migrate to areas just underneath the skin. The adult worm discharges embryos through an opening in the skin. The entire process (from drinking water to embryo) takes about 13 months.

Symptoms and Diagnostic Path

Several hours before the worm's head appears at the skin's surface, there is local itching and burning, followed by an ulcer or blister (usually on the leg or foot) through which the embryos are produced. Other symptoms include nausea and vomiting, fever, and generalized itching. As the blister forms and ruptures, the symptoms disappear.

Uninfected ulcers heal in about six weeks, but secondary infection is common.

Treatment Options and Outlook

Once the worm emerges from the wound, it is pulled out a few centimeters a day and wrapped around a small stick; this process usually takes weeks or months.

No medication can end or prevent infection, but the worm can be surgically removed before an ulcer forms. Painkillers such as aspirin or ibuprofen can help ease swelling, and antibiotic ointment can help prevent bacterial infections. Patients should stay in bed with affected limbs elevated during recovery.

Risk Factors and Preventive Measures

It is important for travelers to purify drinking water, boiling any water that appears impure. Uncooked food washed with contaminated water should be avoided.

dysentery An infection of the intestinal tract that causes severe bloody diarrhea. Amebic dysentery (AMEBIASIS) is caused by the protozoan *Entamoeba histolytica* and causes ulcers in the intestines and sometimes abscesses in liver, heart, brain, or testes. Bacillary dysentery (SHIGELLOSIS) is caused by bacteria of the genus *Shigella* that is spread by contact with a patient or carrier or through contaminated food or water.

The term *dysentery* was invented by Hippocrates to describe a disease known since earliest history. It was written that Horus, the son of the Egyptian gods Osiris and Isis, had dysentery. Known widely as "campaign fever," dysentery has hobbled warriors from the Peloponnesian War through Napoleon's time on to the great struggles of this century, claiming more victims than have died on all the battlefields of all the world's wars. Dysentery has plagued a variety of great historical figures, including William the Conqueror, Edward I, and Henry V of England (the latter two both died of the disease). George Washington also suffered from dysentery that was exacerbated by hemorrhoids so painful that he sometimes had to ride on pillows over his saddle.

It still appears today in the United States, in places that are overdeveloped or where wells have been dug too close to septic systems. It also may crop up in day care centers and preschools, on cruise ships with poor hygiene, and in underdeveloped countries with poor sanitation facilities.

Drug-resistant strains of *Shigella dysenteriae* have appeared since the 1960s in underdeveloped countries, where the fatality rate is very high. Four-fifths of all children living in the tropics will get bacillary dysentery before age five.

In the United States, new strains of *Shigella* have been isolated in undercooked hamburgers served at fast-food restaurants.

See also ANTIDIARRHEAL DRUGS; DIARRHEA AND INFECTIOUS DISEASES; TRAVELER'S DIARRHEA.

dysentery, amebic See AMEBIASIS.

ear infection The common name for *otitis media,* an infection involving the middle ear (the cavity between the eardrum and the inner ear). A middle-ear infection can produce pus or fluid and cause severe earache and hearing loss. While an ear infection is annoying, it is not terribly serious; it is easily treated and there are not usually any long-term complications.

Ear infections are most common in children because of their short eustachian tubes (the passage that connects the back of the nose to the middle ear). This makes it easier for bacteria to enter the back of the throat. Almost all children have had at least one ear infection by the time they are six years old; youngsters are most susceptible to ear infections during the first two years of life.

Some children (especially babies with ear infections within two months of birth) have recurrent ear infections. They seem to run in families and are characterized by persistent fluid in the middle ear and short-term hearing loss. These conditions may require long-term antibiotics or surgery.

During a cold, the eustachian tube can swell and become blocked, allowing fluid to accumulate in the middle ear. The fluid produced by the inflammation cannot drain off through the tube and instead collects in the middle ear, where it can allow bacteria and viruses drawn in from the back of the throat to breed.

The usual cause of a middle-ear infection is bacteria that are normally present in a child's throat, including *Streptococcus pneumoniae, Haemophilus influenzae,* and *Moraxella catarrhalis.*

Risk factors for the development of an ear infection include being male, bottle-fed, Native American or Hispanic, and younger than two. Other risk factors include living in crowded conditions, going to day care, having allergies, and inhaling household cigarette smoke.

Symptoms and Diagnostic Path

Acute middle-ear infection causes sudden, severe earache, deafness, ringing of the ear (tinnitus), sense of fullness in the ear, and fever. Occasionally, the eardrum can burst, which causes a discharge of pus and relief of pain. In a baby or young child, parents may notice a cold with thick discharge, irritability, pulling or tugging at the ear, crying in the middle of the night, head shaking, and poor appetite. There may be fluid draining from the ear, although this isn't always the case. The fever is not usually high; the worst symptom is ear pain.

Chronic middle-ear infection is usually caused by repeated attacks of acute otitis media, with pus seeping from a perforation in the eardrum together with some degree of deafness. Complications include otitis externa (inflammation of the outer ear), damage to the bones in the middle ear, or a matted ball of skin debris that can erode the bone and cause further damage (called a "cholesteatoma"). Rarely, infection can spread *inward* from an infected ear and cause a brain ABSCESS.

Middle-ear infection can be detected by examining the ear with an instrument called an otoscope. A sample of discharge may be taken to identify the organism responsible for the infection, but it is not often done.

Treatment Options and Outlook

Acute middle-ear infection usually clears up completely with antibiotic drugs (usually amoxicillin), although sometimes there may be continual production of a sticky fluid in the middle ear known as "persistent middle-ear infection." A doctor may also remove pus and skin debris and prescribe antibiotic ear drops. Ephedrine nose drops can help establish draining of the ear in children.

One recent study found that one shot of ceftriaxone cured ear infections just as well as 10 days of amoxicillin. Since the mid-1980s, some strains of bacteria have developed resistance to amoxicillin and some other antibiotics. In areas with resistant strains, the child may need cefixime or another broad-spectrum antibiotic. Some children may not improve after 10 days of antibiotics and may need three or four more weeks of drug treatment.

Acetaminophen may be given to relieve pain or to reduce fevers above 101°F. A warm towel or hot water bottle over the sore ear, or an ice pack wrapped in a towel, may ease pain. The child should lie with infected ear down to help drain the fluid.

Rarely, a middle-ear infection can lead to bacterial MENINGITIS or MASTOIDITIS (a serious infection of the air cells behind the middle ear). Warning signs of mastoiditis include high fever, severe ear pain, puslike drainage and redness, swelling and tenderness behind the ear.

Risk Factors and Preventive Measures

Breast-feeding prevents ear infections during the first six months. Bottle-fed babies should not drink with the bottle propped or while lying on their back. Adults should not smoke around an infant, since the smoke irritates the lining of the nose and throat. Early treatment prevents most problems.

The vaccine *H. influenzae* type b (Hib) given to prevent meningitis also may prevent some ear infections that are caused by this bacterium.

eastern equine encephalitis See ENCEPHALITIS, EASTERN EQUINE.

Ebola (hemorrhagic fever) An often-fatal disease caused by one of the deadliest known viruses, which kills from 60 percent to 80 percent of everyone who contracts the disease. The virus was discovered in 1976 in Zaire and in a nearby western equatorial province of the Sudan, where it killed almost all of the 600 people who were infected. An isolated case appeared in Tandala, Zaire, in 1977, and another outbreak in the Sudan appeared in

1979, again killing 90 percent of its victims. An epidemic in the Bandundu Region of Zaire in 1995 killed 245. Outbreaks in the Sudan ended in 2004, but outbreaks in the Congo continue. Other cases have been reported in the Ivory Coast, Uganda, and Liberia. No case of human disease has been reported in the United States.

Still, despite fears of a modern-day plague, there has been little spread of the deadly Ebola infection in developed countries. A primary reason for the spread of the disease in poorer countries appears to be the lack of clean water and adequate hospital supplies, requiring, reuse of needles and syringes. In the 1976 Zaire epidemic, every person with Ebola cause by contaminated syringes died.

Infection with Ebola virus in humans is incidental—humans do not "carry" the virus. Because the natural reservoir of the virus is unknown, the manner in which the virus first appears in a human at the start of an outbreak has not been determined. However, researchers suspect that the first patient becomes infected through contact with an infected animal.

After the first case appears in an outbreak setting, humans can transmit the virus in several ways. People can be exposed to Ebola virus from direct contact with the blood or secretions of an infected person, which is why the virus has often been spread through the families and friends of infected persons. In the course of feeding, holding, or caring for family members, others come into close contact with secretions. People can also be exposed to Ebola virus through contact with objects (such as needles) that have been contaminated with infected secretions.

In African health-care facilities, workers often care for patients without using mask, gown, or gloves, and exposure to the virus has occurred when treating patients with Ebola. In addition, needles or syringes may not be disposable, or may not have been sterilized, but only rinsed before re-insertion into multi-use vials of medicine. If needles or syringes become contaminated with virus and are then reused, many people can become infected.

The Ebola-Reston outbreak that appeared in a primate research facility in Virginia may have been transmitted from monkey to monkey through the air in the facility. While all Ebola virus species have displayed the ability to be spread through airborne particles in the lab, this type of spread has not been documented among humans in a real-world setting, such as a hospital or household. The four currently identified Ebola viruses are known as filoviruses for their long, filamentlike appearance under a microscope.

The virus is also sometimes present in sweat glands and air sacs in the lungs. Its incubation period is between two and 21 days (and averages less than 10). Transmission of the virus may also occur via semen up to seven weeks after clinical recovery.

Scientists strongly suspect that the virus is carried by an insect, such as mosquitoes, but they have so far failed to find such a carrier in more than 1,600 tests they have done on insects. Monkey virus closely resembling Ebola filovirus was isolated from monkeys imported into the United States from the Philippines in 1989; a number of the monkeys died, and at least four people were infected, although none of them suffered symptoms.

Past studies have shown that the greatest risk of spreading Ebola virus is to those who have closest contact with an infected person, such as health care workers and spouses.

Symptoms and Diagnostic Path

Ebola hemorrhagic fever is characterized by the sudden onset of fever, weakness, muscle pain, headache, and sore throat. This is followed by vomiting, abdominal pain, diarrhea, rash, kidney and liver failure, and massive internal and external bleeding. Researchers do not understand why some people are able to recover from Ebola HF and others are not. However, it is known that patients who die usually have not developed a significant immune response to the virus at the time of death.

Diagnosing Ebola in an individual who has been infected for only a few days is difficult because early symptoms, such as red and itchy eyes and a skin rash can be related to many diseases. If Ebola is suspected, several lab tests should be done promptly, including a blood film examination for MALARIA and a blood culture. If the suspected patient has bloody diarrhea, a stool culture should also be performed.

A variety of tests can be used to diagnose a case of Ebola within a few days of the onset of symptoms. Patients tested later in the course of the disease or after recovery can be tested for antibodies to the virus; the disease can also be diagnosed retrospectively in deceased patients.

Treatment Options and Outlook

There is no specific treatment or vaccine that exists for Ebola hemorrhagic fever, although general good hygiene and medical precautions have helped stop the spread of the disease. Severe cases require intensive supportive care, yet there are still few survivors.

Risk Factors and Preventive Measures

Transmission can be prevented by washing hands, and wearing gloves and masks around infected patients, and avoiding reuse of needles. Suspected cases should be isolated. Since the primary method of transmitting the virus is through person-to-person contact with blood, secretion, or body fluids, anyone who has had close personal contact with patients should be kept under strict surveillance.

In 2005, Canadian and U.S. scientists reported that they have developed vaccines against both the Ebola and MARBURG viruses that have been shown to be effective in nonhuman primates. Scientists report that the vaccines are 100 percent effective in protecting monkeys against infection from these often deadly viruses. Monkeys are known to develop hemorrhagic fever symptoms that are similar to those observed in humans infected by these viruses. Demonstrating that these vaccines are safe and effective in monkeys suggests that there may be real potential for use in humans. However, scientists caution that it will be some time before the vaccines will be available for human use. Still, this is the first vaccine system that has protected nonhuman primates from both Ebola and Marburg.

EBV   See EPSTEIN-BARR VIRUS.

echinococcosis   A tapeworm infection found throughout the world, most frequently in the sheep- and cattle-raising areas of South America, South Africa, the Soviet Union, and the Middle East.

The infection is caused by the larval stage of a tapeworm (*Echinococcus granulosus*) whose eggs are transmitted to humans in contact with infected dogs or other canines, or by ingesting soil, vegetables, or water contaminated by feces of infected animals.

In humans, the larval phase of the adult worm forms fluid-filled sacs mostly in the liver and lungs but also in other organs. The incubation period varies from months to years.

Symptoms and Diagnostic Path

Many people in the early stages of infection do not exhibit any symptoms. After many years, however, victims who develop cysts in the liver may experience abdominal discomfort, nausea, and vomiting; a ruptured cyst can cause sudden pain, fever, and possibly death. Liver cysts are most often seen in middle-aged or elderly patients. Patients with cysts in the lung may spit up blood, cough, and have shortness of breath. A rupture of the cyst in a lung can cause an acute PNEUMONIA and lung ABSCESS. These lung cysts are more often found in children and younger patients.

Because many of the early infections cause no symptoms, the disease may not be detected until a routine X-ray, medical exam, or autopsy reveals the infestation.

Treatment Options and Outlook

Surgical removal of the cysts, when possible. Mebendazole and albendazole are two antiinfectives that can destroy the living organisms inside the cysts.

A very serious form of the disease is called alveolar hydatid disease and occurs throughout the world—but most often in Europe, Russia, Japan, Alaska, Canada, and the United States. The disease is transmitted to man through infected feces of fox and domestic cat and dogs. When infected, a person develops multiple cysts that spread rapidly; usually occurring in the liver, the disease is often fatal.

ECHOvirus A type of picornavirus associated with many infections, including MENINGITIS, colds, UPPER RESPIRATORY TRACT INFECTION, CONJUNCTIVITIS, and infantile DIARRHEA. ECHOvirus, which is an acronym for Enteric Cytopathogenic Human Orphan virus, includes 31 types.

Symptoms and Diagnostic Path

Most ECHOvirus infections are mild; symptoms vary from mild to lethal and acute to chronic. Other infections with which the virus is associated include muscle weakness and paralysis, pericarditis, myocarditis, the common cold, and acute febrile respiratory illnesses.

The virus is found throughout the world, and peaks in summer and fall. Outbreaks are common in day-care centers as transmission is believed to occur via airborne particles or body secretions.

Treatment Options and Outlook

The effectiveness of antiviral medication is uncertain, although experts hope that the new antiviral drug pleconaril may be effective. Pleconaril interferes with the binding of the ECHOvirus particle to the cell membrane. Further clinical trials are currently under way.

E. coli infection   See ESCHERICHIA COLI.

ecthyma A shallow ulcerative bacterial skin infection that often causes scarring. Similar to IMPETIGO, it usually occurs on the legs and protected areas of the body.

The infection is caused by group A streptococci or *Staphylococcus aureus*.

Symptoms and Diagnostic Path

The condition begins with one lesion, which enlarges and encrusts; beneath this crust is a pus-filled punched ulcer. Children are more commonly affected with ecthyma, which is usually associated with poor hygiene and malnutrition and minor skin injuries from trauma, insect bites, or SCABIES.

Treatment Options and Outlook

Antibiotics plus meticulous skin care are the treatments of choice.

ectoparasite A parasite that lives on the skin, getting nourishment from the skin by sucking the host's blood; various types of ticks, lice, mites, and some types of fungi may occasionally be ectoparasites on humans. (Parasites living *inside* the body are called "endoparasites.")

ectothrix   A fungus that grows outside the hair shaft.

eczema, herpeticum   A rare skin condition caused by the HERPES simplex virus characterized by an extensive rash of blisters in a patient with a preexisting skin condition. The disease is also called Kaposi's varicelliform eruption.

Symptoms and Diagnostic Path

This condition is characterized by clusters of vesicles on the skin that spread over a period of a week or two, eventually evolving into discrete punched-out small erosions. Other symptoms include fever, malaise, and swollen lymph glands. The vesicles may break down into large erosions that often become infected. The condition may last from two to six weeks and may recur in a milder form.

Treatment Options and Outlook

Treatment includes the antiviral drug acyclovir, along with Burow's solution soaks two or three times daily for vesicles. Early and aggressive antibiotic treatment of secondary infection is vital. Hospitalization with intravenous acyclovir or antibiotics may be required, especially in infants with high fever and dehydration.

Ehrlichia   A genus of bacteria that includes several well-known species infecting domestic animals. The genus is in the same family (*Rickettsia*) as the bacterium that causes another tick-borne human disease, ROCKY MOUNTAIN SPOTTED FEVER. The species were first reported in dogs in 1935 but were only documented to cause human disease in 1953 in Japan. In the United States, human diseases caused by *Ehrlichia* species have been recognized since the mid-1980s.

Currently three species of *Ehrlichia* in the United States cause disease in humans.

Ehrlichiae are small, gram-negative bacteria that primarily invade white blood cells, the same cells that fight disease by destroying invading microorganisms. Ehrlichiae typically appear as minute, round bacteria ranging from one to three micrometers in diameter.

The genus *Ehrlichia* is currently classified as a member of the family Rickettsiaceae, in the order Rickettsiales. The genus includes seven recognized species: *E. canis, E. chaffeensis, E. equi, E. phagocytophila, E. risticii, E. ewingii,* and *E. sennetsu.* A number of other named ehrlichiae, such as *E. platys, E. bovis, E. ovina,* and *E. ondiri* also cause disease in animals.

Ehrlichia chaffeensis   A type of bacterium in the genus EHRLICHIA that causes an illness similar to human granulocytic EHRLICHIOSIS and has been responsible for several deaths.

Ehrlichia chaffeensis primarily infects white blood cells, but also may be seen occasionally in the granulocytes of some patients with severe disease.

Ehrlichia chaffeensis is principally transmitted by the lone star tick (*Amblyomma americanum*). White-tailed deer are a major host of lone star ticks and appear to represent one natural reservoir for *E. chaffeensis.* Antibodies have been found throughout deer populations in the southeastern and midwestern United States, and the organism has been cultured from deer blood.

E. chaffeensis infections are most frequently reported from southeastern and midwestern states with abundant lone star tick populations, especially Arkansas, Florida, Georgia, Missouri, North Carolina, Oklahoma, Tennessee, Texas, and Virginia. Cases have been reported from almost every state in the United States, although some of these may have been imported from states where the disease is highly endemic.

See also EHRLICHIOSIS, HUMAN MONOCYTIC.

Ehrlichia ewingii   A type of bacterium that causes EHRLICHIOSIS. The potentially fatal disease caused by *E. ewingii* has been limited to a few patients in Missouri, Oklahoma, and Tennessee, most of whom have had underlying impaired immune systems.

Ehrlichia ewingii is transmitted by the lone star tick (*Amblyomma americanum*), which is also able to transmit the disease among dogs. Other potential carriers of the disease remain to be identified. Canine granulocytic ehrlichiosis caused by *E. ewingii* has been described in south central and southeastern states, including Arkansas, Georgia, Mississippi, Missouri, North Carolina, Oklahoma, Tennessee, and Virginia.

The symptoms of ehrlichiosis resemble the flu, and include fever, headache, and muscle and joint pain appearing seven to 10 days after a tick bite. Although ehrlichiosis can be successfully treated with antibiotics, someone who does not receive treatment can develop serious liver and lung problems that can lead to organ failure.

Scientists do not know whether *E. ewingii* infection in humans is a new phenomenon or merely a newly-recognized one. Because *E. ewingii* is closely related to EHRLICHIA CHAFFEENSIS and both are found in Missouri, it is possible that previous cases of *E. ewingii* have been misdiagnosed as *E. chaffeensis*.

ehrlichiosis A disease first identified in 1990 that is spread by the type of ticks that also carry LYME DISEASE. From 1986 to 1997, health departments and laboratories reported more than 1,200 cases of human ehrlichiosis to CDC. Although ehrlichiosis is a nationally notifiable disease, not all state health departments have reported cases. Most of the recognized cases have originated from states that also have a high incidence of Lyme disease, such as Connecticut, Minnesota, New York, and Wisconsin. This distribution is consistent with the fact that the ticks that transmit ehrlichiosis (*Ixodes scapularis*) also transmits the bacteria that causes Lyme disease (*Borrelia burgdorferi*). Although the disease can be treated with antibiotics, treatment is often delayed because victims confuse it with a summer flu. If it is treated early and properly, the disease is not associated with neurological damage or arthritis.

The CENTERS FOR DISEASE CONTROL AND PREVENTION reported at least two deaths between 1990–93 from the disease in Wisconsin and Minnesota. Some researchers believe ehrlichiosis is not a new disease; New York and New England patients may have had the illness but who were instead diagnosed with Lyme disease.

It is also possible that some patients are infected with both Lyme and ehrlichiosis at the same time, making a proper diagnosis more difficult. For every 12 Lyme-infected ticks a person might find during an hour's walk in tick-infested areas of Nantucket, there are four ehrlichiosis-infected ticks—and two ticks infected with both diseases, which raises the possibility of getting two infections from one bite.

Ehrlichiosis represents a group of clinically similar yet distinct diseases caused by *Ehrlichia chaffeensis, E. ewingii,* and a bacterium extremely similar or identical to *E. phagocytophila*. Human ehrlichiosis caused by E. chaffeensis was first described in 1987, and is found primarily in the southeastern and south central parts of the country. It is primarily transmitted by the lone star tick (*Amblyomma americanum*). Human granulocytic ehrlichiosis (HGE) was first identified in 1994, the second recognized ehrlichia infection of humans in the United States. The name for the species that causes HGE has not been formally proposed, but this species is closely related or identical to the veterinary pathogens *E. equi* and *E. phagocytophila*. HGE is transmitted by the blacklegged tick (*Ixodes scapularis*) and the western blacklegged tick (*Ixodes pacificus*) in the United States. *Ehrlichia ewingii* is the most recently recognized cause of ehrlichiosis, which has been limited to a few immunocompromised patients in Missouri, Oklahoma, and Tennessee.

Most patients are infected in the spring and summer when they are more commonly exposed to disease-carrying ticks. Most ehrlichiosis cases occur between April and September. A history of tick bites or exposure to tick-infested habitats is not reported in all cases.

Symptoms and Diagnostic Path

While Lyme disease often produces a telltale circular rash around the tickbite site, ehrlichiosis does not usually cause visible symptoms. Instead, about 10 days after a person has been bitten, the bacteria multiply inside white blood cells and then suddenly cause fever, chills, headache, and muscle ache. Their flu-like symptoms are far more severe than those associated with Lyme disease.

While many of the symptoms overlap with Lyme disease, ehrlichiosis symptoms tend to peak very quickly, moving from health to severe debilitation in a few hours.

Only a few labs in the nation can perform the test for HGE. Diagnosis is difficult, and testing has not been standardized. Other lab findings that suggest ehrlichiosis include low white blood count, low platelet count, and high liver enzymes. If it is summer and a patient develops sudden, flu-like symptoms without coughing or nasal congestion, ehrlichiosis is a likely suspect—especially if the patient remembers a recent tick bite. (Lyme disease symptoms usually appear more gradually.)

Treatment Options and Outlook

Untreated ehrlichiosis can be a severe illness; as many as half of all patients require hospitalization. Severe symptoms of the disease may include prolonged fever, renal failure, meningoencephalitis, adult respiratory distress syndrome, seizures, or coma. Between 2 percent and 3 percent of patients may die from the infection. Preliminary evidence suggests that infection caused by the *E. Chaffeensis* bacteria may become more severe than other ehrlichia infections.

The severity of ehrlichiosis also may be related in part to the health of the person's immune system. Patients with compromised immunity caused by cortiocosteroids or cancer chemotherapy, HIV infection, or removal of the spleen appear to develop more severe disease, and their cases are more often fatal.

Prompt treatment is essential; the longer a case is untreated, the worse the outcome. Ehrlichiosis responds to doxycycline and other tetracycline antibiotics; it does not respond to amoxicillin and other antibiotics used to treat Lyme disease.

The antibiotic suppresses the growth of microbes but does not kill them, so the immune system must fight off the infection. Coinfection with another type of bacteria at the same time can suppress the immune system, increasing a patient's vulnerability to other infections. In these cases, treatment may need to be longer.

Signs of the disease fade away within two months, and the disease does not appear to cause the chronic, arthritis-like symptoms that haunt Lyme disease patients for years.

Risk Factors and Preventive Measures

The same precautions that prevent Lyme disease should also be taken to prevent ehrlichiosis. Avoiding tick habitats is the best way to prevent tick bites. But ticks may also be found in lawns, gardens, and on bushes adjacent to homes.

When walking in the woods, people should stay on trails and avoid brushing up against low bushes or tall grass. Ticks do not hop or jump but are carried by the wind. To prevent bites, hikers should wear protective clothing (light-colored long-sleeve shirts and light-colored pants tucked into boots or socks). The light-colored clothing allows ticks to be more easily spotted.

Use an insect repellent, preferably containing no more than 30 percent DEET (N-diethylmetatoluamide), on bare skin and clothing. Duranon can be applied to clothing only, but not to the skin. All insect repellent should be used with caution (especially with children) and should not be applied to the hands or face.

Ticks and their hosts (mice, chipmunks, voles, and other small mammals) need moisture, a place hidden from direct sun, and a place to hide. The clearer the area around a house, the less chance there will be of getting a tick bite.

All leaf litter and brush should be removed as far as possible away from the house. Low-lying bushes should be pruned to let in more sun. Leaves should be raked every fall, since ticks prefer to overwinter in fallen leaves. Woodpiles are favorite hiding places for mammals carrying ticks, so woodpiles should be kept neat, off the ground, in a sunny place, and under cover.

Gardens should be cleaned up every fall; foliage left on the ground over the winter provide shelter for mammals that may harbor ticks. Dry stone walls on the property also increase the potential for ticks.

Shady lawns may support ticks in epidemic areas; lawns should be mowed and edges trimmed. Entire fields should be mowed in fall.

Birdfeeders attract birds that carry infected ticks, so they should not be placed too close to the house. Bird feeding should be stopped during late spring and summer, when infected ticks are most active. Building eight-foot fences to keep out deer may significantly reduce the abundance of ticks on large land parcels.

Four pesticides may help; Damminix; chlorpyrifos (Dursban); carbaryl (Sevin); and cyfluthrin (Tempo). One or two applications a year in late

May and September can significantly reduce the tick population.

See also EHRLICHIOSIS, HUMAN MONOCYTIC; EHRLICHIOSIS, CANINE; EHRLICHIOSIS, EQUINE.

ehrlichiosis, canine   A disease caused by the bacteria *Ehrlichia canis* carried by the brown dog tick *Rhipicephalus sanguineus*. This disease of dogs and other canids was identified during the 1930s and is found throughout the world.

See also *EHRLICHIA*.

ehrlichiosis, equine   A disease of horses caused by the bacteria *Ehrlichia equi* found in the eastern United States. No vectors have been identified.

See also *EHRLICHIA;* ERLICHIOSIS, CANINE.

ehrlichiosis, human monocytic   The first type of EHRLICHIOSIS that was discovered in 1985, and which is transmitted by the Lone Star tick (*Amblyomma americanum*). Since 1986, about 400 cases have been confirmed in 30 states, mostly in the southeastern and south-central United States and at least nine people died.

The disease is caused by *EHRLICHIA CHAFFEENSIS*, a type of bacterium in the genus *EHRLICHIA* that was only identified in 1991.

Symptoms and Diagnostic Path

Symptoms are similar to human granulocytic ehrlichiosis, including fever, headache, chills, malaise, sweating, muscle aches, nausea, and vomiting. The infection may range from a mild illness to a severe, life-threatening disease. It may cause reduction of white blood cells and platelets, anemia, or abnormal liver function.

Treatment Options and Outlook

Antibiotics are effective if begun early enough in the disease.

elephantiasis   Massive swelling of the legs also known as lymphatic FILARIASIS. It is caused by obstructed lymph vessels, which prevents drainage of lymph from the surrounding tissues. This causes inflammation and thickening of the vessel walls, eventually blocking them.

More than 120 million people have been affected by elephantiasis: one-third in India, another third in Africa, and most of the rest in southeast Asia, the Pacific, and the Americas. In tropical and subtropical areas where elephantiasis is common, the infection is continuing to increase due to the rapid and unplanned growth of cities, which creates numerous breeding sites for the mosquitoes that transmit the disease.

The parasitic worms *Wuchereria bancrofti* and *Brugia malayi* cause filariasis, which may lead to elephantiasis. These worms lodge in the lymphatic system (the network of nodes and vessels that maintain the delicate fluid balance between the tissues and blood and are an important part of the body's immune system). The worms live for four to six years, producing millions of immature larvae that circulate in the blood. The infestation spreads when mosquitoes bite infected humans and pick up the larvae, which are then passed on into the bloodstream of the next human by the bite of the infected mosquito.

Symptoms and Diagnostic Path

The syndrome gets its name from the appearance of the skin of the legs, which resembles elephant hide. While the legs are most commonly affected, the arms, breasts, scrotum, or vulva also may be affected.

Although the worm infestation is generally acquired early in childhood, the elephantiasis symptoms may take years to manifest itself, and some people never develop symptoms. The worst symptoms of the chronic disease generally appear in adults, and in men more often than in women. Between 10 percent and 50 percent of men suffer from genital damage, especially a fluid-filled balloonlike enlargement of the sacs around the testes, with elephantiasis of the penis and scrotum. Swelling to several times the normal size of the entire leg, arm, vulva, or breast may affect up to 10 percent of the population in some areas.

Treatment Options and Outlook

Both albendazole and diethylcarbamazine (DEC) are effective in killing the adult parasites, which not only can cure the worm infestation but also can improve patients' elephantiasis and scrotal swellings, especially in the early stages of disease. The most significant treatment advance that has helped ease the suffering of those with elephantiasis has come from recognizing that the problem is caused by bacterial and fungal superinfection of tissues as a result of poor immune function due to earlier filarial infection. Therefore, rigorous cleanliness involving affected limbs, minimizing infection, and promoting lymph flow can lead to astonishing improvement of the elephantiasis.

emerging infectious diseases   While some diseases have been effectively controlled with the help of modern technology such as antibiotics and vaccines, new diseases such as avian flu, WEST NILE VIRUS, and SARS are constantly appearing. These are referred to as "newly emerging infectious diseases." Others, such as MALARIA, TUBERCULOSIS, and bacterial pneumonias, are now appearing in forms that are resistant to drug treatments. Still others are constantly evolving such as various forms of influenza.

Infectious diseases are a continuing danger to everyone, no matter what a person's age, gender, lifestyle, ethnic background, or economic status. These diseases are still one of the most common causes of suffering and death, and they impose an enormous financial burden on society.

Ominously, experts now are warning that emerging infectious diseases today pose a global threat to human and animal health, and the problem is likely to get much worse. Of the germs now causing emerging infectious diseases, 75 percent are able to be transmitted from animals to humans (these are called zoonotic diseases). The apparently rapid increase in the emergence of new zoonoses is a direct result of closer contact with wildlife as humans encroach on wildlife habitat. For example, Ebola virus outbreaks are linked to increased mining or hunting for "bushmeat," and the AIDS pandemic began as humans moved out into the African forests for food.

The increase in international travel is also responsible for the surge in emerging diseases. For example, the spread of West Nile virus into North America, and AIDS and SARS around the world, is a direct result of this globalization. Emerging infectious diseases are not only a problem for human health but are also a major threat to animal welfare, domesticated species, and to wildlife species conservation.

encephalitis   Inflammation of the brain usually caused by a viral infection. Often, the membranes covering the brain (meninges) are affected. An attack may be very mild, but in many cases it is a serious condition.

The most common strains of mosquito-borne encephalitis in North America include St. Louis encephalitis (SLE), eastern equine encephalitis (EEE), California encephalitis (CE), western equine encephalitis, La Crosse encephalitis, West Nile encephalitis, Venezuelan equine encephalitis, and Powassan encephalitis (the only one spread by ticks, not mosquitoes). Japanese encephalitis does not occur in the United States, but it is very common throughout Asia and poses a risk to international travelers.

Most of the time, the virus responsible is the HERPES simplex virus type I, which also causes COLD SORES. There is no insect cause. In the United States, encephalitis is commonly caused by a virus transmitted to humans via a mosquito bite. More and more cases are related to infection with HIV, the organism responsible for AIDS. Occasionally, encephalitis is a complication of other viral infections such as MEASLES or MUMPS.

Symptoms and Diagnostic Path

Usually, symptoms begin with headache, fever, and prostration, often with hallucinations, confusion, paralysis of one side of the body, and disturbed behavior, speech, memory, and eye movement. There is a gradual loss of consciousness and sometimes a coma; seizures may develop. If the meninges are affected, the neck is usually stiff and the eyes are unusually sensitive to light.

Central nervous system symptoms include some (not all) of the following:

- abnormal reflexes
- changes in consciousness
- confusion

- disorientation
- dizziness
- inability to speak
- irritability
- listlessness
- loss of balance
- odor hallucinations
- seizure
- sleepiness
- spasticity
- tremor
- weakness

Symptoms, signs, and a spinal tap to study the cerebrospinal fluid will help diagnose the disease. CT scans and MRIs are used to rule out other causes of headache, fever, and changes in the senses.

Treatment Options and Outlook

The antiviral drug acyclovir administered intravenously is an effective treatment for encephalitis caused by the herpes virus. If the disease is caused by another virus, there is no known effective treatment. Depending on the virus causing the problem, some patients will die, and some who recover will have brain damage, with mental impairment, behavioral disturbances, epilepsy, and deafness.

See also ENCEPHALITIS, CALIFORNIA; ENCEPHALITIS, EASTERN EQUINE; ENCEPHALITIS, JAPANESE; ENCEPHALITIS LETHARGICA; ENCEPHALITIS, ST. LOUIS; ENCEPHALITIS, TICK-BORNE; ENCEPHALOMYELITIS; ENCEPHALITIS, WEST NILE.

encephalitis, California A rare group of viruses that cause ENCEPHALITIS first discovered in Central Valley, California, in 1943.

Since the original virus was isolated, other closely related viruses were found now classified as the California serogroup. The La Crosse virus also belong to the California serogroup. Although little human disease was associated with these viruses until 1960, now the California serogroup virus infections are the most commonly reported cause of mosquito-transmitted encephalitis in the United States. From 1996 to 1998, approximately three times as many reported human cases of mosquito-borne encephalitis were caused by the California serogroup viruses as were reported for western equine encephalomyelitis virus, St. Louis encephalitis, and eastern equine encephalitis viruses combined.

The California virus belongs to a group of viruses called BUNYAVIRUS carried by many different types of mosquitoes, which catch the virus from and give it to both squirrels and chipmunks.

The infected mosquitoes remain infected for life. It is not possible for humans to transmit the virus to one another.

Most adults who live in areas where the mosquitoes exist are immune because they have antibodies produced when they were bitten as children. Elderly people may be susceptible, because the immunity appears to wear off with age.

When an infected mosquito bites a human, the virus passes into the person's bloodstream and then travels to the brain and spinal cord. It multiplies in the central nervous system, inflaming and damaging nerve cells, interfering with signals sent from the brain to other parts of the body.

Symptoms and Diagnostic Path

Only a small percentage of patients with the disease exhibit any symptoms, which usually begins with fever, irritability, drowsiness, headache, nausea/vomiting, and sensitivity to light. This can lead to convulsions or seizures. Most people recover completely.

A spinal tap (lumbar puncture) will reveal antibodies to the specific encephalitis virus in cerebrospinal fluid. The actual virus may be found in brain tissue from those who have died from the disease. Only the antibodies will appear in blood or spinal fluid, not the virus itself.

Treatment Options and Outlook

There is no cure for viral encephalitis. When a person's immune system produces enough antibodies to destroy the virus, the person recovers. Generally, a person with the symptoms of encephalitis is admitted to the hospital for treatment in a darkened room and given medication to reduce fever and treat the severe headache.

Less than 1 percent of the children who contract the disease will die. Some may experience occasional seizures or behavioral changes (such as reduced attention span).

Risk Factors and Preventive Measures

There are no drugs that prevent the California encephalitis.

See also ENCEPHALITIS, JAPANESE; ENCEPHALITIS, ST. LOUIS; ENCEPHALITIS, TICK-BORNE; ENCEPHALITIS, WESTERN EQUINE; ENCEPHALITIS, WEST NILE; ENCEPHALITIS LETHARGICA; ENCEPHALOMYELITIS.

encephalitis, eastern equine (EEE) The least common and most deadly of all the arborvival infections; about 60 percent of its victims die. This type of ENCEPHALITIS primarily affects horses, donkeys, and mules along the eastern seaboard of the United States, but it also infects about four humans each year. There were about 220 confirmed human cases in the United States between 1964 and 2004.

Outbreaks of the disease in horses have occurred along the East Coast since 1831. The first human to die of the disease was a Massachusetts baby in 1938. EEE is related to a similar virus that infects horses and humans in the western states called western equine encephalitis (WEE).

In addition to eastern equine encephalitis and western equine encephalomyelitis, there is a third type: Venezuelan equine encephalitis. Eastern equine encephalitis is a severe form of equine encephalitis; it lasts longer and causes more deaths and problems than either the western or Venezuelan versions. Venezuelan equine encephalitis occurs in Central and South America, Florida, and Texas.

Four different types of mosquitoes carry the virus responsible for EEE. The virus enters the bloodstream via the mosquito bite, traveling directly to the spinal cord and brain. As the virus multiplies in the central nervous system, it damages the nerve cells, interfering with the signals the brain sends to the body. Despite its name, the primary natural hosts of the viruses of eastern and western equine encephalitis are birds, not horses.

Because the virus is not present in the blood of humans, it is not transmitted between people, most people who live in areas where the mosquito carries the virus are immune, since they were bitten as children and developed antibodies without ever becoming sick. Since the disease is transmitted primarily by mosquitoes, it occurs most often during the insect season, especially in low marshy areas.

Symptoms and Diagnostic Path

Unlike St. Louis encephalitis in which only a few patients have symptoms, most people with EEE get symptoms, which begin five to 15 days after a mosquito bite. Symptoms begin with headache, fever, chills, muscle aches, and nausea, followed by paralysis, convulsions, and coma.

In humans, the elderly are most at risk for serious cases; almost 60 percent of older patients die. Infants and young children are also at risk. Those who are sick for a few days before the paralysis and convulsions appear will probably recover completely. Chances for a complete recovery without any permanent damage are best in adults over 40 and under 80.

Signs of the disease in horses include fever, loss of appetite, discomfort, mental deterioration, head pressing, circling, and blindness. Death occurs two to three days after infection, caused by the sudden inability to breathe.

Rapid tests to identify antibodies to the EEE virus in blood and cerebrospinal fluid are now available.

Treatment Options and Outlook

There is no cure for encephalitis. Pain medication for fever and headache may be given.

Long-term damage may include facial palsy, weakness, seizures, or mental problems such as confusion and hallucinations. Children younger than five have a poor outlook for recovery.

Risk Factors and Preventive Measures

A vaccine can prevent the disease in horses and should be given in areas where EEE is prevalent. All foals must be vaccinated, and older horses must be revaccinated during the EEE season. An experimental human vaccine is available for those who work in labs with the virus.

See also ENCEPHALITIS, CALIFORNIA; ENCEPHALITIS, ST. LOUIS; ENCEPHALITIS, JAPANESE; ENCEPHALITIS, TICK-BORNE; ENCEPHALITIS, WESTERN EQUINE; ENCEPH-

ALITIS, WEST NILE; ENCEPHALITIS LETHARGICA; ENCEPH-
ALOMYELITIS.

encephalitis, Japanese A mosquito-borne version
of ENCEPHALITIS that is primarily a rural disease of
the Orient, fewer than one case a year is reported in
American citizens and military personnel traveling
to Asia. It is found primarily in China and Korea,
India, Bangladesh, Nepal and Sri Lanka, and southeast Asian countries. It occurs less often in Japan,
Taiwan, Singapore, Hong Kong, and eastern Russia.
It is the leading cause of viral encephalitis in Asia.

Japanese encephalitis is a zoonosis, a disease that
primarily infects animals but sometimes moves into
the human population. It belongs to a group of
viruses called flavivirus (which includes St. Louis
encephalitis).

The chance that a U.S. traveler to Asia will contract the disease is small; only 11 cases among
Americans traveling or working in Asia are known
to have occurred between 1981 and 1992, eight of
whom were military personnel or their families.

The disease is transmitted by the *Culex* mosquitoes, usually during the summer and fall as the
mosquito season occurs. The mosquitoes breed in
ground pools and flooded rice fields and become
infected after biting infected domestic pigs and
wading birds who are raised near the rice paddies.
However, in areas infested with mosquitoes, only a
small portion of the insects are actually infected
with the virus.

After the mosquito bites, the virus enters the
bloodstream and travels directly to the brain and
spinal cord, where it multiplies, causing inflammation and damage to nerve cells. This damage interferes with the signals the brain sends to the body,
thus causing the symptoms of encephalitis.

Because the virus is not present in human blood,
it can not be transmitted between humans. Most
adults who live in an area where the mosquitoes
carry the disease are immune because they were
infected as children.

Symptoms and Diagnostic Path
Most people who are infected with the virus have
only mild symptoms or no symptoms at all. However, those who develop encephalitis as a result of

the virus are usually gravely ill. Within six to eight
days after the bite, the disease begins with a flu-like
illness, with headache, fever, and stomach problems. Confusion and behavior problems appear
early; in one third of cases, the encephalitis is fatal.
Another third survive with serious types of brain
damage, including paralysis. The last third recover
without any further problems.

Infection during the first and second trimesters
of pregnancy have been associated with miscarriages. Most deaths occur in children aged five to
nine, and in people over age 65. The fatality rate
ranges from 0.3 percent to 60 percent.

The disease can be diagnosed by a rapid test that
looks for antibodies to the virus in the blood and
cerebrospinal fluid. Sometimes the actual virus is
found in brain tissue from patients who have died.

Treatment Options and Outlook
There is no treatment for this viral disease. Anyone
with the symptoms of this disease is admitted to the
hospital and given pain relievers and medicine to
lower the fever. Intensive care is often necessary.

Up to one quarter of survivors have long-
term nervous system damage; the rest recover
quickly. Children have a better chance of long-term
recovery.

Risk Factors and Preventive Measures
There is a vaccine for Japanese encephalitis currently available in the United States through most
traveler's health clinics. It is about 85 percent effective in anyone over age one. The U.S. CENTERS FOR
DISEASE CONTROL AND PREVENTION recommends the
vaccine only to those Americans who work in or
visit at risk rural areas for more than four weeks. In
some cases it is recommended for those visiting
endemic areas for 30 days. The risk is low to most
travelers who stay in cities or who travel through
the country only for short periods. People over age
55 may be at higher risk and should consider vaccination if they travel to areas of risk.

The vaccine is given in three doses, and protection begins about 10 days after the last dose. A
booster shot may be required in two years. Serious
allergic reactions (hives and dangerous swelling of
mouth and throat) have been reported in a few
people, which may not appear until several days

after vaccination. Patients with multiple allergies (especially to bee stings and drugs) appear to be at higher risk for side effects. Fever and local redness and swelling are reported in about 10 percent of those vaccinated.

The vaccine is also available in many Asian countries; travelers should contact the local U.S. embassy or consulate for a list of reputable clinics that may have the vaccine. With or without the vaccine, it is important to try to avoid mosquito bites while traveling.

See also ENCEPHALITIS, CALIFORNIA; ENCEPHALITIS, ST. LOUIS; ENCEPHALITIS, TICK-BORNE; ENCEPHALITIS, WESTERN EQUINE; ENCEPHALITIS, WEST NILE; ENCEPHALITIS LETHARGICA; ENCEPHALOMYELITIS.

encephalitis, La Crosse A major type of ENCEPHALITIS in the eastern United States, this disease is caused by the La Crosse virus in the family Bunyaviridae. The encephalitis caused by this virus is most common in children and young adults under the age of 19. The 30 to 180 annual cases of La Crosse encephalitis represent between 8 percent to 30 percent of all cases of encephalitis. There is no preventive vaccine.

Symptoms and Diagnostic Path

Patients may have all or some of the following symptoms: fever, vomiting, stiff neck, headache, lethargy, seizure, and coma.

Treatment Options and Outlook

There is no specific therapy, but most patients recover. The disease is fatal in fewer than 1 percent of cases.

See also ENCEPHALITIS, CALIFORNIA; ENCEPHALITIS, JAPANESE; ENCEPHALITIS, ST. LOUIS; ENCEPHALITIS, TICK-BORNE; ENCEPHALITIS, WESTERN EQUINE; ENCEPHALITIS, WEST NILE; ENCEPHALITIS LETHARGICA; ENCEPHALOMYELITIS.

encephalitis, St. Louis An ARBOVIRAL INFECTION causing ENCEPHALITIS or MENINGITIS that is transmitted from birds to humans by the bite of an infected mosquito. It is found most often in the central and southern United States and can sometimes be fatal.

Areas with open drainage ditches, old tires, or stagnant water are most likely to experience an outbreak.

More than 3,000 people were infected in a 1933 outbreak in St. Louis, from which this version of the disease was named. Since then, it has caused similar major outbreaks. The last large outbreak in 1975 sickened 2,800 people in 31 states. Los Angeles has experienced outbreaks every year since 1984. Outbreaks usually occur in August and September. Since 1964 there have been 4,478 reported human cases of St. Louis encephalitis with about 128 cases reported each year. The last major epidemic occurred in the Midwest between 1974 and 1977. The most recent outbreak occurred in New Orleans in 1999, with 20 cases.

St. Louis encephalitis is a disease that primarily affects animals, but as the above numbers indicate, it occasionally crosses the species barrier.

Most adults who live in mosquito-prone areas are immune because they were bitten as children, and their immune systems produced antibodies that protect them later. By old age, however, these antibodies have usually disappeared, and the elderly are once again susceptible to infection.

The virus enters the human bloodstream from the bite of an infected *Culex* mosquito, where it travels to the brain and spinal cord, multiples in the nervous system and inflames and damages nerve cells.

Symptoms and Diagnostic Path

Only a few people (1 percent) who have this type of encephalitis ever develop symptoms. Most of those who do report a flu-like illness characterized by headache, malaise, fever, stiff neck, delirium, and convulsions. There may be visual and speech problems, walking difficulty, and personality changes. Symptoms typically appear between five and 15 days after a mosquito bite.

Elderly patients are most at risk for serious symptoms; 20 percent of them die. Those at risk include patients with high blood pressure or heart disease, but most people—even those who are seriously ill—recover completely. The fatality rate is 3 percent to 30 percent.

A doctor may perform either EEG or CT brain scan, which will reveal abnormalities but will not pinpoint the cause of the brain inflammation. Antibodies can be found in the blood and cerebrospinal fluid, and sometimes the virus itself is found in brain tissue of those who have died from the disease.

Treatment Options and Outlook

There is no cure for this viral disease. Public health officials monitor the mosquito activity and infection rates in birds; when rates are high, a mosquito alert is issued.

After an infection, a few patients will experience long-term damage such as weakness, seizures, facial palsies, or mental deterioration. These symptoms may improve gradually.

See also ENCEPHALITIS, CALIFORNIA; ENCEPHALITIS, EASTERN EQUINE; ENCEPHALITIS, JAPANESE; ENCEPHALITIS, LA CROSSE; ENCEPHALITIS, TICK-BORNE; ENCEPHALITIS, WESTERN EQUINE; ENCEPHALITIS, WEST NILE; ENCEPHALITIS LETHARGICA; ENCEPHALOMYELITIS.

encephalitis, tick-borne   A viral infection of the central nervous system caused by a tick bite, usually in people who visit or work in forested areas. Tick-borne ENCEPHALITIS occurs in eastern Europe, Russia, and the former Soviet republics from April through August, when the ticks are alive.

In addition to the bite of ticks, this type of encephalitis can be transmitted by consuming unpasteurized dairy products from infected animals.

Symptoms and Diagnostic Path

Symptoms appear between one to two weeks after the bite of an infected tick or after ingesting infected dairy products and resemble symptoms of mosquito-borne encephalitis.

Treatment Options and Outlook

Treatment is symptomatic. There is no cure.

Risk Factors and Preventive Measures

Vaccines have been developed and are available in most endemic areas; no such vaccine is available for use in the United States.

See also ENCEPHALITIS, CALIFORNIA; ENCEPHALITIS, EASTERN EQUINE; ENCEPHALITIS, JAPANESE; ENCEPHALITIS, LA CROSSE; ENCEPHALITIS, ST. LOUIS; ENCEPHALITIS, WESTERN EQUINE; ENCEPHALITIS, WEST NILE; ENCEPHALITIS LETHARGICA; ENCEPHALOMYELITIS.

encephalitis, western equine   Similar to eastern equine ENCEPHALITIS, this virus affects horses and humans; this version affects humans primarily in the central and western plains of the United States. It is much rarer than its eastern cousin, with more than 639 confirmed cases since 1964. Human infections are usually first detected in June or July.

The disease is caused by the western equine encephalitis virus, which is closely related to the eastern and Venezuelan equine encephalitis viruses. Virus flourishes in birds that live near irrigated fields and farming areas.

Symptoms and Diagnostic Path

Symptoms, which appear between five to 10 days after being bitten, range from mild flu-like illness to full-blown encephalitis, coma, and death. While western equine encephalitis is less often fatal than its eastern cousin, it is still serious and can lead to brain damage and other major complications in about 13 percent of people infected with the disease. About 3 percent of those who develop severe symptoms will die.

Treatment Options and Outlook

Treatment is supportive.

See also ENCEPHALITIS, CALIFORNIA; ENCEPHALITIS, EASTERN EQUINE; ENCEPHALITIS, JAPANESE; ENCEPHALITIS, LA CROSSE; ENCEPHALITIS, ST. LOUIS; ENCEPHALITIS, TICK-BORNE; ENCEPHALITIS, WEST NILE; ENCEPHALITIS LETHARGICA; ENCEPHALOMYELITIS.

encephalitis, West Nile   An infection of the brain caused by the WEST NILE VIRUS, a flavivirus commonly found in Africa, West Asia, and the Middle East and now also common in the United States. It is closely related to St. Louis encephalitis virus found in the United States. The West Nile virus first appeared in the United States in 1999.

West Nile virus infections first appeared in the United States in 1999, when 62 cases of severe disease (with seven deaths) occurred in New York and quickly began spreading across the country. By

October 2002, the nation's death toll from the virus had risen to 160, with almost 3,000 cases. Between January 1, 2004, and January 11, 2005, West Nile virus caused 2,470 cases of disease, including 88 death, according to the CENTERS FOR DISEASE CONTROL AND PREVENTION (CDC). Human cases have now been reported from coast to coast and in Canada. No reliable estimates are available for the number of cases in other parts of the world.

In the temperate parts of the world, West Nile encephalitis occurs most often in late summer and early fall, although the virus can be transmitted all year in warm climates. In addition to West Nile encephalitis, the virus also may cause West Nile mengitis (an inflammation of the covering of the brain) and the less serious West Nile fever (with no evidence of brain involvement).

West Nile encephalitis is transmitted primarily via mosquitoes. It is not possible to get the disease from touching or kissing a person who has the disease, or from a health-care worker. However, the disease is believed to have infected the nation's blood supply. The CDC has received reports that 15 patients were diagnosed after receiving blood products. The disease also may be rarely transmitted via breast milk.

After the bite of an infected mosquito, West Nile virus multiplies in the blood and crosses the blood-brain barrier to reach the brain. There, the virus interferes with normal central nervous system functioning and inflames brain tissue. Everyone who lives in an area where the virus has been identified is at risk of getting West Nile encephalitis, but those over age 50 have the highest risk of severe disease.

Although ticks infected with West Nile virus have been found in Asia and Africa, their role in the transmission and maintenance of the virus is uncertain. However, there is no information to suggest that ticks played any role in the cases identified in the United States.

Symptoms and Diagnostic Path

Most infections are mild, and symptoms include fever, headache, and body aches, occasionally with skin rash and swollen lymph glands. More severe infection may be marked by headache, high fever, neck stiffness, stupor, disorientation, coma, trem-

ors, convulsions, muscle weakness, paralysis, and, rarely, death. Less than 1 percent of people infected with West Nile virus will develop severe illness; the disease is most likely to become severe in older people and those with weakened immune systems. Symptoms generally appear within five to 15 days of being bitten by an infected mosquito. Death rates range from 3 percent to 15 percent.

If a patient is at high risk and has symptoms of West Nile encephalitis, the doctor will send a blood sample to a commercial or public health laboratory for confirmation.

Treatment Options and Outlook

There is no specific therapy. Patients who are severely ill may require hospitalization, intravenous fluids, airway management, a ventilator, prevention of secondary infections, and good nursing care.

See also ENCEPHALITIS, CALIFORNIA; ENCEPHALITIS, EASTERN EQUINE; ENCEPHALITIS, JAPANESE; ENCEPHALITIS, LA CROSSE; ENCEPHALITIS, ST. LOUIS; ENCEPHALITIS, TICK-BORNE; ENCEPHALITIS, WESTERN EQUINE; ENCEPHALITIS LETHARGICA; ENCEPHALOMYELITIS.

encephalitis lethargica An epidemic form of ENCEPHALITIS that has not occurred in the United States in mass numbers since 1920, although an occasional sporadic case occurs now and then. The symptoms in this case are the same as for other encephalitis, with the addition of extreme lethargy and drowsiness.

During major epidemics, about 40 percent of the patients died. Many of those who survived later developed a movement disorder known as post-encephalitic parkinsonism, characterized by tremors, rigidity, immobility, and disturbed eye movements.

A few survivors of the last epidemic were still alive in the 1970s when a new antiparkinsonism drug (levodopa) remarkably improved their condition. Unfortunately, after almost 50 years of immobility, most sufferers did not appear to be able to cope with their awakening and lapsed back into their former stupor.

See also ENCEPHALITIS, CALIFORNIA; ENCEPHALITIS, EASTERN EQUINE; ENCEPHALITIS, JAPANESE; ENCEPHALITIS, LA CROSSE; ENCEPHALITIS, ST. LOUIS; ENCEPHALI-

TIS, TICK-BORNE; ENCEPHALITIS, WESTERN EQUINE; ENCEPHALITIS, WEST NILE; ENCEPHALOMYELITIS.

encephalomyelitis Also called equine encephalitis (ENCEPHALITIS, EASTERN EQUINE), this disease is characterized by an inflammation of the brain and spinal cord (as opposed to ENCEPHALITIS, which refers to inflammation of the brain alone). There are various applications of the terms *encephalitis* and *encephalomyelitis*. *Encephalomyelitis* is now the usual term in animal diseases.

While encephalomyelitis is now also called "sleeping sickness," it should not be confused with African sleeping sickness (TRYPANOSOMIASIS) caused by a protozoan.

The agents most often involved in human infections are the viruses of St. Louis encephalitis (ENCEPHALITIS, ST. LOUIS), western equine encephalomyelitis, California encephalitis (ENCEPHALITIS, CALIFORNIA) and MUMPS virus, ECHOVIRUSes, and COXSACKIE VIRUS.

Encephalomyelitis also sometimes occurs in domestic animals. Avian encephalomyelitis (also called "crazy chick disease" or "epidemic tremor") is a viral disease of young chickens, characterized by profound weakness, paralysis, and head and neck trembles. Sporadic bovine encephalomyelitis ("Buss disease") is an uncommon infection of cattle by the bacterium *Chlamydia*. Porcine encephalomyelitis is a viral infection of pigs that does not usually cause symptoms.

Symptoms and Diagnostic Path
The most common symptoms of encephalomyelitis in humans and horses is mental impairment. In humans, symptoms include weakness, discomfort, headache, nausea before drowsiness, confusion, stiff neck, and seizures. Permanent complications are common in infants and children who survive. Signs of the disease in horses include fever, loss of appetite, discomfort, mental deterioration, head pressing, circling, and blindness. Death occurs two to three days after infection, caused by the sudden inability to breathe.

Treatment Options and Outlook
There is no specific treatment for viral encephalomyelitis in animals or humans. Disease caused by

bacteria, fungi, or protozoa—which is much more rare—involves cause-specific therapy.

Risk Factors and Preventive Measures
Horses and poultry can be vaccinated against viral Venezuelan equine encephalomyelitis.

See also ENCEPHALITIS, CALIFORNIA; ENCEPHALITIS, EASTERN EQUINE; ENCEPHALITIS, JAPANESE; ENCEPHALITIS, LA CROSSE; ENCEPHALITIS LETHARGICA; ENCEPHALITIS, ST. LOUIS; ENCEPHALITIS, TICK-BORNE; ENCEPHALITIS, WESTERN EQUINE; ENCEPHALITIS, WEST NILE.

endometritis An inflammation of the lining of the uterus (endometrium) usually caused by infection with chlamydia, GONORRHEA, or TUBERCULOSIS. Endometritis also may occur after surgery, childbirth, abortion, or intrauterine device (IUD) insertion. Other risk factors may include a history of fallopian tube or cervical infection, or other pelvic infections.

Symptoms and Diagnostic Path
General discomfort, fever, lower abdominal or pelvic pain, abnormal vaginal bleeding or discharge, discomfort with bowel movement, constipation, or abdominal distention.

Physical exam plus tests including a white blood count, cultures for sexually transmitted diseases, and often a biopsy of the uterine lining.

Treatment Options and Outlook
Most cases of endometritis respond to antibiotics, but more complicated cases may require hospitalization and intravenous antibiotics. The simultaneous treatment of sexual partners and the use of condoms throughout the course of treatment is essential.

Untreated, endometritis can lead to more serious infection and result in complications with pelvic organs, reproduction, and general health.

See also CHLAMYDIAL INFECTIONS.

endothrix A superficial fungus whose growth and spore production are confined primarily within the hair shaft, without forming conspicuous spores on the outside of the hair.

endotoxin shock See SEPTIC SHOCK.

Entamoeba histolytica A species of amoeba that cause amoebic dysentery and hepatic AMEBIASIS in humans.

Human cases are diagnosed by finding cysts in the stool. In most cases, amoebas remain in the gastrointestinal tract of the hosts. Severe ulceration of the stomach and intestinal surfaces occur in less than 16 percent of cases. Occasionally, the parasite invades the soft tissues, most commonly the liver. Only rarely are masses formed (amoebomas) that lead to intestinal obstruction. Fatalities are rare.

The most dramatic incident of infection with this type of amoeba in the United States occurred during the Chicago World's Fair in 1933, when drinking water was contaminated with sewage from defective plumbing. More than 1,000 cases occurred, with 58 deaths. In recent times, food handlers are suspected of causing many scattered infections, but there has been no single large outbreak.

enteric fever See TYPHOID FEVER.

enteritis Inflammation of the lining of the intestine from a variety of causes, including bacterial or viral infections. If both the large and small intestines are involved, the problem is known as enterocolitis. Gastroenteritis, on the other hand, refers to an inflammation of the stomach and intestines and accompanies a variety of disorders.

enterobiasis A parasitic infestation of the intestines by the common pinworm (*Enterobius vermicularis*).

Pinworm is believed to be the most common worm infection in the United States. School-age children and preschoolers have the highest rates of infection. It is also common for more than one family member to be infected, although adults are less likely to have pinworm infection symptoms. Pinworms are about an inch long and since they live in the human rectum, acquired the nickname "seatworm."

People can become infected after accidentally swallowing pinworm eggs from contaminated surfaces or fingers. Once the worms have infected a human, the female pinworms leave the intestines through the anus and deposit eggs on the surrounding skin. Pinworm eggs are infective within a few hours after being deposited on the skin, and can survive up to two weeks on clothing, bedding, or other objects.

Symptoms and Diagnostic Path
Symptoms include itching and sleeplessness caused by the presence of the worm crawling in the perianal area to lay its eggs.

Tape is applied to the skin around the perianal area and then examined under a microscope for the presence of worm eggs.

Treatment Options and Outlook
An entire household may need to be treated to make sure all pinworms are destroyed. Therapy may include treatment with one of a variety of medications: piperazine, pyrantel pamoate, pyrvinium pamoate, or thiabendazole.

Risk Factors and Preventive Measures
Disinfection procedures in the home do little good in preventing infection.

To reduce continuous self-infection, bathing upon awakening can help reduce the egg contamination. Underwear, nightclothes, and sheets should be changed and washed daily. Because the eggs are sensitive to sunlight, blinds or curtains should be opened in bedrooms during the day. Personal hygiene should include washing hands after going to the toilet, before eating, and after changing diapers, and fingernails should be trimmed. Nail-biting and scratching bare anal areas should be avoided, which can be difficult because the anus is intensely itchy at night.

Cleaning and vacuuming the entire house are probably not necessary or effective. Children may return to day care after the first treatment dose, after bathing, and after trimming and scrubbing nails.

Enterobius vermicularis A common parasitic nematode (known also as pinworm, seatworm, or threadworm) that resembles a small, thin white thread.

These tiny parasitic worms live in the large intestine. The female worms lay their eggs around the anus at night. The worms are spread when a person touches the anal area of an infected individual, then touches the mouth, transferring and swallowing the eggs. Pinworms can be spread as long as either worms or eggs are present, and eggs can survive up to two weeks away from a human host.

See also ENTEROBIASIS.

Enterococcus   The former term for 12 species of *Streptococcus*-like bacteria that inhabit the human gastrointestinal tract. The bacteria are now grouped in their own genus, since they differ from more traditional strep germs.

Enterococcus faecium and *E. faecalis* are two that are particularly dangerous, since they are now becoming highly resistant to antibiotics. These antibiotic-resistant organisms first appeared in the 1980s in New York City hospitals, where they led to the death of 19 out of 100 patients infected with the bacteria.

In 1997, 52 percent and 83 percent of *Enterococcus*-related illness were resistant to vancomycin and ampicillin respectively. Vancomycin-resistant enterococcus (VRE) is a mutant strain of Enterococcus that originally developed in patients who were exposed to vancomycin. VRE was first identified in Europe in 1986 and in the United States two years later. VRE is not dangerous in healthy people with an intact immune systems, because the healthy bacteria in the digestive tract helps control VRE. However, VRE is dangerous because it cannot be controlled with antibiotics and can cause life-threatening infections in people with impaired immune systems, including the very young, the very old, and the very sick.

VRE is particularly dangerous because it can easily transmit its "resistance genes" to more dangerous bacteria such as streptococcus and staphlococcus.

enterotoxin   A type of bacteria-released poison that inflames the lining of the intestine, causing vomiting and diarrhea. Staphylococcal food poisoning is caused by eating food contaminated with an enterotoxin produced by staphylococci bacteria. The toxin is resistant to heat and is not destroyed by cooking. The severe diarrhea and vomiting associated with CHOLERA is also caused by an enterotoxin produced in the intestine by the cholera bacteria.

enterovirus   A group of viruses that multiply primarily in the intestinal tract. This group includes the COXSACKIE VIRUS, ECHOVIRUS, and polio virus. Others can trigger MENINGITIS, ENCEPHALITIS, respiratory illness, diarrhea, CONJUNCTIVITIS, and a host of other diseases, including the common COLD.

Any one of the enteroviruses can produce a wide variety of symptoms that may mimic symptoms produced by other enteroviruses. They are very difficult to kill and are not affected by antibiotics or most disinfectants. They can survive temperatures of up to 122°F and are found throughout the Tropics and subtropics; however, they appear to prefer late summer or early fall in cooler climates. While they can be inactivated in the presence of chlorine, the smallest amount of organic matter will protect them so that they can survive most attempts at public water purification.

Most children are infected with some types of enteroviruses at a young age; in general, these viruses cause older people to suffer more serious symptoms, with infection.

Enteroviruses have been found along beaches miles from the nearest offshore dump site; swimmers are at high risk for infection, since the easiest way into the human body is through the mouth.

See also ANTIDIARRHEAL DRUGS; DIARRHEA AND INFECTIOUS DISEASE; TRAVELER'S DIARRHEA.

epidemic   The occurrence of more cases of disease than one would expect under normal circumstances. The term also describes the pattern of certain diseases that markedly ebb and flow over a short period of time. (For example, prior to the development of the measles vaccine, large numbers of measles cases would occur in waves.)

When a disease sweeps over broad geographic areas at one time, creating widespread epidemics, the disease is referred to as being *pandemic*. The INFLUENZA virus of 1918 was a pandemic, as HIV is today.

In Europe during the Middle Ages at least one-fourth of all deaths were caused by epidemic diseases.

Major epidemics have included AIDS, EBOLA, PLAGUE, CHOLERA, polio, TYPHUS, SMALLPOX, and YELLOW FEVER. Some epidemics, such as the yearly sweep of flu viruses, are relatively harmless if the patient's immune system is healthy and patients have been properly vaccinated. Other epidemics have become more of a concern, including the AIDS outbreak, the 1993 outbreak of HANTAVIRUS, and regular outbreaks of a new and deadly strain of *ESCHERICHIA COLI*. Since 1985, TUBERCULOSIS has been more prevalent in the United States due in part to drug-resistant forms of the disease. Mutated forms of pneumococcal PNEUMONIA have become resistant to antibiotics and are a rising epidemic concern.

epidemiology The scientific discipline that seeks to detect disease causes and to determine preventive measures. The focus of epidemiology is on diseases as they occur in defined groups, rather than as they affect individuals.

epiglottitis Inflammation of the epiglottis, a thin flap of cartilage lying behind the root of the tongue that covers the entrance to the larynx during swallowing. Acute epiglottitis is a severe, life-threatening form of the condition that usually affects children.

In the past, epiglottitis was caused by *Haemophilus influenzae* type B, an aggressive bacterium that at one time caused many serious infections in children under age five. The vaccine against this bacteria has essentially wiped out all cases of *H. influenzae* epiglottitis, MENINGITIS, CELLULITIS, and PNEUMONIA, diseases that used to kill or cripple several thousand children a year. Rare cases of epiglottitis still occur, now caused by other bacteria such as *Staphylococcus aureus*, *Streptococcus pneumoniae*, and *Streptococcus pyogenes*.

Symptoms and Diagnostic Path
The severe form is characterized by sore throat, fever, noisy breathing, croupy cough, and a swollen epiglottis. The patient may turn blue and require an emergency tracheostomy to maintain breathing.

Treatment Options and Outlook
Securing an airway with either a breathing tube or tracheostomy followed by antibiotics, rest, oxygen, and supportive care.

Epstein-Barr virus (EBV) One of the most common universal human viruses, the EBV causes infectious MONONUCLEOSIS. A member of the HERPES family, EBV was named for the two scientists who discovered it in 1964.

It infects most people sometime during their lives, usually after childhood; as many as 95 percent of American adults between ages 35 and 40 have been infected. In the United States and other developed countries, many children are not infected by the virus; if they are, they will not usually have any symptoms. If a child becomes infected during adolescence, the virus causes infectious mononucleosis. About 10 percent of high school and college students become infected each year in the United States, of whom more than half develop infectious mononucleosis. In poor countries with lower standards of hygiene, however, most children are infected by the time they are six years old, when the disease is mild and almost unnoticeable.

Transmission of the EBV is not understood but is believed to require contact with saliva of an infected person, since the virus is not normally transmitted through air or blood. EBV does not leave the body. It establishes a lifelong dormant infection in some of the body's immune system cells. A very few carriers will go on to develop Burkitt's lymphoma and head and neck cancer. EBV appears to play a major role in the development of these cancers, but it is not considered to be the only cause.

During the 1980s, the virus was linked to a syndrome featuring severe fatigue diagnosed as CHRONIC FATIGUE SYNDROME (CFS), because some sufferers had above-average levels of Epstein-Barr virus antibodies in their blood. Scientists suspected that the virus's ability to reactivate after long periods of time could mean it had something to do with the debilitating condition of CFS. This theory has since been abandoned.

Risk Factors and Preventive Measures
At least one drug company is currently testing a vaccine against the EBV.

equine morbillivirus (EM) The former name for HENDRA VIRUS.

erysipelas Contagious infection of the facial skin and subcutaneous tissue caused by group A beta-hemolytic streptococci and marked by rapid-spreading redness and swelling. The bacteria are believed to enter the skin through a small lesion. Although this disease is contagious, it does not produce EPIDEMICS.

Before the advent of antibiotics, this disease could be fatal (especially for infants and the elderly). Today, it is quickly controlled with prompt treatment. However, since the late 1980s an increasing incidence of this condition has been noted.

Symptoms and Diagnostic Path

After a five- to seven-day incubation period, the patient experiences a sudden high fever with headache, malaise, and vomiting. The skin feels tight, uncomfortable, itchy, and red, with patches appearing most often on the face, spreading across the cheeks and bridge of the nose. It also occurs on the scalp, genitals, hands, and legs. Within the inflammation, pimples appear, blister, burst, and crust over.

Treatment Options and Outlook

PENICILLIN will cure the infection within seven days. Bed rest, hot packs, and aspirin for pain and fever may also help. Erysipelas is fatal in less than 1 percent of treated cases, usually among the very young, old, and immuno compromised.

erythema annulare centrifugum This is one of a group of "reactive erythemas" characterized by expanding ring-shaped plaques. The lesions, which are usually found on the trunk, enlarge slowly. Although the disorder can occur at any age, most patients are young adults when stricken. Symptoms may last for only a short time, or they may persist for decades, depending on the cause.

This type of erythema may be caused by a DERMATOPHYTE infection, fungus infection (*CANDIDA ALBICANS*), blue cheese ingestion, cancer, parasitic bowel disease, or autoimmune disorder.

Symptoms and Diagnostic Path

The lesions of this condition may appear as chronic ring-shaped, reddened skin eruptions that may appear at any time from infancy to old age. The lesion usually begins as a small, raised, pink-red spot that slowly enlarges and forms a ring, as the central area flattens and clears. Occasionally, the lesions grow into irregular shapes that do not look like rings. The lesions, which may appear alone or in groups, most often occur on the thighs and legs but also may be located on the face, trunk, and arms. Some patients may experience mild itching. The disease can be diagnosed by lab studies of skin scrapings and a biopsy sample.

Treatment Options and Outlook

Treating the underlying cause (such as fungus or parasite) will effectively cure the redness.

erythema chronicum migrans A skin lesion that is the initial sign of LYME DISEASE. It begins as a small papule and spreads, extending by a raised red margin and clearing in the center. It marks the site of a deer tick bite.

erythema infectiosum See FIFTH DISEASE.

erythema nodosum An inflammatory skin disease associated with an infectious agent or drug sensitivity to sulfonamides, PENICILLIN, salicylates, or others. The eruption of reddish-purple swellings on the skin also may be a result of another illness, such as inflammatory bowel disease, collagen disease, lymphoma, leukemia, or some other condition. It occurs most often in women between ages 20 and 50, although the disease can appear in both sexes at any age.

Pain may be severe and disabling, but permanent problems from this disease are rare. Lesions usually disappear within one or two months, although the disorder can recur.

Streptococcal throat infection is the most common underlying cause, although this disorder is also associated with TUBERCULOSIS. About 30 percent of the time no cause can be found. The exact mechanism behind the disease is not known, although it is believed to be some type of immune reaction around large blood vessels in the subcutaneous fat.

Symptoms and Diagnostic Path

Shiny, tender swellings of up to four inches across appear suddenly on shins, thighs, and sometimes arms. There is usually also fever and pain in muscles and joints, and there may be other symptoms including chills, malaise, headache, or sore throat.

Treatment Options and Outlook

The underlying illness should be treated. Bed rest with the legs raised is important; for ambulatory patients, support stockings may help. Warm water compresses may be soothing, and tenting the bedcovers may relieve discomfort from lesions rubbing against material. Otherwise, treatment may include painkillers or sometimes nonsteroidal anti-inflammatory drugs to reduce inflammation. While corticosteroids may also be used, they reduce the patient's resistance if the erythema is caused by infection; the drugs may also interfere with diagnostic tests. Even when the cause is not known, the prognosis for recovery is good.

erythrasma A bacterial infection of skin folds, including the groin and underarms, that causes mild burning and itching. It is more common in warmer climates and among diabetics.

The infection is caused by *Corynebacterium minutissimum.* Recurrences are common.

Symptoms and Diagnostic Path

Erythrasma does not usually cause any symptoms. It presents as a slowly enlarging area of pink or brown dry skin. The diagnosis can be confirmed by a swab or scraping for microscopy and culture.

Treatment Options and Outlook

C. minutissimum is very sensitive to a wide variety of antimicrobial drugs; extensive cases may also require oral administration of erythromycin. Tolnaftate and Whitfield's ointment also are beneficial.

Escherichia A genus of gram-negative rodlike bacteria that may infect in the intestines of humans and other animals.

Escherichia coli (E. coli) A species of coliform bacteria of the family Enterobacteriaceae that is normally found in the intestines, milk, water, and soil.

Part of its potential danger is that its many different strains are capable of reproducing at extraordinary rates, doubling its population every two hours. (If enough food was available, one *E. coli* cell could reproduce into a mass bigger than the Earth in three days). Fortunately, most of the strains are harmless to the majority of people most of the time.

Named for the 19th-century German physician Theodor Escherich who identified it, the bacterium is the most frequent cause of urinary tract infections and is commonly found in wounds. *E. coli* blood poisoning can be rapidly fatal as a result of shock because of the action of an endotoxin released by the bacteria.

There are five groups of *E. coli* whose toxins can cause TRAVELER'S DIARRHEA. The most severe is *ESCHERICHIA COLI* O157:H7 that can cause kidney failure and a fatal bloody diarrhea.

See also ANTIDIARRHEAL DRUGS; COLIFORM COUNT; DIARRHEA AND INFECTIOUS DISEASE.

Escherichia coli (E. coli) O157:H7 One of the most deadly of the hundreds of strains of the bacterium *ESCHERICHIA COLI.* Although most strains of *E. coli* are harmless and live in the intestines of both humans and animals, the rare O157:H7 strain produces a powerful toxin that can cause severe illness. It has emerged during the past 10 years as a cause of food-borne illness that can lead to kidney failure and death.

This mutation, which was discovered in 1982, has at least 62 subtypes. The combination of letters and numbers in the name of this bacterium refers to specific markers found on its surface and distinguishes it from other types of *E. coli.* This type of *E. coli* food poisoning cases appears to be increasing, as has the frequency of complications from infection.

An estimated 73,000 cases of infection and 61 deaths occur in the United States each year, most associated with eating undercooked, contaminated ground beef. This is part of an estimated total of about 7 million cases of food-borne illness in general.

The disease was first recognized as a cause of illness in 1982 during an outbreak of bloody diarrhea that was traced to contaminated hamburgers. During this outbreak, scientists discovered that the *E. coli* O157:H7 strain had somehow acquired the gene for Shiga toxin, caused by the organism *Shigella dysenteriae.* This strain of *E. coli* caused three outbreaks in 1982 among scores of patients who came down with an alarming type of bloody diarrhea.

The strain continued to appear sporadically until, in 1993, four children died and hundreds more became sick after eating *E. coli*—tainted hamburger in a fast-food restaurant in Washington. The incident set off a furor throughout the country as consumer safety groups urged the government to improve its meat inspection system.

The Washington outbreak was followed within months by more outbreaks of food-borne illness caused by *E. coli,* forcing the closing of two other restaurants and sickening 60 more consumers. Annually, the U.S. CENTERS FOR DISEASE CONTROL AND PREVENTION (CDC) estimates that *E. coli* alone is responsible for 20,000 cases of food poisoning, although these estimates may not be accurate, since physicians are not required to report these poisonings.

A study by the Western States Meats Association found the common bacteria *Escherichia coli (E. coli)* was present in 1.5 percent of ground pork and also in poultry, and 3.7 percent in beef.

In the past, people got *E. coli* food poisoning by drinking tap water in foreign countries. In the wake of the reported mass poisonings and deaths from *E. coli,* the government vowed to revamp the federal meat inspection system, which had relied on visual inspections. In related action, the USDA issued new labels for raw meat and poultry that discussed safe handling and cooking methods.

The Shiga gene has continued to spread, and has now been found in other strains of *E. coli,* as well as other bacteria common to the human intestine (such as *Enterobacter*).

Recent EPIDEMICS have included the September 1999 case of 10 children hospitalized with *E. coli* 0517:H7 infection after attending the Washington County Fair.

Outbreaks have been traced to many different types of food. It has been found to survive in dry fermented meat despite production standards that meet federal and industry food processing requirements, scientists say. It has been found in salami, where the bacteria may have been present on raw meat that was brought into a plant and subsequently survived the fermentation and drying steps involved in salami production.

Primarily, the organism is found in cattle farms, since it lives in the intestines of healthy cattle. Meat becomes contaminated during slaughter, and organisms can be mixed with beef when it is ground in huge vats. Alternatively, bacteria on a cow's udders or on milking equipment can find its way into raw milk.

Since contaminated meat looks and smells normal, it is possible to eat tainted meat unknowingly. Although the number of organisms needed to cause disease is not known, it is believed to be very small.

The problem is not with steak; a bit of bacterial contamination on the surface of a steak is not much of a threat because it is quickly killed when the surface of the meat is cooked. It is the practice of grinding the meat that gives bacteria its chance. When a contaminated steak is minced up and mixed with other beef from other animals, the bacteria become widely distributed—not just on the surface, but throughout the meat. Contaminated and undercooked hamburger is suspected of causing more than half of all outbreaks of bloody diarrhea. Many outbreaks have begun in fast-food restaurants, but since the large chains have begun to sample their meat, the real problem today lies in grocery store hamburger, according to experts. The meat in grocery stores, the experts say, goes largely untested.

The toxin-making bacteria are killed only if the hamburger is cooked to an inside temperature of 155°F, hot enough to eliminate all meat pinkness.

Drinking unpasteurized milk or swimming in or drinking sewage-contaminated water can also cause infection. In July 1991, 80 people were infected while swimming in an Oregon lake. In July 1993, 35,000 New Yorkers had to boil their water because the specific *E. coli* strain eluded chlorination and appeared in New York's tap water.

The disease can also be transmitted from person to person through contact with contaminated stool, if hygiene or handwashing is not adequate. This is especially common in day-care centers and among toddlers who are not yet toilet trained.

Symptoms and Diagnostic Path
The *E. coli* O157:H7 bacterium produces toxins that cause hemorrhagic colitis, with severe cramps and

then watery or bloody diarrhea, lasting for several days. Other symptoms include nausea and vomiting appearing within hours to a week after eating; there is usually no fever. Most people recover quickly and completely, but the complications are what make this a serious disease.

In certain people at risk (such as among the very young or old), the bacteria may cause HEMOLYTIC UREMIC SYNDROME (HUS), in which the red blood cells are destroyed and the kidneys fail. Up to 15 percent of infections lead to this complication. In the United States, HUS is the main cause of kidney failure in children; most cases are caused by infection with this type of E. coli.

In the elderly, HUS plus fever and neurologic symptoms may be fatal in as many as 50 percent of patients.

Patients are infectious for about six days while bacteria are being excreted in the stool. There is no solid evidence, but it appears that victims can get this infection more than once.

The infection is diagnosed by identifying the bacterium in stool. Most labs that culture stool do not test for E. coli O157:H7, so it is important to request that the stool be tested for this organism or its toxin. Everyone with sudden diarrhea and bleeding should have the stool checked for this bacterium.

Treatment Options and Outlook

Most patients recover within 10 days without need of specific treatment. There is no evidence that antibiotics help, and there is some evidence to suggest it may set off kidney problems. Antidiarrhea medicine should also be avoided.

HUS, on the other hand, is a life-threatening condition that is treated in a hospital intensive care unit, with blood transfusions and kidney dialysis. With intensive care, the death rate from this complication is between 3 and 5 percent. There is no cure for HUS.

Patients who have had only mild infection, with diarrhea, usually recover completely. Of those who develop HUS, one third have abnormal kidney function years later and a few need long-term dialysis. Another 8 percent suffer with other complications, including high blood pressure, seizures, blindness, and paralysis for the rest of their lives.

Adults may get an extremely serious bleeding disorder called thrombotic thrombocytopenic purpura, in which blood stops clotting; small red spots and large bruises appear all over the body, and blood oozes through the mouth. The outlook is not promising for patients with this complication.

Risk Factors and Preventive Measures

To protect against this type of food poisoning, travelers should not drink untreated water and ice or eat salads, raw fruits and vegetables that cannot be peeled, and unpasteurized milk products. Diners should always make sure hamburgers are well done.

Consumers can prevent infection by thoroughly cooking ground beef, avoiding unpasteurized milk and washing hands carefully. Undercooked ground beef should not be served to young children, the elderly, or anyone with an impaired immune system.

When caring for an infected patient, hand washing is crucial to avoid person-to-person spread of the disease. About 38 states now ask doctors to report outbreaks of the disease but none regularly test for other strains of E. coli that produce the toxin.

See also ANTIDIARRHEAL DRUGS; DIARRHEA AND INFECTIOUS DISEASE.

European swamp fever   See LEPTOSPIROSIS.

exanthem subitum   See ROSEOLA.

exogenous infection   An infection that develops from bacteria normally found outside the body, which is not usually part of the normal human bacterial population.

eye infections   The most common infection of the eye is CONJUNCTIVITIS, also known as pinkeye. Most of these infections are caused by bacteria (such as staphylococci) or by viruses associated with a cold, sore throat, or illness such as MEASLES. Viral conjunctivitis is the version that often appears in schools, sweeping through classrooms in massive EPIDEMICS.

Newborns may contract a type of conjunctivitis from their mothers during birth. This type of infection may be caused by common bacteria, organisms responsible for GONORRHEA or genital HERPES, or by a CHLAMYDIAL INFECTION and may cause blindness in the newborn infant unless treated.

Keratoconjunctivitis is an inflammation of both the conjunctiva and the cornea; it is often caused by a virus. Corneal infections are more serious and can lead to blurry vision or perforation if not treated.

Infection within the eye (endophthalmitis) may make it necessary to remove the eyeball. This can occur after a penetrating injury to the eye, or from infections elsewhere in the body.

F

Fasciola hepatica   The name of the type of liver fluke that causes FASCIOLIASIS.

fascioliasis   Infection with a liver fluke (also called the giant intestinal fluke) found throughout the world, especially the southern and western United States. It is also a common parasite in humans and pigs in central and south China, Taiwan, Southeast Asia, Indonesia, India, and Bangladesh.

The disease is caused by the liver fluke *Fasciola hepatica* and *F. gigantica* acquired by swallowing encysted forms of the fluke in water plants such as raw watercress, water chestnuts, or bamboo shoots. The eggs of the infective fluke are shed in fecal material into water; when they hatch, they produce larvae that penetrate and develop in the flesh of snails. These organisms then escape and develop cysts on various water plants. Humans are infected by eating these plants uncooked; the immature flukes are released from the cysts and develop into adult worms in the small intestine.

Symptoms and Diagnostic Path

Symtoms include pain, fever, jaundice, hives, and diarrhea. Prolonged infection may be related to fibrosis of the liver.

Treatment Options and Outlook

Triclabendazole is the drug of choice; bithionol is an alternative. Most infected people do not have any symptoms, but severe infections occur in very small numbers of people who are infected with large numbers of flukes.

fever   An abnormal internal temperature of the body above "normal" due to disease, although the normal range depends on when and how the temperature is taken. Right after activity, for example, the temperature may rise to 99°F. Rectal temperatures are up to a degree higher and under-the-arm temperatures are usually up to a degree lower than 98.6°F. In addition, normal body temperature is lower in the morning and higher in the late afternoon and evening.

The thermal regulatory center in the brain is responsible for controlling the body's temperature. This setting rises during an infection, resulting in a fever, when white blood cells release certain proteins as part of the immune response that trigger the brain to release a chemical called prostaglandin. This causes the nerve cells to produce a feeling of coldness, which is why a patient experiences chills during the development of fever.

In response to infection, the brain increases the body's temperature, speeding up the activities of the immune system against the invading germs. What this means is that a fever is actually not a bad thing—it can actually help the body fight disease.

However, a very high fever can be uncomfortable and eventually—if it goes high enough—can lead to seizures and death.

A temperature may be taken with an oral, digital, or rectal thermometer. Those who find a traditional thermometer hard to read may find a digital readout thermometer easier. While some doctors rely on this type of instrument, others insist that digital thermometers are not as accurate. A rectal thermometer is used for infants and young children who cannot hold an oral thermometer in their mouths. An oral thermometer should not be used to take a rectal temperature. After each use, the thermometer should be cleaned using lukewarm soapy water and rinsed well with cold water or the thermometer may be rinsed with alcohol followed by cold water. Hot water will break a traditional thermometer.

The course of a fever depends on its cause. The degree of the fever does not really indicate how serious the illness is, however, since severe infections may only cause a low fever, and some mild infections can cause a high fever.

Medicines called antipyretics will bring down a fever; aspirin and acetaminophen work by slowing the production of prostaglandins. Because fevers are beneficial, however, one should only take antipyretics for fevers over 101°F. Anything lower than this is considered to be a low-grade fever. In an infant younger than three months of age, however, any fever over 100.4°F requires medical evaluation. Treating a fever in children lessens the risk of seizures, which tend to run in families and occur in less than 3 percent of normal children up to six

years. Febrile seizures last less than 15 minutes and do not cause brain damage or epilepsy.

Aspirin should not be given to anyone under age 18 because it has been associated with the development of Reye's syndrome in children who have the flu or CHICKEN POX. (Reye's syndrome is a very serious condition affecting the brain and liver.)

If the fever is very high, a cooling tub bath, wet sheet, or ice packs may be ordered.

Children should not be rubbed with alcohol, since the fumes can be dangerous and there is evidence that the alcohol can be absorbed through the skin. A child should not be immersed in cold water, which will reduce the body temperature too quickly.

fever blisters   Another name for COLD SORE.

fifth disease   A viral infection that often affects red blood cells. Fifth disease is also known as "slapped cheeks" disease because of its dramatic bright red rash across the cheeks. Named in 1899 as the fifth of six common childhood illnesses that cause a rash (after MEASLES, MUMPS, CHICKEN POX, and GERMAN MEASLES), it is the least well known of them all.

Among healthy children the disease is mild; once the rash appears they are not contagious and may return to school.

The disease is caused by the parvovirus B19, (not the same parvovirus common in dogs). It usually occurs in small outbreaks among young children in the spring. The virus itself was discovered in England in 1975, but it was not until 1983 that scientists realized it caused fifth disease.

In much the same way as a cold spreads, fifth disease is transmitted via mouth and nose secretions or from contact with contaminated objects. It also may travel through the air in small droplets, and is found in the blood of infected people, so that a blood transfusion could transmit the disease. Outbreaks occur from late winter through spring among school-age children. Adults who have already been infected with the virus are immune.

People with fifth disease appear to be contagious during the week before the rash appears; by the time the rash occurs, the person is probably beyond the contagious period.

WARNING SIGNS FOR FEVER

Any child under age three months with a rectal temperature higher than 100.4°F must see a health care practitioner as soon as possible. A doctor should be called if older infants and children have a fever above 102°F that lasts longer than three days, increases after two days, or if any of the following warning signs develop:

- unusual irritability, screaming, tense or stiff arms or legs
- extreme drowsiness (child hard to wake)
- confusion, delirium, hallucinations
- breathing problems (wheezing, crackling, high-pitched sounds)
- neck pain, stiff neck, holding neck in odd way
- seizures
- sunken or bulging soft spot on head (especially in front)
- vomiting after attempt to give fluids
- dry lips, tongue, and mouth
- no wet diaper or urination in six hours

Arrange doctor's appointment if a fever is accompanied by any of the following symptoms:

- stomach pain
- sore throat, difficulty swallowing
- ear pain; pulling, tugging, or rubbing ear

Symptoms and Diagnostic Path

In children, the illness begins with a headache, slight tiredness, or muscle pain, followed in two or three days by a rash of rosy red spots on the cheeks. Within a few days, the rash has spread over the body, buttocks, and arms and legs. There is often a mild fever in addition to the skin rash. About half the time, the rash will be itchy.

Adults will notice fever and joint pain (especially in the knees) that mimics arthritis and may be severe, flaring up in wet weather and in the morning.

Most babies born to mothers with the disease are normal and healthy, although the virus is able to cross the placenta and infect the fetus. Studies suggest that about 2.5 percent of pregnant women infected with parvovirus have spontaneous abortions or stillbirths.

Those who have sickle-cell disease do not get fifth disease, but when infected with the virus they come down with a more serious infection called aplastic crisis (their bone marrow stops making red blood cells). They require hospitalization and blood transfusions.

Pregnant women can have a test for immunity to parvovirus. These antibody tests are available through state health departments.

In most cases, the disease is diagnosed based on the appearance of typical symptoms. A specific blood test to confirm the diagnosis has recently become available but is not necessary in healthy children.

Treatment Options and Outlook

There is no treatment for fifth disease. With bed rest, clear fluids, and acetaminophen to lower fever, the rash usually clears within 10 days. Red blood cells are given to sickle-cell patients. Fevers over 101°F should be treated; calamine lotion will ease the itch of the rash. Adults may take ibuprofen or another nonsteroidal anti-inflammatory drug (NSAID) for the joint pain.

Those in high-risk groups who contract fifth disease may experience chronic anemic conditions afterward. Those at high risk include anyone with sickle-cell anemia or red blood cell abnormalities, or who is undergoing immunosuppressive treatment for cancer, an organ recipient, or as HIV patient.

While there is no evidence that parvovirus B19 is a significant cause of birth defects, some studies have shown that infection may increase the risk of miscarriage or spontaneous abortion.

Risk Factors and Preventive Measures

As yet there is no way to control the spread of fifth disease.

filariasis A group of tropical diseases caused by a range of parasitic roundworms and larvae that transmit disease to humans. About 200 million people are affected by filariasis, which occurs in tropic and subtropic areas of southeast Asia, South America, Africa, and the Pacific. Mosquitoes inject the worm larvae when they bite, which migrate to the lymph nodes where they develop into mature worms in about a year.

Some of the species live in the lymphatic vessels and block them, causing ELEPHANTIASIS (swelling of limbs with thickened, coarse skin). Another type of worm can be seen and felt just underneath the skin, which produces irritating and painful swellings called calabar swellings.

Bancroftian filariasis (*Wuchereria bancrofti* filarial nematode) is spread widely throughout Africa, southern and southeastern Asia, the Pacific, and the tropical and subtropical regions of South America. Malayan filariasis (*Brugia malayi* filarial nematode) is found only in southern and southeastern Asia. Imported cases of the filariases may be found in the United States, especially among immigrants from the Caribbean and Pacific islands.

Bancroftian and Malayan filariases are transmitted to humans by the bite of an infected mosquito. The infective larvae that are transmitted into humans via the bite pass into the human lymph system, where they develop to maturity during a six- to 12-month period. Fertilized mature female worms release embryos that develop into moving larvae (microfilariae), which appear in the human blood system at night only.

Symptoms and Diagnostic Path

Initial inflammatory symptoms occur between three months to a year after the mosquito bite, with episodes of chills, headache, and fever. The fever is often associated with inflammation of the lymphatic system. There is swelling, redness, and pain in arms, legs, or scrotum.

An ABSCESS may occur as a result of dying worms and secondary bacterial infection. Repeated episodes of inflammation lead to obstruction of the lymphatic system, especially in the genital and leg areas. Chronic swelling stimulates the growth of connective tissue in the skin, causing massive permanent enlargement and deformity (elephantiasis). In Bancroftian filariasis the legs and genitalia are most often involved; in the Malayan variety the portion of the legs below the knees are affected, but genitals are usually spared.

Blood specimen examination for filaria antigen, patient history, and appearance of the patient.

Treatment Options and Outlook

The prognosis is good in early or mild cases, and if the patient can avoid reinfection. Three weeks of diethylcarbamazine cures the infection. However, reactions to large numbers of dying parasites are common (fever, malaise, nausea, and vomiting), so doses are usually low at first. Oral antihistamines may help control hives, and elastic stockings may help control swelling. However, no treatment can reverse elephantiasis. Surgery may ease massive enlargement of the scrotum.

Risk Factors and Preventive Measures

In infested areas, filariasis can be controlled by taking diethylcarbamazine or ivermectin preventively, and by using insecticides, repellents, nets, and protective clothing.

fish and infectious disease The danger of fish contamination is not just with the contaminants they ingest. Because bacteria that live on fish are adapted to withstand the cool and cold waters of lakes and oceans, they can thrive in temperatures cold enough to normally preserve food. These microbes will quickly spoil the fish, unless it is kept at temperatures close to freezing. Even under the best conditions, fish lasts only seven to 12 days; but it often takes seven days for fish to get from the water to the supermarket, where it may sit for several more days. Bacterial decomposition of tuna, mackerel, mahimahi, bluefish, or albacore can cause immediate gastrointestinal problems, rash, and abdominal pain, although symptoms subside after a day or two.

At the fish counter, the word *fresh* is supposed to mean never frozen or heated. In many cases, however, *fresh* means anything the store wants it to mean.

Risk Factors and Preventive Measures

Seafood should look and smell fresh, with vivid skin and bright eyes and no fishy or ammonia odor. It is best to select fish from the bottom of the refrigerator case where it is coldest. At home, it should be kept very cold and eaten within one or two days. Although it is important to cook fish thoroughly, no amount of cooking will destroy contaminants.

The fatty skin should be scraped off before cooking. Pregnant women, nursing mothers, and young children should limit consumption of fish that might have high levels of mercury and PCBs.

After weeks, months, or years of eating contaminated fish, methyl mercury poisoning affects the central nervous system, causing numbness or tingling of mouth, lips, tongue, and extremities; visual disturbances; hearing problems; speech disorders; difficulty swallowing; weakness; fatigue; concentration problems; emotional changes and instability; inability to write, read, or remember simple things; stumbling gait. In severe cases, stupor, coma, and death.

flatworms Any species of worm that has a flat shape (as opposed to a roundworm or nematode, which is shaped cylindrically). There are two types of flatworms that affect humans—cestodes (TAPEWORMS) and trematodes (FLUKES and schistosomes).

See also SCHISTOSOMIASIS.

fleas Throughout history, the bite of the flea has been notorious for causing disease. These wingless bloodsucking insects may transmit ARBOVIRUSES to humans. Certain species of fleas can transmit PLAGUE, murine TYPHUS, and possibly TULAREMIA. Flea bites cause irritation and inflammation, and allergy in those sensitive to flea bites. Fleas can also spread tapeworms from dogs, cats, rats, and mice to humans.

The flea life cycle has four stages: eggs, larvae, pupae, and adults. Female fleas lay as many as 50 eggs a day, starting a life cycle that can be completed in as little as three weeks, depending on temperature and humidity. The eggs hatch into larvae, which feed on flea excrement of partially digested blood. Larvae grow and spin cocoons, where they grow to pupae and then adults. The adult remains in the cocoon until vibrations indicate a host is nearby. This waiting can extend the life cycle. Six-legged adults emerge and attach to a host to feed and breed, beginning the cycle all over again.

flesh-eating bacteria   The popular name for "necrotizing fasciitis," a severe but rare invasive group A strep infection of the skin that can destroy deep muscle in a matter of hours. This type of severe skin infection spreads with an invasive speed that is truly incredible.

Several cases of the disease occurred in 1994 in parts of the northeastern United States, the United Kingdom, and Ontario, Canada. It is more likely to attack adults than children, as well as patients who have just undergone surgery. The cases in Great Britain set off a wave of hysteria about this so-called new disease, and drew massive media attention—even the venerable London *Times* trumpeted that the public should not panic as "death toll rises to 12."

In fact, the country was *not* being gripped by some deadly, new and unknown infection; necrotizing fasciitis appears in about 1,500 to 2,000 cases each year in the United States, killing about 30 percent of those affected. It was described in China as long ago as 1924.

The bacterium releases a toxin that invades the skin, destroying fat and muscle. Scientists believe that the toxin is able to trick the body's immune system so that instead of attacking the bacteria, the cells of the immune system join forces with the toxin to destroy fat and muscle.

Certain strains of group A strep are more likely to cause this invasive disease.

Symptoms and Diagnostic Path
Onset of symptoms is typically rapid; symptoms often begin at the site of a minor wound (or no obvious wound at all) or with breathing problems. There may be swelling of an arm or leg, and the skin is very painful, red, and hot. This may be followed by the appearance of blisters filled with clear fluid, which quickly turn deep red or red-violet, followed by tissue death. The toxins can produce shock and infection throughout the body, with rapid heartbeat and organ failure; onset of illness to hospitalization may take only a day or two. In the most serious cases, death may occur within hours. Reduced blood flow may lead to GANGRENE. Severe pain at the site of infection is an early, and striking, symptom.

The infection is diagnosed with blood cultures or aspiration of pus; surgical exploration may be needed. The clinical appearance is unmistakable as tissue dies and liquefies so quickly.

Treatment Options and Outlook
Prompt medical attention is critical to survival. PENICILLIN is the drug of choice. Surgery (removal of infected tissue and limb amputation) is essential to stop the spread of bacteria. Even with treatment, about one-third of patients stricken with this lethal bacteria will die, and many are significantly disfigured.

flies and infection   Flies are capable of transmitting at least 65 different diseases, including TYPHOID FEVER, DYSENTERY, CHOLERA, and TUBERCULOSIS. They feed on fecal matter, discharge from wounds and sores, and decayed matter such as spoiled food, spreading the disease organisms they pick up by regurgitating and excreting wherever they land. Because the fly's mouth parts are adapted for sponging up liquids, they are able to feed on solid food only by vomiting on it; the saliva liquefies the solid food, which the fly then soaks up.

Houseflies live only about two and a half weeks during the summer, but they can survive up to three months at lower temperatures. Female flies deposit from 100 to 150 eggs in decaying matter (like grass clippings, garbage, or human/animal waste). Depending on the temperature, the eggs hatch into maggots between eight hours and two days later. Mature maggots burrow for protection into dry surrounding areas, where they eventually mature into adult houseflies. Within two days of maturity, adult flies mate again, and the cycle begins anew.

To control the spread of houseflies, it is important to limit their food sources by controlling sanitation. Homeowners should not allow garbage, grass clippings, weed piles, or other decaying organic matter to build up. (Compost piles are not usually a fly-breeding site unless the compost is wet.) Trash cans should be clean and covered tightly. Window and door screens can keep flies outside. Since flies can enter buildings through ventilation holes, screening should keep them out. Ultraviolet light traps, fly traps, fly swatters, baited fly traps, and other devices can eliminate flies within the home. Chemical control should be the last resort and used only for severe infestations.

flu See INFLUENZA.

fluke A parasitic flatworm of the class Trematoda, including the genus *Schistosoma*.
See also SCHISTOSOMIASIS.

folliculitis Inflammation of hair follicles by *Staphylococcus* bacteria.

Symptoms and Diagnostic Path

Although this condition can occur anywhere on the skin, it is most often found on bearded areas of the face, neck, armpits, thighs, or buttocks. Folliculitis on the face may lead to pustules; in the armpits, it may cause a BOIL.

Treatment Options and Outlook

Antibiotics, drainage, and clean linen help cure the infection.

Risk Factors and Preventive Measures

Because the infection may be spread from one person to the next in the same household, each family member should use separate towels and washcloths, bathe often, and wash clothing well.

fomites Nonliving material (such as bed linens) that may convey disease-causing organisms.

Foodborne Diseases Active Surveillance Network, The (FoodNet) The primary food-borne disease component of CDC's Emerging Infections Program (EIP) designed to determine the frequency and severity of food-borne diseases. FoodNet conducts active surveillance for infections caused by seven bacterial and two parasitic organisms: CAMPYLOBACTER, ESCHERICHIA COLI O157:H7, LISTERIA, SALMONELLA, SHIGELLA, VIBRIO, and YERSINIA; and CRYPTOSPORIDIUM and Cyclospora. Each year, millions of people become sick with food-borne illnesses; however, only a fraction seek medical care and an even smaller number submit laboratory specimens.

FoodNet, begun in 1996, represents a collaborative project in conjunction with the U.S. Department of Agriculture (USDA) and the Food and Drug Administration.

food-borne infections Infectious diseases spread through tainted food or beverages are common and sometimes life-threatening problems for millions of people in the United States and around the world. As many as 76 million people suffer food-borne illnesses each year in the United States, according to the CENTERS FOR DISEASE CONTROL AND PREVENTION (CDC), accounting for 325,000 hospitalizations and more than 5,000 deaths. Moreover, in the wake of terrorism in the beginning of the 21st century, public health, agricultural, and environmental officials worry about keeping the nation's food and water supply safe from terrorists. This bioterrorism threat is being studied by a number of U.S. agencies, including the CDC, Food and Drug Administration, Department of Agriculture, Environmental Protection Agency, and National Institutes of Health.

More than 250 different diseases caused by contaminated food or drink have been identified. Most food items that carry disease are raw or undercooked foods of animal origin, such as meat, milk, eggs, cheese, fish, or shellfish. About 400 to 500 food-borne disease outbreaks are reported each year, but not all diseases are likely to be reported and many cases are sporadic.

Any illness that appears suddenly and causes stomach pain, vomiting, and diarrhea should be a suspected case of food poisoning. Estimates of the number of food-borne illnesses vary between a low of 6 million to a high of 81 million cases yearly, with 9,100 deaths, according to the Centers for Disease Control and Prevention. At least one-third of the cases have been traced to poultry and meat.

SYMPTOMS OF FOOD POISONING	
Abdominal pain, fever, nausea, vomiting, and diarrhea one week after poisoning	Anisakiasis
Diarrhea, nausea/vomiting appearing one–six hours after meal	*Bacillus cereus*
Slurred speech, double vision, muscle paralysis four–36 hours after meal	Botulism
Cramps, fever, diarrhea, nausea/vomiting appearing two–five days after eating and lasting up to 10 days	Campylobacteriosis
Explosive watery diarrhea, abdominal cramps, dehydration; symptoms begin suddenly one–five days after infection	Cholera
Nausea, vomiting, and diarrhea within six–12 hours after eating fish, followed by low blood pressure and heart rate, severe itching, temperature reversal, numbness/tingling of extremities (may last months)	Ciguatera
Watery diarrhea, nausea/vomiting appearing within two days to a week after eating; severe cases include blood diarrhea; enterhemorrhagic infection includes bloody diarrhea and kidney failure	*E. coli*
Diarrhea and gas from eight hours to 24 hours after eating and usually lasting a day	Clostridium perfringens
Explosive diarrhea; foul-smelling, greasy feces; stomach pain; gas; appetite loss; nausea; and vomiting; incubation period one–two weeks	Giardiasis
Fever, headache, diarrhea, meningitis, conjunctivitis, miscarriage appearing within 12 hours to three weeks after ingestion	Listeriosis
Burning mouth/extremities, nausea, vomiting, and diarrhea *within hours* after ingestion	Neurotoxic shellfish poisoning
Burning mouth/extremities, nausea/vomiting, diarrhea, muscle weakness, paralysis, breathing problems *within minutes* after ingestion	Paralytic shellfish poisoning
Diarrhea, rumbling bowels, fever, vomiting, cramps eight–72 hours after ingestion, and may last one or two days	Salmonellosis
Gastroenteritis, diarrhea, nausea/vomiting 12 hours–50 hours after eating	Shigellosis
Explosive diarrhea, cramps, vomiting not longer than a day, between 30 minutes–six hours after eating	Staphylococcal food poisoning
Diarrhea, nausea/vomiting, fever followed by muscle pain and stiffness two–three weeks after ingestion	Trichinosis
Gastroenteritis, explosive diarrhea, nausea/vomiting, cramps (*V. vulnificus* can lead to fatal blood infection) eight–30 hours after eating	*Vibrio* food poisoning (*V. parahaemolyticus, V. vulnificus*)

According to the U.S. Food and Drug Administration, just about everyone experiences a food-borne illness at least once a year, and between 21 and 81 million cases of diarrhea related to food-borne illness are treated in the United States each year. Some food-borne diseases such as BOTULISM or TRICHINOSIS are becoming less common, whereas others such as SALMONELLOSIS or *ESCHERICHIA COLI* are becoming more common.

CAMPYLOBACTER was reported more often than any other pathogen: almost one case out of 108, or 2.5 million Americans a year.

Other common types of food-borne illness are Salmonellosis and *E. coli* infection, as well as infection with NORWALK VIRUS.

Some common diseases are sometimes caused by tainted food, although they are usually transmitted by other routes. These include infections caused by *SHIGELLA*, HEPATITIS A, and the parasites *GIARDIA LAMBLIA* and *CRYPTOSPORIDIA*. Even strep throat may be transmitted via food.

In addition to direct infection, some food-borne diseases are caused by a toxin that is produced by germs in the food. For example, the bacterium

Staphylococcus aureus can grow in some foods and produce a toxin that causes intense vomiting. BOTULISM occurs when the bacterium *CLOSTRIDIUM BOTULINUM* produces a powerful toxin.

Some of the changes in rates of food-borne illnesses may reflect changes in meat and poultry processing as mandated by the USDA's Pathogen Reduction and Hazard Analysis and Critical Control Point Systems rule. The program was implemented in January 1998 in the largest plants.

The greatest danger from food poisoning is not the toxin itself but the body's natural response to poison—vomiting and diarrhea—that robs the body of vital fluids. If dehydration becomes serious, food poisoning victims need to be hospitalized and given fluids intravenously. Poisoning from *E. coli* bacteria can lead to severe infection that can include bloody diarrhea, leading to kidney failure. It is this type of food poisoning from improperly cooked hamburgers that killed several young children in 1993.

Symptoms and Diagnostic Path

While the time between ingestion and onset of symptoms varies according to the cause of poisoning, symptoms usually develop with some types of shellfish poisoning between one and 12 hours for bacterial toxins and between 12 and 48 hours for viral and *Salmonella* infections. Symptoms also vary depending on how badly the food was contaminated, but there will often be similar symptoms

---

HOW TO PREVENT FOOD POISONING

Meat, poultry, and eggs are most vulnerable to contamination during storage, preparation, cooking, and serving. To stay healthy, observe the following proper food handling and kitchen safety tips:

- *Proper refrigeration* Temperature in the refrigerator must be 40°F or below (0°F in the freezer). Cooling does not kill bacteria, but it stops their growth. Air should circulate around refrigerated items. Food in refrigerator should be wrapped to keep off bacteria in the air.
- *Wash hands* To avoid contamination by bacteria or other organisms when preparing food, hands should be washed thoroughly with soap and water *before* and *after* handling food.
- *Wash utensils* Wash cutting board and utensils with hot soapy water before touching any other food.
- *Thawing* Meat should not be thawed at room temperature; thaw meat or poultry in a microwave oven or in the refrigerator and then cook immediately.
- *Marinades* Used marinade should not be served unless it has been cooked at a roiling boil for several minutes.
- *Serving* Meat and poultry should be served on a clean plate with a clean utensil to avoid contaminating the cooked food with its raw juices.
- *Leftovers* Poultry and meat should be cooled quickly when refrigerating leftovers; stuffed poultry should not stand for long periods. The stuffing should be removed after cooking and promptly refrigerated.
- *Eggs* Cracked eggs should never be used because they may contain *Salmonella* bacteria. Because even an uncracked egg may contain bacteria, eggs should be cooked thoroughly. Raw eggs (such as in Caesar salad dressing, homemade eggnog, or hollandaise sauce) should be avoided. Eggs should be refrigerated in their cartons in the coldest part of the refrigerator (*not* on the refrigerator door).
- *Mold* Any food with mold should be discarded (except for cheese, which may be eaten after the mold is trimmed off).
- *Microwave* A turntable should be used to rotate dishes as they cook; because microwave ovens heat food unevenly, cold spots in a food may harbor dangerous bacteria.
- *Cleaning* Wooden salad bowls should not be seasoned with oil; it can become rancid. Can opener and blender should be free from food. The sink should be scrubbed after working with poultry or meat. Sponges in the kitchen for wiping dishes or countertops should be discarded after one week. (They should never sit in water, which encourages bacterial growth.) Sink and counters should be cleaned with detergent containing bleach to kill harmful bacteria.

For more information about food safety, call the U.S. Department of Agriculture's Meat and Poultry Hot Line at 1-800-535-4555 (in Washington, D.C., call 1-202-477-3333 between 10:00 A.M. and 4:00 P.M.

For more questions about storing or handling fish, call the help line of the Rhode Island Seafood Council at 1-800-EAT-FISH between 8:00 A.M. and 5:00 P.M. ET.

regardless of the cause: nausea and vomiting, diarrhea, stomach pain, and—in severe cases—shock and collapse.

A doctor should be called if severe vomiting or diarrhea appear suddenly, if the victim collapses, or if there is a suspicion of food poisoning and the victim is a child, an elderly person, or someone with a chronic illness or otherwise compromised immune system.

Treatment Options and Outlook
In all cases of food poisoning, symptoms should be treated much like a bout of flu, including drinking fluids (water, tea, bouillon, and ginger ale) to replace fluid loss. Mild cases may be treated at home, with clear liquids, including some salt and sugar. If the person cannot retain fluids because of vomiting, IV fluids are needed. Most cases of food poisoning are not serious (except for botulism), and recovery is usually within three days. If possible, samples of any food left from recent meals should be saved for testing.

Governmental overview began in 1906 with the passage of the Pure Food and Drug Act and the Meat Inspection Act, designed to make American food as safe as possible. In addition, three different governmental agencies are responsible for regulating and monitoring the safety of the U.S. food supply. The Food and Drug Administration is responsible for ensuring the safety and wholesomeness of all food except meat, poultry, and eggs. The Department of Agriculture monitors the safety of poultry, meat, eggs, and egg products and conducts inspections nationwide.

However, because of a range of regulatory loopholes, the governmental safety net does not always work effectively.

Risk Factors and Preventive Measures
To prevent the spread of food-borne diseases, the consumer should do the following:

- Food from animal sources should be thoroughly cooked or pasteurized; foods should not be eaten raw or undercooked.
- Juices or drippings from raw meat, poultry, shellfish, or eggs should not contaminate other food.

- Potentially contaminated food should not be left for extended periods of time at temperatures that allow bacteria to grow.
- Promptly refrigerate leftovers and food prepared in advance.

SAFE FOOD STORAGE

Food	Where	How Long
Poultry		
Raw	Refrigerator	1–2 days
	Freezer	9 months
Cooked	Refrigerator	3–4 days
	Freezer	4–6 months
Seafood		
Lean, fish, raw	Refrigerator	1–2 days
	Freezer	6–8 months
Fatty fish, raw	Refrigerator	1–2 days
	Freezer	4 months
Raw shrimp	Refrigerator	1–2 days
	Freezer	9 months
Cooked seafood	Refrigerator	3 days
	Freezer	2 months
Meat		
Ground meat	Refrigerator	1–2 days
	Freezer	3–4 months
Chops (all)	Refrigerator	3–5 days
Frozen lamb chops	Freezer	6–9 months
Frozen pork chops	Freezer	4–6 months
Roasts (all)	Refrigerator	3–5 days
Frozen beef roasts	Freezer	6–12 months
Frozen veal/pork roast	Freezer	4–6 months
Frozen lamb roast	Freezer	6–9 months
Steak	Refrigerator	3–5 days
Cooked leftovers	Refrigerator	3–4 days
	Freezer	2–3 months
Vacuum-sealed packages		
(unopened)	Refrigerator	2 weeks
(opened)	Refrigerator	3–5 days
	Freezer	1–2 months
Ham		
country dry-cure	Cupboard	1 year
soaked/cooked	Refrigerator	7 days
Dairy		
Raw eggs in shell	Refrigerator	3 weeks
Hard-boiled (in shell)	Refrigerator	1 week
Milk	Refrigerator	5 days
	Freezer	1 month
Mayonnaise (opened)	Refrigerator	1 year

Guidelines provided by the USDA and the Food Marketing Institute

The single most important way to prevent food-borne illness is thorough cooking, which kills most food-borne bacteria, toxins, viruses, and parasites. In addition, proper food preparation—washing hands, cutting board, and knife with soap and water before and right after handling raw meat, poultry, seafood, or eggs will help stop the spread of contamination. Anyone who is sick with diarrhea or vomiting should not prepare food for others.

It is also important to monitor the food supply. The United States imports 30 billion tons of food a year, including fruit, vegetables, seafood, and canned goods, which often come from developing countries where food hygiene and basic sanitation is poor.

FOOD SAFETY AT PICNICS

Picknickers should

- Use an insulated cooler with an ice or frozen gelpack on top, with foods that need to be kept coldest on the bottom
- Pack food right from the refrigerator
- Wrap food separately in plastic, and do not place directly on ice that is not drinking-water quality
- Separate raw fish, meat, or poultry so drippings do not contaminate other food
- Keep cooler in the shade, not the trunk, with the lid on
- Keep utensils and food covered when not in use
- Keep hot foods hot in an insulated dish or vacuum bottle
- Take along disposal wipes to clean hands before and after food preparation
- Not leave food unrefrigerated longer than two hours (one hour if temperature is above 85°F)

HOW TO REPORT CASES OF SUSPECTED FOOD POISONING

According to the U.S. Department of Agriculture's Safety and Inspection Service, consumers should report possible food poisoning in three situations:

- If the food was eaten at a large gathering
- If the food was from a restaurant, deli, sidewalk vendor, or other kitchen that serves more than a few people
- If the food is a commercial product (such as canned goods or frozen food), since contaminants may have affected an entire batch

When making a report, officials need to know the following:

- Consumer's name, address, telephone number
- A detailed explanation of the problem
- When and where the food was eaten
- Who ate it
- Name and address of the place where the food was obtained

If the food is a commercial product, the consumer should

- Provide the manufacturer's name and address
- Provide product's lot or batch number
- Look for the USDA inspection stamp on the wrapper of meat or poultry, which will identify the plant where the food was made or packaged.

The centralization of the food industry means that a single contaminated product may appear in different foods and different forms, potentially infecting a great number of people. In addition, new and emerging food-borne pathogens are constantly being identified, which cause diseases that were not recognized 50 years ago. These include bacteria, parasites, viruses, and toxins.

Food Safety and Inspection Service The public health agency of the U.S. Department of Agriculture responsible for ensuring that the nation's commercial supply of meat, poultry, and egg products is safe, wholesome, and correctly labeled and packaged. The service follows the law as required by the Federal Meat Inspection Act, the Poultry Products Inspection Act, and the Egg Products Inspection Act.

The FSIS inspects all raw beef, pork, lamb, chicken, and turkey, as well as processed meat and poultry products, including hams, sausage, soups, stews, pizzas, and frozen dinners (generally, products that contain 2 percent or more cooked meat and poultry or 3 percent or more raw meat and poultry). Examples of processed egg products regulated by FSIS include dried egg yolks, scrambled egg mix, dried egg powder, and liquid eggs.

FSIS also inspects all meat, poultry, and egg products sold in interstate commerce and reinspects imported products. More than 7,600 inspection personnel verify that regulations regarding food safety and other consumer protection concerns are met in nearly 6,500 meat, poultry, and egg processing plants.

In slaughter plants, inspection involves examining, before and after slaughter, birds and animals intended for use as food. In egg processing plants, inspection involves examining, before and after breaking, eggs intended for further processing and use as food.

In addition to these inspection activities, the agency sets requirements for meat and poultry labels and for certain slaughter and processing activities, such as plant sanitation and thermal processing. FSIS tests for microbiological, chemical, and other types of contamination and conducts epidemiological investigations in cooperation with the CENTERS FOR DISEASE CONTROL AND PREVENTION based on reports of food-borne health hazards and disease outbreaks.

To ensure the safety of imported products, FSIS maintains a comprehensive system of import inspection and controls, and each year reviews inspection systems in all foreign countries eligible to export meat and poultry to the United States to ensure that they are equivalent to those under U.S. laws.

In an effort to improve the safety of meat, poultry, and egg products, the agency is taking a "farm-to-table" approach by improving the safety of meat, poultry, and egg products at each step in the food production, processing, distribution, and marketing chain. These steps are designed to focus attention on the risk of microbial contamination—the nation's most significant food safety problem. The agency's goal is to reduce contamination as much as possible by building the principle of prevention into the production and inspection processes and fostering the development and use of new technology.

In 2000, FSIS completed implementation of its Pathogen Reduction and Hazard Analysis and Critical Control Point (HACCP) systems. Under the regulations, each meat and poultry plant must develop and implement a written plan for meeting its sanitation responsibilities and develop and implement a HACCP plan that systematically addresses all significant hazards associated with its products. In addition, all slaughter plants must regularly test for generic *E. coli* to verify their procedures for preventing and reducing fecal contamination—the main source of bacteria that cause human foodborne illness. Raw products from slaughter plants and plants that grind meat and poultry are subject to Salmonella testing by FSIS. These efforts are directed at reducing microbial contamination over time.

With the Pathogen Reduction and HACCP final rule, FSIS has shifted its regulatory approach for meat and poultry. The expanded approach includes not only the product but also the process. A system under which potential food safety problems are identified and prevented is replacing a system that focused largely on detecting problems at the end of the production line.

As FSIS proceeds with HACCP implementation, it has also developed new inspection models for use in plants that slaughter young and generally healthy animals. In this pilot project, FSIS inspectors focus on public health concerns rather than on sorting carcasses, which is left to the plant to do. The project is an effort to determine whether integrating HACCP, a science-based, preventive food safety system into all aspects of slaughter operations, will result in the production of product that is at least as good as that produced under the traditional inspection system. To date, the data show that it is resulting in product with fewer food safety and non-food safety defects.

FSIS is working with federal, state, and local agencies to ensure food safety at all stages of the farm-to-table chain. This includes developing federal standards for the safe handling of food during transportation, distribution, and storage. FSIS also is working with producers and others to develop and implement voluntary food safety measures that can be taken on the farm and before animals enter the slaughter facility to reduce the risk of harmful contamination of meat and poultry products.

FSIS is relying more heavily on risk assessments as a means of guiding food safety policy decisions. The agency has conducted risk assessments for *Salmonella enteritidis* in eggs and egg products, *E. coli* O157:H7 in ground beef, and, with the FDA, a risk ranking for *Listeria monocytogenes* in a variety of foods. Risk assessment is a structured process for determining the risks associated with any type of hazard—biological, chemical, or physical.

FSIS is also working to improve the surveillance of food-borne illness. The FOODBORNE DISEASES ACTIVE SURVEILLANCE NETWORK (FoodNet), operated by CDC, USDA, FDA, and State health departments, provides more precise information on the incidence of food-borne disease in the United States.

food safety and natural disasters Before a natural disaster or weather emergency occurs, there are a number of preparations consumers can make to keep their food safe from bacterial decomposition, according to the U.S. FOOD SAFETY AND INSPECTION Service (FSIS). Using an appliance thermometer in the refrigerator and freezer, make sure the freezer is at or below 0°F and the refrigerator is at or below 40°F. If there is a risk of power loss, consumers can freeze containers of water to help keep food cold in the freezer, refrigerator, or coolers. Leftovers, milk, and fresh meat and poultry should be frozen to help maintain a safe temperature longer. Grouping food together in the freezer helps items stay cold longer. If possible, buy block or dry ice ahead of time. Consumers whose homes are at risk of flooding should store food on high shelves and in coolers.

After the disaster or weather emergency, consumers should keep the refrigerator and freezer doors closed as much as possible to keep the food cold, according to the FSIS. An unopened refrigerator can keep food safely cold for about four hours, and an unopened, full freezer will keep items frozen for about 48 hours (this drops to 24 hours if it is only half full). It is possible to safely refreeze food if it still contains ice crystals or is at 40°F or below.

Dry or block ice can keep items in a refrigerator and freezer cold if the power is out for a long period of time; 50 pounds of dry ice can keep an 18-cubic-foot full freezer cool for two days. Beyond that time, the temperature of the freezer should be checked with an appliance thermometer or food thermometer; if it is still at 40°F or below or still contains ice crystals, the food is safe.

If a thermometer has not been kept in the freezer, check each package of food to determine its safety. If the food still contains ice crystals, the food is safe. However, after four hours without power, consumers should throw out perishable food such as meat, poultry, fish, soft cheeses, milk, eggs, leftovers, and deli items.

After a flood, residents should drink only bottled water and throw out all food that has come in contact with flood waters (even canned goods), along with wooden cutting boards, plastic utensils, pacifiers, and baby bottle nipples. Metal pans, ceramic dishes, and utensils that came in contact with flood water can be washed with hot, soapy water and then be sanitized by boiling in clean water or by soaking for 15 minutes in a solution of one teaspoon of bleach per quart of water.

Fort Bragg fever Another name for LEPTOSPIROSIS, an infection caused by the organism of the genus *Leptospira*, associated with the urine of a variety of wild and domestic animals. The disease was first identified in recruits at Fort Bragg, North Carolina, during the summer of 1942.

See also WEIL'S SYNDROME.

Francisella tularensis The name of the bacteria that causes TULAREMIA, an infectious disease of wild animals occasionally found in humans. The bacterium was formerly known as *Pasteurella tularensis*.

fungal infection A disease of the skin (also called mycoses) caused by the spread of FUNGI that may range from a mild to a fatal condition. Fungal skin infections are either considered "superficial" (affecting skin, hair, nails) or "subcutaneous" (beneath the skin).

The *superficial* fungal infections include THRUSH (candidiasis), RINGWORM and ATHLETE'S FOOT). *Subcutaneous* infections are rare; the most common is SPOROTRICHOSIS, occurring after a scratch becomes contaminated with a certain species of fungus. Examples of this type of condition occur in tropical climates.

Harmless fungi are always present on the skin, but they do not multiply because of bacterial competition or because the body's immune system fights them off. Fungal infections of the skin are most common in those taking long-term antibiotics or corticosteroid or immunosuppressant drugs, or in patients with an immune system disorder such as AIDS.

Symptoms and Diagnostic Path
The symptoms and appearances of a fungal skin infection depend on what type of fungus is causing the problem and where on the body the fungus appears. In general, fungal infections cause a rash that may be either itchy, red, and scaly or a fine scale that looks just like very dry skin. A fungal infection may affect just one part of the body or several different areas.

Athlete's foot (TINEA PEDIS) causes itchy, scaling, and soggy skin in the web spaces between the toes. Nail infections (onychomycosis) may cause malformed, thickened, and crumbly nails. Jock itch (TINEA CRURIS) causes an itchy red rash in the groin and surrounding area. Ringworm on the body (TINEA CORPORIS) causes red patches with scaly edges and clear skin at the center. Ringworm of the scalp (TINEA CAPITIS) affects young children, causing inflammation and hair loss. Pityriasis versicolor (also called TINEA VERSICOLOR) causes increased dark patches on pale skin and light patches on darker skin. THRUSH (*CANDIDA ALBICANS*) can affect the mouth, tongue, and vagina, causing small, white patches. In adults, vaginal thrush can cause itchiness and a thick, white discharge. Although some cases of fungal infection are clear cut, in others it may be difficult to tell the difference between fungal rashes and skin conditions such as psoriasis and eczema. Most fungal infections are easy to spot by appearance and location alone. However, to make sure, a doctor may send a skin scraping or a hair or nail fragment to the laboratory for analysis.

Treatment Options and Outlook
Physicians use three classes of drugs to fight fungal disease, but in the past five years fungi have begun to grow resistant to common drugs, just as some types of bacteria. Strains of fungi resistant to each of the three types of drugs are now common in hospitals that care for the sickest patients—especially patients with cancer and AIDS. This growing resistance appears to have developed for the same reasons that bacteria have grown impervious: the overuse of drugs to combat fungal infections.

Extensive use of antifungal medications occurred because of the large number of people with impaired immune systems due to AIDS and chemotherapy. Between 5 to 10 percent of AIDS patients now have resistant fungi that cause oral CANDIDIASIS, a common mouth infection.

fungi   A phylum of plants (including yeasts, rusts, slime molds, smuts, mushrooms, and so on) characterized by the absence of chlorophyll and the presence of a rigid cell wall. There are more than 100,000 different species of fungi around the world, most of which are harmless or beneficial to human health (such as molds used to produce antibiotics, yeasts used in baking and brewing, edible mushrooms and truffles).

However, some fungi can invade and form colonies in the skin or underneath the skin, leading to disorders ranging from a mild skin irritation and inflammation to severe or fatal systemic infections.

Fungi reproduce by sending out spores (cells that resemble plant seeds). When a spore lands in a moist place, it sends out small threads from which the fungus feeds. These moist places that support fungi include dead plant and animal matter and BACTERIA.

See also FUNGAL INFECTION.

fungicide   A drug that kills FUNGI.

furuncle   Another name for a BOIL, this is a skin infection caused by bacteria that enter through the hair follicle, forming a painful pus-filled nodule.

The boil is most often caused by a *Staphylococcus*, which multiplies in a skin gland or hair follicle. Patients must not irritate or squeeze the lesion or they will spread the infection into adjacent tissue.

Symptoms and Diagnostic Path
Pain, redness, and swelling, with tissue death deep in the center of the inflamed area, which forms a core of dead tissue.

Treatment Options and Outlook
Local care, moist heat, and incision and drainage.

gangrene Death of tissue generally associated with loss of blood supply, followed by bacterial invasion and putrefaction. It may affect either a fairly small area of skin or an entire limb. It also can occur in the intestines or gallbladder. Internally, gangrene may be a complication of strangulated hernia, appendicitis, or cholecystitis, or impaired blood supply.

In *dry gangrene,* an area of the skin dies because of blocked blood supply, without bacterial infection; this type does not spread to other tissue. It may be caused by arteriosclerosis, diabetes mellitus, a stroke, blood clot, or frostbite. *Wet* (or *moist*) *gangrene* follows bacterial infection of dry gangrene or the obstruction of blood flow following a wound. This form of gangrene has an offensive odor, spreads rapidly, and may be fatal in a few days.

Gas gangrene is a particularly virulent form of wet gangrene caused by a deadly type of bacteria (usually various species of CLOSTRIDIUM, particularly C. perfringens) that destroy skin and muscle while producing a foul odor. Gas gangrene is responsible for millions of deaths during war and is also known as anaerobic myositis and necrotizing fasciitis (FLESH-EATING BACTERIA).

Symptoms and Diagnostic Path

Symptoms include pain in the dying skin tissue that becomes numb and black once the tissue dies. If bacterial infection occurs, the gangrene will spread, giving off a noxious odor with redness, swelling, and oozing pus around the blackened area.

Gas gangrene causes pain, swelling, and tenderness of the wound area, with moderate fever, rapid heartbeat, and low blood pressure. The skin around the wound may be pale, bronze, or red and begins to die and rupture, revealing muscle. As large, bloody blisters form, the wound may develop a sweet smell and leak brown, bloody, or pale yellow fluid. As the infection worsens, symptoms begin to affect the entire body, including fever, sweating, quickened pulse, and an abrupt plummeting blood pressure.

Gas gangrene is diagnosed by observing the infected wound, noting its sweet odor, and evaluating the extent of injury.

Treatment Options and Outlook

In all types of gangrene, surgical removal of the dead tissue is required. Improving circulation to the affected area can improve dry gangrene if it is begun early enough. Once the tissue becomes infected, antibiotics are given to prevent the spread of infection.

Once wet gangrene is diagnosed, amputation of the affected part is required, along with neighboring healthy tissue, in order to save the patient. Untreated gas gangrene may lead to severe blood problems, kidney failure, coma, and death.

Risk Factors and Preventive Measures

Gangrene of an extremity with no blood supply (such as vascular disease of toes and feet) cannot be prevented once the tissue has lost its oxygen supply.

If possible, wound gangrene is best avoided by meticulous wound care, removal of dead tissue, and maintaining blood supply and cleanliness. Gangrene is a natural process that occurs in the presence of dead tissue; therefore, removing dead tissue helps prevent gangrene. Gangrene can be quickly fatal in certain conditions where the infection itself corrodes and destroys healthy skin in a rapid, catastrophic way.

Emergency surgery to remove all of the affected tissue must be done to save the patient's life. This surgery is often radical and deforming.

Gardnerella vaginalis   See VAGINITIS.

gas bacillus   One of several species of bacillus that produce a gas as a byproduct of metabolism. Examples of gas bacilli include *ESCHERICHIA COLI* and the clostridial species that produce gas gangrene.

gastroenteritis, bacterial   Inflammation of the stomach and intestines as a result of bacterial infection.

It can be caused by bacteria such as *E. coli, SALMONELLA, SHIGELLA,* and others.

Symptoms and Diagnostic Path
Between two to five days after eating, patients experience fever, cramps, headache, nausea, diarrhea, and a sickness often mistaken for the flu. It is common in children but also appears in adults.

Treatment Options and Outlook
Mild cases can be treated at home. Bed rest, sedation, and IV fluids can be given if the patient is severely dehydrated. Antibiotic or antimicrobial therapy is usually not necessary unless the infection has begun to affect the whole body. However, the use of antibiotics may actually create a carrier state. Antidiarrheal medications are not usually prescribed because they may prolong the infectious process. After the symptoms subside, water may be given by mouth; if this is not followed by nausea, clear fluids may be added followed by a bland diet. In most cases, the illness subsides slowly without any special treatment.

Risk Factors and Preventive Measures
Preparing food carefully with attention to hygiene can reduce the chances of gastroenteritis. Those who care for patients with this condition must be meticulous about their own hygiene in order not to further spread the infection.

See also ANTIDIARRHEAL DRUGS; DIARRHEA AND INFECTIOUS DISEASE; TRAVELER'S DIARRHEA.

gastroenteritis, viral   Inflammation of the stomach and intestines caused by viral infection.

Viral gastroenteritis is often called the "stomach flu," although it is not caused by the influenza virus.

People who get viral gastroenteritis almost always recover completely, but it can be a serious illness for those who cannot drink enough fluids to replace what they lose through vomiting or diarrhea. Infants, young children, and the disabled or elderly are at risk for dehydration from loss of fluids and may need to be hospitalized for treatment to correct dehydration.

Viral gastroenteritis affects people in all parts of the world. In the United States, ROTAVIRUS and astrovirus infections occur during the cooler months of the year from October to April, whereas ADENOVIRUS infections occur throughout the year. Viral gastroenteritis outbreaks can occur in schools, child care facilities, and nursing homes, or in other group settings such as banquet halls, cruise ships, dormitories, and campgrounds.

Many different viruses can cause gastroenteritis, including rotaviruses, adenoviruses, caliciviruses, astroviruses, Norwalk virus, and a group of NORWALK-LIKE VIRUSES. Viral gastroenteritis is not caused by bacteria or parasites, or by medications or other medical conditions, although the symptoms may be similar. The viruses that cause gastroenteritis are contagious, and are spread through close contact with infected persons by sharing food, water, or eating utensils.

Individuals may also become infected by eating or drinking foods or beverages that have been contaminated by food handlers with viral gastroenteritis, especially if they do not wash their hands regularly after using the bathroom. Shellfish may be contaminated by sewage; people who eat raw or undercooked shellfish harvested from contaminated waters may get diarrhea. Drinking water can also be contaminated by sewage.

While viral gastroenteritis can strike anyone of any age, some viruses tend to cause diarrheal disease primarily among people in specific age groups. Rotavirus infection is the most common cause of diarrhea in infants and young children under five, while adenoviruses and astroviruses cause diarrhea mostly in young children. Norwalk and Norwalk-like viruses are more likely to cause diarrhea in older children and adults.

Symptoms and Diagnostic Path

Symptoms include lack of appetite and sudden and violent onset of vomiting and nausea, abdominal discomfort, and diarrhea. Symptoms begin one or two days after infection with a virus, and may last for one to 10 days, depending on which virus causes the illness.

Treatment Options and Outlook

Treatment includes bed rest, sedation, and IV fluids if the patient is severely dehydrated. After the symptoms subside, water may be given by mouth; if this does not cause nausea, clear fluids may be added, followed by a bland diet.

Risk Factors and Preventive Measures

Consumers can reduce their chance of getting infected by frequent handwashing, prompt disinfection of contaminated surfaces with household chlorine bleach-based cleaners, and prompt washing of soiled clothes. There is no vaccine or medicine currently available that prevents viral gastroenteritis. A vaccine that had been developed to prevent severe diarrhea from rotavirus infection in infants and young children was withdrawn from the market because it was linked to intestinal intussception.

See also ANTIDIARRHEAL DRUGS; DIARRHEA AND INFECTIOUS DISEASE; TRAVELER'S DIARRHEA.

genital herpes See HERPES, GENITAL.

genital papilloma virus See PAPILLOMAVIRUS, HUMAN.

genital warts See WARTS, GENITAL.

genitourinary tract infection See URINARY TRACT INFECTION.

germ The popular term for any microorganism that causes disease. Either a virus or a bacterium is an example of a germ.

German measles The common name for rubella, a viral infection is not very similar to MEASLES, although it also causes a rash on the face, trunk, and limbs. German measles is a mild illness in children and a slightly more problematic one in adults, but it is really serious only when contracted by women in the early months of pregnancy. An infection at this time may infect the fetus, which can lead to a range of serious birth defects known as rubella syndrome.

Although rubella occurred throughout the world, it is now much less common in most developed countries because of successful vaccination programs. The United States has tried to eradicate the disease by vaccinating all school-age children. In 1969 when the vaccine became available, at least 60,000 Americans contracted rubella. By 1993, the number dropped to 192.

Rubella is caused by the rubella virus, which is transmitted by particles in the air when an infected person coughs or sneezes. It also can be transmitted on contaminated objects; the virus can survive for a short period of time on tissues, doorknobs, phones, and so on.

Before the development of the vaccine, rubella was common in spring and winter, and peaked every six to nine years. There were huge rubella epidemics in the United States in 1935, 1943, and 1964. The last major U.S. epidemic occurred during 1964–65. Since country-wide vaccination began, no large rubella epidemics have occurred. Isolated outbreaks do continue amid people who do not get vaccinated because of religious or philosophic reasons. Most reported cases in the United States since mid-1900s have occurred among Hispanic young adults who were born in areas where rubella vaccine is not usually given.

Symptoms and Diagnostic Path

The infection usually affects youngsters between the ages of six and 12 with a rash that starts on the face and spreads downward and out to arms and legs. The rash may run together to make large patches, but it does not itch. It lasts for a few days, with a slight fever and enlarged lymph nodes; some children may have a mild cough, sore throat, or runny nose before the rash appears. Sometimes the entire infection comes and goes without notice; at least 30 percent of children with rubella have no symptoms at all, although they are infectious to others.

Adolescents and adults may have slightly more pronounced symptoms, including headaches, fever, body aches, eye infections, or a runny nose, which occurs about one to five days before the rash. Swollen glands in the neck and behind the ear typically appear seven to 10 days before the rash. The virus may be transmitted from a few days before the symptoms appear until a day after symptoms fade.

Incubation period ranges from 14 to 23 days; the average is 16 to 18 days.

Rubella may be confused with other conditions characterized by rashes, such as SCARLET FEVER or drug allergy.

A lab test to confirm rubella is important, since the symptoms can be so mild they may be overlooked or mistaken for something else. This is especially true if a pregnant woman may be exposed.

Blood tests are available that reveal rubella immunity or an active rubella infection. If a person has been vaccinated, the blood test will show that the person is immune. Pregnant women need a rubella immunity test at the first prenatal visit; if not immune, the woman will receive rubella vaccine in the hospital after delivery.

If a pregnant woman gets an infection resembling rubella during pregnancy and she is not immune, blood tests must be done to determine whether rubella is the cause of the illness.

Treatment Options and Outlook

There is no specific treatment for rubella, although acetaminophen may reduce the fever.

Congenital rubella is the most serious complication of rubella infection, since it can cause fetal death or miscarriage. The risk is highest when the pregnant woman is infected in the first 12 weeks of pregnancy (miscarriage rate is as high as 85 percent during this time). At 14 to 16 weeks, the risk drops to just 10 to 24 percent, and after 20 weeks the risk is almost nonexistent.

Infants who survive infection in the womb may be born with a variety of birth defects, including deafness, eye problems (including blindness), heart defects, mental retardation, growth retardation, and bleeding disorders.

Rare complications in adults include bleeding disorders or ENCEPHALITIS.

Risk Factors and Preventive Measures

Any child with rubella must be kept at home until well past the infectious stage; babies born with rubella may retain the infection virus in their nose, throat, and urine for as long as a year.

Vaccination can provide long-lasting immunity. It is given in the United States to all infants as part of the measles and mumps vaccine. There is not usually any reaction to the vaccine. The vaccine is a live attenuated virus that provides complete protection to more than 95 percent of those who receive it. Rubella infection itself also provides immunity.

The recommended vaccine, MMR (measles, mumps, rubella), is not effective when given earlier than 12 months because the baby may have maternal antibodies that will interfere with the vaccine's action. A first dose is given at 12 to 15 months; a second booster is given at age four to six, before the child starts school. Older children who missed these shots should receive one dose of MMR by the 11–12-year-old visit.

Women of childbearing age can be given the vaccine if they are not already immune. Anyone who is not sure of having received the vaccine or having rubella should be vaccinated. There is no risk to receiving the vaccine if a person is already immune.

Rubella is common in many countries; anyone who travels abroad should be sure they are immune to rubella or receive the vaccine before leaving. The national recommendations for rubella elimination are as follows:

- vaccination for all children
- premarital screening, vaccination for those who need it
- prenatal screening and postpartum vaccination if needed
- routine vaccination in a medical setting
- proof of immunity for hospital workers and college students

There are some people who should not receive the vaccine. These include pregnant women or women who plan to become pregnant within the next three months; or anyone with a high fever or who has a severe allergy to neomycin. There is no PENICILLIN in rubella vaccine, and it is safe for those allergic to eggs.

germicide   A drug that kills microorganisms.

Giardia lamblia   A type of protozoa found in the intestinal tract and in feces of humans, sheep, cattle, and beaver that causes foul-smelling, explosive diarrhea called GIARDIASIS. The protozoa was named for the 19th-century French biologist Alfred Giard, who discovered it.

The protozoa are most often found in tropical areas, and in those who travel to the Tropics. Recently, it has become more common in developed countries, where it is especially common in preschools and among people living in institutions.

See also ANTIDIARRHEAL DRUGS; DIARRHEA AND INFECTIOUS DISEASE.

giardiasis   The most common cause of waterborne intestinal infection in the United States, giardiasis is an infection of the small intestine caused by the *GIARDIA LAMBLIA* protozoa, which is found in the human intestinal tract and in feces. In recent years, outbreaks of giardiasis have been common among people in institutions, preschool children, at catered affairs, and large public picnic areas. Since the 1990s, *Giardia* infection has become one of the most common causes of human water-borne disease (both drinking and recreational water) the United States. *Giardia* are found worldwide and within every region of the United States.

Giardiasis is spread by contaminated food or water or by direct personal hand-to-mouth contact. Children can spread the infection by touching contaminated toys, changing tables, utensils, or their own feces. For this reason, the infection spreads quickly through a day-care center or institution for the developmentally disabled. Unfiltered streams or lakes that may be contaminated by human or animal feces are a common source of infection to campers.

Symptoms and Diagnostic Path

Giardiasis is not fatal, and about two-thirds of infected people have no symptoms. When they do occur, uncomfortable symptoms appear about one to three days after infection. The infection interferes with the body's ability to absorb fats in the intestinal tract, so the stool is filled with fat. Symptoms include explosive diarrhea, foul-smelling and greasy feces, stomach pains, gas, loss of appetite, nausea, and vomiting. In some cases, the infection can become chronic.

Giardiasis is diagnosed by examining three stool samples for the presence of the parasites. Because the parasite is shed intermittently, half of the infections will be missed if only one specimen gets checked. Stool collection kits are available for this purpose.

A different test looks for the proteins of *Giardia* in the stool sample.

Treatment Options and Outlook

Acute giardiasis usually runs its course and then clears up, but antibiotics will help relieve symptoms and prevent the spread of infection. Medications include metronidazole, furazolidone, and paromomycin.

Occasionally, treatment fails; in this case, the patient should wait two weeks and repeat the medication. Anyone with an impaired immune system may need to combine medications. Healthy carriers do not need to be treated.

Some children get chronic infection and suffer with diarrhea and cramps for long periods of time, losing weight and growing poorly. Those most at risk for an infection are people with impaired immune function, malnourished children, people with low stomach acid, and older people.

Risk Factors and Preventive Measures

Giardia can be very contagious. The best way to avoid giardiasis is to stay away from drinking untreated surface water. While chlorine in water treatment will not kill the cysts, filtered public water supplies eliminate it. Also, giardiasis can be prevented by

- maintaining good personal hygiene
- not eating unwashed fruit or vegetables unless they can be peeled

• boiling water if in doubt; campers should boil stream water for three minutes before drinking

If an outbreak occurs in a child-care center, the director should notify the local health department. Children with severe diarrhea must stay at home until the stool returns to normal.

See also ANTIDIARRHEAL DRUGS; DIARRHEA AND INFECTIOUS DISEASE; TRAVELER'S DIARRHEA.

gingivitis See GUM DISEASE.

glanders An endemic infection found in Asia, Africa, and South America that afflicts horses and donkeys, and that may occasionally be transmitted to humans. The disease has been eradicated in Europe and North America; human infection has not occurred in the United States since 1945. However, so few organisms are necessary for infection it is considered a potential agent for biological warfare.

The infection is caused by the bacterium *Burkholderia mallei* transmitted to humans from horses or other domestic animals.

Symptoms and Diagnostic Path
Glanders causes an ulcer or ABSCESS where it enters a wound in the skin. If untreated, it may spread to the bones, liver, central nervous system, and other tissues, and may be fatal.

Symptoms depend on how the person was infected, but may include localized, pus-forming skin infections, pulmonary infections, bloodstream infections, and chronic suppurative infections of the skin.

Generalized symptoms of glanders include fever, muscle aches, chest pain, muscle tightness, headache, excessive tearing of the eyes, light sensitivity, and diarrhea.

If there is a cut or scratch in the skin, a localized infection with ulcers will develop within one to five days, together with swollen lymph nodes. Infections involving the mucous membranes in the eyes, nose, and respiratory tract will cause increased mucus production from the affected sites. Pulmonary infections will cause PNEUMONIA, pulmonary abscesses, and pleural effusion. Bloodstream infections are usually fatal within seven to 10 days. The chronic form of glanders involves multiple abscesses within the muscles of the arms and legs or in the spleen or liver. The disease is diagnosed by identifying *B. mallei* from blood, sputum, urine, or skin lesions.

Treatment Options and Outlook
Because human cases of glanders are rare, experts do not know a great deal about the effectiveness of antibiotic treatment in humans. Studies of sulfadiazine have suggested it may be effective in animals and humans. *B. mallei* is usually sensitive to tetracyclines, ciprofloxacin, streptomycin, novobiocin, gentamicin, imipenem, ceftrazidime, and the sulfonamides; resistance to chloramphenicol has been reported.

Risk Factors and Preventive Measures
There is no vaccine available for glanders. In countries where glanders is endemic in animals, eliminating the infection in animals is the only way to protect humans.

gonorrhea The most commonly reported communicable disease in the United States, most often affecting the genitourinary tract; sometimes the pharynx, eyes, or rectum are affected. Since 1980 the number of people with gonorrhea has been declining; still, in 2002, 351,852 Americans were infected. Many more cases go unreported.

People are at risk if they have more than one sex partner or do not use condoms. Most patients are between the ages of 15 and 24. Gonorrheal infections must be reported to local health departments in the United States.

The disease is caused by a spherical bacterium, NEISSERIA GONORRHOEAE, that is always grouped in pairs. It is passed from one person to the next during sex. It is not possible to get gonorrhea from toilet seats or swimming pools.

A woman who has unprotected sex with an infected man has an 80 to 90 percent chance of being infected herself—a much higher rate than with other STDs. But a man who has unprotected sex with an infected woman has only a 20 to 25 percent chance of becoming infected, because it is harder for bacteria to enter the body through the penis than through the vaginal.

Symptoms and Diagnostic Path

Between three to five days after exposure, symptoms will appear in the genital or rectal area, or in the throat (depending on the sexual practice). Up to 80 percent of infected men experience painful urination, frequent urge to urinate, and white or yellow thick pus from the penis. About half of infected women have swelling of the vagina, abnormal green-yellow vaginal discharge, vaginal bleeding between periods, pelvic discomfort (itching and burning), and pain when urinating.

As the infection spreads—which is more common in women than in men—there may be nausea and vomiting, fever, and rapid heartbeat, or peritonitis. Inflammation of the tissues surrounding the liver also may occur, causing pain in the upper abdomen. Severe cases of gonorrhea are also more common in women and are characterized by signs of blood poisoning, with tender lesions on the skin of the hands and feet and inflammation of the tendons of the wrists, knees, and ankles. If the disease spreads to the conjunctiva of the eyes, there may be scarring and blindness.

In both men and women, infection in the throat causes a mild, red, sore throat.

Culture of the organism from body fluids.

Treatment Options and Outlook

For many years, PENICILLIN was the drug of choice, but in the late 1970s the bacteria became resistant. The most resistant strains are found in New York, California, and Florida, but resistance is seen in all states and most of Canada.

Today, treatment involves two antibiotics: a shot of ceftriaxone and doxycycline pills. The pills will also cure chlamydia (see CHLAMYDIAL INFECTIONS), which has similar symptoms to gonorrhea (many people have both infections). Alternatively, instead of a shot a doctor may give a single dose of cefixime, ciprofloxacin, or ofloxacin. Pregnant women get a shot of ceftriazone and erythromycin pills.

An infant born with the symptoms of gonorrhea must be hospitalized and given ceftriaxone.

PELVIC INFLAMMATORY DISEASE develops in almost 40 percent of untreated women, causing scars in the tubes, infertility, and tubal pregnancies. Untreated pregnant women may experience an infection in the amniotic fluid, smaller babies, or premature birth.

Babies born to infected mothers develop MENINGITIS or gonorrhea conjunctivitis at birth; untreated infants can become blind. For this reason, drops are placed in all babies' eyes at birth to prevent gonorrhea and chlamydia conjunctivitis. In males, gonorrhea can spread to the epididymis (the structure attached to the testicles that helps transport sperm), causing pain and swelling that can ultimately lead to infertility.

More uncommon, in either males and females, gonorrhea can affect other areas, including the throat, eyes, heart, brain, joints, and skin.

Gonyaulax catanella A species of plankton protozoa that produces a toxin ingested by shellfish along the North American coasts. Eating these contaminated shellfish can lead to SHELLFISH POISONING.

These protozoa also cause RED TIDE, which refers to large numbers of protozoa in such dense concentrations that it colors the water red, brown, orange, purple, or yellow.

Treatment Options and Outlook

There is no known antidote for shellfish poisoning caused by toxin-producing plankton. Administration of prostigmine may be effective, together with artificial respiration and oxygen as needed.

gram-negative shock See SEPTIC SHOCK.

granuloma Grouping of cells associated with chronic inflammation that can occur in any part of the body. Granulomas are usually a reaction to certain infectious agents, although they may occur with no known cause.

Certain infections, such as LEPROSY and SYPHILIS, can lead to infective granulomas in many different organs of the body. A pyogenic granuloma is a common benign skin tumor that develops after a minor injury. Pyogenic granulomas can be surgically removed or treated with cryosurgery.

See GRANULOMA, INFECTIOUS; GRANULOMA INGUINALE.

granuloma, infectious A lumpy lesion of GRANULOMA tissue that may develop in diseases such as

TUBERCULOSIS, SYPHILIS, ACTINOMYCOSIS, LEPROSY, or other tissue-invading organisms.

granuloma inguinale A chronic bacterial infection of the genitals that is usually assumed to be a sexually transmitted disease. This relatively rare disease occurs most often among men living in tropical and subtropical areas. There are about 100 cases a year in the United States.

In the United States, homosexuals are at greater risk; it is relatively rare in heterosexual partners of those affected. Men are affected more often than women, but children and the elderly are rarely affected. Past infection does not confer immunity, and there is no evidence of natural resistance.

The disease is caused by the bacteria *Calymmatobacterium granulomatis*, a small gram-negative rod-shaped bacillus. It is spread by anal sexual contact with an infected individual. Granuloma inguinale is communicable as long as the infected person remains untreated and bacteria from the lesions are present.

Symptoms and Diagnostic Path
Within eight to 80 days after infection, lumps or blisters in the genital area appear, becoming a slowly widening sore. Untreated, the lesions will spread, deepen, multiply, and may become infected. Untreated lesions can destroy genital tissue.

Microscopic examination and identification of a smear taken from a lesion and stained.

Treatment Options and Outlook
Several antibiotics will cure the disease; the sores usually will completely heal within five weeks. All patients who are suspected of having this disease are also tested for SYPHILIS, since infection with both diseases is common.

If left untreated, granuloma inguinale can cause extensive destruction of the genitals and may spread to other parts of the body. In this event, the resulting heart failure or PNEUMONIA may be fatal.

group A strep See STREPTOCOCCUS, GROUP-A.

group B strep See STREPTOCOCCUS, GROUP-B.

guinea worm disease See DRACUNCULIASIS.

Gulf War syndrome (GWS) A term that has been used to describe a collection of chronic signs and symptoms reported by U.S., British, Canadian, Czech, Danish, Saudi, Egyptian, and Australian coalition soldiers who were deployed in Operation Desert Storm in 1991. More than 100,000 American veterans of Desert Storm/Desert Shield returned from the Persian Gulf and within six to 24 months, began to complain of a variety of complex symptoms. These included disabling fatigue, intermittent fevers, night sweats, short-term memory problems, headaches, skin rashes, intermittent diarrhea, and abdominal bloating. Some patients have other symptoms including neurotoxicity and brainstem dysfunction that can result in autonomic, cranial, and peripheral nerve demyelination, possibly due to complex chemical exposures.

About 40 percent of these soldiers have transmittable infections, including mycoplasmal and possibly other chronic bacterial infections, that have spread to immediate family members and civilians in the Gulf region.

The origin of Gulf War syndrome is not yet understood. Some experts believe that GWS may be caused by a variety of exposures, including

- bacteria, viruses, and toxins, before, during, and after the conflict
- chemical mixtures, such as organophosphates, antinerve agents, and possibly nerve agents
- depleted uranium and fallout from destroyed nuclear reactors

Some studies have suggested that about half of the sickest Gulf War patients have chronic invasive infections involving certain uncommon mycoplasmas, such as *Mycoplasma fermentans* (incognitus strain). Others appear to have microorganism infections, such as those caused by *Brucella* or other bacteria.

Other experts insist stress could be the cause of these health problems.

gum disease Infection at the roots of the teeth cause bleeding and receding gums that—if unchecked—can lead to tooth loss. More than 75 percent of Americans over age 35 have some form of gum disease, characterized by swollen, bleeding gums.

Gingivitis is an early, reversible stage of gum disease characterized by inflammation of the gums. At this stage it can usually be eliminated by daily brushing and flossing. Mild gum disease is very common in young adults; it is especially common among pregnant women and diabetics because of their changing hormone levels. In the more advanced stages of gum disease, called periodontitis, the gums and bone that support the teeth can become seriously damaged. The teeth can become loose, fall out, or have to be removed by a dentist.

Gingivitis occurs when plaque, a sticky film of bacteria, collects around the base of the teeth. Experts believe that toxins produced by bacteria within the plaque irritate the gums, causing them to become infected, tender, and swollen.

Symptoms and Diagnostic Path

Bleeding gums are nearly always a symptom of gingivitis. Other symptoms include a reddish purple color of the gums, and a soft, shiny, swollen appearance.

Untreated gum disease may lead to periodontitis, the advanced stage of gum disease, in which infected pockets form between the gums and the teeth. As the infection spreads, the supporting tissues of the teeth and the surrounding bone erode, loosening the teeth.

Acute necrotizing ulcerative gingivitis (trench mouth) may develop following infection with anaerobic bacteria in those with chronic gingivitis, especially those with lowered resistance to infection. This is a serious condition that can destroy gum tissue; it requires antibiotics.

Treatment Options and Outlook

Good oral hygiene is the main way to both treat and prevent gum disease. In cases of periodontitis, the dentist will surgically remove part of the gum margin (a technique called gingivectomy) as a way of removing the pockets of infected gums. It is performed in the dentist's office using local anesthetics.

Risk Factors and Preventive Measures

Up to 30 percent of the U.S. population may be genetically susceptible to gum disease, according to the American Academy of Periodontology (AAP). Genetic testing to identify these people can help by encouraging early treatment that may help them keep their teeth for a lifetime.

See also VINCENT'S DISEASE.

Haemophilus A genus of gram-negative bacteria often found in the respiratory tract of humans and animals. The genus includes *H. influenzae,* which causes respiratory tract infections and one form of MENINGITIS; *H. haemolyticus* affecting upper respiratory tracts; and *H. ducreyi,* which causes CHANCROID.

The *Haemophilus* genus can be treated with cephalosporins, tetracyclines, sulfonamides, quinalones, and monobactanes as well as penicillinase-resistant PENICILLINS.

Haemophilus B See HAEMOPHILUS INFLUENZAE TYPE B (HIB).

Haemophilus ducreyi A type of bacteria that causes CHANCROID.

Haemophilus influenzae type b (Hib) A type of rod-shaped bacterium that can cause serious diseases. It is the leading cause of bacterial MENINGITIS in children, a serious infection characterized by inflammation of the brain and spinal cord that may be fatal. More than two-thirds of all bacterial meningitis victims are children younger than age five; until 1992, most of them were infected with *Haemophilus influenzae* type b (usually shortened to *H. flu* or "Hib"). It is serious because nearly one child in every 20 who gets meningitis dies, and up to 35 percent develop permanent brain damage.

According to the CENTERS FOR DISEASE CONTROL AND PREVENTION, from the 1980s more than half of the estimated 20,000 Americans aged five years or younger who became infected with the Hib bacterium each year developed bacterial meningitis. This disorder was the leading cause of acquired mental retardation in the United States, leaving many youngsters blind, deaf, or paralyzed.

However, widespread use of a Hib vaccine licensed for infants in 1990 has dramatically reduced the incidence of the deadly disease. According to the Centers for Disease Control and Prevention, the incidence of invasive Hib infection has dropped by almost 98 percent among infants and children since the introduction of the vaccine. Although Hib meningitis is not yet completely eradicated, the vaccine has been stunningly effective.

The *Haemophilus influenzae* type B bacterium has several different strains, each with a different capsule around the bacterium. Type b was the most common cause of meningitis in children before the vaccine; the other types are rare. However, the bacteria causes other diseases besides meningitis; one strain is a common cause of ear infections in children. Other illnesses caused by *H. influenzae* type B bacteria include EPIGLOTTITIS, septic arthritis, CELLULITIS, BACTEREMIA, and PNEUMONIA.

The bacteria enter a person's body through the nose; meningitis results if the bacteria travel through the blood into the membrane covering the brain (the meninges). Healthy children can carry the bacteria in their nose and throat secretions; the infection is spread by kissing or sharing possessions, drinks, and food. Child care workers also can spread the bacteria.

Symptoms and Diagnostic Path

Symptoms appear within two weeks after exposure. All types of meningitis may appear in children either gradually or suddenly. The gradual type is harder to diagnose because the symptoms (at least at first) are vague. Much more common is the abrupt onset variety of meningitis, in which symptoms appear in less than 24 hours, with a sudden high fever (100°F to 106°F) chills, vomiting, stiff neck, intense headache in the front of the head, or a seizure. The neck hurts when the child tries to touch his chin to the chest. There may be muscle spasms and sensitivity to light.

Some children exhibit unusual behavior as the infection begins, including aggressiveness, irritability, agitation, delirium, or screaming, followed by lethargy or coma. Others may experience a cold or an ear infection before the onset of meningitis.

A baby from age three months to two years may exhibit fever, vomiting, irritability, seizures, and a high-pitched cry. The baby may suddenly become rigid, and the soft spot on the front of the head may become hard or bulging.

A lumbar puncture (spinal tap) is necessary to sample the fluid around the spinal cord and check for bacteria, white cells, sugar, and protein. This will help determine what is causing the meningitis. Bacterial meningitis causes cloudy fluid, with a high amount of certain types of white blood cells, low sugar, and high protein. Bacteria will grow in blood culture or spinal fluid culture in 24 to 48 hours; rapid tests on fluid or blood give results in just a few hours and are often helpful in identifying the type of bacteria.

Recent antibiotic treatment prior to getting meningitis may make diagnosis more difficult. Lumbar puncture is a safe procedure when done in a large emergency room or in an experienced pediatrician's office and is imperative in correctly diagnosing meningitis.

Treatment Options and Outlook

Without treatment, a child can die from Hib meningitis; with antibiotics, about 95 percent of children recover. Any child with possible *H. flu* meningitis will be admitted to the hospital for IV antibiotics. A baby or child would also receive dexamethasone with the antibiotic and continue to take it for two to four days to prevent swelling of the brain and subsequent hearing problems. Children should rest in a darkened, quiet room; any fever higher than 101°F should be treated with acetaminophen and sponge baths.

A child with *H. flu* meningitis is considered to be infectious until after receiving 24 hours of antibiotics; however, even after recovery some children will carry bacteria in nose and mouth. Rifampin is given to eliminate this bacteria. Healthy carriers are infectious for a few weeks to a few months.

Children who recover from this type of meningitis, as well as those who are vaccinated, are immune to subsequent bacterial exposure.

Increased pressure on the brain from fluid buildup is a serious complication; signs of this include changes in head size activity, vision, breathing, pupils' reactivity or decrease in urine.

The most common long-lasting complication is hearing impairment. Recent studies suggest that children over six weeks of age who received dexamethasone immediately had less hearing loss than those who did not.

Other less common complications include blindness, hydrocephalus, arthritis, seizures, and permanent developmental delays.

Risk Factors and Preventive Measures

The best prevention for Hib infection is vaccination for all infants. The Hib vaccine is one of the safest of all vaccine products and cannot cause meningitis. About one in every eight children who receive the vaccine may have some slight redness, swelling, or tenderness at the injection site. About one in every 140 children will develop a fever higher than 102°F. The reactions begin within 24 hours of the shot and quickly pass.

Before the vaccine, as many as 5 percent of healthy preschoolers carried *H. flu* type b but did not get sick. Vaccinated children cannot become carriers.

An antibiotic called rifampin is used to prevent cases of Hib after exposure; if all babies and young children in a home or child care group are vaccinated, preventive medicine after an exposure is not necessary. Rifampin will temporarily get rid of *H. flu* from the noses and throats of healthy carriers about 95 percent of the time. It helps prevent any exposed child in a day care center or a family from getting *H. flu* meningitis.

hand, foot, and mouth disease   A common infectious disease of toddlers that produces blistering of palms, soles, and the inside of the mouth. The condition often sweeps through day-care centers in the summer. There is no connection between this condition and the hoof-and-mouth disease found in cattle.

An infected child can pass on the disease wherever the rash or sores appear; the virus will be present in the stools and the digestive tract for several weeks. Infected children do not need to be isolated, however, because most adults are immune and the illness is not severe.

The disease is caused by the COXSACKIE VIRUS which is spread by contact with nose and mouth secretions.

Symptoms and Diagnostic Path

Many children are infected but do not exhibit symptoms; they develop immunity without experiencing the illness. It is possible, however, to get this disease again from a different strain of the virus. The mild illness usually lasts only a few days.

Symptoms usually appear within four to six days after infection, and include ulcers inside the cheeks, gums, or tongue, together with a fever, achiness, sore throat, headache, and poor appetite. Two days later, a rash on palms, fingers, soles, and diaper area appear; this is the signal that the virus is abating.

Tests are unnecessary. If the child is very ill, and the diagnosis is not clear, samples can be taken for culture from the lesions or stool.

Treatment Options and Outlook

There is no treatment other than painkillers to relieve blister discomfort. Acetaminophen is given for fever above 101°F or for headaches. Small sips of soothing foods and fluids will ease mouth sores, such as frozen or diluted juice, lukewarm broth, soft noodles, or gelatin desserts.

Complications are extremely rare.

Risk Factors and Preventive Measures

Hand washing is the only way to prevent this disease. This is especially important in a day-care or nursery school. Family members can be protected by washing the towels, washcloths, and bedding used by a sick child.

Hansen's disease See LEPROSY.

hantavirus A group of viruses carried by rodents (mice, rats, and voles) responsible for a variety of diseases, including HANTAVIRUS PULMONARY SYNDROME and hemorrhagic fever. The virus is transmitted when humans breathe air contaminated by affected rodents' droppings, urine, or saliva and is not passed directly from human to human.

All of the viruses in this group trigger the leakage of blood from a patient's capillaries, causing rapid organ failure before the immune system can react. Each hantavirus infects primarily one type of rodent.

The Hantaan, Seoul, Puumala, Prospect Hill, and Porogia strains are five viruses within the hantavirus genus within the BUNYAVIRIDAE virus family. The newest strain is the SIN NOMBRE (no-name) VIRUS, which first appeared in the Four Corners area of the western United States. (It was originally called Muerto Canyon [Valley of Death] virus for the spot on a New Mexico Navajo reservation where it was isolated. Because this name offended the Navajo, the virus was renamed Sin Nombre.) Deer mice were the rodents responsible in this outbreak.

The *Hantaan* virus was the first of the group to be identified in a Korean lab in 1976 from the lungs of a striped field mouse. This variety causes a bleeding disease called Korean hemorrhagic fever, a problem during the Korean War. Named for the Hantaan River in South Korea, the virus infected 2,500 U.S. troops and killed between 5 and 10 percent of its victims. The related *Seoul virus* infects domestic rats, and causes a similar (but less deadly) type of fever. Because it is carried by rats, it is more common. *Puumala virus* affects the bank vole and is found most often in Scandinavia and western Europe.

hantavirus pulmonary syndrome A rare respiratory illness caused by a strain of HANTAVIRUS (a group of viruses carried by rodents) that causes patients to gasp for air as their lungs fill with fluid. It kills about half the people it infects, usually within a week. The syndrome was first diagnosed in the United States in 1993 at a Navajo reservation in the Four Corners area of New Mexico, Colorado, Utah, and Arizona, and has been identified throughout the United States. After the initial outbreak, physicians across the country were asked to report any illness with symptoms similar to those of HPS that could not be explained by any other cause.

Since 1993, researchers have discovered that there are several hantaviruses that cause HPS. In June 1993, a Louisiana man who had not visited the Four Corners area developed HPS. The patient's tissues revealed another hantavirus, named the Bayou virus, which was linked to the rice rat (*Oryzomys palustris*). In late 1993, a 33-year-old Florida man was diagnosed with HPS caused by yet another hantavirus, named the Black Creek Canal virus; its carrier is the cotton rat (*Sigmodon hispidus*). And yet another case occurred in New York, caused by a Sin Nombre–like virus named New York-1; the white-footed mouse (*Peromyscus leucopus*) is believed to be the carrier.

In addition, cases of HPS from related hantaviruses have been documented in Argentina, Brazil, Canada, Chile, Paraguay, and Uruguay.

Hantaviruses can be found throughout the world, where more than 170 names have been given to the hantavirus infections, including the often-fatal hemorrhagic fever. Until 1993, hantaviruses had been linked to the development of hemorrhagic fever. But the strain that was discovered in Four Corners caused a new disease, with debilitating flu-like symptoms and respiratory failure.

There appears to be an increasing risk of human exposure to viruses that cause hantavirus pulmonary syndrome (HPS). Between January and May, 1999 there was a dramatic increase in human cases of HPS. By May 28, 1999, 217 cases in 30 different states had been confirmed by the U.S. CENTERS FOR DISEASE CONTROL AND PREVENTION (CDC) since the initial outbreak in 1993.

In the Arizona, Colorado, and New Mexico region there were at least eight confirmed cases during the five-month period from January to May 1999. During the same five-month period in the years 1995 through 1998 there were only about two cases per year—a dramatic fourfold increase.

One key finding that may explain the rise in HPS cases is the fact that the prevalence of antibodies for hantavirus in rodents dramatically increased between the spring of 1998 and 1999, which indicates that the prevalence of the virus also increased despite the fact that the number of rodents remained relatively unchanged.

HPS is caused by a hantavirus first named Muerto Canyon (Valley of Death) virus for the spot on a New Mexico Navajo reservation where it was isolated. Because this name offended the Navajo, the virus was renamed SIN NOMBRE (or "no name") virus. The disease can be spread by several common rodent species (deer mice, white-footed mice, and cotton rats) and has been found in 23 states; it is most common in New Mexico, which has had 28 cases; in Arizona, with 21 cases; and in California, with 13 cases. Doctors believe patients become infected by breathing in the dried urine or feces of infected deer mice; about 30 percent of the deer mice in the Four Corners area carry the Sin Nombre agent. Infected rodents have been found in other parts of the country as well.

Oddly enough, some patients have contracted the illness after little or no contact with rodents. Studies also have shown that the virus does not trigger infection in everyone it infects. In fact, the CDC acknowledges that the link between rodents and victims is unclear. Scientists do not know why some people become infected and others do not.

Even more worrying, some people have exhibited symptoms of hantavirus pulmonary syndrome but do not have the virus. In fact, there were half a dozen recent incidents in California where young and healthy people died suddenly of acute respiratory failure, yet did not test positive for hantavirus or any other microbe.

Scientists believe the U.S. outbreak was triggered by climate irregularities associated with the most recent El Niño (the occasional warming of waters in the tropical Pacific). While it is believed that the mice who carry the virus were probably infected for years, the climate-induced explosion in the deer mouse population may have fueled the spread of the disease in humans.

In addition to contact with contaminated urine or droppings, people can become infected with the virus after being bitten by rodents. Many people who have developed the disease live in mice-infested homes. One woman who developed the disease was exposed to rodents her cat dragged into the house, and another died after cleaning a rodent-infested barn.

The hantavirus does not appear to be highly infectious, and it is almost always found in isolated cases. There were only four instances in which more than one case occurred at the same time and place.

The types of hantavirus that cause HPS in the United States cannot be transmitted from one person to another. It is not possible to get the virus from touching or kissing a person who has HPS, or from a health care worker who has treated someone with the disease. In addition, the virus is not transmitted via blood transfusions.

Symptoms and Diagnostic Path

Hantavirus pulmonary syndrome begins as a flu-like illness with fever and chills, muscle aches, and cough; it can be easily misdiagnosed as HEPATITIS or an inflamed pancreas. The virus goes on to damage the kidneys and lungs, causing an accumulation of fluid that can drown the victim. The disease is fatal in almost half of all cases.

Treatment Options and Outlook

The antiviral drug Virazole (ribavirin) has reduced fatalities in clinical studies.

Risk Factors and Preventive Measures

Army scientists developed a vaccine against hantavirus infection in 1995. While it is experimental, it is available to protect military personnel in South Korea and other areas of the world where the infection is common, according to the army's Medical Research Institute of Infectious Diseases in Ft. Detrick, Maryland. Such a vaccine does not need the approval of the Food and Drug Administration to be used among military personnel, if they give informed consent.

The CDC cautions homeowners to be careful around rodent excretion, even though hantavirus is a rare disease. People should assume that all rodent excretions are infected, and should handle the droppings only after spraying them with disinfectant and wearing gloves.

See also HEMORRHAGIC FEVER WITH RENAL SYNDROME.

Haverhill fever   A febrile disease transmitted by rat bite, first diagnosed in Haverhill, Massachusetts, in 1925.

The disease is caused by one of two bacteria: *STREPTOBACILLUS MONILIFORMIS* or *Spirillum minus*. *Spirillum minus* causes a common disease often found in Asia, particularly Japan, where it is called *sodoku*. This form of rat-bite fever typically causes a unique skin rash characterized by red or purple plaques; the previously healed wound at the site of the bite may reactivate and open. Joint involvement is rare.

Symptoms and Diagnostic Path

Within 10 days of a rat bite, the patient experiences fever, chills, vomiting, headache, muscle, and joint pain, and a rash appears.

Lab analysis of blood or pus can reveal the bacteria that cause the disease.

Treatment Options and Outlook

Antibiotics are effective against Haverhill fever.

head lice   See LICE.

hearing loss and infectious disease   Hearing loss affects about three and a half percent of children up to age 17. Although ear infections are the most common cause of hearing loss in the United States, there are other infectious causes—many of which can be treated successfully. The most common of these are bacterial MENINGITIS and CYTOMEGALOVIRUS INFECTION, but there is a long list of other infectious agents (viruses, bacteria, and parasites) that can lead to hearing problems. In addition, hearing loss can be a side effect of antibiotics (such as the aminoglycosides).

Bacterial meningitis   Hearing loss related to this disease can be caused by *STREPTOCOCCUS PNEUMONIAE* (18 to 30 percent), *Neisseria meningitidis* (10 percent), and *HAEMOPHILUS INFLUENZAE* (6 percent). In pneumococcal meningitis, the incidence and severity of hearing loss is strongly linked to the length of time the disease lasts. Because of vaccination, *H. influenzae* is no longer a major cause of meningitis in the United States, although it remains a serious problem in other parts of the world.

The hearing loss with this disease is related either because of direct damage to the eighth cranial nerve (the hearing nerve) or to inflammation of the interior parts of the hearing mechanism itself.

Although steroids can prevent hearing loss related to *H. influenzae*, steroids do not help prevent hearing loss in meningitis caused by *S. pneumoniae* or *N. meningitidis.*

Syphilis Scientists have known for a long time that congenital syphilis is a cause of hearing loss, but only recently have experts understood that syphilis acquired at any time can lead to hearing problems. There are no controlled studies on treatment, but benzathine PENICILLIN in combination with steroids offers the best hope for improvement.

Borrelia burgdorferi The agent that causes LYME DISEASE has been linked to hearing loss in about 2 percent of patients with the disease, usually involving low-frequency sound waves. The reason behind the deafness is not clear, but researchers suspect the loss occurs as a result of damage to the auditory center or the hearing nerve. Doxycycline or amoxicillin can be given to patients over age nine; younger children should receive amoxicillin or penicillin V. Those with hearing loss in the high frequencies are more likely to see improvement with antibiotic treatment.

Mycobacterium tuberculosis While it is uncommon to find TB infecting the middle ear, it may sometimes be the first symptom of the disease. Such infection causes multiple perforations of the eardrum and chronic ear inflammation. Anti-TB drugs should be given to treat this condition.

Cytomegalovirus (CMV) Each year in the United States, about 4,000 children acquire hearing loss linked to CMV, which may interfere with the fetal development of the ear. The hearing loss usually centers in the high-frequency sounds, with equal loss in both ears. There is no known treatment. Of all children born with CMV, 95 percent do not show any symptoms. Among those who do, 60 percent will develop hearing loss. Those who do not have symptoms rarely develop neurologic problems, but 10 percent of these infants remain at risk for hearing loss.

Measles About one in every 1,000 cases of measles causes hearing loss. Sensorineural hearing loss associated with measles is usually sudden and occurs in both ears, primarily of the higher frequencies; there also may be vertigo and ringing in the ears. This hearing loss tends to be permanent.

Mumps Hearing loss as a result of mumps occurs in about five of every 10,000 cases; there have been a few cases in the United States since vaccination was introduced in 1967. While scientists do not fully understand the link between mumps and deafness, they suspect the virus may cause the atrophy of the organ of Corti (part of the hearing mechanism) as well as a loss of hair cells within the hearing mechanism.

The onset of hearing loss is quick and occurs in only one ear in 80 percent of the cases; the deafness is usually profound and permanent and usually occurs in the higher frequencies. There may also be ringing of the ears, sensation of fullness in the ear, vertigo, nausea, and vomiting.

Rubella In the United States, rubella among pregnant women is rare; when it does occur it often leads to deafness (between 25 percent and 51 percent of the time) in the infant. Hearing loss related to rubella is profound in 55 percent of the cases; severe in 30 percent; and mild to moderate in 15 percent. The hearing loss affects all frequencies, but the middle frequencies cause the most problems.

Research suggests that congenital rubella is progressive and continues to damage the ears even after infancy.

Varicella-zoster Infection with this virus can lead to a syndrome involving facial palsy, herpes of the ear, and hearing loss, first described in 1907. This Ramsay-Hunt syndrome (also called herpes zoster oticus) can produce several patterns of hearing loss, together with ringing of the ears in 48 percent of cases. A patient who also experiences vertigo is not likely to recover from the hearing loss. Prompt treatment with acyclovir seems to be effective.

HIV Studies have reported up to 49 percent of HIV-infected patients have some degree of sensorineural hearing loss, as a possible result of infection of the cochlea, the hearing center in the brain, or both. Patients with HIV-associated hearing loss also may experience vertigo and facial nerve palsy. Drug treatment does not seem to affect the hearing loss.

Fungal infections Fungal infections of the ear can cause either a conductive or sensorineural hearing loss. The most common organisms responsible for the loss include the *Candida* and *Aspergillus* species. Among those with impaired immune systems, *Cryptococcus neoformans* and *Zygomycetes* are a particular problem. A variety of antifungal drugs can be used to treat the problem, but there are no studies that prove their efficacy.

Toxoplasma gondii   Congenital infection with this organism has been related to hearing loss, although the reason behind the problem is not well understood. Treatment with pyrimethamine, sulfadiazine, or spiramycin is effective.

Visceral leishmaniasis   While this disease is not common in the United States, it is endemic in many other areas of the world, where it causes a type of hearing loss, probably by affecting the covering of the hearing nerve. Treatment with stibogluconate sodium is effective and can frequently cure the hearing loss.

Flukes   Infestation with the intestinal FLUKE *Fasciola hepatica* can produce hearing loss. Rarely seen in the United States, it is more common in Latin America, Asia, and Africa. A patient is infected by eating raw aquatic plants contaminated with the flukes. Bithionol is the treatment of choice.

heart disease and infection   Bacteria may be another important risk factor in the development of heart disease. There is no question that heredity and diet play a role in the clogging of arteries, but there is mounting evidence that infection may trigger the inflammatory process that swells the lining of an artery. One possible explanation, according to researchers, is that infections may cause inflammation of the arteries, which can be measured by testing for a substance called C-reactive protein (CRP).

Separate research studies have suggested that sinusitis, bronchitis, and urinary tract infections could play a role in heart disease.

Some studies have identified infection with specific types of bacteria: HELICOBACTER PYLORI, which causes ulcers, and *Chlamydia pneumoniae*, which causes pneumonia (a different strain is responsible for the sexually transmitted disease chlamydia) (see CHLAMYDIAL INFECTIONS). *C. pneumoniae* has often been found in the artery-clogging plaque that builds up in atherosclerosis. Indeed, when rabbits fed an artery-clogging diet high in fat and cholesterol were infected with the germ, their plaques grew faster than those of animals fed just the unhealthy diet.

Research suggests that prescribing antibiotics immediately after a heart attack or episode of severe chest pain might significantly reduce the chances of further attacks. At least one study has found that the risk of further heart problems was 40 percent less in the group getting antibiotics than among those getting fake pills. Moreover, statistics show that frequent users of antibiotics have a lower risk of heart attack than those who have not used the drugs.

Despite these studies, the government does not recommend that heart patients be treated with antibiotics. Heavy use of antibiotics can not only increase the risk that everyone will have more resistant infections, and the heart patient is more likely to carry resistant organisms later on.

***Helicobacter pylori* infection**   Infection with this bacterium causes most stomach ulcers and almost all duodenal ulcers, and represents one of the most common chronic infections in humans. The bacteria infect two-thirds of all people around the world. In the United States it is most common among older adults, African Americans, Hispanics, and lower socioeconomic groups.

Since the 1950s doctors knew that family members of ulcer patients were three times more likely than the general population to have ulcers as well. But the link was not firmly established until 1983, when Australian gastroenterologist Barry J. Marshall identified the bacterium in stomach tissue of ulcer patients, when it was first called *Campylobacter pylori*. In an attempt to prove the link between bacteria and ulcers, he swallowed the bacteria and developed an ulcer. Before that time, physicians had believed that ulcers were a noninfectious disease. Before this bacterium was discovered, the major causes of ulcers were believed to be spicy food, acid, stress, and lifestyle. Most patients were given long-term medications that relieved ulcer-related symptoms and may have healed the ulcer but did not treat the underlying infection. As a result, ulcers recurred. Today, doctors know that most ulcers are caused by *H. pylori*, and appropriate antibiotic regimens can successfully eliminate infection in most patients.

Ulcers are found in one out of every 10 Americans, and *H. pylori* is implicated in 90 percent of those cases. Virtually everyone with the bacteria has chronic gastritis (a mild inflammation of the stomach lining).

Although the human stomach is filled with acids, this bacterium manages to thrive there by nestling into the stomach's mucous lining. How the bacteria spread is unclear. Studies suggest the bacteria are passed via person-to-person contact, but are probably not sexually transmitted. If one family member is infected, it is likely that the rest of the family also harbor the bacteria. The bacteria are also common in areas of poor sanitation and crowded living conditions, and among families with multiple children (especially where children share beds). Scientists suspect the infection may be spread by swallowing infected food or water in addition to person-to-person contact. *H. pylori* is not naturally found in animals.

Symptoms and Diagnostic Path

Following infection, patients experience nausea and stomach pain, vomiting and fever, which lasts between three and 14 days. If not treated, patients will develop chronic gastritis that can last for decades. While half the world's populations are believed to be infected (including an estimated 40 million Americans), for some reason the bacteria only causes ulcers in between 10 to 20 percent of their hosts. Although ulcers do not always occur, bacteria always produce inflammation of the stomach lining. Some people with the infection do not have ulcers but do experience nausea, gas, bloating, and burning stomach pain. These symptoms occur twice as often in people with *H. pylori* as in those without the bacteria.

Blood tests can determine the presence of antibodies to the bacteria. This test tells if a patient has ever had the infection, but cannot determine if the infection is active. It is not 100 percent accurate, however. A punch biopsy of the stomach can be examined under a microscope for the presence of *H. pylori*.

There is also a rapid breath test to identify *H. pylori*. This test involves swallowing a harmless substance that will be broken down in the stomach if bacteria are present. The breakdown products are detected in the breath. This Urea Breath Test probably provides the most accurate assessment as to whether or not *H. pylori* is in the stomach, and it is very useful in proving whether treatment has eradicated the infection.

Treatment Options and Outlook

About 90 percent of *H. pylori* infections can be cured with a combination of anti-ulcer medication (Pepto Bismol, Biaxin) and specific antibiotics (metronidazole, clarithromycin and omeprazole, tetracycline, or amoxicillin). Because the treatment may not be completely successful, follow-up testing at least four weeks after completing treatment may be needed to make sure the bacteria are no longer present. If tests reveal no bacteria, the patient is not likely to be reinfected ever again. Persistent infection may require a different medication for longer period of time.

The National Institutes of Health has recommended that all patients with stomach or duodenal ulcers who also have *H. pylori* be treated for both the ulcer and the infection.

While there appears to be a relationship between the bacteria and stomach cancer, these cancers are becoming less common in the United States, and therapy for *H. pylori* has not been recommended as a preventive measure.

There is no solid evidence that diet affects *H. pylori* or ulcer healing. With proper medical treatment, ulcers heal as well on a regular diet as with a bland diet. Still, it is wise to avoid smoking, nonsteroidal antiinflammatory drugs (NSAIDs), aspirin, excessive alcohol, and caffeine.

The organism has also been found in a disproportionately large number of patients with certain kinds of stomach cancer. Some scientists suggest the infection may triple the risk of this rare cancer.

Risk Factors and Preventive Measures

In 1996, the National Institutes of Health has urged U.S. doctors to test all ulcer patients for the bacterium and to treat the infected with antibiotics for two weeks. However, the treatment is not easy; it involves taking 12 to 16 pills for two weeks and carries the risk of some side effects, such as fatigue and dizziness.

Careful personal hygiene (thorough handwashing, using separate personal items such as glasses and toothbrushes) is probably the best way to prevent person-to-person spread.

Since scientists have succeeded in immunizing mice, a human vaccine may be developed in the future.

helminth   A parasitic worm.

helminthiasis   An infestation by any species of parasitic worms. Ascariasis, FILARIASIS, HOOKWORM disease, and TRICHINOSIS are all common types of worm disease.

hemolytic uremic syndrome (HUS)   One of the most common causes of sudden kidney failure in children, usually the result of an infection by *ESCHERICHIA COLI* bacteria in contaminated foods such as rare hamburger, dairy products, and juice. Some people have contracted HUS after swimming in pools or lakes contaminated with feces.

E. coli infects the digestive tract (GASTROENTERITIS), but most children with gastroenteritis recover fully in two or three days and do not develop HUS. However, a few children develop HUS if the bacteria in the digestive system produce toxins that enter the bloodstream and start to destroy red blood cells.

Non-diarrheal HUS is more rare and tends to occur in older or very young children. It can occur after *Streptococcus pneumoniae* infection.

Symptoms and Diagnostic Path
Gastrointeritis is characterized by vomiting, stomach cramps, and bloody diarrhea. Symptoms of HUS may not become apparent until a week after the gastroenteritis problems have begun. With HUS, the child remains pale, tired, and cranky and may have small, unexplained bruises or bleeding from the nose or mouth. This bleeding is the result of toxins that destroy the platelets (cells that normally help clotting in the blood).

As HUS progresses, a child's urine output decreases because the damaged red blood cells clog the tiny blood vessels in the kidneys, making them work harder to remove wastes and extra fluid from the blood. This inability to get rid of excess fluid and wastes may trigger high blood pressure or swelling of the face, hands, feet, or the entire body. The progression to acute kidney failure occurs in about half the cases of HUS.

Treatment Options and Outlook
HUS is treated by maintaining normal salt and water levels in the body so as to ease the symptoms and prevent further complications. Blood transfusions of packed red blood cells may be necessary, and high blood pressure may need to be treated. Only the most severe cases require dialysis to help filter wastes from the blood. Some children may sustain significant kidney damage that slowly develops into permanent kidney failure and will then require long-term peritoneal dialysis or hemodialysis or a kidney transplant, but most children recover completely with no long-term consequences.

Risk Factors and Preventive Measures
Washing and cooking foods adequately, avoiding rare hamburger, and avoiding unclean swimming areas are the best ways to avoid this disease.

hemorrhagic fever with renal syndrome (HFRS)   An infectious disease caused by HANTAVIRUSes that trigger a group of symptoms including fever, kidney malfunction, and low platelet count. Because platelets are important in proper clotting, low numbers of circulating platelets can result in spontaneous heavy bleeding, or hemorrhage.

This infection occurs predominantly in the Eastern Hemisphere, and is spread to humans by exposure to virus-infected rodents or their droppings. Infection usually occurs when someone inhales airborne virus-contaminated particles from rodent droppings.

Before 1951, HFRS was relatively unknown to Western physicians, but in Asia HFRS had been recognized for centuries. However, it was not until 3,200 cases occurred among United Nations forces in Korea between 1951 and 1954 that Western doctors became familiar with the disease. In 1993, in the southwestern United States, an outbreak of respiratory illness caused by the SIN NOMBRE VIRUS belonging to the Hantavirus genus occurred and is described as the Hantavirus pulmonary syndrome (HPS).

Rats that carry the Seoul virus (*Rattus norvegicus*) live in many port cities of the eastern United States and were introduced from Europe by cargo ships. Improved surveillance for hantavirus infection in humans suggests that HFRS caused by Seoul infection does occur in a few reported American cases. There are about 150,000 to 200,000 hospitalizations in China each year caused by HFRS. The severe form of HFRS also occurs in Japan and Singapore. The milder form of HFRS (nephropathic epidemica) occurs in the Scandinavian countries of Sweden, Finland, Norway, and Denmark.

The disease is caused by five different hantaviruses: Hantaan, Puumala, Belgrade, Seoul, and Muerto Canyon viruses. The striped field mouse, yellow-neck mouse, Norway rat, and the bank vole are the principal reservoirs for viruses that cause hemorrhagic fever with renal syndrome. Human to human transmission of the virus has not yet been documented.

Symptoms and Diagnostic Path

The onset of hemorrhagic fever with renal syndrome is often sudden, and begins with an intense headache, backache, fever, and chills. It then progresses in five overlapping waves, starting with the fever, low blood pressure, lack of urine, diuretic, and convalescent stages. Often one or more of the stages may not cause symptoms. Hemorrhage, if it occurs at all, usually appears during the fever stage and appears as a facial flushing or reddish appearance in the eyes and mucous membranes, together with a rash on the palate and skin folds.

After the febrile stage ends, low blood pressure may develop and last between hours and days. The patient may experience nausea and vomiting, which in severe cases may lead to death as a result vascular leakage and acute shock. Half of all deaths occur during the oliguric phase because of an increase in blood volume. As the patient recovers, kidney function improves, although death may still occur as a result of shock or lung problems. The last stage of the illness (the convalescent phase) may last between weeks and months before the patient fully recovers.

Treatment Options and Outlook

Treatment of hantavirus infection is primarily supportive, since there are not any drugs that will kill the virus. However, the antiviral drug ribavirin has reduced some fatalities caused by hantavirus.

Because HFRS worsens so quickly, supportive treatment should be started at the first sign of symptoms. Low blood pressure can be treated with medications; blood transfusions are given for hemorrhage and shock; hemodialysis can be helpful in the case of kidney failure.

The fatality rate depends on which virus has caused the illness. In general, HFRS caused by Puumala virus is less severe and is only fatal in about 0.1 percent of all cases. Disease caused by the Hantaan virus is usually more severe, and can be fatal in about 5 percent to 10 percent of all cases.

Risk Factors and Preventive Measures

Since transmission of the viruses is almost entirely from rodent to human, the best way to prevent disease is to prevent rodent infestation. Rodent trapping, poisoning, or cats are often recommended in situations where rodent infestation of the home poses a serious health risk.

See also HANTAVIRUS PULMONARY SYNDROME.

Hendra virus A rare virus causing an emerging infectious disease formerly known as equine morbillivirus. In the first known outbreak, the virus surfaced in Australia, in the fall of 1994. It killed 13 of 17 infected horses and one of two humans before it was identified. Comparison with other viruses showed that the mystery virus was most closely related to a group known as morbilliviruses, which includes viruses such as MEASLES. It had not been reported before anywhere in the world.

The virus was initially called equine morbillivirus, but genetic analysis of the entire virus later showed that its most appropriate classification was in a new genus within the Paramyxoviridae family. The name Hendra virus is now currently used, after the Brisbane suburb in which the outbreak occurred.

In October 1995, Hendra virus was associated with a second death when an Australian farmer died in Brisbane. The farmer, who tested positive for Hendra virus, had close contact with two horses in August 1994, both during their clinical illness and while they were being autopsied. Subsequent tests on tissue from the dead horses revealed the presence of Hendra virus. In January 1999, another Australian horse died from Hendra disease.

NIPAH VIRUS, also a member of the family Paramyxoviridae, is related to, but not identical to, Hendra virus. Nipah virus was first identified in 1999 during an outbreak of encephalitis and respiratory illness among adult men in Malaysia and Singapore.

Unlike other viruses in the family, Hendra virus can infect more than one animal species. Scientists believe fruit bats are the natural host of the virus. Although Hendra virus is not highly contagious, if an infection occurs it can be fatal. Horses can be infected by eating material contaminated with the virus, and transmission from cat urine to horses can occur.

The virus is extremely virulent, killing 70 percent of infected horses. The virus induces cells lining the blood vessels to clump, creating holes in the vessel walls, allowing fluid to leak into the lungs and tissues. As the fluid pours into the lungs, the patient (horse or human) drowns in these fluids. There is no known treatment.

Symptoms and Diagnostic Path

Only three human cases of Hendra virus disease have been recognized. Two of the three individuals known to be infected had a respiratory illness with severe flu-like signs and symptoms.One of the three Hendra virus infections was marked by a delayed onset of progressive encephalitis.

Treatment Options and Outlook

The drug ribavirin has been shown to be effective against the viruses, but controlled drug studies have not been performed and the usefulness of the drug is uncertain. Hendra virus infection appears to have a high fatality rate; two of the three human patients infected with Hendra virus died.

Risk Factors and Preventive Measures

Hendra virus infection can be prevented by avoiding animals known to be infected and by using appropriate personal protective equipment devices when it is necessary to come into contact with potentially infected animals.

hepatitis   Inflammation of the liver. Although generally caused by a virus, alcoholism or certain drugs also can damage the liver and lead to hepatitis.

When the liver is damaged, it cannot excrete the blood breakdown substance called bilirubin, which then builds up in the blood. This causes a yellow tinge to skin and eyes (called jaundice). The appearance of jaundice is more or less a warning sign that

the liver is no longer able to cleanse the blood. In severe cases of hepatitis, the liver fails altogether, resulting in death unless a liver transplant is done.

Hippocrates was the first to mention epidemics of jaundice, and the disease went on to become a factor in many large military campaigns. During the Civil War, for example, hepatitis affected more than 70,000 soldiers. By the time World War II began, scientists were able to differentiate between two types of hepatitis—what was then called "infectious" hepatitis, spread by contaminated food or water, and "serum," hepatitis, spread by infected blood.

By the 1960s, scientists learned that the disease was caused by specific unrelated viruses and gave them alphabetical names to distinguish them. The alphabet of hepatitis viruses all belong to different genuses.

The various hepatitis viruses differ in their likelihood of producing chronic infection. About 70 percent of those infected with HEPATITIS C becomes a carrier of the virus. HEPATITIS A causes only temporary liver damage, which is reversed as the body produces antibodies. HEPATITIS B or hepatitis C, however, can cause long-term complications. Delta, or D, virus, is always a coinfection with hepatitis B; HEPATITIS E does not occur in North America. Although the viruses are unrelated to one another, they act in similar ways, attacking and damaging only the liver.

Hepatitis B and C may quickly develop into fulminant hepatitis, in which the liver cells are completely destroyed. As the liver function stops, toxic substances build up and affect the brain, causing lethargy, confusion, combativeness, stupor, and coma. This can often lead to death, although with aggressive treatment the patient may live. If the victim does not die, the liver is often able to regenerate and resume function, and the brain recovers.

See also HEPATITIS A, HEPATITIS B, HEPATITIS C, HEPATITIS D, HEPATITIS E, HEPATITIS G.

hepatitis A   The most common and least dangerous type of hepatitis, this is the first hepatitis virus that scientists were able to identify. A food-borne virus, it looks much like a poliovirus with just one bare strand of RNA within a 20-sided shell that can replicate only in the liver. It infects only humans and a few primates, primarily via contaminated feces. Formerly known as "infectious hepatitis," hepatitis A is fairly common; during EPIDEMICS, the number of reported cases reaches 35,000, but thousands of cases go unreported. About 100 people die each year.

While there is not a typical "season" for hepatitis A, it occurs in cycles. In the United States, cases peaked from 1961 to 1971, declined, and then peaked again from 1983 to 1991; numbers dropped again after 1992. Foods have been implicated in more than 30 outbreaks since 1983. The most recent include north Georgia frozen strawberries, Montana frozen strawberries, and Baltimore shellfish—all in 1990.

The illness is caused by lack of sanitation and occurs most often among school-age children and young adults. In overcrowded areas in developed countries and many developing countries, it is so common that 90 percent or more of 10-year-olds are healthy carriers and immune as adults. It is estimated that 40 percent of healthy adults in the United States are immune to hepatitis A as a result of previous infection and have lifelong immunity.

The virus dates from 400 B.C.E., when it afflicted armies in every war; it is believed to have played a role in Napoleon's defeat.

Other former names for hepatitis A include epidemic hepatitis, epidemic jaundice, catarrhal jaundice, infectious icterus, Botkins disease, and MS-1 hepatitis.

Hepatitis A belongs to the ENTEROVIRUS GROUP of the PICORNAVIRUSES, which include poliovirus, COXSACKIE VIRUS, ECHOVIRUS, and RHINOVIRUS. Hepatitis A is spread by eating food or drinking water contaminated with the hepatitis A virus (HAV), which is shed in the stool.

The virus enters through the mouth, multiplies in the body, and is passed in the feces; it can then be carried on an infected person's hands and spread by direct contact, or by eating food or drink handled by that person. Anyone can get hepatitis A, but it occurs most often among children. Most people get it either from close personal contact between family members, sex partners (especially homosexual men), and in nursery schools or child care centers.

The virus is hardy and spread easily. Unlike many other viruses, it can live for more than a month at room temperature on kitchen countertops, children's toys, and other surfaces. It can be maintained indefinitely in frozen foods and ice. To inactivate the virus, food must be heated at 185°F for one minute.

A food handler with hepatitis A can spread the disease if he or she touches food that is not cooked before it is eaten (usually sandwiches or salads). Well water contaminated by improperly treated sewage has also been implicated, since hepatitis A can live for a long time in water and it is difficult to test water for hepatitis A. People who drink treated municipal or county water supplies are not at risk.

It is possible to get hepatitis A from eating raw or undercooked foods, such as shellfish (especially oysters). When they eat, shellfish filter large amounts of water; if it is contaminated with hepatitis A, the virus will be concentrated in the shellfish. Even though federal regulations and posting of contaminated waters offer some protection, there is still a risk of contracting viruses when eating raw shellfish. In 1990, an infected Missouri dish washer who prepared lettuce infected 110 people who had eaten at the restaurant; two died.

Symptoms and Diagnostic Path

One-quarter of all people with hepatitis A will not have any symptoms. Infants and young children tend to have very mild cases; three-quarters of children have no symptoms and the rest have low fever and achiness, but rarely jaundice.

The disease in older patients can be more serious, characterized by fever (100–104°F), extreme tiredness, weakness, nausea, stomach upset, pain in the upper right side of the stomach, and loss of appetite. Within a few days, a yellowish tinge appears in the skin and the whites of the eyes. Urine will be darker than usual, and the stool is light colored. Anyone over age 12 may become quite sick for a week or two. Once the jaundice appears, patients begin to feel better. The disease is rarely fatal, and most people recover in a few weeks without any complications.

The incubation period ranges from 15 to 50 days. Patients are most infectious in the two weeks before symptoms develop. Food handlers who know they are infected should not work until they are past the infectious stages, which ends one week after first becoming jaundiced.

Blood tests showing acute antibodies to hepatitis A are the best diagnosis. Symptoms of hepatitis A are so similar to other diseases that a doctor needs a test to make the correct diagnosis.

Treatment Options and Outlook

There is no drug treatment for hepatitis A. While symptoms appear, patients should rest and eat well—low-fat, high-carbohydrate, easily digested foods in small amounts are good choices. These could include crackers, noodles, rice, or soup. Antinausea medicine can be prescribed for severe nausea. Headaches or body aches may respond to acetaminophen. Normal activities may be resumed when the acute illness is over. Infection confers lifelong immunity.

Very rarely, hepatitis A can also develop into fulminant hepatitis in which the liver cells are completely destroyed. As the liver function stops, toxic substances build up and affect the brain, causing lethargy, confusion, combativeness, stupor, and coma. This can often lead to death, although the patient may live with aggressive treatment. If the patient does not die, the liver is able to regenerate and resume function, and the brain recovers.

Risk Factors and Preventive Measures

The hepatitis A vaccine is 100 percent effective after a single primary dose. Available since 1996 in the United States, more than 99 percent of people become immune after two doses; a booster is recommended for this vaccine between six and 12 months after the first dose.

In addition, workers in child-care centers where there are diapered children must maintain strict rules about frequent hand washing and procedures for diaper changing.

Since cooking tainted food kills the virus, shellfish from contaminated areas must be cooked (boiled) for at least eight minutes to be considered safe for eating.

Those who are exposed to hepatitis A can prevent infection by getting a shot of immune globulin (IG), which is pooled human blood plasma that contains protective antibodies against the disease. People who need a shot of IG include the following:

- all household members and sex partners of hepatitis A patients
- close friends of an infected school-age child
- restaurant staffers where one food handler has hepatitis A; patrons of the restaurant need IG within two weeks of exposure only if the infected food handler handles uncooked food and has poor hygienic practices, or has diarrhea
- staff and residents of prisons, institutions, homes, when two or more residents have hepatitis A
- all staff in child-care centers or homes where one or more children or employees have hepatitis A; if three or more children or their families have hepatitis A, family members of the other children need IG as well
- unimmunized travelers to developing countries

hepatitis B   Formerly known as serum hepatitis, this is the most common preventable infectious disease in the United States. The virus, which is far more complex than HEPATITIS A, can destroy the liver and is 100 times more transmissible than the AIDS virus. The number of new infections per year has declined from an average of 260,000 in the 1980s to about 73,000 in 2003. The highest rate of disease occurs in 20- to 49-year-olds, and the biggest decline has been among children and adolescents, as a result of routine hepatitis B vaccination. Nevertheless, there are an estimated 1.25 million chronically infected Americans, of whom 20 to 30 percent acquired the infection in childhood.

The hepatitis B virus (HBV) is carried in the blood and is also found in saliva, semen, and other bodily fluids. It is transmitted much the same as the AIDS virus, but hepatitis B is even easier to catch: One drop of blood infected with hepatitis B contains millions of viral particles. Still, hepatitis B is not spread by casual contact. The virus must get into a person's blood to cause infection. It enters the blood via sexual contact, blood transfusions, dirty needles, or by sharing toothbrushes, razors, or utensils. Unfortunately, the virus is very stable and can survive on dried surfaces (even thorns or stones) for days. More than half of all cases are linked to sexual intercourse with infected partners.

Many health-care workers have become infected from needle sticks, lab accidents, or splashing blood; dentists have caught the infection from patients and gone on to infect other patients. A health-care worker with a needle stick from a patient with hepatitis B has between a 6 percent and 30 percent chance of becoming infected. By comparison, the chance of contracting AIDS this way is only about 0.5 percent.

It is possible for infected mothers to pass the virus to their babies during the final three months of pregnancy, during delivery, or during nursing. There is less danger of passing on the infection if the mother contracts the disease in the early stages of pregnancy. All pregnant women should be tested for hepatitis B.

Many millions of people around the world are chronically infected with hepatitis B, and can give the virus to others (unlike those who have had hepatitis A). Because the germ can induce liver cancer, it is believed to be the world's most common viral cause of cancer.

Symptoms and Diagnostic Path

It can take up to six months after exposure before symptoms of hepatitis B appear, as compared to only six weeks for hepatitis A. Many people have few symptoms. If they do appear, they appear gradually and include tiredness, nausea, joint and muscle aches, mild abdominal pain in upper right side, poor appetite, hives or rash, and mild diarrhea for three to 10 days. This may be followed by jaundice in about half of those who become infected. Nausea is usually not associated with hepatitis B (it is more common with hepatitis A). Other symptoms may include light-colored stools, dark urine, and itchy skin. After jaundice appears, symptoms may improve.

Infants infected by their mothers may have no symptoms at first, but they are at high risk for developing cirrhosis and liver cancer in the second decade of life.

In about one-third of cases, people are not terribly sick; another third have no symptoms at all. In fact, the chance of becoming a carrier are greater if symptoms do not develop. About 25 percent of carriers do suffer chronic symptoms and are at greatest risk of developing cirrhosis. A few may be quite ill for several weeks. Those over age 40 may be more severely ill; children have few symptoms.

The virus can be found in blood and body fluids several weeks before symptoms appear and several months after. The appearance of certain antibodies indicate resolution of disease. People who are chronic carriers (about 10 percent of those infected) are always infectious, although they do not appear to be ill. Those who recover are immune for life.

Hepatitis B can be diagnosed by blood tests; other tests (that look for markers) can differentiate hepatitis B from other types of hepatitis. Liver function tests can measure enzymes produced by the liver that will be elevated in all forms of hepatitis.

Treatment Options and Outlook

Chronic active hepatitis B is treated with alpha-interferons and antiviral compounds. Many people report short-term side effects from interferon, such as fever, chills, appetite loss, vomiting, muscle aches, and sleep problems that disappear after a few weeks.

For acute hepatitis, there is no treatment beyond bed rest and a high carbohydrate, low-fat diet. After recovery, patients need a blood test to see if they have retained the E antigen. Those who do are extremely infectious and are at higher risk of developing complications. About 10 percent of these chronic carriers lose the antigen each year. A high percentage of patients go on to develop chronic hepatitis, leading to chronically poor liver function.

Most people recover from the infection entirely and are not at risk for long-term complications. On the other hand, babies, children, and the 5 percent of adult carriers are of more concern.

Between 10 and 85 percent of babies born to infected mothers will develop hepatitis themselves; of those, 90 percent develop chronic hepatitis, at high risk for eventually developing cirrhosis or liver cancer as adults. Twenty-five percent of them will die of liver disease as adults.

Risk Factors and Preventive Measures

While hepatitis B is completely preventable, thousands continue to be infected with the disease each year. The vaccine introduced in 1983 was made from blood plasma; a few years later a vaccine from synthetic products was introduced; a third synthetic vaccine was produced in 1991. The last two vaccines are given in three doses.

Anyone at risk for the disease, including all medical and nursing personnel, should have the vaccine. As of November 1991, the vaccine was recommended for all infants; boosters are not currently recommended.

Unlike some vaccines, there is no apparent risk of serious side effects from the hepatitis B vaccine. Reactions are limited to a sore arm at the site of injection or a slight fever.

Those who are not immunized but have been exposed may receive immune globulin HBIG for 90 percent protection if they receive the dose within seven days of exposure and begin the hepatitis B vaccine series at the same time.

Babies born to infected mothers receive HBIG within 12 hours after birth. The vaccine series must be started at the same time.

Carriers should follow standard hygienic procedures to make sure their close contacts are not directly contaminated. Carriers must not share razors, toothbrushes, or any other object that may become contaminated with blood. In addition, household members (especially sexual partners) should be immunized with hepatitis B vaccine. It is important for carriers to inform their dentist and health care providers of their status.

hepatitis C   A blood-borne type of hepatitis that can live quietly in the body for years. First identified in 1974, it was called non-A, non-B hepatitis. Until recognized in 1989 as hepatitis C. About 4 million Americans have been diagnosed with the conditions (one out of every six people).

Until the virus starts to attack the liver, most people do not know they are infected. Many do not know how they got the disease, and even after it is diagnosed, virtually nothing will get rid of it. The disease can be far more deadly than its cousins hepatitis A and B, both of which can be avoided with a vaccine.

In the United States, hepatitis C virus is linked to 20 percent of all clinical hepatitis cases and is the leading cause of chronic hepatitis. It is also the primary reason for liver transplants in the United States. Hepatitis C can lead to liver cancer, killing up to 10,000 Americans a year and causing almost half of all deaths from liver failure, according to the National Center for Infectious Diseases.

Not everyone with hepatitis C will get sick; however, about a third of those with chronic hepatitis C will develop either cirrhosis or cancer of the liver.

Between 55 to 85 percent of infected people develop chronic infection, and up to 70 percent develop chronic liver disease. Those who are able to fight off the infection are more likely to be younger, female, and have certain types of complex genes. African-American men appear to be least likely to spontaneously clear the virus.

There is little evidence that the amount of virus in the blood or its viral genotype significantly affect the risk of progression of liver disease. However, many other factors increase this risk, including older age at time of infection, male gender, and a weakened immune system, such as infection with human immunodeficiency virus (HIV). Coinfection with chronic hepatitis B also appears to increase the risk of progressive liver disease. Higher alcohol use (two beers, glasses of wine or alcoholic drinks a day in men) also plays an important role in promoting the development of progressive liver disease. Lower amounts of alcohol also may increase the risk of liver damage associated with HCV. Other factors, including iron overload, nonalcoholic fatty liver disease, medications harmful to the liver, and environmental contaminants, also may have important effects.

The CENTERS FOR DISEASE CONTROL AND PREVENTION estimates that 35,000 Americans are newly infected each year; long-term liver damage in chronic patients kills between 10,000 to 12,000 Americans a year. Because most people with chronic HCV infection have yet to be diagnosed but are likely to come to medical attention in the next decade, a fourfold increase in the number of adults diagnosed with chronic HCV infection is projected through 2015. Currently, people aged 40 to 59 years have the highest prevalence of HCV infection, and in this age group, the prevalence is highest in African Americans (6.1 percent).

The number of newly diagnosed patients (those who were infected years ago and are just now being diagnosed) is clearly rising, especially among baby boomers who were IV drug abusers. Intravenous drug users make up about 30 percent of the HCV-infected population; experts believe that almost all such users are ultimately infected by the lethal virus.

The hepatitis C virus is a member of the Flaviviridae family. There are six HCV genotypes and more than 50 subtypes. Genotype 1 accounts for 70 to 75 percent of all HCV infections in the United States and is associated with a lower rate of response to treatment.

Hepatitis C is spread primarily through blood-related sources, such as IV drug use, transfusions, and kidney dialysis; it is the cause of most cases of post-transfusion hepatitis. The risk of sexual transmission appears to be small, and there is no evidence that this type of hepatitis can be spread by casual contact, by eating tainted food, or by coughing or sneezing. In rare cases, an infected mother can pass the disease to a newborn. Some people carry the virus in their bloodstream and may remain contagious for years.

Before 1989, the infection was spread through transfusions; about 300,000 patients may have contracted the disease this way, before the nation's blood banks began testing for the virus in 1990. Transmission from blood products and organ transplants was virtually eliminated by the introduction of a more sensitive test for antibody to HCV (anti-HCV) in mid-1992.

In about half of cases the patients have done nothing that would put themselves at risk, and the source of the infection cannot be identified.

The virus is related to the YELLOW FEVER virus.

Symptoms and Diagnostic Path

About 20 percent of those infected with the virus will develop symptoms, including appetite loss, fatigue, nausea and vomiting, stomach pain, and jaundice within two weeks to six months after exposure. Usually, symptoms appear by two months. Half of these patients may go on to develop chronic liver disease.

After initial exposure, the RNA from the virus can be detected in blood within one to three weeks. Antibodies to HCV are detected by enzyme immunoassay (EIA) in only 50 to 70 percent of patients at the onset of symptoms, increasing to more than 90 percent after three months. Within an average of four to 12 weeks, liver cell injury can be detected by high levels of alanine aminotransferase (ALT) in the blood. People who have no symptoms usually find out they have hepatitis C when they give blood or get a liver function test when applying for life insurance. A variety of liver function tests, plus liver biopsy, can detect the disease.

Treatment Options and Outlook

There is no known cure for hepatitis C. The current best treatment involves combination therapy with ribavirin and the introduction of pegylated interferons. Genotype determinations influence treatment decisions. Overall, pegylated interferon plus ribavirin is more effective than standard interferon-ribavirin combination or pegylated interferon alone. Patients who do not respond to the first round of treatment may benefit from retreatment with pegylated interferon-based regimens. Combination therapy can get rid of the virus in up to five out of 10 people for genotype 1 and in up to eight out of 10 people for genotypes 2 and 3.

Between 10 to 14 percent of patients taking pegylated interferon and ribavirin discontinued treatment because of severe side effects. Major side effects of combination therapy include influenza-like symptoms, blood abnormalities, and neuropsychiatric symptoms. Psychological conditions (particularly depression) are common among people with hepatitis C and are frequent side effects of interferon. Patients' mental health should be assessed before beginning antiviral therapy and monitored regularly during therapy. Antidepressants may help manage the depression associated with antiviral therapy.

Risk Factors and Preventive Measures

At the present time, there is no hepatitis C vaccine. Hope for such a vaccine faded, according to the National Institute of Allergy and Infectious Diseases, when studies showed that exposure to the virus does not protect against reinfection.

Since 1990, U.S. blood donation centers have routinely used a blood-donor-screening test for hepatitis C. Widespread use of this test has significantly reduced the number of transfusion-associated cases of hepatitis C. People who have had hepatitis C should understand that their blood and possibly other body fluids are potential sources of infection. They should avoid sharing toothbrushes, razors, needles, and the like.

In addition, infected patients should not donate blood and should inform health care workers. Limits on sexual activity with steady partners may not be needed; however, those with acute illness and multiple sex partners may be at higher risk and should use condoms to reduce the risk of acquiring or transmitting hepatitis C as well as other infections.

The risk of transmitting the infection from mother to child before birth is between 2 and 7 percent for infants of infected women. Higher levels of virus in the blood appears to be associated with a greater risk. HCV transmission increases up to 20 percent in women who are infected with both HCV and HIV. There are no studies evaluating the use of cesarean section to prevent mother-to-infant transmission of HCV. However, avoiding fetal scalp monitoring and prolonged labor after rupture of membranes may reduce the risk of transmission to the infant. There are currently no data to determine whether antiviral therapy reduces transmission of the virus before birth, and both the antiviral drugs ribavirin and interferons are contraindicated during pregnancy.

Children should be screened for HCV if they are born to HCV-infected women, received transfusions prior to 1992, or have high-risk behavior. Children and adolescents with chronic HCV infection generally have no symptoms.

Little is known about the treatment of children and adolescents, but research suggests that children respond to treatment better than adults. Some patients may benefit from treatment even if the liver disease is mild. Given the long life expectancy of children and their better tolerance to drugs, the long-term safety of these medications needs to be studied in children.

hepatitis D   An uncommon version of the HEPATITIS virus in the United States, HDV infects about 15 million people around the world. Because the virus requires the presence of HEPATITIS B virus (HBV) to produce infection, the frequency of hepatitis D closely parallels HBV. In southern Italy, parts of Russia, and Romania, more than 20 percent of HBV carriers with no symptoms and more than 60 percent of those with chronic liver disease due to HBV are also infected with hepatitis D.

The major way hepatitis D is spread through contaminated needles (primarily IV drug abuse and exposure to blood products). Sexual transmission of hepatitis D is less efficient than for hepatitis B, but non-IV drug-using male homosexuals, female prostitutes, and institutionalized mentally retarded people are at higher risk for developing hepatitis D.

Transmission from mother to child has not been documented in the United States.

Symptoms and Diagnostic Path

Hepatitis D cannot be distinguished from other causes of hepatitis. The development of a new episode of acute hepatitis in a patient with known chronic hepatitis B infection should prompt a search for evidence of a new hepatitis D infection. Hepatitis D can increase severity of symptoms associated with hepatitis B.

Symptoms include jaundice, fatigue, abdominal pain, loss of appetite, nausea and vomiting, joint pain, and dark urine.

In patients with acute hepatitis D infection, anti-HDV antibody may be detected. The disease can be diagnosed by detecting HDV antigen in liver biopsies or antibodies in blood.

Treatment Options and Outlook

Hepatitis B vaccine should be given to prevent HBV/HDV coinfection. Treatment of the acute infection is supportive; treatment of chronic HDV infection includes administration of interferon-alfa and a liver transplant, if necessary.

Risk Factors and Preventive Measures

The hepatitis B vaccine can prevent hepatitis D, since hepatitis B infection is required for hepatitis D infection to occur.

hepatitis E   A form of HEPATITIS that is clinically indistinguishable from HEPATITIS A and that is endemic in most of the world. It does not often occur in the United States. The disease exists in both epidemic and sporadic forms and is usually associated with contaminated drinking water and poor hygiene. Major water-borne EPIDEMICS have occurred in Asia, North Africa, and East Africa. Rarely, U.S. cases have been diagnosed in people who did not travel to endemic areas. There is no evidence for immunity against this virus in the American population, so in theory it could become a problem in this country.

The disease is most often seen in young to middle-aged adults between ages of 15 and 40.

Pregnant women appear to be extremely susceptible to severe disease, and high rates of death have been reported in this group.

Also known as enterically transmitted non-A, non-B hepatitis (ET-NANBH), it is also called fecal-oral non-A, non-B hepatitis or A-like non-A, non-B hepatitis. It should not be confused with HEPATITIS C, also called parenterally transmitted non-A, non-B (PT-NANBH) or B-like non-A, non-B hepatitis.

Major outbreaks have occurred in India (1955 and 1975–76), the USSR (1955–56), Nepal (1973), Burma (1976–77), Algeria (1980–81), the Ivory Coast (1983–84), in refugee camps in Eastern Sudan and Somalia (1985–86), and most recently in Borneo (1987).

The hepatitis E virus is transmitted by the fecal-oral route. The virus has been transmitted via water and person-to-person; the potential exists for transmission via contaminated food.

Symptoms and Diagnostic Path

Between two to nine weeks after infection, symptoms of malaise, jaundice, anorexia, abdominal pain, dark urine, and fever appear. The disease is usually mild and fades away within two weeks. The fatality rate is very low; less than 1 percent of non-pregnant patients progress to fatal fulminant hepatitis, but in pregnant women the fatality rate rises to 20 percent.

Symptoms and epidemiological characteristics of the disease, and by excluding hepatitis A and B by blood tests. Confirmation requires identification of certain viruslike particles by immune electron microscope in the feces of acutely ill patients.

Treatment Options and Outlook

No antiviral treatment has been proven effective against hepatitis E, although preliminary studies suggest ribavirin and alpha-interferon may be effective. Treatment is supportive.

Risk Factors and Preventive Measures

Good sanitation and personal hygiene are the best preventive measures. There is no current vaccine, and it is not yet clear whether infection with hepatitis E confers lifelong immunity. Several recombinant HEV vaccines are being tested, but none are currently available for commercial use.

hepatitis G   A distant cousin of HEPATITIS C, hepatitis G was first identified in 1995. It apparently causes a mild acute hepatitis but is not a clinically significant chronic disease. However, the precise effects on the liver and an individual's health over time remain unknown. However, recent evidence suggests that HGV improves the outlook for patients also infected with HIV. Patients infected with HIV alone have a poorer prognosis than do patients infected with both HGV and HIV. Researchers have no idea why.

Very similar to hepatitis C, hepatitis G is also called hepatitis GB virus C or HGBV-C. Coinfection with hepatitis B or C—or both—is common. However, hepatitis G infection does not seem to worsen coinfection with hepatitis B or C.

Hepatitis G has at least five subtypes, depending on the part of the country where it occurs. It appears to be primarily a monkey virus that was transferred from one monkey to another until it infected humans via contaminated blood. Researchers have found the virus in blood in the United States, Canada, Peru, Egypt, West Africa, and Europe. About 1.5 percent of Japanese hepatitis patients who do not have the A through E varieties are infected with the G virus. About 18 percent of similar West African patients have the same virus in their blood.

Healthy people in the United States may carry the G virus since research suggests it was present in the nation's blood supply 25 years ago. And experts suggests that between 1 and 2 percent of the nation's blood donors have a previously undetected hepatitis G infection—higher than the rate for either hepatitis B or C.

There is an estimated 900 to 2,000 new infections each year; most have no symptoms.

In 0.3 percent of cases of community-acquired acute viral hepatitis, hepatitis G is the only identified virus. This strain of viral hepatitis was previously thought to be transmitted only through infected blood; now it is known to be transmitted sexually as well. Researchers in Sweden and Honduras found a surprisingly high rate of infection with the virus in healthy individuals without known risk factors (such as injection drug use and treatment for hemophilia). It was the high rates of infection in homosexual men and in healthy volunteers that led the authors to question the possibility of transmission via sexual contacts. It is known that HGV can be transmitted from an infected mother to her infant during childbirth, but now they believe HGV might be transmitted by "other routes yet to be defined."

There is an increased prevalence of hepatitis G genetic material among groups with frequent exposure to blood or blood products (such as people with hemophilia, patients on hemodialysis, and injection drug users). Other modes of transmission are possible but have not been well documented.

About 10 percent to 20 percent of cases of community-acquired hepatitis and transfusion-associated hepatitis are not associated with the known major hepatitis viruses (A, B, C, D, or E). The fairly recent identification from patients with hepatitis G, which is about 25 percent identical to the hepatitis C virus, has implicated it as a cause of non-A-E hepatitis.

Symptoms and Diagnostic Path

After a brief attack, the virus may remain in the body for years, scientists speculate. They believe the virus may replicate in the liver for years, eventually revealing liver damage. Japanese studies suggest that some hepatitis patients whose liver failed were indeed infected with hepatitis G.

At this time, HGV infection can be identified only through special liver function tests that indicate current infection. An antibody test for HGV is under development and, when available, should explain the origins of infection more fully than HGV RNA testing can.

It appears that once antibodies are found, the virus is usually no longer present in the blood.

Treatment Options and Outlook

There is no proven treatment for HGV infection; at this point, guidelines for its investigation and management cannot be developed.

The nature and frequency of HGV infection is unclear. Although caution and vigilance must be maintained, there is a growing consensus that HGV is "a virus looking for a disease" and may in fact prove not to be a cause of viral hepatitis. Acute HGV infection is generally reported to be clinically and biochemically mild and transient. Although the viral genetic material can be detected for years after infec-

tion in perhaps a minority of people who have been infected, there is no compelling evidence that HGV infection can lead to serious consequences. However, the role of HGV in a more virulent form of hepatitis (fulminant hepatitis) is unknown.

Risk Factors and Preventive Measures

Blood banks do not screen for hepatitis G. Some healthy blood donors may have hepatitis G, and transmission through transfusion has been documented. Donors already infected with hepatitis B or C will largely be excluded already; and the hepatitis G infection seems largely benign.

herd immunity A situation that occurs when a large segment of the population is vaccinated against a particular germ. This, in turn, makes the odds of infection among unvaccinated individuals low.

herpes Any of a variety of inflammatory skin diseases characterized by spreading or creeping small clustered blisters caused by the herpes simplex virus. Forms of the virus cause COLD SORES and the sexually transmitted disease genital herpes, characterized by blisters on the sex organs. The virus also causes many other conditions affecting the skin.

There are two forms of the herpes simplex virus— type 1 and type 2. Herpes simplex, type 1 (HSV1) is usually associated with infections of the lips, mouth, and face, whereas herpes simplex, type 2 (HSV2) is usually associated with infections of the genitals, and in congenital herpes.

However, there is a certain amount of overlap between the two viruses; conditions usually caused by HSV2 may be caused by HSV1, and vice versa. Both types are highly infectious, spread by direct contact with the lesions or by the fluid inside the blisters.

Most people have been infected with HSV by the time they reach adulthood. While the first infection with this virus may cause no symptoms at all, there may be a flu-like illness in addition to ulcers on the skin around the mouth; afterward, the virus remains in the nerve cells of the face. Many people experience recurrent reactivations of the virus, suffering with repeated attacks of cold sores, especially during a fever or prolonged sun exposure.

Sometimes the virus infects the finger, causing painful blisters called herpes whitlow. In patients with a preexisting skin condition (such as DERMATITIS), the virus may cause an extensive rash of blisters called ECZEMA HERPETICUM.

A person suffering an immunodeficiency disorder (such as AIDS) or someone taking immunosuppressant drugs who is exposed to the virus may experience a severe generalized infection that can be fatal.

A close cousin of the herpes simplex virus, the VARICELLA-ZOSTER VIRUS, is responsible for two other skin blistering disorders—CHICKEN POX and SHINGLES. Like the herpes simplex virus, the varicella-zoster virus can affect the eyes or the brain, in addition to the skin. Herpes gestationis and dermatitis herpetiformis are among other conditions in which herpes-like groups of blisters may appear on the skin, but neither is related to the herpes simplex or varicella-zoster virus infections.

Treatment of HSV varies according to its site and severity. The antiviral drug acyclovir (taken internally or applied topically to the blisters) is effective in shortening the symptoms during a primary attack, and there is some indication the drug taken prophylactically may lessen future attacks.

See also HERPES, GENITAL.

herpes, genital   One of the most common sexually transmitted diseases in the country, striking young, single men and women. The medical community has always considered genital herpes to be more of a discomfort rather than a dangerous or life-threatening situation. This nonlethal but incurable disease invades the body and remains for a lifetime, appearing often several times a year with painful sores in the genital area. At least 45 million Americans ages 12 and older (or one out of five teens and adults) have genital herpes infection. Between the late 1970s and the early 1990s, the number of Americans with genital herpes infections increased 30 percent.

Genital HSV-2 infection occurs more often in women (about one out of four women) than in men (almost one out of five), probably because male-to-female transmissions are more likely than female-to-male transmission, according to the CENTERS FOR DISEASE CONTROL AND PREVENTION.

Herpes simplex, type 2 causes most of the genital herpes cases. HSV1 causes most herpes infections above the waist. The virus can infect any skin or mucous membrane surface on the body. For example, a person with a cold sore who engages in oral sex can transmit herpes to a partner's genitals.

The infection is spread by contact with the genital secretions of a person with an active lesion. It is possible, however, for a person in the latent phase (with no active lesion) to shed virus and infect a sex partner. Genital herpes can also be acquired by infants as they pass through the birth canal of infected mothers. Neonatal herpes simplex infection can cause serious damage to the brain and many other organs; even with therapy, more than 20 percent of the 1,500 infants infected each year in the United States will die, and many of the survivors are seriously impaired. Because of this, thousands of women in the United States with a history of genital herpes are advised to undergo a Cesarean section when prenatal cultures or exams suggest an active infection near the time of delivery.

HSV2 infection can also lead to serious or fatal complications in adults who have a weakened immune system because of AIDS or who are undergoing drug therapy for organ transplants.

Symptoms and Diagnostic Path

Many people who are infected have no symptoms at all; only about 40 percent of patients ever have symptoms. When they do, the primary (or first) appearance of herpes lesions is the worst, with severe local symptoms and many painful lesions. These last up to 10 days, and it may take two to three weeks to completely recover from this first attack. When the sores fade away, the virus remains behind. The virus is now *latent*. During the first attack, some people have a generalized sick feeling, with swollen glands in the pelvic area and fever, fatigue, headache, muscle ache, and nausea. People with no antibodies to herpes (cold sores) usually will be sicker during a first attack. Women usually have lesions on the cervix or vulva. Recurrences may appear on the vulva, skin between vagina and anus, upper thighs, anal area, or buttocks. Men get lesions on the head or shaft of the penis and the anus.

Most people have a recurrence within six months of their first attack. This recurrence begins with a tingling, itching, or prickling sensation in the area where the virus entered the body. This is followed in a few days by a raised cluster of small painful blisters; there may be several groups of blisters. Eventually, the sores will crust over and dry up. Most people do not have the generalized sick feeling with recurrent infections.

Patients are infectious until the sores heal completely, usually up to 12 days; recurrent infections usually remain infectious for up to a week. Recent studies have shown that it is quite possible to shed virus without symptoms, which is how it is possible to infect a partner when no sores are present.

Neonatal herpes can take many different forms. About one third of babies will have skin, eyes, or mouth lesions before any other symptoms; another third will have a brain infection (ENCEPHALITIS), PNEUMONIA, or infection of other organs. The other third will have both. Respiratory distress, fever, skin lesions, or convulsions are common herpes symptoms in newborns.

Doctors may diagnose genital herpes by symptoms alone, but there are also several lab tests that can confirm the infection. A specimen from the base of a lesion can identify the type of cell called giant cells, which usually indicates a herpes virus. Herpes also grows rapidly in tissue culture; specimens from a new lesion can be identified within 48 hours in the lab. Blood tests can look for antibodies to herpes; the newest blood tests can tell the difference between type 1 and 2, but differentiation is not clinically important as they both behave and are treated in the same way.

Treatment Options and Outlook

The antiviral drugs acyclovir, famciclovir and valacyclovir became available in the 1980s to reduce the number and severity of attacks, but these drugs are not a cure, since they do not kill the virus. Available in ointment, capsule, liquid, and IV forms, capsules are usually used to treat primary genital herpes or a severe recurrence, or to suppress frequent recurrences. Taking one of these drugs at the first sign of a recurrence—that is, dur-ing the tingling phase before lesions begin—can shorten the healing time from four to five days to one day.

People with more than six recurrences in a year can take daily antiviral drugs to prevent recurrence; but most patients do not take them for more than three years. Very few people report side effects with these drugs. Daily oral medication can reduce the number of recurrences by at least 75 percent in people with frequent episodes.

IV antiviral drugs are given for severe primary herpes for hospitalized patient, or for babies born with or exposed to herpes during birth.

Frequent sitz baths in lukewarm water following by drying sores with a hair dryer on cool can ease the pain. A small amount of petroleum jelly on the sores can reduce the irritation during urination. Very painful sores may be eased with an anesthetic ointment. While sores are present, women should wear loose cotton underwear, avoiding panty hose and tight pants.

Rarely, herpes MENINGITIS (infection in the lining of the brain or spinal cord) or herpes ENCEPHALITIS (infection in the brain) follows an initial infection. In the past, it was believed that there could be a link between herpes and cancer of the cervix; new studies show that genital herpes probably has no role in cervical cancer.

Risk Factors and Preventive Measures

Several vaccines are currently being tested in clinical trials, but no vaccine is currently available to prevent genital herpes. At least two companies are in the final stages of clinical trials for such a vaccine, however.

herpes simplex virus, type I (HSVI)   One member of the herpesvirus family that is usually associated with infections of the lips, mouth, and face. This virus was first described by the Roman doctor Herodotus around 100 C.E. as "herpetic eruptions" around the mouth during fever. Recurrent episodes can be triggered by stress, ultraviolet light, immune system problems, or exertion. HSVI is very similar to HSVII, with a nearly identical genetic code. Either type can infect the same body sites.

See also HERPES.

herpes simplex virus, type II (HSVII)   A member of the herpesvirus family that is usually associated with infections in the genital area. It may also occur in newborns, who acquire the disease during birth. It is believed to infect one out of every five people in the United States, but only one-third of those experience symptoms.

Like its close cousin HSVI, recurrent episodes of HSVII can be triggered by stress, ultraviolet light, immune system problems, or exertion.

See also HERPES.

herpes zoster   See SHINGLES.

Histoplasma capsulatum   A fungal organism that causes HISTOPLASMOSIS is a single budding yeast at body temperature and a mold at room temperature. The fungus is spread by airborne spores from soil contaminated with bird droppings and is commonly found in the Ohio and Mississippi River Valleys.

histoplasmosis   A lung infection caused by inhaling the spores of the fungus *Histoplasma capsulatum*. Infection confers immunity for life. The disease is endemic in the northern and central United States, Argentina, Brazil, Venezuela, and parts of Africa. However, most people who inhale the spores are not affected by them.

The disease is caused by a type of fungal organism that is a single, budding yeast at body temperature and a mold at room temperature. It is spread by airborne spores from soil contaminated with droppings from infected chickens, pigeons, or bats. In rare cases when infection does occur, it occurs either because a person has been exposed to large quantities of the spores (such as pigeon handlers) or because the patient's immune system is impaired.

Symptoms and Diagnostic Path
The primary form of the disease does not usually produce any symptoms; when it does, they include breathlessness, dry cough, fever, and joint pain. Spontaneous recovery is typical, although small areas of calcification in the lungs and lymph glands may remain.

In a few people (especially those with impaired immune systems), the disease takes a chronic, sometimes fatal, form and spreads throughout the body. Called *progressive histoplasmosis*, the disease resembles TUBERCULOSIS and is characterized by ulcerating sores in the mouth and nose; enlarged spleen, liver, and lymph nodes; and severe infiltration of the lungs, with fever, malaise, and a cough. Between 50 to 100 people a year die from this form of disease.

Examination of tissue or sputum and history will help confirm disease.

Treatment Options and Outlook
The severe form of histoplasmosis is treated with the antifungal drug amphotericin B.

Risk Factors and Preventive Measures
In contaminated, enclosed environments (such as chicken coops) people should avoid exposure to the dust and surrounding soil. A protective mask, and spraying areas with water, may help minimize exposure.

HIV   The acronym for HUMAN IMMUNODEFICIENCY VIRUS.

Hong Kong flu   See INFLUENZA.

hookworms   Small round blood-sucking worms that usually cause diarrhea or cramps, and that can penetrate the skin (usually the feet), causing a red itchy rash. The worms, which belong to the species *Necator americanus* (New World hookworm) or *Ancylostoma duodenale* (Old World hookworm), infest 1 billion people in tropical and Third World countries. There is some risk of contracting hookworms in the United States.

Hookworm larvae live in the soil and infect humans by penetrating the skin. Once inside the body, they travel to the lungs and then inside the small intestine, where they attach themselves and drain blood for nourishment. Heavy hookworm infestation can cause considerable damage to the intestinal wall, causing serious problems for newborns, children, and pregnant women. While one hookworm extracts only a fraction of a teaspoon of blood from the circulation every day, more severe infestations can be more serious; an infestation of 1,000 worms can drain almost a cup of blood a day. If the patient cannot replace the lost blood quickly enough (as in the case of pregnant women or children), this may cause an iron deficiency and malnutrition. In children, chronic infestation with worms can lead to slowed growth and impaired behavioral, cognitive, and motor development. Occasionally, hookworm disease may be fatal (especially to infants).

One of the most common species, *A. duodenale,* is found in southern Europe, northern Africa, northern Asia, and parts of South America. *N. americanus,* was widespread in the southeastern United States early in this century.

People who have direct contact with soil that contains human feces in areas where hookworm is common are at high risk of infection. Children are at especially high risk because they play in dirt and often go barefoot. Since transmission of hookworm infection requires development of the larvae in soil, hookworm cannot be spread person to person. Contact among children in institutional or child care settings should not increase the risk of infection.

Symptoms and Diagnostic Path

In minor infestations, there may be no symptoms; in more severe cases, the worms can cause abdominal pain, anemia, cough, diarrhea, appetite loss, weight loss, protein deficiency, and pneumonia. The infection can lead to slowed mental and physical growth that may be irreversible. It may be fatal, especially in newborns.

Treatment Options and Outlook

Antihelminthic drugs (such as mebendazole) kill the worms; improved diet and blood transfusions may be necessary. Unfortunately, many areas of the world where infestation is a problem do not have access to drug treatment.

Risk Factors and Preventive Measures

Scientists are trying to develop vaccines using hookworm-produced proteins that would generate antibodies to neutralize the anticlotting proteins and

cut off the worms' food supply. Such a vaccine would be of great help in areas where reinfestation is a problem.

Of course, the best prevention is to improve sanitation so that transmission cannot occur, which is how hookworm disease was eradicated from the southeastern United States. This is more difficult in most Third World countries. It also may be prevented by not walking barefoot or touching soil with bare hands in endemic areas.

See also ANTIDIARRHEAL DRUGS; DIARRHEA AND INFECTIOUS DISEASE.

hordeolum   See STYE.

hospital-acquired infections   Bacteria infections transmitted within hospitals pose one of the greatest and most controllable threats in the United States, where more than 5 percent of hospital admissions and about 14 percent of intensive care patients acquire an infection during their stay. This is about 2 million cases a year. According to some estimates, nosocomial (hospital-acquired) infections rank among the 10 leading causes of death in the United States. These infections today affect about 2 million patients each year in acute care facilities resulting in 90,000 deaths, according to the CENTERS FOR DISEASE CONTROL AND PREVENTION.

While the disease-causing organisms found in hospitals can be virulent, the main problem in these infections is that hospitalized patients usually have an underlying disease or impaired immune function in the first place.

HPV   See PAPILLOMAVIRUS, HUMAN.

HSV   See HERPES.

human granulocytic ehrlichiosis   See EHRLICHIOSIS.

human immunodeficiency virus (HIV)   See ACQUIRED IMMUNODEFICIENCY SYNDROME.

human   papillomavirus See   PAPILLOMAVIRUS, HUMAN.

humidifiers and infectious disease The use of a humidifier during the winter can help keep mucous membranes moist and healthy—but poorly maintained humidifiers can be the source of infection.

The nose, throat, and lungs work best when the air has a relative humidity of about 40 percent. If the air during the winter falls below that level, moisture will be absorbed into the heated air from the mucous membranes. Since dried mucous membranes cannot clean themselves, they become more vulnerable to invasion from cold viruses. A well-maintained humidifier can keep the air moist and nose and throat moist.

But it is imperative that the device is used correctly. If the air becomes too humid, or the machine is not properly cleaned, mold and dust mites can multiply.

To keep the risk of infection from molds or bacteria to a minimum, consumers should not let the humidity rise above 40 percent; the water reservoir in the humidifier should be cleaned *daily* with a vinegar solution.

HUS See HEMOLYTIC UREMIC SYNDROME.

immune response The body's defensive reaction to invading organisms that are recognized as foreign to the body. The response triggers the production of antibodies, lymphocytes (white blood cells), and other substances and cells that destroy the invaders.

See also IMMUNE SYSTEM; IMMUNITY; IMMUNIZATION.

immune system A complex network of highly specialized organs and cells that work together to attack invading substances seen as "foreign" (such as BACTERIA, VIRUSES, and FUNGI) and clear infection from the body. The human body protects itself against invasion from a wide variety of infectious diseases by this intricate combination of organs and cells. The network works most efficiently when a person is well rested, eats a healthy diet, and is not under too much stress. Genetics plays a part as well; some people are born with stronger immune systems than others.

Normally, it is the immune system's responsibility to protect the human body from invaders (such as viruses or bacteria) by producing antibodies—specialized cells that recognize "foreign" invaders and fight them off. The immune system is constantly on duty patrolling the body, distinguishing between substances that *should* be in the body and "foreign" agents that could spell trouble. Anything the immune system detects as "foreign" will be attacked. These foreign substances are called antigens. When a germ enters the body, the immune system goes into action, triggering the white blood cells to attack. White blood cells move throughout the body via the organs of the immune system, including bone marrow, lymph nodes, tonsils, adenoids, thymus gland, blood, and lymphatic vessels.

White blood cells come in two varieties: B cells, which are produced in the bone marrow, and T cells, which mature in the thymus gland. Both of these cells produce antibodies that destroy bacteria and viruses. A third type of white blood cell—the large phagocytes—surround invading microbes and swallow them.

This immune response is often the source of all of the symptoms people experience during an infection—chills, fever, aches, appetite loss, fatigue, inflammation, and rash.

A person whose immune system is not working well—such as someone with AIDS—has more difficulty in fighting off invading germs. This is why anyone with an impaired immune system gets sick more often, and more seriously, with illnesses that might not even harm someone whose immune system is working properly.

See also IMMUNE RESPONSE; IMMUNIZATION.

immunity The quality of being unaffected by a particular disease or condition.

immunization A method of producing immunity to disease through artificial means. This is done through a vaccination, which is an injection of treated antigens to stimulate the body to produce its own antibodies to a specific disease. The material in the vaccination may either be live bacteria or VIRUSES, organisms treated so that they are harmless, or dead organisms or their products that are altered to produce the same effect.

While the United States has produced many vaccinations to deal with a variety of infectious disease, the only infection that has been eradicated throughout the world is SMALLPOX.

Preschoolers are the most vulnerable to communicable disease, which is why infants soon after birth are started on a U.S. government-required series of immunizations. At present there are a series of shots that must be given to protect against childhood diseases, in future scientists predict there may be one vaccine to protect against many diseases.

Immunization is not straightforward, however. Some vaccines are perceived by the public as carrying a risk, especially the pertussis part of the DPT (diphtheria-pertussis-tetanus) vaccine, which had been linked to seizures and other serious side effects. In response to these concerns, a safer acellular version of the pertussis vaccine is now in use.

Still, reports from health departments estimate that less than half of American children are properly immunized by age two; in the inner city, the rate drops to less than a third. Since 1991, most insurance companies cover children's immunizations, and some health departments offer free shots.

While a serious illness means a vaccination must be postponed, minor colds with low fevers do not interfere with immunization. Slight soreness and swelling at the injection site are normal and are not an indication that the child should not finish the series of shots. Antibiotics prescribed for another illness will not interfere with vaccinations except the oral typhoid vaccine.

Children should not be vaccinated if they have had a serious allergic reaction to a previous shot. Anyone who has a severe allergy to eggs should not receive the MMR (measles-mumps-rubella), INFLUENZA, or YELLOW FEVER vaccines. A child with serious illness should be not vaccinated until fully recovered.

immunizations for adults Anyone over age 65 should get several vaccines, including a tetanus diphtheria (Td) every 10 years, an INFLUENZA vaccine each fall, and one dose of pneumococcal polysaccharide vaccine with a booster every six years for transplant recipients, patients without a spleen, or anyone with chronic kidney failure.

See also IMMUNIZATION; VACCINE.

immunizations for chronic disease patients Anyone with chronic heart disease, lung problems, dia-

betes, kidney disease, or sickle-cell disease should have the pneumococcal vaccine and an INFLUENZA vaccine each fall.

See also IMMUNIZATION; VACCINE.

immunizations for health-care professionals Several immunizations are suggested for anyone who works in the health-care field and comes into contact with patients. These include the HEPATITIS B vaccine (Recombivax or EngerixB) in a three-dose series; INFLUENZA vaccine every fall; MMR (measles-mumps-rubella) vaccine unless there is proof of immunity; and tetanus (Td).

See also IMMUNIZATION; VACCINE.

immunizations for homosexual males/heterosexuals with multiple partners Anyone with this sexual history should receive the HEPATITIS B vaccine in a three-dose series, plus routine vaccines recommended for adults.

See also IMMUNIZATION; VACCINE.

immunizations for influenza There are two types of vaccines available to protect individuals against influenza for one season—either an injection or a nasal spray. The ability of flu vaccine to protect a person depends on the age and health status of the person getting the vaccine and how close the vaccine matches the virus strains in circulation.

The flu shot is a vaccine containing killed virus approved for use in people older than six months, including healthy people and people with chronic medical conditions.

The nasal-spray flu vaccine is made with live, weakened flu viruses that do not cause the flu. The spray, approved for use only in healthy people between the ages of five and 49 years and those who are not pregnant, is less effective than the shot.

Each vaccine contains three influenza viruses that change each year based on international surveillance and scientists' best guesses about which types and strains of viruses will circulate in a given year.

About two weeks after an injection or spray is given, antibodies that provide protection against influenza virus infection develop in the body. Although October or November is the best time to get vaccinated to provide protection for that year's flu season, people can still get vaccinated in December and later. Flu season can begin as early as October and last as late as May.

Anyone who wants to reduce the chance of getting the flu can get vaccinated, but people at high risk of having serious flu complications or those who live with or care for those at high risk should get the vaccination. People at high risk for complications from the flu include

- anyone over age 65 and people who live in nursing homes and other institutions
- anyone with chronic heart or lung conditions (including asthma)
- anyone who needed medical care or was hospitalized the previous year because of a metabolic disease (such as diabetes), chronic kidney disease, or an impaired immune system
- children aged six months to 18 years on long-term aspirin therapy
- women pregnant during the influenza season
- all children six to 23 months of age
- people with any condition that makes it hard to breathe or swallow, such as brain injury or disease, spinal cord injuries, seizure disorders, or other nerve or muscle disorders
- people 50 to 64 years of age, since nearly one-third of people in this age group in the United States have at least one medical condition that places them at higher risk for serious flu complications
- anyone in close contact with someone in a high-risk group, including all health-care workers, household contacts and out-of-home caregivers of children 0 to 23 months of age, and close contacts of people over 65
- anyone over age six months displaced by a natural disaster (such as a severe hurricane) and living in crowded group settings

There are some people who should not be vaccinated for flu without first consulting a doctor, including people

- who have a severe allergy to chicken eggs
- who have had a severe reaction to an influenza vaccination in the past
- who developed Guillain-Barré syndrome within six weeks of getting a flu shot in the past
- under six months of age
- who have a moderate or severe illness with a fever (these patients should wait until the fever passes)

Side Effects
Minor side effects from the flu shot include soreness, redness, or swelling where the shot was given; low-grade fever; and aches for a day or two. The flu shot rarely causes any problems; however, on rare occasions flu vaccination can cause serious allergic reactions. Those injured from a flu shot can file a claim for compensation with the National Vaccine Injury Compensation Program (VICP). More information is provided at http://www.hrsa.gov/osp/vicp.

Side effects from the nasal-spray vaccine can include runny nose, headache, vomiting, muscle aches, sore throat, cough, and fever.

immunizations for institutionalized patients Developmentally disabled residents of group-living institutions should receive a HEPATITIS B vaccine in a three-dose series, since these patients have a high rate of hepatitis B. They should also receive an INFLUENZA vaccine each fall.

See also IMMUNIZATION; VACCINE.

immunizations for kidney disease patients Anyone undergoing hemodialysis or who has had a kidney transplant should receive the three-dose series of HEPATITIS B, an INFLUENZA vaccine each fall, and the PNEUMOCOCCAL VACCINE.

See also IMMUNIZATION; VACCINE.

immunizations for patients with impaired immune systems Anyone with an impaired immune system should receive an INFLUENZA vaccine each fall, and a one-time PNEUMOCOCCAL VACCINE with a booster in six years. Those with HIV infection should also receive these two vaccines, plus the primary series of the HAEMOPHILUS INFLUENZAE TYPE B conjugate vaccine (Hib). Also indicated are two doses of the measles-mumps-rubella (MMR) vaccine and the inactivated poliovirus vaccine if not immune or without previous vaccination.

Patients who have had their spleen removed should have both the pneumococcal and meningococcal vaccine.

See also IMMUNIZATION; VACCINE.

immunizations for pregnant women   Pregnant women who are not immune to MEASLES, MUMPS, or rubella should receive these live virus VACCINES right after delivery. Otherwise, pregnant women should receive a booster dose of tetanus (Td) if more than 10 years have passed since the last vaccine, together with a HEPATITIS B vaccine if the woman is at risk of exposure because of lifestyle or contact with a carrier. She should receive an INFLUENZA vaccine if she has medical conditions that warrant this. She should only receive YELLOW FEVER and polio vaccines if she is traveling to an area where there is a high risk of exposure, and travel cannot be put off until after delivery.

See also IMMUNIZATION.

immunizations for public-safety workers   Several immunizations are suggested for anyone who works in the public safety field. These include the HEPATITIS B vaccine (Recombivax or EngerixB) in a three-dose series; INFLUENZA vaccine every fall; MMR (measles-mumps-rubella) vaccine unless there is proof of immunity.

See also IMMUNIZATION; VACCINE.

immunizations for research lab workers   Anyone who handles specimens in research labs, that contain poliovirus should receive inactivated poliovirus VACCINE in the absence of three doses of oral polio vaccine. Anyone who works with PLAGUE bacteria should have a plague vaccine (the three-dose primary series, with boosters every one to two years). Scientists who work with ANTHRAX bacteria (*Bacillus anthracis*) should receive the anthrax vac-

cine. People who work with RABIES virus should have the rabies preventive vaccine.

See also IMMUNIZATION.

immunizations for veterinarians   Vets and animal handlers should receive a RABIES vaccine and blood test every two years, with a booster if necessary. Those working in western states should also receive a PLAGUE vaccine in a three-dose primary series, with boosters every one or two years.

See also IMMUNIZATION.

immunoglobulin   Any of five related proteins that acts as antibodies and that are found in the blood and bodily secretions designed to protect the body against invasion from invading germs. In response to specific antigens, immunoglobulins are formed in the bone marrow, spleen, and all lymphoid tissue of the body (except the thymus). Kinds of immunoglobulins include IgA, IgD, IgE, IgG, and IgM. IgG is the most common; IgG, IgA and IgM are the most important.

impetigo, bullous   Also called staphylococcal impetigo, this superficial skin infection is caused by *Staphylococcus aureus* bacteria.

Symptoms and Diagnostic Path
Symptoms include thin-walled flaccid bullae that rupture easily and contain fluid ranging from clear to pus. After rupture, the base quickly dries to a shiny veneer, which looks different than the thicker crust found in common impetigo. Lesions are usually found in groups in one area.

Treatment Options and Outlook
As with common impetigo, bullous impetigo is treated with antibiotics. Topical treatment is not helpful. Septic complications are rare but can occur.

See also IMPETIGO, COMMON.

impetigo, common   A superficial skin infection most commonly found in children caused by streptococcal bacteria. Impetigo should be treated as soon as possible to avoid spreading the infection to other children and to prevent a rare complication—a form of kidney disease called acute glomerulonephritis.

Impetigo is spread by touching and is usually found on exposed body areas such as the legs, face, and arms. Because impetigo is spread quickly through play groups and day care, children with the infection should be kept away from playmates and out of school until the sores disappear.

Symptoms and Diagnostic Path
The condition starts as tiny, almost imperceptible blisters on a child's skin, usually at the site of skin abrasion, scratch, or insect bite. Most lesions occur on exposed areas, such as the face, scalp, and extremities. The red and itchy sores blister briefly, then begin to ooze for the next few days, leaving a sticky crust. Untreated, the infection will last from two to three weeks. It is most prevalent during hot, humid weather.

Treatment Options and Outlook
This infection should be treated immediately to avoid spreading the infection to other children. Oral antibiotics are effective.

Rarely, impetigo can lead to kidney disease known as acute glomerulonephritis. In this case, the patient's immune system makes antibodies to the strep, which unfortunately are harmful to the patient's own kidneys.

Risk Factors and Preventive Measures
Cleanliness and prompt attention to skin injury can help prevent impetigo. Impetigo patients and their families should bathe regularly with antibacterial soaps and apply topical antibiotics to insect bites, cuts, abrasions, and infected lesions immediately. Impetigo in infants is especially contagious and serious. To prevent spreading, pillowcases, towels, and washcloths should not be shared and should be washed with antibacterial soaps and chlorine bleach.

impetigo, staphylococcal See IMPETIGO, BULLOUS.

impetigo, streptococcal See IMPETIGO, COMMON.

infant botulism See BOTULISM.

infection control The policies and procedures of a health facility aimed at reducing the risk of hospital-acquired or community-acquired infections spreading to others.

See also HOSPITAL-ACQUIRED INFECTIONS.

infectious disease Any illness that is caused by a specific microorganism. Infectious diseases are a large and important group of conditions; they remain the major cause of death throughout the world. According to the World Health Organization, the "world's deadliest diseases" are all infectious. In order, they are PNEUMONIA, DIARRHEA, TUBERCULOSIS, MALARIA, HEPATITIS B, AIDS, MEASLES, TETANUS, WHOOPING COUGH, and ROUNDWORM.

Infectious disease-causing organisms make up a number of well-defined groups: the most important are VIRUSES, BACTERIA, and FUNGI, together with three smaller groups (the rickettsiae, chlamydiae, and mycloplasmas). All of these organisms are fairly simple and can quickly multiply in tissue. In addition, the more complicated parasites (PROTOZOA, worms, and FLUKES) spend only part of their life inside human tissue; colonization of a human being by one of these parasites is usually referred to as an infestation, not an infection.

Symptoms and Diagnostic Path
Symptoms of infectious diseases are caused partly by the damage done to cells and tissues by the microorganisms and the toxins (poisons) they release. Symptoms are also caused by the body itself as it tries to fend off the attack. The strength of a patient's immune system can strongly influence how quickly and how well the infection is fought off. One of the most common signs of infection is fever.

One of the problems with infectious diseases is that there is usually a time lapse (the "incubation period") during which the person has the infection but does not experience symptoms. Often, the patient can transmit the infection during this period; some people may never develop symptoms, but can still pass on the disease. This is how an EPIDEMIC can begin and become established before preventive measures can be taken. This is particularly devastating if the disease has a long incubation period and fatal outcome, such as in AIDS.

Treatment Options and Outlook

Treatment for infectious diseases caused by bacteria often involves antibiotics and other antimicrobial drugs. Because some organisms are susceptible only to certain antibiotics, doctors must carefully choose which medication to prescribe. The "miracle drug" antibiotics such as PENICILLIN and tetracycline have been so often prescribed—and often misused by patients—that they have encouraged the microbes to develop resistance and even immunity. The result: infections that are nearly impossible to treat. Today, doctors are seeing infections that are no longer treatable because the bacterium is resistant to every antibiotic ever developed. Drug companies have begun working on new antibiotics, but these new drugs are years away from approval and widespread use.

Over the past 100 years, many of the developed countries believed they were gradually winning the war against infectious diseases due to better sanitation, pest control, personal hygiene, and quarantines. Effective drugs were developed as were vaccines to provide immunity against certain illnesses. The general health and good nutrition of most people in the developed countries bolstered their immune systems and improved survival. Unfortunately, just as scientists were feeling most complacent, the picture began to change.

During the past 20 years, 30 new diseases have emerged to threaten the health of hundreds of millions of people. For many of these diseases there is no treatment, cure, or vaccine. The mortality rate from infectious disease between 1980 and 1992 increased from 41 to 65 deaths per 100,000. Even discounting AIDS, deaths in the United States from infectious diseases has risen 39 percent over these years. Overuse of medicine, human settlement of uninhabited areas, international travel, and poverty have combined to produce a devastating spread of infectious diseases, according to the World Health Organization.

There are still very few effective medicine against viruses, which do not respond to antibiotics.

As people push farther and farther into the tropical rain forests, they are coming into more frequent contact with deadly microbial diseases that have been circulating among animals for centuries. Diseases have been crossing over from animal to man and back again for years, but only in recent history could germs take advantage of space-age transportation linking countries and continents around the globe. While the deadly yet rare infections are frightening enough, there are diseases today in the United States hospitals that cannot be cured.

Many organizations such as the National Council on International Health and the American Public Health Association are working with governmental agencies like the CENTERS FOR DISEASE CONTROL AND PREVENTION and the U.S. Agency for International Development to develop a plan to meet the growing threat of infectious diseases. The CDC, calling infectious diseases a "global crisis," notes that new diseases are emerging just as old diseases, such as TB and PLAGUE, are returning to kill again. Many of these older diseases have developed resistance to modern drugs. Experts say today that the world will be lucky to make it through the next 30 years without a new pandemic.

Risk Factors and Preventive Measures

Many serious infectious diseases can be avoided by IMMUNIZATION; by using condoms, practicing good hygiene, and avoiding contact with animal feces. For travel outside the developed world, extra immunizations and careful measures to guard against insects can help.

infectious mononucleosis   See MONONUCLEOSIS.

infectious parotitis   See MUMPS.

influenza (flu)   A contagious respiratory infection that often occurs in EPIDEMICS. The disease is most dangerous not in itself, but because it can lead to PNEUMONIA, especially among older people and those with impaired immune systems. When complicated by pneumonia, the flu is the sixth most common cause of death in the United States, killing 20,000 Americans.

Influenza occurs most often in the winter months. Although illnesses like the flu may occur in summer, these are usually caused by other viruses. Every year as winter begins, the flu spreads across the globe; in the United States, up to 50 million people will be infected. The flu is responsible for about three days of lost work per adult, and field studies indicate the attack rate ranges from a low of about 10 percent in people over age 65 to a high of 36 percent in children from ages one to 18. At the peak of a typical epidemic, up to 22 percent of all physician visits are for flulike symptoms.

While more than 90 percent of flu-related deaths occur among the elderly, children under age five and women in the third trimester of pregnancy are also at higher risk for complications. The word *flu* is a slang term that applies to a variety of types of viral GASTROENTERITIS (stomach or intestinal flu), which are not really related to the true respiratory influenza caused by influenza virus.

Influenza is as old as human history; the mysterious 430 B.C.E. deadly plague in Athens may have been caused in part by deadly flu viruses. Historians also suspect that the mighty army of Charlemagne was destroyed by a flu epidemic of 876 C.E. The first true recorded flu pandemic occurred in the 16th century. In 1647, the flu was causing havoc in North America up through New England, where it was known variously as "jolly rant," "grippe," and "the new acquaintance." Its current name was bestowed after the 1732 epidemic in the American colonies, when English doctor John Huxham linked the disease with an old Italian folk word that linked colds, cough, and fever to the "influence" of the stars. About every 20 to 50 years, another pandemic (worldwide epidemic) sweeps across Earth, with yearly local epidemics in between. Major pandemics occurred in 1627, 1729, 1788, 1830, 1847, 1872, 1890, 1918, 1957, and 1968.

Several times in this century, influenza has appeared as a much more serious pandemic; these major episodes occur when the flu virus undergoes an "antigenic shift" in which one flu subtype is replaced by a different strain for which the population has not developed antibodies. Therefore, everyone on Earth is extremely susceptible to infection.

Still, because there were far more deadly diseases to worry about, even in the beginning of this century the flu did not attract much medical attention until the great Spanish flu pandemic of 1918, the worst of the pandemics, killing 10 million more people than did World War I. In the United States alone, 550,000 people died. The Spanish flu of 1918 left about 21 million dead out of about 1 billion cases before it vanished; scientists still do not know where it went and worry that another outbreak could occur. Its name was particularly insulting to Spaniards, since this particular pandemic appeared to have actually begun in the United States.

The 1918 pandemic was not restricted to the big cities, although more than 20,000 New Yorkers were killed in the fall of 1918. Whole Inuit villages in Alaska were decimated, and Samoa lost 20 percent of its people.

Since World War II, vaccines have helped cut the death rate, which was very low in the 1957 pandemic of Asian flu, and in the 1968 pandemic. In 1976, an outbreak of swine flu in Fort Dix, New Jersey, set off alarms throughout the United States, since it was swine flu that was believed to have caused the mass mortality in 1918, although no one knows for sure. Then-president Gerald Ford signed a law providing $135 million for a vaccine campaign that reached about a quarter of the population. The United States and Canada set up a crash mass vaccination program; however, when some people who had been vaccinated developed Guillain-Barre syndrome (a rare type of temporary paralysis) the United States canceled its program. The dreaded pandemic never developed, and the U.S. government eventually paid about $93 million in damages to Guillain-Barre victims.

Public health experts warn that another pandemic can strike at any time and that it could be as vicious as the 1918 episode. In 1997, when a lethal influenza variant called AVIAN FLU (bird flu) afflicted 18 people in Hong Kong, contributing to the death of six, officials feared the next wave had begun. Authorities in the region managed to contain the problem quickly, however, by finding the source—infected chickens, ducks and geese—and then destroying all the poultry in Hong Kong.

Outbreaks of bird flu have continued sporadically ever since. Bird flu is an infection caused by avian influenza viruses that occur naturally among birds. Wild birds worldwide harmlessly carry the viruses in their intestines, but because avian influenza is very contagious among birds, the virus can make some domesticated birds (including chickens, ducks, and turkeys) fatally ill. Infected birds shed the virus in their saliva, nasal secretions, and feces; other birds become infected from contaminated secretions or excretions. Domesticated birds may become infected with avian influenza virus through direct contact with infected waterfowl or other infected poultry or through contact with contaminated surfaces.

Infected domestic poultry may contract one of two main forms of the disease—one of which is not very virulent, but the other is quite deadly. The "low pathogenic" form may cause only mild symptoms, such as ruffled feathers and a drop in egg production. The deadly form spreads faster through flocks, causing disease that affects all of the internal organs and kills almost every bird within 48 hours.

During the 2003 flu season, outbreaks of avian influenza H5N1 occurred in Cambodia, China, Indonesia, Japan, Laos, South Korea, Thailand, and Vietnam, killing more than 100 million birds. By March 2004 the outbreak was under control, but within three months, new outbreaks among poultry were reported by Cambodia, Tibet, Indonesia, Kazakhstan, Malaysia, Mongolia, Siberia, Thailand, and Vietnam. Influenza H5N1 infection also has been reported among poultry in Turkey and Romania and among wild migratory birds in many parts of the world.

As of June 2005, 103 people have been infected with influenza A (H5N1) in Vietnam, China, Indonesia, Thailand, and Cambodia, according to the World Health Organization, and more than half have died, suggesting an unprecedented level of risk for a modern flu.

The World Health Organization conservatively estimates that an avian flu epidemic would kill 7 million people worldwide, and that a pandemic on the scale of the devastating global influenza epidemic of 1918 would kill at least 180 million people today.

Vaccines against any given influenza variant take about six months to produce, test for safety and distribute—too long to do much good in the face of a fast-moving pandemic.

The influenza virus was first named *Hemophilus bacterium influenzae*, but this was never proved conclusively. In the same year, W. Smith, F. W. Andrewes, and P. P. Laidlaw proved the cause of influenza was a virus that was experimentally transmissible to ferrets. This virus is now identified as influenza A. Influenza B virus was discovered in 1940, and influenza C was identified nine years after that. At the moment, the virus exists as one of these three types. However, types A and B mutate quickly; several strains of each of these types now exist. The three basic flu types have variants that are designated according to where they first strike, such as New Jersey (A), Bangkok (A), and so on. The 1957 and 1968 Asian flu pandemics were caused by strains of type A.

The highly contagious infection is spread by direct contact or via droplets and dust in the air over short distances from patients who are coughing or sneezing. The virus can also survive for hours in dried mucus, so dirty tissues should be carefully disposed of. Anyone can catch the flu, regardless of age, sex, or race, but certain groups are more likely to develop complications of the disease. Deaths occur primarily among those over age 65, or those with certain chronic diseases.

The contagious period varies, but it probably starts the day before symptoms appear and extends for about a week.

An attack will confer immunity to the specific strain only. Because the viruses that cause flu are always changing (mutating), people who have been infected or who have gotten a flu shot in other years may become infected with a new strain.

Symptoms and Diagnostic Path

About one or two days after exposure, symptoms of flu develop suddenly, with fever, headache, and body aches. Intestinal symptoms are uncommon. The throat is sore, dry, and red. A cough appears on the second or third day, followed by a drop in fever with drenching sweats by the third to fifth day. As the fever drops, the patient becomes highly susceptible to secondary bacterial invasion. Fatigue and depression may last for weeks afterward.

Although most people are sick for only a few days, some people have a much more serious illness (such as pneumonia) and may need to be hospitalized.

There is no easy way to diagnose influenza. While the virus can be isolated from the throat, and antibodies can be found in the blood, these tests are expensive and slow. Diagnosis is usually made on the basis of the symptoms and the occurrence of other cases in the area.

Treatment Options and Outlook

The antiviral drug Relenza (zanamivir) was approved by the FDA in July 1999 for patients over age seven for the treatment of uncomplicated type A and B influenza, the two types most responsible for flu epidemics. Clinical studies show that for the drug to be effective, patients needed to start treatment within two days of the onset of symptoms. The drug seems to be less effective in patients whose symptoms are not severe or do not include a fever.

Relenza is a powder that is inhaled twice a day for five days from a breath-activated plastic device. Patients with severe asthma or a lung condition called chronic obstructive pulmonary disease should not use Relenza, which may not be effective and which can cause bronchospasm in these patients. Reports of decline in respiratory function in patients without a history of airway disease also have been received. Some adverse events have required immediate hospitalization, and some patients with serious adverse events have died.

Relenza should not be used to prevent influenza and is not a substitute for the influenza vaccine.

Risk Factors and Preventive Measures

The flu vaccine is available as an injection or a nasal spray. How well the flu vaccine protects someone depends on their age and health status, and how closely the vaccine matches the virus strains in circulation.

The flu shot vaccine contains killed virus that has been approved for use in people over age six months, including both healthy people and those with chronic medical conditions. The nasal spray includes live, weakened flu viruses approved for use only in healthy, nonpregnant people between the ages of five and 49 years but is less effective.

Every year, scientists include three influenza viruses in one vaccine, based on their best guesses about which strains of viruses will circulate that year. Influenza antibodies develop in the body about two weeks after the vaccine is given. October or November (the beginning of flu season) is the best time to get vaccinated, but vaccinations are still effective as late as December or January. Flu season can begin as early as October and last as late as May. Routine vaccination against the flu is the most important way to control the disease. Vaccines are available through personal physicians or the local health department. Research has shown that even in years when new strains emerge, people in high-risk groups who get yearly flu shots tend to have milder illnesses and are less likely to be hospitalized with complications due to influenza A.

The first practical vaccination against the flu was developed in 1943 with killed viruses of both types A and B. Because the influenza viruses are constantly evolving, the vaccines must continually be updated; as new strains of the virus appear, they are included in the vaccine.

Each year, scientists at the U.S. CENTERS FOR DISEASE CONTROL AND PREVENTION and the World Health Organization make an educated guess about which kind of flu will predominate during the next winter season. These two groups maintain a global network that collects data required to select strains for the coming flu season's vaccine, and monitor the occurrence of especially severe epidemics. A similar process is undertaken in Europe by the WHO and various national authorities there.

In this country, for example, when developing the flu vaccine for the winter of 1994–95, CDC scientists studied flu viruses from 1,500 samples around the world. They chose in March 1994 to include vaccine made from three strains, A-Texas, B-Panama, and A-Shangdong; four drug companies then manufactured 70 million doses of vaccine.

The government recommends annual vaccinations for people at high risk of having serious flu complications or those who live with or care for those at high risk. People at high risk for complications from the flu include

- anyone over age 65 and people who live in nursing homes and other institutions
- anyone with chronic heart or lung conditions (including asthma)
- anyone who needed medical care or was hospitalized the previous year because of a metabolic disease (such as diabetes), chronic kidney disease, or an impaired immune system

- children aged six months to 18 years on long-term aspirin therapy
- women pregnant during the influenza season
- all children six to 23 months of age
- people with any condition that makes it hard to breathe or swallow, such as brain injury or disease, spinal cord injuries, seizure disorders, or other nerve or muscle disorders.
- people 50 to 64 years of age
- anyone over age six months displaced by a natural disaster (such as a severe hurricane) and/or who is living in crowded group settings.

Minor side effects from the flu shot include soreness, redness, or swelling where the shot was given; low-grade fever; and aches for a day or two. The flu shot rarely causes any problems; however, on rare occasions flu vaccination can cause serious allergic reactions. Those injured from a flu shot can file a claim for compensation with the National Vaccine Injury Compensation Program (VICP). More information is provided at http://www.hrsa.gov/osp/vicp.

Side effects from the nasal-spray vaccine can include runny nose, headache, vomiting, muscle aches, sore throat, cough, and fever.

People who should not be vaccinated for flu without first consulting a doctor include people

- who have a severe allergy to chicken eggs
- who have had a severe reaction to an influenza vaccination in the past
- who developed Guillain-Barré syndrome within six weeks of getting a flu shot in the past
- under age six months
- who have a moderate or severe illness with a fever (these patients should wait until the fever passes)

Because the viruses that cause flu are always changing, people who have been infected or who have gotten a flu shot in other years may become infected immunity from an earlier flu shot can decrease the next ear, people in high-risk groups should be vaccinated each year.

In the fall of 1997, a limited recall of flu vaccine was necessary for the first time since flu vaccines had been distributed because certain batches did not fully protect against the disease. Those who had been immunized with the weakened vaccine were asked to be revaccinated to protect against disease.

insects and disease There are at least 1 million known species of insects in the world, and most are either harmless or helpful to humans. The harmful ones, however, are capable of causing sickness in many ways, such as by becoming parasites to humans, living underneath the skin or on the body surface, or spreading disease on their feet and legs. Biting insects can spread infectious organisms, including WEST NILE VIRUS, MALARIA, FILARIASIS, LEISHMANIASIS, ONCHOCERCIASIS, CHAGAS DISEASE (American TRYPANOSOMIASIS), African trypanosomiasis, and so on.

Insects are found everywhere on the planet, from the poles to the equator, from the highest elevations to the level of the sea. At any one time, there are about 10 quintillion individual insects flying or crawling around on the Earth, as they've been doing for the past 400 million years. In fact, insects are among the most successful life forms that have ever lived, outnumbering humans one billion to one. More than half of all known species—and three-quarters of all known animal species—are insects. But there are plenty of insects out there yet to be classified: anywhere from three to 30 or more unknown species for every one that has been identified. Most insect-carried diseases are confined to the Tropics and subtropics, but some are beginning to appear in the United States.

To cut down on the chance of mosquito bites, travelers should use mosquito nets and wear clothes that cover the body. The most effective repellent is DEET, which should be used carefully and sparingly and is not recommended for children. High concentrations (over 35 percent) should be avoided. Travelers should also buy a flying-insect killing spray to use in living and sleeping quarters during the night. For even more protection, clothing and bed nets can be sprayed with permethrin, an insect repellent licensed for use on clothing only. If used correctly, permethrin will repel insects from clothing for several weeks. Portable mosquito bed nets, DEET, and permethrin can be bought in hardware or backpacking stores.

interferon Natural proteins produced by the human body to fight viruses by boosting the immune system. Interferon is active against many viruses, but specific interferons are effective only against the virus that produced them. There are three types of interferons: alpha, beta, and gamma. This family of proteins is produced by cells in response to a viral infection. In addition, they influence cell growth and increase the body's response to infection. The name comes from the fact that they literally interfere with virus replication. The production of interferon itself causes many of the symptoms people experience with flu.

The substances were discovered in 1957 by two researchers at the National Institute for Medical Research in London. The two (Alick Isaacs and Jean Lindenmann) showed that the protein secreted by infected cells did not interact with viruses directly; instead, the substance induces diseased cells and their neighbors to make still other proteins that could prevent invading viruses from replicating.

For many years the supply of human interferon for research was limited its costly extraction technique in which the first commercially available interferon was made from human white blood cells; the process only resulted in the production of a small, expensive amount of interferon. In 1980, however, the protein became available in greater quantities as a result of genetic engineering. Synthetic interferon is produced in a process known as recombinant interferon.

Researchers have also discovered that interferons are not a single molecule but that there are various forms, all of which are able to interfere with viral infection. These molecules belong to the family of cytokines—small proteins that carry signals from one cell to another.

The important part that interferons play in the immune system cannot be overestimated. Interferons influence the activity of almost every part of the immune system, boosting the body's ability to fight off attacks to most disease-causing microbes, including BACTERIA and PARASITES as well as viruses. Interferons can also inhibit cell division, which may explain in part why they can often impair the growth of cancer cells. One type of interferon has even been found to help maintain early pregnancy in several animal species.

Interferon is usually given by an injection just beneath the skin in the thigh or buttock. Most people find it easy to administer the injections themselves using the same technique as in diabetes treatment.

In the early stages of treatment many people experience flulike symptoms such as fever, chills, tiredness, nausea, and muscle aches and pains. The severity and duration of these symptoms varies and are often helped by taking the injections along with two paracetamol tablets. About 20 percent of people who experience ongoing problems may not be able to tolerate a full course. Rarely other side effects may occur, such as hair loss, mood changes, bacterial infections, and thyroid disease. Everyone on interferon treatment should be monitored regularly and frequent blood tests should be done to check the reduction in the number of blood cells and response rate. Changes in the dose and duration of treatment may be required in the light of these tests.

Because this protein is so important to the body's health, scientists have been concentrating on ways to harness its activity to fight disease. While initial hopes that interferon would prove to be a magic cure for all disease has proved to be unfounded, they have been approved by the U.S. Food and Drug Administration to treat seven diseases, including chronic HEPATITIS C, genital WARTS, Kaposi's sarcoma, and multiple sclerosis.

isolation precautions Procedures (including isolating in a private room) designed to prevent a patient from infecting others or from being infected by them. Complete isolation is used if a patient has a contagious disease, such as TUBERCULOSIS, that can be transmitted to others by direct contact and airborne droplets. All people entering the patient's room must wear masks, gowns, caps, and gloves, which are afterward burned or sterilized. Bed linen, eating utensils, bedpans, and other items that touch the patient also are sterilized. Even though they wear gloves, nurses must wash their hands after each nursing task.

Partial isolation is ordered if a patient's disease is transmitted in a more limited fashion; for example, only by breathing (as in WHOOPING COUGH) or only by contact with infected skin (such as IMPETIGO), blood (as in ACQUIRED IMMUNODEFICIENCY SYNDROME), or feces (as in CHOLERA).

Reverse isolation is used to protect a patient whose resistance to infection is very low or nonexistent. Air entering the room is filtered, and visiting is limited; everyone who visits must wear caps, gowns, masks, and gloves. Bed linen and all items used by the patient are sterilized. In severe cases, such as patients who are undergoing bone marrow transplantation, the patient is placed in an isolator or in a room ventilated with special purified air.

jail fever A nickname for TYPHUS.

Japanese encephalitis See ENCEPHALITIS, JAPANESE.

Jarisch-Herxheimer reaction A reaction following treatment for SYPHILIS (and other intracellular infections) caused by the widespread death of antigens. The syndrome is named for the 19th-century Austrian dermatologist Adolph Jarisch, who first described it.

The reaction is often accompanied by headache and fever and is more common in those with early syphilis. There are no proven ways to prevent the reaction.

jock itch The common term for TINEA CRURIS, a common fungal infection of the groin and upper thighs. It is most common among males.

The infection is caused by certain fungi of the species *Trichophyton, Microsporum,* or *Epidermophyton floccosum* that live on skin tissue, hair, and nails. Jock itch occurs when the groin area becomes sweaty, allowing fungi to thrive. The FUNGI are transmitted by sharing towels, benches, or shower stalls in locker rooms. Since fungi grow best in warm, moist environments, they thrive in hot, humid weather and among men who sweat a lot, wear tight clothing, or who are obese.

Symptoms and Diagnostic Path

Jock itch is a mild but annoying infection characterized by reddened, itchy, scaly areas spreading from the genitals outward to the inner thighs. The rash may be dry, crusted, bumpy, or moist; the scrotum is not usually affected. Some people are prone to jock itch and are often reinfected.

A fungal culture from skin scrapings will provide a definite diagnosis. However, it may be difficult to differentiate jock itch from other yeast infections in the groin. It is important to have the condition correctly diagnosed.

Treatment Options and Outlook

Antifungal drugs (such as miconazole and clotrimazole) are often prescribed as a lotion, cream, or ointment to ease the itchy rash.

The area should be bathed well with soap and water, removing all scabs and crusts, followed by application of antifungal cream on all lesions. Treatment should be continued for some time after the symptoms have passed to make sure the fungi has been eliminated and to prevent recurrence. Mild infections on the skin surface may require treatment for up to six weeks.

In very severe cases, or if there is no improvement with the cream after a few days, oral medication may be required.

Scratching the rash can lead to additional skin infection.

jungle fever The common name for YELLOW FEVER.

Kawasaki disease A serious yet relatively rare condition found mostly in infants and young children that is one of the leading causes of acquired heart disease in children. It occurs more often among boys and those of Asian descent. It is known medically as mucocutaneous lymph node syndrome. While it is possible to experience the syndrome more than once, recurrence is extremely rare.

Little is known how the syndrome is spread or how a person contracts it, although it does not appear to be transmitted from one person to another. Since outbreaks occur, it is suspected to be related to an infectious agent such as a virus, but a genetic predisposition also has been identified.

Symptoms and Diagnostic Path
Most patients experience a high fever (lasting more than five days) that does not respond to antibiotics. There may also be irritability; swollen lymph nodes; swollen hands and feet; and red eyes, lips, throat, and tongue. The rash may cover the entire body and may be followed by peeling of the skin on hands and fingers.

Treatment Options and Outlook
Most patients are treated in the hospital, where they can be watched and given aspirin and immunoglobulins to reduce the risk of heart problems.

The most common complication is a ballooning of the vessels of the heart, followed by blood clot formation that may block the artery, leading to a heart attack. Other complications include inflammation of the heart muscle or its sac, or abnormal heart function. Other organs may also be involved. Between 1 and 2 percent of patients die of the disease and its complications.

Risk Factors and Preventive Measures
There are no known ways to prevent the disease.

kerion An inflamed area of the skin that develops as an immune reaction to a fungus (usually scalp RINGWORM).

Symptoms and Diagnostic Path
A kerion is characterized by a red, pustular swelling that lasts for up to two months and may leave a scar and permanent loss of hair.

Treatment Options and Outlook
While the swelling may heal without treatment, applications of ichthamnol paste and antifungal agents are also used.

See also TINEA.

kidney disorders, infectious Infection of the kidney is called PYELONEPHRITIS. The infection often occurs when there is an obstruction of the flow of urine through the urinary tract, leading to stagnation of urine. The cause of the obstruction may be a kidney defect present at birth, a kidney stone, bladder tumor, or enlarged prostate. Pyelonephritis also can result from spread by the blood stream.

TUBERCULOSIS of the kidney is caused by infection carried by the blood from elsewhere in the body (usually the lungs).

kitchen infections The dirtiest area of the home is the kitchen, which is teeming with unseen microbes and deadly organisms. Disease-causing organisms are found everywhere in the average American kitchen—in the sponges, dish towels, sink, and countertops. The diseases they cause kill more than 9,000 Americans every year, primarily the very young, the very old, and those with impaired immune systems. And, food-borne infections occur far more often in food prepared in the home kitchen than in commercial restaurants.

While state and federal agencies compile statistics about widespread infections traced to food and food-preparation areas, many cases of individual illness are never reported. Studies that have looked at this area have discovered that household exposure to food-borne pathogens is the primary source of illness.

Bacteria tend to concentrate in the sink, the drain, and kitchen sponges, according to researchers. In one study, most of the dishcloths and sponges sampled from home kitchens contained large numbers of virulent bacteria, including *ESCHERICHIA COLI* and strains of *Salmonella*, *PSEUDOMONAS AERUGINOSA*, and *Staphylococcus*. If a sponge remains moist, the number of live microbes does not decrease for two weeks. Bacteria can survive for at least two days in a damp sponge that gradually dries in the air. On dry surfaces, however, bacteria can survive for no more than a few hours. They can colonize even stainless steel, which is not really as smooth as it looks.

If they are not removed immediately, microbes produce an organic substance that allows them to survive sprays of water, light rubbing, and even weak detergent solutions. As other types of microbes appear, they form a biofilm that further protects them.

Cutting boards are another source of contamination in the kitchen. While there have been conflicting reports about whether plastic or wooden cutting boards were more likely to contain germs, recent research suggests that the differences between the two depend on how moist they are. A dry wooden board absorbs moisture and draws the bacteria into its pores.

Fortunately, it is possible to remove these germs from kitchen surfaces. A brisk scrubbing with detergent dissolves food and microbes on metal surfaces. A follow-up rinse with dilute bleach will remove even the most tenacious organisms.

Wood, because of its organic building blocks, will react with bleach, neutralizing its ability to kill germs. Instead, it is possible to hand scrub microbes from the surface of new wooden or plastic cutting boards using soap and water. However, it is not possible to decontaminate plastic boards that are scarred by knives, and bacteria below the surface of a wooden board are not removed by hand scrubbing, and can remain alive for several hours. Microwave heating has successfully killed both *E. coli* and *Staph* microbes on cutting boards. After 10 minutes on high heat in an 800-watt home microwave oven in one study, a medium-sized board emerged bone dry and free of live microbes both on and below the surface. Wetting the board first sped up the time it took to kill microbes, suggesting that the microbes probably boiled to death.

The microwave can be used to disinfect other kitchen items, including dry cellulose sponges (30 seconds); wet sponges take longer (1 minute). Dry cotton dishcloths require only 30 seconds, but take three minutes when wet.

No amount of microwaving can disinfect plastic boards, since their surfaces never get hot enough to kill the microbes. However, studies have shown that the normal cycle in a dishwasher can sterilize even well-used plastic boards.

Today consumers can buy sponges with bacteria-killing compounds in the cellulose, and antimicrobial cutting boards.

Klebsiella   A genus of bacteria that normally lives inside a person's colon. However, when the bacteria escapes the colon, it can lead to fatal infections such as PNEUMONIA.

The most clinically important species of this genus is *Klebsiella pneumoniae*, a large bacterium that can produce a heat-stable enterotoxin. *K. pneumoniae* infections are common in hospitals where they cause pneumonia and urinary tract infections in catheterized patients. In fact, *K. pneumoniae* is second only to *E. coli* as a urinary tract pathogen. The bacteria also can cause surgical wound infections and infections of the blood. All of these infections can progress to shock and death if not treated early and aggressively. In addition, to pneumonia, *Klebsiella* can also cause less serious respiratory infections, such as bronchitis, which is usually a hospital-acquired infection. Typically, *Klebsiella* infections tend to occur in people with a weakened immune system or who have underlying diseases, such as alcoholism, diabetes, chronic lung disease, and advanced age.

Klebsiella infections occur much more often today, probably due to the bacterium's growing ability to resist antibiotics such as the PENICILLINS. Often, two or more powerful antibiotics are used to help eliminate a *Klebsiella* infection.

The bacteria was named for the 19th-century German bacteriologist Theodore A. E. Klebs, who first identified it.

La Crosse encephalitis   See ENCEPHALITIS.

Lassa fever   A viral infection found in the tropical regions of the world, especially West Africa; epidemics have occurred in Nigeria, Sierra Leone, Guinea, and Zaire. The disease is a major public health concern because it is highly contagious and can cause a severe or fatal illness. The rapid spread of the infection has been clearly identified in the case of hospital outbreaks.

In areas of Africa where the disease is endemic, Lassa fever is a significant cause of illness and death. While the disease is mild or has no observable symptoms in about 80 percent of infected patients, the remaining 20 percent have a severe disease that affects all the systems of the body. Lassa fever is also associated with occasional EPIDEMICS with a 50 percent fatality rate.

In West Africa, there are about 100,000 to 300,000 infections a year, with about 5,000 deaths. In some areas of Sierra Leone and Liberia, between 10 percent to 16 percent of all patients admitted to hospitals have Lassa fever.

The Lassa virus was discovered in 1969 and named after the town in Nigeria where the first two cases originated. The virus, a member of the viral family Arenaviridae, is a single-stranded RNA virus that has been found in one species of rodent. The virus can be transmitted through direct contact with rodent droppings and urine, by touching objects or eating food contaminated with droppings or urine, or through cuts or sores. It is also possible to inhale tiny particles in the air contaminated with rodent excretion. Because these rodents are sometimes used as food in Africa, infection may occur by direct contact when they are caught and prepared for eating.

Lassa fever also may spread through person-to-person contact. This type of transmission occurs when a person comes into contact with virus in the blood, tissue, secretions, or excretions of an individual infected with the Lassa virus. A person may also become infected by breathing in small airborne particles coughed out by an infected person. While the virus cannot be spread by casual skin-to-skin contact without exchange of body fluids, person-to-person transmission is common. In health care settings the virus may be spread via contaminated medical equipment, such as reused needles.

Symptoms and Diagnostic Path
Between one to three weeks after infection, symptoms appear, including fever, pain behind the chest wall, sore throat, back pain, cough, abdominal pain, vomiting, diarrhea, conjunctivitis, facial swelling, protein in the urine. Neurological symptoms may include hearing loss, tremors, and ENCEPHALITIS.

If a person has traveled to West Africa and has a severe fever within three weeks after returning, the illness should be reported to a physician who would test for Lassa fever.

Treatment Options and Outlook
The antiviral drug ribavirin has been used successfully, especially when given early in the disease. Symptoms are treated and patients should be made as comfortable as possible.

The most common complication of Lassa fever is varying degrees of deafness, which occur in about a third of all cases; often, hearing loss is permanent. Deafness may develop in mild as well as in severe cases. Spontaneous abortion is another serious complication.

Between 15 percent to 20 percent of patients hospitalized for Lassa fever die, but overall only about 1 percent of infection with the Lassa virus is fatal. The death rates are particularly high for women in the third trimester of pregnancy, and for unborn babies; about 95 percent of infected fetuses die before birth.

Risk Factors and Preventive Measures

Lassa fever can be prevented in the community by discouraging rodents from entering homes and by storing grain in rodent-proof containers, disposing of garbage at a distance from homes, keeping the house clean, and keeping cats to control mice. Caregivers should avoid contact with blood and bodily fluids while caring for anyone with Lassa fever. Routine barrier nursing precautions probably protect against transmission of Lassa virus in most circumstances, but to be safe, caregivers should also wear protective clothing such as masks, gloves, gowns, and face shields. Contaminated equipment also should be sterilized.

Legionella pneumophila   A small gram-negative bacterium that causes LEGIONNAIRES' DISEASE.

Legionellosis   Another name for LEGIONNAIRES' DISEASE.

Legionnaires' disease   A bacterial infection that can take one of two distinct forms: Legionnaires' disease, and the milder Pontiac fever.

An estimated 8,000 to 100,000 people are diagnosed with Legionnaire's disease each year; an additional unknown number are infected with the *Legionella* bacterium but rarely have any symptoms. Cases have been identified throughout the United States and in several foreign countries, and is believed to occur worldwide.

Outbreaks usually occur in the summer and early fall, but cases may occur year-round. Between 5 and 30 percent of known cases of Legionnaires' disease have been fatal.

The disease was named for its first identified outbreak, which occurred in 1976 during a Legionnaire convention at the Bellevue-Stratford Hotel in Philadelphia; 182 Legionnaires became ill and 29

died. Most of them had pneumonia, and because doctors did not know what the men had, they called it "legionnaire's disease." In January, 1977, scientists identified the bacterium that causes the disease and realized it had also caused outbreaks before 1976; nevertheless, the name remained.

Throughout the spring of 1994, about 30 passengers on weekly cruises from New York City to Bermuda came down with the disease; after the cruise ship stopped sailing, the source of infection was discovered to be sand filters used in the whirlpool baths.

People of any age may contract the disease, but it usually affects middle-aged or older people (especially those with chronic lung disease and smokers). Anyone with an impaired immune system or who takes drugs that impair the immune system are at higher risk.

Pontiac fever, on the other hand, commonly occurs in healthy individuals and resembles a flu-like illness more than pneumonia.

Legionnaires' disease is caused by the bacterium *Legionella pneumophila* transmitted by breathing in bacteria carried in water droplets through the air. The bacteria live in warm water; once they enter air-conditioning cooling towers, they circulate throughout a building.

Outbreaks have occurred after people have inhaled spray from a contaminated water source (such as air-conditioning cooling towers, whirlpool spas, or showers) in workplaces, hospitals, or other public places. Infection is not spread from one person to another, and there is no evidence of people becoming infected from auto air conditioners or household window air conditioners.

Legionella can be found in many different water systems, but the bacteria reproduce best in warm, stagnant water such as is found in some plumbing systems and hot water tanks, cooling towers and condensers of large air-conditioning systems, and whirlpool spas. New research suggests the bacterium can spread up to six kilometers by air.

Symptoms and Diagnostic Path

Between two and 10 days after exposure, symptoms of fever, chills, and cough appear. The cough may be dry or produce sputum; some patients may also experience muscle aches, headache, fatigue, loss of appetite, and diarrhea.

It is difficult to distinguish Legionnaires' disease from other types of pneumonia by symptoms alone. Lab tests may show decreased kidney function; chest X-rays reveal pneumonia.

A diagnosis requires special tests not normally performed on suspected cases of pneumonia: looking for bacteria in sputum, finding antigens in urine, and comparing antibody levels in two blood samples three to six weeks apart. Experienced doctors are the most important diagnostic tool, since lab tests take several days to months.

Treatment Options and Outlook

Erythromycin is the recommended antibiotic for Legionnaires' disease; sometimes, rifampin may be used in severe cases.

Risk Factors and Preventive Measures

Outbreaks must be reported to the health department. The disease can be prevented by better design and maintenance of cooling towers and plumbing systems in order to limit the growth and spread of bacteria. A person diagnosed with Legionnaires' disease is not a threat to others who share office or living space with him or her.

After the 1994 outbreaks on a cruise ship, public health officials met with industry representatives and issued more strict health guidelines. The new rules require changing hot tub filters more often, testing the water hourly, raising the chlorination level, and improving maintenance intervals. Consumers booking a cruise can ask their booking agent whether the cruise ship adheres to the new guidelines. It is also possible to find out how a ship scored on its most recent sanitary inspection by writing to the U.S. Public Health Service, 1015 N. America Way, Ste. 107, Miami, FL 33132. A score of more than 86 is acceptable.

Leishmania A genus of protozoan parasite transmitted to humans by any of several species of sand flies. Infestation causes one of a variety of diseases called LEISHMANIASIS.

leishmaniasis A variety of diseases that affect the skin and mucous membranes transmitted by the bite of some types of sand fly. More than 350 million people in 90 countries of the world are presently at risk; 12 million people are already affected by the disease, which is fatal in one form. The disease is most often characterized by a skin form or an internal organ form. Up to 75 percent of the cases of leishmaniasis that are evaluated in the United States and that are not related to the military are cases of cutaneous leishmaniasis acquired in Latin America.

At least three types of the disease affect the skin, one is common in the Middle East, North Africa, and the Mediterranean; the others are found in Central and South America. It does not occur in Australia, the South Pacific, or Southeast Asia.

The parasites that transmit the infection belong to the genus LEISHMANIA, a protozoa transmitted by the bite of a tiny insect called the phlebotomine sand fly. Of 500 known species, only 30 of them carry the disease, and only the female sand fly transmits the protozoan, infecting itself with the parasites contained in the blood it sucks from its host. During a period of four to 25 days, the parasite continues its development inside the sand fly, where it is transformed. When the infectious female sand fly feeds on a fresh source of blood, its sting inoculates its new victim with the parasite.

The sand fly is found throughout the tropical and temperate regions of the world. The female lays its eggs in the burrows of rodents, in the bark of old trees, ruined buildings, cracks in house walls, and in rubbish.

Symptoms and Diagnostic Path

There are several types of this disease, with a wide range of symptoms. The *visceral* (internal organ) type characterized by irregular bouts of fever, weight loss, swelling of spleen and liver, and anemia. Untreated, this form of leishmaniasis is fatal almost 100 percent of the time.

In *mucocutaneous* leishmaniasis, lesions can partially or completely destroy the mucous membranes of the nose, mouth, and throat and can cause severe disfigurement. The *cutaneous* (skin) form of the disease produces skin ulcers on exposed parts of the body such as the arms, legs, and face, causing many lesions (sometimes up to 200) and severe disability. Most of the time the patient is permanently scarred.

Treatment Options and Outlook

It is essential to understand the geographic strains of the different parasites in order to properly treat the disease. All forms of this disease can be treated effectively with drugs (such as sodium stibogluconate or glucantime) given by injection. All types of this disorder with secondary bacterial infection also should be treated with antibiotics.

There are no vaccines or drugs to prevent infection. Travelers can reduce the risk of infection by avoiding contact with sand flies, which are most active during outdoor activities from dusk to dawn. Although sand flies are primarily night-time biters, infection can be acquired during the day if resting sand flies are disturbed. Sand fly activity in an area can easily be underestimated because sand flies are noiseless fliers, and bites might not be noticed.

Travelers should wear protective clothing and use insect repellent with N,N-diethylmetatoluamide (DEET); repeated applications may be necessary under conditions of excessive perspiration, wiping, and washing. Although putting permethrin on clothing can give added protection, it does not eliminate the need for repellent on exposed skin.

Contact with sand flies indoors can be reduced by using bed nets, and screening on doors and windows. Fine-mesh netting (at least 18 holes to the linear inch) is required for an effective barrier against sand flies, which are about a third of the size of mosquitoes. Spraying bed nets and window screens with permethrin aerosol can provide some protection, as can spraying dwellings with insecticides.

Risk Factors and Preventive Measures

People of all ages are at risk for leishmaniasis if they live or travel where the sand flies live. The disease is more common in rural areas, although it occurs in the outskirts of some cities. The risk is highest for travelers who are outdoors in leishmaniasis-endemic areas between dusk and dawn. Adventure travelers, Peace Corps volunteers, missionaries, ornithologists, people who do research outdoors at night, and soldiers are all at higher risk for leishmaniasis (especially the skin form of leishmaniasis).

leprosy A chronic bacterial infection (also called Hansen's disease) that damages nerves in the skin, limbs, face, and mucous membranes. Untreated leprosy can lead to severe complications, including blindness and disfigurement, but leprosy can be cured with proper medication. Contrary to popular belief, it is not highly contagious. While the disease still carries significant stigma, patient care has become integrated with routine health care. Anti-leprosy organizations have fought to repeal stigmatizing laws and practices; patients should not be referred to as "lepers."

Although leprosy is one of the oldest diseases in human history, it was not until 1873 that Armauer Hansen first identified the bacilli under a microscope. There were 407,791 new cases detected in 2004, and 286,063 cases at the beginning of 2005. The number of new cases detected around the world fell by about 107,000 cases (a 21 percent decrease) during 2004 compared with 2003. Since the beginning of the 21st century, the number of new cases detected has continued to decrease dramatically by about 20 percent each year.

In the United States, there are about 108 cases diagnosed each year, primarily in California, Florida, Hawaii, Louisiana, New York, and Texas. Approximately 16 percent of the new cases of leprosy are children.

History

Leprosy was first mentioned as a curse in Shinto prayers of 1250 B.C.E.; it was also mentioned in some Egyptian legends to explain the exodus of the Hebrews. For hundreds of years, those with leprosy were taken to a priest, not a doctor, and were found "guilty," not sick.

These customs led to the forcible confinement of patients in "leprosaria" or leper colonies; their children, whether infected or not, were denied an education in community schools. In eighth-century France, leprosy was considered grounds for divorce, and the Roman empire enforced banishment. Some countries passed legislation providing for the compulsory sterilization of leprosy patients because of fears that the condition was hereditary. Others would not permit patients to handle the nation's currency. Others "steam treated" patients' letters before allowing them in the mail, and some countries did not allow patients to vote. In medieval Europe, leprosy patients had to carry a "clapper" to warn others that a person with leprosy was approaching. Even as late as 1913, state Senator G. E. Willett of Montana was forced to give up his seat after he was diagnosed with leprosy.

Religious customs also affected many treatments for leprosy. In 250 B.C.E., Chinese leprosy patients pricked their swollen limbs to let out the "foul air." Ramses II of Egypt believed that people with leprosy who used his water wells would be cured. And in medieval Europe, it was believed that leprosy could be cured by the touch of a king.

Historically, topical treatments ranged from turtle soup, whiskey, and various poultices (such as onion, sea salt, and urine in Egypt; arsenic and powdered snake bones in China; water mixed with blood of dogs and infants under age two in Scotland; elephants' teeth; the flesh of crocodiles, snakes, lions, and bears). Other ingredients used to treat leprosy ranged from carbolic acid, creosote, phosphorus, mercury, and iodine, and plant extracts included madar or cashew-nut oil.

The idea of caring for patients with leprosy became popular among missionaries following biblical directives and the teachings of Jesus. This service became fashionable about 1100 C.E. in Europe, when many Crusaders (including a king) returned with the disease. Special hospitals were built, operated, and supported by cathedrals, but when the outbreak of bubonic PLAGUE in the 1300s wiped out entire populations, patients with leprosy began to be segregated again. Some countries seized the property of those with leprosy before burning them alive.

Leprosy is erroneously associated with the Old Testament, where references to *tsara'ath*, a term that closely translates to "leprosy," actually refers to a broad spectrum of problems that affected cloth, leather, linen, and house walls as well as humans. Most medical historians doubt that leprosy even existed among the Hebrews in Moses' time. Biblical scholars also have problems with the translation of the Greek term *lepra* partly because the Greeks had a specific term for leprosy. The Greek word *lepra* was most likely used to mean a variety of severe skin diseases. Greek medical writings later than the third century B.C.E. provide the earliest clinical references to modern leprosy. No mention of leprosy occurs in the New Testament after the Gospels.

Leprosy is caused by a rod-shaped bacterium, *MYCOBACTERIUM LEPRAE*, that is spread in droplets of nasal mucus. A person is infectious only during the first phase of the disease, and only those living in prolonged close contact with the infected person are at risk. Leprosy is probably spread by droplet infection through sneezing and coughing. In those with untreated leprosy, large amounts of bacteria are found in nasal discharge; the bacteria travel through the air in these droplets. They can survive three weeks or longer outside the human body, in dust or on clothing.

Although relatively infectious, leprosy is still one of the least contagious of all diseases. This—together with the fact that only 3 percent of the population are susceptible to leprosy—means that there is no justification for the practice (still prevalent in some countries) of isolating patients. Only a few people are susceptible because most people acquire a natural immunity when exposed to the disease.

Most of the body's tissue destruction is caused not by bacterial growth but by a reaction of the body's immune system to the organisms as they die. In *lepromatous leprosy,* damage is widespread, progressive, and severe. *Tuberculoid leprosy* is a milder form of the disease.

Symptoms and Diagnostic Path

Damage is first confined to the nerves supplying the skin and muscles, destroying nerve endings, sweat glands, hair follicles, and pigment-producing cells. It first causes a lightening (or darkening) of the skin, with a loss of feeling, and sweating. Some types of the disease produce a rash of bumps or nodules on the skin. As the disease progresses, bacilli also attack peripheral nerves; at first patients may feel an occasional "pins and needles" sensation or have a numb patch on the skin. Next, patients become unable to feel sensations such as a light touch or temperature, and gradually, hands, feet, and facial skin become numb. Delicate connections between nerve cells and nerve endings are severed, and whole sections of the body become totally numb. For example, if the nerve above the elbow is affected, part of the hand becomes numb and small muscles become paralyzed, leading to curled fingers.

When a patient can no longer sense pain, the body loses the automatic withdrawal reflex that protects against trauma from sharp or hot objects, leading to extensive scarring or even loss of fingers and toes. Muscle paralysis can lead to further deformity, and damage to the facial nerve means eyelids cannot close, leading to ulceration and blindness. Direct invasion of bacteria also may lead to inflammation of the eyeball, also leading to blindness.

Treatment Options and Outlook

Several antibiotic agents are effective against leprosy and are best used in combinations of two or three, including dapsone, clofazimine, and rifampin. Multidrug therapy was developed as leprosy bacilli became resistant to the single sulfone drug dapsone. The most powerful of these three drugs is rifampin, a drug first used against TUBERCULOSIS and found to be effective against leprosy in 1968. Particular combinations of these drugs were recommended in 1984 by the World Health Organization as standard treatment for mass campaigns against leprosy.

The three drugs are often distributed in blister packs containing a month's supply of pills; dapsone is taken daily, clofazimine is taken every other day, and rifampin is taken monthly. Now there are more than 1 million people receiving these drugs worldwide, and more than 1 million others who have already completed treatment.

While the medication can usually cure leprosy within six months to two years, patients are no longer contagious within a few days after treatment begins. To prevent a relapse, treatment needs to be administered for at least two years after the last signs of the disease have disappeared. In the United States, patients are eligible for treatment by the Public Health Service at special clinics and hospitals, or at the Gillis W. Long Hansen's Disease Center in Louisiana, the only institution in the United States devoted primarily to treatment, research, training, and education related to leprosy. Eleven regional centers, located primarily in major urban areas, treat those with leprosy on an outpatient basis.

No vaccine for leprosy is available because scientists have not been able to grow cultures in lab environments. However, about 95 percent of the population is immune to leprosy, which occurs naturally in armadillos.

After leprosy is cured, patients must learn to watch for wounds and injuries they cannot feel; they must wear special shoes to protect insensitive feet.

leptospirosis A bacterial disease characterized by a skin rash and flu-like symptoms caused by a spirochete bacterium excreted by rodents. Also known as autumn fever, there are between 100 and 200 cases and a few deaths reported in the United States each year. Leptospirosis is considered to be a disease that is reemerging in this country and is possibly the most common disease that rats transmit to humans in the United States. There are several strains of the organism; infection with one usually provides immunity to that organism alone, but not to other strains.

Although the disease is not new in the United States, it is hard to diagnose and its prevalence is unknown. Those especially at risk are urban patients who complain of flulike symptoms (especially during the summer) and who could have been exposed to rat urine or to pools of infected water in alleys and parks of the inner city.

Unrecognized leptospirosis might be common in city dwellers; one 1992 Baltimore study found 16 percent of blood samples taken at an STD clinic were positive for leptospirosis. An earlier study found that about a third of children tested in Detroit also had been exposed. None of the inner-city patients had been diagnosed with leptospirosis.

The infectious disease is caused by the spirochete *Leptospira interrogans* transmitted in the urine of wild or domestic animals, especially rats, livestock, and dogs. People get the disease when broken skin or mucous membranes contact the infected urine or water, soil, or vegetation. The bacteria survive best in warm water (72°F) that is stagnant; most cases have been reported from swimming, wading, or splashing in pools, streams, or puddles that were contaminated with animal urine.

In addition to urban dwellers, leptospirosis is an occupational disease of farmers, sewer workers, or others whose job requires contact with animals (especially rats). Most patients are male teenagers and young adults. Leptospirosis is not usually transmitted from person to person.

Symptoms and Diagnostic Path

Leptospirosis has two phases. After an incubation period of up to three weeks, the first phase begins with an acute illness of sudden headache, fever and chills, severe muscle aches, and skin rash appears. Up to 10 percent of infected patients develop a serious systemic form of the illness, called Weil's syndrome. This phase starts a few days after the fever drops; fever will return and bacteria may spread to the brain, causing MENINGITIS. Other serious symptoms include jaundice, confusion, depression, or decreased urine. The kidneys are often affected, and liver damage is common. People infected with this potentially fatal form of leptospirosis are usually very ill and are often hospitalized.

Leptospirosis is often mistaken for viral meningitis or HEPATITIS, but its two distinct phases separate it from those infections.

The disease is diagnosed using specific blood, urine, or fluid tests available through state public health laboratories. If positive, results are sent to the CENTERS FOR DISEASE CONTROL AND PREVENTION lab for confirmation. However, it takes up to a month to make a final determination. A physician must request such testing; it is not routinely done, and local labs do not ordinarily perform these tests. However, researchers have developed an experimental test that can detect within 24 hours tiny amounts of the bacterium's genetic material. The test has not yet been validated.

Treatment Options and Outlook

Tetracycline and erythromycin are effective, and in about one-third of cases patients improve rapidly. Fluid replacement is essential if jaundice or other signs of severe illness occur. Kidney dialysis may be needed in some cases.

Untreated patients may develop WEIL'S SYNDROME, a severe form of leptospirosis that can cause permanent kidney and liver damage; most patients recover, but sometimes the disease is fatal.

Risk Factors and Preventive Measures

The disease can be prevented by good sanitation practices, including using boots and gloves in hazardous places and practicing rodent control. It is common practice to immunize livestock and dogs against the disease, but even vaccinated animals can shed the bacteria in urine for a long time and infect humans.

lice Small wingless insects about the size of a sesame seed, with six legs and claws for grasping the hair; they feed on human blood. Lice are crawling insects that cannot jump or fly. Lice are divided into three species: *Pediculus humanus capitis* (head louse), *Pediculus humanus corporis* (body louse), and *Phthirius pubis* (the crab, or pubic louse). All three have flat bodies that measure up to three mm across.

Head lice live on and suck blood from the scalp, leaving red spots that itch intensely and can lead to skin inflammation and skin infection. The females lay a daily batch of pale eggs, called "nits" that attach to hairs close to the scalp; the nits hatch in about a week, and the adults can live for several weeks.

Head lice are not simply a plague of the poor, but are found among people of all walks of life. Between 6 and 12 million cases of head lice occur each year among U.S. schoolchildren between ages three and 12, even among those who shampoo daily. Children are most often affected by contracting the lice through direct contact, usually at school by sharing hats, brushes, combs, or headrests. Pets cannot get head lice.

Symptoms and Diagnostic Path

Because lice move so quickly, it is usually the nits that will be seen on the hair shaft. Nits are the tiny eggs of a louse that are yellow when newly laid, turning to white once they hatch. Nits are small, oval-shaped eggs that are "glued" at an angle to the side of the hair shaft. They hatch within eight days, and the empty eggshells are carried outward as the hair grows. Both head and pubic lice lay eggs at the base of hairs growing on the head or pubic area. Nits can be seen anywhere on the hair, especially behind the ears and at the back of the neck.

Nits should not be confused with hair debris, such as fat plugs or hair casts. Fat plugs are bright white irregularly shaped clumps of fat cells stuck to the hair shaft. Hair casts are thin, long cylinder-shaped segments of dandruff encircling the hair shaft; they are easily dislodged.

Lice infestations are diagnosed by the presence of nits; by calculating the distance from the base of the hair to the farthest nits, it is possible to estimate the duration of infestation.

All nits must be removed, according to the NATIONAL PEDICULOSIS ASSOCIATION. Since no lice pesticide kills all nits, any nits left on the hair can be confusing; thorough nit removal will reduce or eliminate the need for more treatments.

Nits can be removed with a special nit removal comb, with baby safety scissors, or with the fingernails.

Head lice and their nits can also be found on eyebrows and eyelashes. If one person in a family has head lice, all family members should be checked. However, only those who are infested should be treated with lice pesticide.

Body lice live and lay eggs on clothing next to the skin, visiting the body only to feed. Body lice affect people who rarely change their clothes.

Crab lice live in pubic hair or (rarely) armpits and beards. Pubic lice are commonly known as "CRABS" because they resemble a crab under the microscope. Crab lice cause incessant itching, are visible to the naked eye, and are easily transmitted during sex. It is also possible to pick them up from sheets or towels. They can live away from the host's body for up to one day, and the eggs can survive for several days. Affected patients who do not wash underwear, sheets, and towels in hot enough water are likely to be reinfected.

Treatment Options and Outlook

For *head lice,* lotions containing malathion or carbaryl kill lice quickly; the lotion should be washed off 12 hours after application, followed by combing the hair with a fine-tooth comb to remove dead lice and nits. Shampoos containing malathion or carbaryl are also effective if used repeatedly over several days. Combs and brushes should be plunged into very hot water to kill any attached eggs. The National Pediculosis Association discourages the use of lindane products (such as Kwell), because they appear to be potentially more toxic and no more effective than other treatments. Still, no product kills 100 percent of nits. Lice medications are not intended to be used on a routine or preventive basis.

All lice-killing medications are pesticides, and therefore should be used with caution. A pharmacist or physician should be consulted before using or applying pesticides when the person is pregnant, nursing, or has lice or nits in the eyebrows or eye-lashes or has other health problems (such as allergies). Head lice pesticides can be absorbed into the bloodstream; therefore, they should not be used on open wounds on the scalp or on the hands of the person applying the medication. These pesticides should not be used on infants and should be used with caution on children under age two. Instead, lice and nits can be removed manually or mechanically.

The product should be used over a sink (not a tub or shower) to minimize pesticide absorption and exposure to the entire body. Eyes of the affected individual must be kept covered while administering the pesticide.

All nits must be removed from the hair shaft. Bedding and recently worn clothing should be washed in hot water and dried in a hot dryer. Combs and brushes should be cleaned and then soaked in hot (not boiling) water for 10 minutes. Lice sprays should not be used, according to the National Pediculosis Association. Vacuuming is the best way to remove lice and attached nits from furniture, mattresses, rugs, stuffed toys, and car seats.

Neighborhood parents and the child's school, camp, or child care provider should be notified of the infestation. Children should be checked once a week for head lice.

Body lice can be killed by placing infested clothing in a hot dryer for five minutes, by washing clothes in very hot water, or by burning.

Pubic lice can be treated with an over-the-counter treatment.

Listeria monocytogenes A species of bacteria that infect many domestic and wild animals and in humans cause MENINGOENCEPHALITIS and sometimes infections of the womb.

See also LISTERIOSIS; PREGNANCY AND INFECTIOUS DISEASE.

listeriosis A food-borne illness that may cause no symptoms in healthy people but that is particularly dangerous to a fetus or newborn, the elderly, and people with damaged immune systems. The illness is also common among cattle, pigs, and poultry.

There are about 2,500 cases of serious listeriosis each year; of these, 500 patients die. Once thought to be exclusively a veterinary problem, it was identified as a human disease in 1981 when a Canadian outbreak was linked to tainted cole slaw made from cabbage grown in soil fertilized with *Listeria*-infected sheep manure. Four years later, another outbreak was traced to Mexican-style soft cheese in California. This outbreak sickened 150 people, including many pregnant women, and resulted in newborn deaths.

Over the past 10 years the government recalled cooked products contaminated with *Listeria,* including hot dogs, bologna and other luncheon meat, chicken and ham salad; sausages; chicken; sliced turkey breast; and sliced roast beef.

Listeriosis is caused by one species in a group of bacteria called *LISTERIA MONOCYTOGENES,* found in cow's milk, animal and human feces, soil, and leafy vegetables. In the past 10 years, there have been several outbreaks that seem to have been linked to the ingestion of soft cheeses (such as feta, some types of Mexican cheeses, Camembert, blue-veined cheeses) and deli-type lunchmeats. One recent study found that 20 percent of hot dogs tested contained the bacterium *L. monocytogenes.* Those with impaired immune systems may catch the disease from undercooked chicken.

The bacteria is remarkably tough, resisting heat, salt, nitrite, and acidity much better than many other organisms. It can survive on cold surfaces and can multiply slowly at temperatures as low as 34°F. (Refrigeration at 40°F or below stops the multiplication of many other food-borne bacteria.) Freezing the food will stop the bacteria from multiplying, and commercial pasteurization will eliminate the organism in dairy products. *Listeria* does not change the taste or smell of food.

When *Listeria* is found in processed products, the contamination probably occurred after processing (rather than due to poor heating or pasteurizing).

Listeriosis also can be spread through sexual contact, although it is not known how common this is.

Babies can be born with listeriosis if their mothers eat contaminated food during pregnancy. Pregnant women are 20 times more likely than other healthy adults to get listeriosis; about one-third of all cases happen during pregnancy. However, it is newborns rather than their mothers who suffer the most serious effects of infection during the pregnancy.

Patients with AIDS are 300 times more likely to get listeriosis than healthy people. Others at increased risk include persons with cancer, diabetes, kidney disease, those who take glucocorticosteroid drugs, or the elderly. While healthy adults and children sometimes become infected, they rarely become seriously ill.

Symptoms and Diagnostic Path

Healthy adults may not have any symptoms at all or may experience a flu-like illness with fever, muscle aches, and nausea or diarrhea. If infection spreads to the nervous system, it can cause a type of MENINGITIS, leading to symptoms including headache, stiff neck, confusion, loss of balance, or convulsions.

If a pregnant woman develops the infection, she may experience fever, tiredness, headache, sore throat, dry cough, or back pain. After a few days she will feel better but notice that the fetus is not moving; she may miscarry up to the sixth month or go into labor prematurely; some infants may be stillborn.

There is no routine screening test for susceptibility during pregnancy as there is for rubella and some other infections. A blood or spinal fluid culture will reveal the infection. During pregnancy, a blood test is the most reliable way to diagnose the infection.

Treatment Options and Outlook

Antibiotics are most helpful in pregnant women to prevent disease in the fetus. Babies with listeriosis receive the same antibiotics as adults, although a combination of antibiotics may be used until diagnosis is certain. Even with prompt treatment, some infections result in death, especially those with other serious medical problems.

If the fetus is affected early in the pregnancy, the baby will probably be born prematurely. Such an infant is usually very ill, with breathing problems, blue skin, and low body temperature. If the baby survives, there may be a bloodstream infection or meningitis. Still, half of these babies die, even if treated. Fetuses affected later in the pregnancy may be carried to term with normal birth weight; if infected during delivery, they may develop meningitis; 40 percent may die. Some surviving babies may have permanent brain damage or mental retardation.

Adults with impaired immune systems who contract listeriosis may develop meningitis with fever, intense headache, nausea, and vomiting. This is followed by delirium, coma, collapse, and shock; sometimes, ABSCESSES and skin rash appear.

Risk Factors and Preventive Measures

While most people do not have to worry about the disease, scientists at the CENTERS FOR DISEASE CONTROL AND PREVENTION warn that pregnant women, the very old, and those with damaged immune systems might want to avoid deli-counter foods and soft cheeses (there is no risk for hard cheese, processed slices, cottage cheese, or yogurt). Those at risk are advised to cook hot dogs to a steaming 160°F for several minutes to avoid contamination; hot dogs at restaurants or ball parks, should be avoided, since cooking temperatures cannot be verified. One study found that garlic inhibits the growth of this harmful bacteria in the intestine, probably because of a sulfur compound found in fresh garlic.

liver fluke   See FLUKE; SCHISTOSOMIASIS.

lockjaw   See TETANUS.

loiasis (loaisis, loaiasis)   A form of the tropical parasitic disease FILARIASIS caused by an infestation of the *Loa loa* worm, which may travel for 10 or 15 years underneath the skin and causes an inflammation known as a calabar swelling.

Sometimes the migrating worms can be seen underneath the conjunctiva in the eye. Commonly called the eye worm, the name *loa loa* actually means "worm worm." The disease is limited to the region of the rain forests in the Congo River area in central and western Africa and equatorial Sudan; it is especially common in Cameroon and on the Ogowe River. An estimated 20 million people are infected with the worm; in the Congo River basin, up to 90 percent of villagers in some areas are infected.

The disease is acquired through the bite of an infected African deer fly. Once inside the body, the infective larvae develop slowly into a mature adult (the process takes about a year). During this period, it lives and moves around underneath the skin. In periods of growth and development, *Loa loa* makes frequent excursions through the connective tissues, where it is often noticed by the patient. Adult worms (which live for up to 15 years) move in the subcutaneous tissues where the female deposits the microfilariae. Microfilariae may become apparent in the patient's blood within five to six months of infection and may remain in the blood for as long as 17 years. They move into peripheral blood during the day and into the lungs at night.

Symptoms and Diagnostic Path

Symptoms of loiasis generally do not appear until several years after the bite of the infected fly, although they have been known to appear within four months. Most of the symptoms observed in people infected with *Loa loa* occur during periods when the migrating adults appear near the surface of the skin. The worms often appear near the eye, where they can be easily seen and extracted before they damage the conjunctiva.

Allergic reactions to the migrating worms can cause calabar swellings in the arms and legs, triggered by metabolic products from the worm that sensitize the patient. The painful swellings develop quickly and last three to five days, appearing when the worms are quiet and disappearing when the worms move on. Recurrent swelling can create painful cystlike enlargements of the connective tissues around the tendons.

Occasionally, the adult worm migrates into the conjunctiva and cornea, causing pain and swelling. Dying worms can cause chronic ABSCESSES.

Lab diagnosis is based on finding microfilariae during the day, or adults in the subcutaneous tissues.

Treatment Options and Outlook

Diethylcarbamazine has been the preferred drug for the past 40 years, and usually cures the disease, and may also be useful as a preventive measure. The drug kills both worms and microfilariae. However, it should be used with caution in patients with heavy infestations of worms, since this can provoke eye problems. Antihistamines and prednisone may be needed to ease allergic reactions due to the disintegration of microfilariae.

Some individual may experience a strong allergic response, causing giant hives and swelling of the mucous membranes accompanied with fever. Evidence of heart or kidney problems may be found in up to 20 percent of these cases.

Risk Factors and Preventive Measures

Repellents containing DEET or dimethyl phthalate, wearing long pants, and sleeping in well-screened areas are important ways to protect against bites.

lower respiratory tract infections   See RESPIRATORY TRACT INFECTIONS.

lung fluke   See FLUKE; SCHISTOSOMIASIS.

Lyme disease   A tick-borne illness causing more than 16,000 infections each year in the United States. Untreated, Lyme disease can cause a host of problems, including arthritis and disorders of the heart and central nervous system. It is most commonly found in the northeast coastal states from Maine to Maryland, in the upper Midwest, and on the Pacific coast. Typically individuals contract Lyme disease in the late spring or early summer when ticks are abundant, or whenever the temperature is above 40°F for several consecutive days.

The number of new cases of Lyme disease has doubled in the United States since 1991, according to the U.S. CENTERS FOR DISEASE CONTROL AND PREVENTION (CDC), from more than 9,000 cases in 1991 to nearly 18,000 new cases in 2000. Not all cases are reported to the health department, however. In 2000, Lyme disease cases increased by 8 percent compared to 1999, in which 16,273 cases were reported. The doubling in new cases may be partly due to increased awareness and better reporting of Lyme disease, but also because more people were exposed to ticks in densely populated areas.

Most of the new cases in 2000—about 95 percent—were reported by 12 states in the northeastern, mid-Atlantic, and north-central United States, including Connecticut, Rhode Island, New

Jersey, New York, and Delaware. The highest number of cases was reported by Columbia County, New York. Only six states reported no cases of Lyme disease in 2000: Colorado, Georgia, Hawaii, Montana, New Mexico, and South Dakota. Children aged five to nine years and adults 50 to 59 years are the hardest hit groups, because they have a higher exposure to infected ticks and less frequent use of protective measures than other age groups.

While the disease has been portrayed in sometimes frightening fashion in the media, most of the time it is easily treated and does not progress to the chronic stage. It probably causes severe long-term effects in less than 10 percent of untreated patients; moreover, recent studies indicate that many people who think they have Lyme disease actually have other conditions.

In the United States, the disease was first recognized in Lyme, Connecticut, after two mothers were told in 1975 that their children had juvenile rheumatoid arthritis. This type of arthritis is a disabling condition of children in which joints are swollen and painful. When the women discovered many others in the area had the disease—which does not normally occur in clusters—they took their concerns to Yale University.

By the late 1970s, Yale researchers Allen Steere and Stephen Malawista found that many patients they studied were afflicted with a mysterious disease that produced a variety of symptoms, in addition to the joint swelling. They determined the cause was apparently a microorganism transmitted by at least one species of tick found widely in the woods around Lyme. In 1982, it was identified by Willy Burgdorfer of Rocky Mountain Labs in Hamilton, Montana, who discovered the spiral-shaped bacterial species that today bears his name: BORRELIA BURGDORFERI.

Now that scientists knew the cause, they could confirm that a group of skin conditions and neurological syndromes identified in Europe were also manifestations of Lyme disease. Since then, researchers have identified the disease throughout the world. It also occurs in almost every state in the United States, although it remains concentrated in the northeast, Minnesota, and northern California.

Only recently identified in the United States, Lyme disease is not a new affliction. German scientists have found evidence of the disease in 19th-century ticks, making these insects the bacteria's earliest-known hosts. The ticks came from the Vienna Natural History Museum in Austria, which supplied 21 ticks pickled in alcohol to the scientists. The genetic material in two matched that of *Borrelia garinii,* one of three forms of the bacteria that can induce Lyme disease. The 21 ticks had come from a Hungarian cat in 1884, and from a fox caught in Austria in 1888. Scientists suspect that the disease may have occurred even earlier, but finding even older ticks to study has been difficult.

European victims of Lyme disease suffer slightly different forms of the disease, probably because there are differences in the strains of *B. burgdorferi* active in different parts of the world. Europeans patients experience long-term neurological complications, such as cognitive deficits and dementia; up to 10 percent of untreated Europeans also suffer for many years with a skin condition in which affected areas of the skin become red, thin, and wrinkled. In the United States, these symptoms are rare.

The disease is caused by *Borrelia burgdorferi,* a spirochete form of bacteria. It is transmitted primarily by the deer tick, the tiniest of which is about the size of the period at the end of this sentence, which are found on deer, birds, filed mice, and other rodents. The tick must be attached to its victim for between 36 to 48 hours before an infectious dose of *B. burgdorferi* can be transmitted. For this reason, simply by checking often for ticks, most people can avoid becoming infected.

Most people are diagnosed in the spring, summer, or early fall because this reflects the life cycle of the infected tick. In the northeastern United States, about half of all adult *Ixodes scapularis* ticks are infected. On Block Island and Nantucket Island the numbers are even higher. Even so, in most sections of the Northeast, only between one and three percent of people have contracted Lyme disease.

The tick (*Ixodes pacificus*) that transmits Lyme diseases in California relies on intermediate hosts (such as lizards) that are resistant to infection; for this reason, ticks—and consequently humans—in the West are infected much less often than in the Northeast. The same is true for species that transmit Lyme in some areas of Europe and Asia.

Symptoms and Diagnostic Path

Most people who do become infected will usually display one or more symptoms. Between three days and a month after becoming infected, about 60 percent of patients will notice a small red spot that expands over a period of days or weeks, forming a circular, triangular, or oval-shaped rash called ERYTHEMA CHRONICUM MIGRANS. The reddened area, which usually appears at the bite site, neither itches nor hurts. Sometimes the rash resembles a red raised bull's-eye rash with a clear center at the site of the bite.

The rash can range in size from a dime to the entire width of a person's body. As the infection spreads, several rashes can appear at different sites on the body. Without treatment, the rash begins to disappear within days or weeks.

As the spirochetes move through the body via the bloodstream, other symptoms affecting other parts of the body may appear. These may include flu-like symptoms (such as headache, stiff neck, appetite loss, body aches, and fatigue). Although these symptoms may resemble those of common viral infections, Lyme disease symptoms tend to persist or may occur intermittently.

Early neurological problems may also appear in about 20 percent of patients. Some patients may experience Bell's palsy in one or both sides of the face, which may become paralyzed for weeks or months before returning to normal. Other symptoms may include MENINGITIS, ENCEPHALITIS, or numbness and tingling of other parts of the body.

Lyme disease is not easy to diagnose because its symptoms and signs mimic those of many other diseases, such as viral infections or MONONUCLEOSIS. Joint pain can be misdiagnosed as inflammatory arthritis, and neurologic signs may be misidentified as a primary neurologic disease such as MULTIPLE SCLEROSIS.

Diagnosis of Lyme disease includes history of exposure to ticks (especially in endemic areas), symptoms, and the result of blood tests confirming that the patient has antibodies to Lyme bacteria. There are a number of tests that can be used to diagnose the presence of Lyme disease; the best-known combination is the ELISA and Western blot.

Enzyme-linked immunoassay (ELISA) This test is widely accepted and routinely performed as the first step in confirming Lyme disease in patients with symptoms, especially if symptoms did not include the expanding rash typical of early disease. The ELISA checks for higher blood levels of antibodies produced in response to *Borrelia burgdorferi*, the bacteria that cause Lyme disease. If performed at least four weeks after a tick bite, this test will identify virtually all patients with Lyme disease, but there is a 5 to 7 percent risk of false positives. Therefore, ELISA is used only as a preliminary screening; all positive results must be confirmed by a second test—the Western blot.

Western blot This is a more accurate test for Lyme disease that can identify specific Lyme-associated antibodies in the blood. It is routinely used to confirm (or in some cases contradict) positive ELISA results. A positive ELISA followed by a negative Western blot usually means that the patient does not have Lyme disease. The Western blot is not foolproof and should not be used to diagnose Lyme disease in patients without symptoms, but the ELISA/Western blot combination is considered the most reliable testing method currently available.

Polymerase chain reaction (PCR) This very sensitive test can detect the DNA of *B. burgdorferi*. However, this test has problems that limit its widespread use. *B. burgdorferi* bacteria do not persist in easily obtainable fluids such as blood or joint or spinal fluid, but typically bind to joint and nerve tissues. A PCR on spinal fluid may be positive in a patient with Lyme meningitis, but is usually negative in a patient with long-term disease. In addition, a PCR can be easily contaminated and produce false-positive results.

Prevue B This fast Lyme antibody-detection screening assay provides color results using serum or whole blood samples and can be performed in a physician's office. While results are quick, a positive result must still be confirmed by a laboratory-performed Western blot.

There are a number of experimental tests that are currently being studied, including

C6 Lyme Peptide ELISA (C6LPE) This simple, sensitive and specific antibody titer may very well significantly improve the reliability of Lyme disease testing.

Lyme urine antigen test (LUAT) This antigen capture assay is designed to detect certain proteins exhibited by *B. burgdorferi*. However, although heavily marketed on the Internet, it is of no proven value in the diagnosis or management of Lyme disease and has not been FDA-approved for commercial use or recommended by the Centers for Disease Control and Prevention. Because the LUAT has not yet been independently validated, it can lead to misdiagnosis and unnecessary treatment.

Treatment Options and Outlook

Antibiotics within three days of a tick bite (doxycycline, cefuroxime, or amoxicillin) kill the bacteria. Most patients who are treated in later stages of the disease also respond well. Pregnant women may require hospitalization. Azithromycin, erythromycin, or clarithromycin are slightly less effective against Lyme disease and should be used only as alternative treatments for patients who have allergies or unpleasant side effects to the preferred medications. More aggressive intravenous antibiotic treatment with cefotaxime or ceftriaxone is recommended in patients who have severe heart or brain involvement.

Either oral or IV treatment should be given for between two and four weeks, depending on the stage of disease, symptoms, and their severity. After the first treatment, a second four-week course of oral medication, or a two- to four-week course of IV antibiotics, may be necessary in patients who have recurrent arthritis.

There is currently no scientific evidence that any other treatment approaches, such as repeated or prolonged medication, higher doses, or combining or alternating antibiotics, are any more effective in curing the disease than the standard methods. Moreover, excessive treatment can raise the risk of unpleasant side effects or drug reactions such as rash, diarrhea, gallbladder disease, and bone marrow damage.

Unfortunately, cases that are not diagnosed soon enough may resist a antibiotic therapy. In a few patients, symptoms of persistent infection may continue or the disease may recur, so that physicians prescribe repeated long courses of antibiotic therapy. The value of this approach, which can have serious side effects (such as inducing formation of gallstones) remains controversial.

Patients with late chronic Lyme disease may exhibit varying degrees of permanent damage to joints or the nervous system. In general, this occurs among patients who were not diagnosed in the early stages of the disease, or for whom early treatment was not successful. Deaths from Lyme disease have been reported only very rarely.

A vaccine was taken off the market in 2002.

After several months of being infected, slightly more than half of those people not treated with antibiotics develop recurrent attacks of painful and swollen joints that last a few days to a few months. The arthritis can shift from one joint to another; most often, the knee is infected. About 10 to 20 percent of untreated patients who experience temporary arthritic symptoms will go on to develop chronic Lyme arthritis. In contrast to many other forms of arthritis, Lyme arthritis typically is not symmetrical.

One out of 10 Lyme patients develop heart problems (such as irregular heartbeat) for a few days or weeks, generally appearing several weeks after infection. Most people will not be aware of this problem unless a physician detects it, although some patients might realize they cannot exercise as they once did. This condition usually lasts only for a week to 10 days and almost never requires a pacemaker. Other nervous system complications include subtle changes such as memory loss, difficulty with concentration, and change in mood or sleeping habits. Nervous system abnormalities usually develop several weeks, months, or even years after an untreated infection. These symptoms often last for weeks or months, and may recur. Less often, Lyme disease causes eye inflammation, HEPATITIS, or severe fatigue. Pregnant women who contract the disease run the risk of miscarriage, stillbirth, or birth defects.

Post-Lyme syndrome   Many people experience persistent symptoms after Lyme disease treatment, called post-Lyme syndrome. Some physicians and patients believe that this condition arises from recurring active infection, although studies of patients who had been treated following recommended guidelines have not substantiated this argument. However, the original infection can recur if treatment was not long enough, doses were too low, inappropriate antibiotics were prescribed, or patients did not take medication correctly.

Preliminary evidence suggests that relapsing symptoms in patients who had been properly treated may be the result of tissue damage from the original infection. Another possibility is the recent discovery of yet another spirochete similar to *B. burgdoferi*, which may cause later-stage symptoms.

Risk Factors and Preventive Measures

In some cases, antibiotics given after a tick bite but before symptoms develop can prevent Lyme disease.

A vaccine is also available for field dogs at risk for developing the disease because of the area in which they live.

Experts at the U.S. Centers for Disease Control do not recommend preventive treatment with antibiotics after all tick bites. It is better to avoid tick bites in the first place; avoiding their habitat is the best way to prevent tick bites, but ticks may also be found in lawns, gardens, and on bushes adjacent to homes.

When walking in the woods, hikers should stay on trails and avoid brushing up against low bushes or tall grass. Ticks do not hop, jump, fly, or descend from trees, although they may blow in a strong breeze. To prevent bites, hikers should wear protective clothing (light-colored, long-sleeve shirts and light-colored pants tucked into boots or socks) so that ticks can be more easily spotted.

An insect repellent preferably containing no more than 30 percent DEET (N-diethylmetatoluamide) may be used on bare skin and clothing. Duranon can be applied to clothing only, but not to the skin. All insect repellent should be used with caution (especially on children) and should not be applied to the hands or face.

Ticks and their hosts (mice, chipmunks, voles, and other small mammals) need moisture, a place hidden from direct sun, and a place to hide. Therefore, the clearer the area around a house, the less chance there will be of getting a tick bite. All leaf litter and brush should be removed as far as possible away from the house. Low-lying bushes should be pruned to let in more sun. Leaves should be raked every fall, since ticks prefer to overwinter in fallen leaves. Woodpiles are favorite hiding places for mammals carrying ticks; woodpiles should be neat, off the ground, in a sunny place, and under cover.

Gardens should be cleaned up every fall; foliage left on the ground over the winter provide shelter for mammals that may harbor ticks. Stone walls on the property increase the potential for ticks.

Shady lawns may support ticks in epidemic areas; lawns should be mowed and edged. Entire fields should be mowed in fall, preferably with a rotary mower.

Birdfeeders attract birds that carry infected ticks so feeders should not be placed close to the house. The ground under the feeder should be cleaned regularly. Bird feeding should be stopped during late spring and summer, when infected ticks are most active. Building eight-foot fences to keep out deer may significantly reduce the abundance of ticks on large land parcels. Pets allowed outside on a daily basis should be examined regularly; tick collars and/or dips may be needed.

Three pesticides may help: chlorpyrifos (Dursban), carbaryl (Sevin), and cyfluthrin (Tempo). One or two applications a year in late May and September can significantly reduce the tick population.

lymphangitis Infection of the lymph node channels that cause tender red streaks to appear on the skin. The infection may spread to the bloodstream. This condition is a clear indication of serious infection and requires immediate treatment with antibiotics.

The infection is caused by a spread of bacteria (usually STREPTOCOCCUS or *Staphylococcus*) from an infected wound into the lymphatic channels.

Symptoms and Diagnostic Path

The red streaks extend from the site of infection toward the nearest lymph nodes; there is usually a fever, pain, chills, headache, and general feeling of illness.

An examination will reveal infected lymph nodes or lymph vessels. A biopsy and culture of the affected area or node may reveal the cause of the inflammation. Blood cultures may identify spread of infection to the bloodstream.

Treatment Options and Outlook

Antibiotics together with warm, moist compresses, usually clear up the infection without complication. Because lymphangitis may spread within hours,

prompt treatment is essential. Specific antibiotics should control the underlying infection; painkillers may be needed. Anti-inflammatory medications may help reduce inflammation and swelling, and hot, moist compresses may ease inflammation and pain. An ABSCESS may need to be surgically drained.

Prompt treatment with antibiotics should clear the infection, but it may take weeks or months for the swelling to fade. The length of the recovery period depends on the underlying cause.

lymphocytic choriomeningitis virus (LCMV) A virus carried by hamsters and wild or lab mice that is not harmful to adults but that can cause birth defects in unborn children whose mothers contract the virus.

LCMV was first identified in 1933 in a woman who was thought to have a form of ENCEPHALITIS. In 1955, it was first recognized in the United Kingdom as a virus that could cause congenital disease. Since then, individual cases of congenital LCMV infection have been identified in Germany, France, Lithuania, and across the United States. Mice and hamsters are the primary sources of LCMV infections. Humans acquire this virus by direct contact with infected rodents or by inhaling the virus.

So far, more than 49 infants around the world have been diagnosed with LCMV, including three cases of congenital LCMV in Arizona. Experts really do not know how many infants have been affected by LCMV before birth because doctors do not routinely look at LCMV as a possible cause of congenital blindness or retardation. In one instance, twin girls from Cochise County were born to a mother who had unknowingly contracted LCMV during pregnancy. One girl has vision problems and the other is severely developmentally delayed and has seizures. More than 90 percent of the babies who have contracted the LCMV virus before birth have had adverse effects, the most common of which were vision problems. Other problems include neurological problems such as cerebral palsy, mental retardation, seizures, and decreased visual acuity.

A pregnant woman with a pet hamster should have someone else take care of it during the pregnancy. If cleaning up after wild mice, the woman should wear gloves and spray the area with water to avoid the possibility of wafting the virus into the air. Pregnant women who work with mice in a laboratory setting should have the mice tested for LCMV.

lymphogranuloma venereum (LGV) A serious SEXUALLY TRANSMITTED DISEASE involving the lymph glands in the genital area caused by an aggressive strain of CHLAMYDIA TRACHOMATIS. The incidence of the disease is highest among sexually active people.

Symptoms and Diagnostic Path
The first symptom is a small, painless pimple on the penis, female external genitalia, or vagina, that appears from three to 30 days after exposure; it is so small it often goes unnoticed. The infection then spreads to the lymph nodes in the groin, and from there it moves to surrounding tissue. An individual remains infectious as long as there are active lesions.

Treatment Options and Outlook
The disease responds to certain antibiotics such as tetracycline or sulfamethoxazole.

Risk Factors and Preventive Measures
There are several ways to prevent the spread of LGV, including using condoms, washing genitals after sex, avoiding sexual contact if infected, notifying all partners in case of infection, and reducing the number of sex partners.

mad cow disease The common name for BOVINE SPONGIFORM ENCEPHALOPATHY (BSE), a fatal infectious disease of the brain and spinal cord in cows that causes microscopic holes in brain tissue. Scientists believe there is a link between mad cow disease and a similar fatal brain disease in humans known as variant-CREUTZFELDT-JAKOB DISEASE (vCJD).

Mad cow disease is the bovine form of a condition that began appearing in British cows in the 1980s. Some were pathologically nervous, others bizarrely aggressive, but when the "mad cows" died, as they inevitably did, their brains were discovered to be shot through with holes.

While the exact cause of mad cow disease is unknown, the most accepted theory is that it is caused by a mutant form of a protein called a PRION, first identified by California neurologist Stanley B. Prusiner. In 1982, Prusiner identified the radical new infectious particle that was neither virus nor bacteria, but that somehow can pass its mutated shape by nudging up against a healthy cell's normal prions to alter the cell shape. Not all scientists agree, however that prions cause the disease; some still insist that the prion is a result of the disease, and that some new virus may be responsible.

Mad cow disease can arise out of nowhere and lie dormant for years, which the British government believes is how it started in England. Perhaps only one cow spontaneously developed the disease. To become an epidemic it needed an "amplifier," which in Britain turned out to be the practice of feeding cattle the ground-up remains of others of their species. This was amplified by feeding rendered cow meat-and-bone meal to young calves.

While the mad cow disease was disturbing enough, it became even more serious when scientists realized it was probably causing a similar brain-wasting disease in humans. While at first emphatically denying a link, eventually British pathologists confirmed a connection between mad cow disease and a new variety of Creutzfeldt-Jakob disease (CJD), a degenerative brain illness that strikes about one elderly person per million per year. The new variety of CJD, called variant-CJD, (vCJD) attacks very young patients—some as early as their teens—compared with classic form of the disease, which strikes only the elderly. VCJD is caused by eating or inhaling particles of beef contaminated with mad cow disease. Mad cow and vCJD are assumed to be related because both attack and destroy the brain in the same fatal way. The disease starts with mood swings, numbness, and uncontrolled body movements; eventually the brain is destroyed. The vCJD usually kills in about 18 months after symptoms appear, compared to four to six months for classic CJD. There is no treatment and both diseases are uniformly fatal. Eventually, the British government acknowledged that eating mad cow–contaminated beef was the "most likely explanation" for vCJD.

With that realization, the British government changed their rules on animal feed, preventing the "feeding like to like" system that had perpetuated the epidemic. The control measures worked, and mad cow is disappearing from British herds. Since the EPIDEMIC began, more than 80 Britons have died from exposure to mad cow meat. Three people in France died of vCJD, also presumably contracted from eating meat from diseased animals.

The mad cow epidemic in Europe is largely being contained because of the energetic efforts—and the power—of the European Union, which regulates the situation for all of Europe. After the detection of 25 mad cows, Germany announced plans to slaughter and destroy 400,000 elderly animals, which are most prone to the disease. Beef consumption in Germany plunged 50 percent, and 34 countries banned German beef imports. Italian farmers have protested in Rome, demanding government compensation for losses caused by Italy's country's mad cow scare. Beef sales have dropped in Spain, where 12 cows showed characteristic holes in their brains. Mad cow has also appeared in Portugal, Switzerland, the Netherlands, Belgium, Denmark, Ireland, Luxembourg, Liechtenstein, and Hong Kong. Recently, patients have been identified with vCJD in Greece and Hong Kong.

In response to the British experience, the United States enacted import restrictions and tests of diseased cattle and people performed at the National Prion Disease Pathology Surveillance Center. The last imports of British beef occurred in 1989, and only 32 British animals entered the food chain during the 1980s. By 1990, the United States had prohibited the entry of live sheep and cattle, and rendered animal protein, from Britain. In 1997 the Food and Drug Administration (FDA) banned the feeding of ruminant offal to ruminants. Since then, federal regulators have banned imports of beef and byproducts from all of Europe and Brazil, which imported British cows in the 1980s.

From 1986 through 2001, more than 98 percent of all mad cow cases in the world were reported from the United Kingdom, where the disease was first described. During this same period, the number of European countries reporting at least one case increased from four to 18 through 2001. During 2001–03, Canada, Japan, and Israel reported their first cases, and others followed.

The identification in 2003 of a mad cow case in Canada, and the subsequent identification later that year of a case in the United States that had been imported from Canada led to the concern that transmission of mad cow may be occurring in North America. As a result, safeguards to minimize the risk for human exposure to mad cow were implemented in the United States by the Department of Agriculture. However, a second case of mad cow was found in the United States in Texas in 2005.

From 1995 through August 2004, 147 human cases of vCJD were reported in the United Kingdom, seven in France, and one each in Canada, Ireland, Italy, and the United States. The patients from Canada, Ireland, and the United States had lived in the United Kingdom during a key exposure period

of the UK population to the mad cow agent. The incidence of vCJD in the United Kingdom appears to have peaked in 1999, and it has been dropping ever since. However, the future pattern of this epidemic is uncertain.

Transfusion of blood contaminated with the vCJD agent is believed to have been responsible for a few cases of disease in the United Kingdom, which prompted the FDA to outline a geography-based donor deferral policy to reduce the risk of bloodborne transmission of vCJD in the United States. One deferral criterion was living for five or more years in continental Europe from 1980 onward.

Mad cow disease is just one of a group of illnesses known as transmissible spongiform encephalopathies (TSE). A similar illness among deer and elk in the United States has gotten much less fanfare. This TSE is called chronic wasting disease, and it has been found for decades in two western states. Less than 1 percent of Rocky Mountain elk, and 4 percent to 6 percent of mule deer and white-tailed deer in southeast Wyoming and northeast and north-central Colorado have chronic wasting disease. The disease is also present in captive herds in five or six states, and could spread either from mother to offspring, or horizontally from one animal to another, probably by having one animal consume forage contaminated with fecal matter from an infected deer or elk.

Colorado and Wyoming both recommend that hunters limit their exposure to spinal cords and brains by using rubber gloves while cleaning kills. No humans have been known to have been sickened directly by chronic wasting disease, and there is no evidence that cattle have been infected. However, there is some evidence that this prion could infect people more or less as readily as the BSE prion does.

Risk Factors and Preventive Measures

In the United Kingdom, the risk of acquiring vCJD from eating beef and beef products appears to be extremely small, about one case per 10 billion servings. In the other countries of the world, the current risk would not be expected to be any higher than that in the United Kingdom.

To reduce the risk of acquiring vCJD from food, travelers outside the United States may consider either avoiding beef and beef products altogether or choosing solid pieces of muscle meat (rather than brains or beef products like burgers and sausages). Milk and milk products from cows are not believed to pose any risk for transmitting the mad cow agent.

malaria An infectious disease caused by a parasitic protozoa within the red blood cells, now believed to be one of the major reemerging infections of the world. Each year, there are between 300 million and 500 million new cases; 2.7 million will die. It is so serious that every 30 seconds somewhere in the world a child dies of the disease.

Malaria is one of the oldest known infections. First mentioned in ancient Sanskrit and Chinese documents, malaria was described in detail by Hippocrates who discriminated among different types of malarial fever in the fifth century B.C.E., early physicians thought the illness was carried by hot, wet air, which is where it got its name—from the Italian word for "bad air." Long the scourge of the ancient world, it is believed that the army of Alexander the Great was probably wiped out by malaria during its march across India.

Among Africans, it is believed that the neverending pressure of the illness led to the rise of the sickle-cell trait common in that population. The slight deformity of the red blood cells in sickle-cell anemia discourages the infiltration by the malarial parasite.

It is believed that malaria was introduced into the United States by European colonists and African slaves in the 16th and 17th centuries, where it then became endemic in many areas of the country, following the migration of the colonists. It was a particular problem in warm, wet areas of the United States such as the Chesapeake Bay region and the Mississippi Valley. It is believed that Andrew Jackson, Ulysses S. Grant, and George Washington all at various times suffered from malaria.

The first treatment against the disease was begun as early as 1630, when "Jesuit's bark" (the bark of the chinchona tree) was used to ease the fever of a Spanish magistrate in Peru. News of the treatment spread to Europe, where the chinchona bark cure was enthusiastically adopted—except by the profoundly anti-Catholic Oliver Cromwell, who refused to take Jesuit's bark for malaria and died of the disease. Eventually, quinine was isolated from the bark, leading to the development of the synthetic version (chloroquine) of the bark. This cheap, effective drug almost won the world's battle with malaria until resistant strains of the disease began appearing in the 1960s.

The incidence of the disease peaked in 1875, but it is estimated that more than 600,000 cases were reported in 1914. By 1934, the number of cases dropped to 125,556, and by the 1950s, experts concluded that malaria had been eliminated in this country, through the efforts of spraying, removing breeding sites, accurate assessment, and focused control. It was still understood that international travel could reintroduce the disease into this country. Since 1957, nearly all cases diagnosed in the United States have been acquired by mosquito transmission in areas where malaria is known to exist. In the United States, there are an average of 1,300 new cases a year. Most cases in the United States occur in travelers and immigrants returning from malaria-risk areas, especially in sub-Saharan Africa and the Indian subcontinent.

Environmental changes, the spread of drug resistance, and increased air travel could lead to the reemergence of malaria as a serious public health problem in the United States, according to the U.S. CENTERS FOR DISEASE CONTROL AND PREVENTION. Recent outbreaks of mosquito-transmitted diseases in densely populated areas of New Jersey, New York, Texas, and Michigan are evidence that the risk exists.

Indeed, the parasite that causes malaria has become resistant to the usual antimalarial drugs. Only 10 percent of the world's population was at risk of catching this disease in 1960, but today that number has grown to 40 percent.

Malaria is caused by four different species of the *Plasmodium* parasite transmitted by the *Anopheles* mosquito. The deadliest parasite causing the sometimes-fatal version of malaria is *Plasmodium falciparum;* others are *P. vivas, P. malariae,* and *P. ovale.*

The malaria parasite is genetically more diverse and much older (at least 100,000 years old) than some scientists have thought, according to new data uncovered by National Institutes of Health researchers. The new information suggests that creating vaccines to control the deadly disease poses a greater challenge than experts had imagined.

The experts also found that parasites resistant to the primary antimalarial drug chloroquine occurred in several geographic locations and rapidly spread across continents. This finding destroys the long-held notion that chloroquine resistance developed independently in only two areas in the mid-20th century and slowly spread to other countries from those sites. The new information implies that resistance to chloroquine and other antimalaria drugs can arise and spread more completely than had been thought and underscores the need for careful drug-use monitoring programs.

Parasites in the blood of an infected person are taken into the stomach of the mosquito as it feeds; when the mosquito bites a person, parasites are injected into the person's bloodstream, migrating to the liver and other organs. After an incubation period from 12 days to 10 months (depending on the variety), parasites return to the bloodstream and invade the red blood cells. At this point, symptoms appear. Rapid multiplication of the parasites destroys the red cells and releases more parasites capable of infecting other red blood cells. This leads to the shivering, fever, and sweating that is the hallmark of the disease; the loss of healthy red cells causes anemia.

The mature parasites remain in the blood and do not reinvade the liver, although a few may remain behind in the liver in a dormant state. These can be released months or years later, causing a relapse of malaria in people who thought they were cured.

Symptoms and Diagnostic Path

Symptoms vary and may appear from eight to 12 days after a bite in falciparum malaria to as many as 30 days for other types. Early signs may mimic the flu, causing fever, chills, headache, muscle ache, and malaise. As each new batch of parasites is released, symptoms of shivering and fever reappear. The interval between fever attacks is different in different types of malaria; in quartan malaria caused by *P. malariae* it is three days; in tertian malaria (*P. ovale* or *P. vivax*) it is two days; in malignant tertian (or quotidian) malaria (*P. falciparum*)—the most severe kind—from a few hours to a few days.

In the most serious form of malaria (falciparum malaria), red blood cells become sticky and block the small blood vessels to the brain, kidney, and lungs,

damaging these organs. Patients with this variety can die within several days without antibiotics. Irreversible complications can come on suddenly.

Malaria is more severe in children; more than 10 percent of untreated children will die. If infection occurs during pregnancy, there is a risk of premature delivery, abortion, and stillbirth.

Anyone who becomes ill with chills and fever after being in an area where malaria is endemic must see a doctor. Delaying treatment of falciparum malaria can be fatal. Because malaria is often misdiagnosed by North American doctors, travelers to malaria-ridden areas must be tested with a specific blood test for malaria, which requires direct microscopic exam of red blood cells to look for the parasite.

Blood smears are necessary for a diagnosis; the parasite can be specifically identified on blood smears on slides. Antibody tests are not always helpful because many people have antibodies from past infections.

Treatment Options and Outlook

People who become ill with fever during or after being in a high-risk area should seek prompt medical attention. Malaria can be treated effectively in the early stages, but delaying treatment can have serious consequences. Effective drugs include chloroquine, quinacrine, and chloroguanide.

The need for a different drug is imperative, since the parasite is becoming resistant to quinine and chloroquine.

There are side effects with the standard treatment. Quinine increases the risk of low blood sugar and ABSCESSES at the injection site. Patients treated with artemether are slower to come out of their malaria-induced coma, and more likely to have convulsions. Other animal studies suggest brain stem damage is related to high doses of artemether.

Falciparum malaria requires hospitalization, with IV fluids, red blood cell transfusions, kidney dialysis (if kidneys fail), and assisted breathing.

Risk Factors and Preventive Measures

There is no vaccine against malaria. The World Health Organization has been trying to eradicate malaria for the past 30 years by killing mosquitoes that carry the parasite, but as the mosquitoes and parasites became resistant to insecticides, prevention now aims at avoiding bites and taking preventive medicine (such as mefloquine or lariam).

Malaria can often be prevented by the use of antimalarial drugs and use of personal protection measures against mosquito bites. While the risk of malaria is slight in the United States, people traveling to high-risk areas should take precautions. The risk for tourists who stay in air-conditioned hotels on tourist trips in urban or resort areas is lower than that for backpackers, missionaries, and Peace Corps volunteers. Decisions on whether to use antimalarial drugs depends on the traveler's itinerary, duration of travel, and the place where the traveler will spend each night.

More recently, a series of bisphosphonate drugs already approved to treat osteoporosis and other bone disorders carry potent antiparasitic activity, and offer a new approach to the treatment of malaria. The drugs (Fosamax, Actonel, and Aredia) target and inhibit a specific enzyme in the parasites.

In addition, the CDC advises those traveling for less than three weeks to areas with chloroquine-resistant malaria carry with a dose of Fansidar, a combination of pyrimethamine and sulfadiazine. Fansidar should be used only if the traveler develops symptoms and will not be able to reach a doctor immediately. Although Fansidar effectively combats many strains of chloroquine-resistant malaria, the CDC generally does not recommended it for regular preventive use because it sometimes causes severe or even fatal skin reactions. For want of a proven alternative, health-care workers may advise some long-term travelers to high-risk areas to take prophylactic doses of Fansidar as well as chloroquine. Such travelers must carefully monitor themselves for any signs of a bad reaction, especially of the skin or mucous membrane. In addition, people who know they are sensitive to sulfa drugs should not take Fansidar.

Researchers are studying possible vaccines, but the parasite's complex life inside its human host makes a vaccination difficult.

Anyone who has been diagnosed with *P. malariae* should not give blood because it is possible to transmit the infection to others for 40 years after the initial infection.

Before going on a trip, travelers may want to check the CDC Travelers Hotline at (404) 332-4559 or the Malaria Hotline at (404) 332-4555 to find out current recommendations.

Mantoux test See TUBERCULIN TEST.

Marburg virus An exotic virus found primarily in Africa that causes an infection with grotesque symptoms and that carries a 25 percent fatality rate. The discovery of this genetically unique animal-borne virus led to the creation of the filovirus family. The four species of EBOLA virus are the only other known members of this family.

The virus first appeared in the late summer of 1967, when three employees at a vaccine factory in Marburg, Germany, came down with what doctors thought was the flu. By the next day, symptoms became bizarre, including unusual rashes, severe diarrhea, peeling skin, bloody vomit, and hemorrhaging from every orifice. The number of infected people grew, including household members of patients and the physicians who treated them, until 37 people were ill; seven died by the end of the year, and others experienced liver failure, impotence, and psychosis. The infections were confined to three cities, but centered in Marburg. Several nearly identical cases were identified in lab workers in Frankfurt at the same time, and in Belgrade in September. Of the 31 patients, 25 had directly handled monkey blood, either while dissecting the animals and working with their organs or cells or while cleaning culture containers.

Spouses and health-care providers in contact with the lab workers got sick with exhaustion, weight and hair loss, sweats, and psychiatric problems for weeks afterward. The three outbreaks were traced to several shipments of vervet monkeys from the same area of Uganda, although there was no evidence of that illness among monkey trappers. Experts believe the monkeys became infected while enroute—probably while in London, where they were kept for some hours together with other species of birds and animals; half of these monkeys died before reaching Europe.

In the monkey's tissues, scientists discovered a large new rod-shaped virus, which turned out to be remarkably similar to the Ebola virus.

Nearly a quarter of a million vervet monkeys had been imported into Europe and the United States by the late 1960s because researchers had found their kidney cells ideal for growing viruses. Although the total number of Marburg virus cases were few, the EPIDEMIC created alarm because the mortality rate was so high, the symptoms were horrific, and there was no effective treatment.

Because of the epidemic, labs began to use other species of animals for experiments, and the Marburg virus seemed to disappear. However, in 1975 an Australian tourist most likely exposed in Zimbabwe died of the disease in a hospital in Johannesburg, South Africa. A traveling companion of the patient and a nurse who had cared for them both became ill as well, but they eventually recovered.

Nine years after the first Marburg outbreak, a similar illness struck in Zaire and Sudan but with much more severe symptoms—the dreaded Ebola virus, close cousin to the Marburg. Scientists there discovered that the virus was shaped like a question mark. This virus was named after a river near the epidemic's starting point—Ebola-Zaire.

Just how the Marburg virus is transmitted to humans is unknown, but experts do know that humans who become ill with Marburg hemorrhagic fever may spread the virus to other people by close contact, often in a hospital. Droplets of body fluids or direct contact with patients, equipment, or other objects contaminated with infectious blood or tissues may transfer the disease.

Symptoms and Diagnostic Path

After an incubation period of five to 10 days, symptoms of fever, chills, and headache appear suddenly. About five days later a rash on the chest, back, and stomach may occur, followed by nausea, vomiting, chest pain, sore throat, abdominal pain, and diarrhea. Symptoms become increasingly severe and may include jaundice, inflammation of the pancreas, severe weight loss, delirium, shock, liver failure, massive hemorrhaging, and multi-organ dysfunction.

Because many of the symptoms of Marburg hemorrhagic fever are similar to those of other infectious diseases such as MALARIA or TYPHOID FEVER, diagnosis can be difficult. A variety of lab tests are used to diagnose the disease, including ELISA testing, polymerase chain reaction (PCR), and virus isolation.

Treatment Options and Outlook

There is no specific treatment other than easing symptoms by providing fluids and electrolytes, maintaining oxygen and blood pressure, replacing lost blood and clotting factors, and treating any complicating infections. Sometimes transfusion of fresh-frozen plasma and other preparations to replace the blood proteins important in clotting is effective. One controversial treatment is the use of heparin (which blocks clotting) to prevent the consumption of clotting factors. Some researchers believe the consumption of clotting factors is part of the disease process.

Recovery from Marburg hemorrhagic fever may be prolonged and accompanied by recurrent HEPATITIS and inflammation of the testis, spinal cord, or eyes. The fatality rate for Marburg hemorrhagic fever is between 23 percent and 25 percent.

Risk Factors and Preventive Measures

In 2005, Canadian and U.S. scientists reported that they have developed vaccines against both the Ebola and Marburg viruses that have been shown to be effective in nonhuman primates. Scientists report that the vaccines are 100 percent effective in protecting monkeys against infection from these often deadly viruses. (Monkeys are known to develop hemorrhagic fever symptoms that are similar to those observed in humans infected by these viruses.)

Demonstrating that these vaccines are safe and effective in monkeys suggests that there may be real potential for use in humans. However, scientists caution that it will be some time before the vaccines will be available for human use. Still, this is the first vaccine system that has protected nonhuman primates from both Ebola and Marburg.

mastitis   An infection of the breast that usually occurs during breast-feeding. Acute mastitis is most common during the first two months of nursing.

The infection is usually caused by either streptococcal or staphylococcal bacteria.

Symptoms and Diagnostic Path

The breast is painful, with swelling and redness and swelling of nearby lymph nodes, together with fever and fatigue. If untreated, an ABSCESS may form.

Treatment Options and Outlook

Antibiotics, rest, painkillers, and warm soaks will cure the problem. In most cases, breast-feeding may continue.

mastoiditis An infection of one of the mastoid bones (the prominent bones behind the ear), usually as a result of an EAR INFECTION. Mastoiditis usually affects children, and sometimes causes hearing loss. This disease has become uncommon since the widespread use of antibiotic drugs to treat ear infections.

The disease occurs when infection spreads from the middle ear to a cavity in the mastoid bone, and from there to a honeycomb of air cells in the bone itself.

Symptoms and Diagnostic Path

Severe earache, headache, and fatigue. Swelling behind the ear is often enough to actually move the external ear. Symptoms also may include fever, a creamy discharge from the ear, and progressive hearing loss.

Mastoiditis can be identified during a physical exam. Early diagnosis is essential because of the potential serious complications.

Treatment Options and Outlook

This infection is not easy to treat and often requires intravenous antibiotics for several days. If the infection persists, an operation called a mastoidectomy may be required. In this procedure, the surgeon makes an incision behind the ear to open up the mastoid bone and remove the infected air cells. A drainage tube is left in place and removed several days after the operation.

The infection may spread to inside the skull, causing MENINGITIS, BRAIN ABSCESS, or a blood clot in veins inside the brain. Or the infection may spread outward, affecting the facial nerve and causing a facial paralysis.

measles A childhood viral illness causing a widespread red rash and fever considered to be the most contagious disease in the world. One infected person in a crowded room is able to transmit the illness to almost every unvaccinated person in the room. The medical name for measles is rubeola. It is sometimes called "red measles" to distinguish it from the much milder disease known as rubella (GERMAN MEASLES). While measles was once commonly found throughout the world and was not normally considered dangerous, complications can lead to death.

Doctors have known about measles for centuries; it was first described by the 10th-century Persian physician al-Rhazes, who called the illness by its Arabic name, *hasba* (meaning "eruption"). It was so common that he thought measles was a natural occurrence of childhood, like losing baby teeth, instead of an infectious illness. In fact, its present name did not appear until the 14th century, where it was derived from the Arabic word *miser,* used to describe the unhappiness of lepers.

It spread quickly across North Africa into Europe, where it was introduced by explorers to the New World with tragic results. In central Mexico, the native population was decimated, dropping from about 30 million to 3 million in just 50 years by *pequeña* (little leprosy).

In populations who have never been exposed to it, the disease can be a killer; 800 children died of measles during an epidemic in the Charlestown area of Boston in 1772. And a hundred years later, within three months of the arrival of a foreign ship, a quarter of the inhabitants of Fiji—some 30,000 people—died from measles. It is so remarkably virulent that in 1951 a single person with measles landed in Greenland and within six weeks, all but five of the 4,300 never-before-exposed Greenland natives came down with the disease.

Although measles was known to be a viral disease since 1911, it was not until 1954 that two Harvard researchers isolated the actual measles virus in the lab. When a vaccine was finally licensed in 1963, experts thought the disease would be eradicated by 1982. When this did not occur, the target date was revised to 1990. But instead of disappearing, measles cases began to rise again from only 1,500 cases in 1983 to 28,000 cases in 1990. Half of those reported cases occurred in children under age five. Because many high schools and colleges experienced measles outbreaks in the late 1980s and early 1990s, most schools now require older students to be re-immunized.

Since 1991, measles cases have again been decreasing; there were 963 cases in 1994 and just 301 in 1995; by 2003, there were only 56 cases. It is still a killer in developing countries, where more than 1 million deaths a year are recorded—especially among malnourished children with impaired immunity. Indeed, two-thirds of reported cases in the United States were traced to international importation.

One case of measles confers lifelong immunity; the vaccine also confers lifelong immunity. Anyone who received two doses of vaccine during childhood will not get measles.

The measles virus is spread by airborne droplets from nasal secretions. Symptoms appear after an incubation period of between nine to 11 days, and the patient is infectious from shortly after the beginning of this period until up to a week after symptoms have developed. Infants under six months of age rarely contract measles because they still harbor some immunity from their mothers.

The virus survives best in low humidity; it can survive in the air for several hours. It is so infectious, it is capable of traveling down a hall on air currents and into other rooms where healthy people are located, infecting them as well. It is also possible to contract the disease from touching bedding or towels touched by an infected person, or by directly touching secretions from a patient's nose, mouth, eyes, or cough.

A milder form of the disease can occur among people who do not develop adequate immunity from just one dose of vaccine, who were immunized too early, or who had received an older less effective variety of the vaccine. As their immunity wears off, these people become susceptible to measles, which causes a low fever and rash on face and trunk.

Symptoms and Diagnostic Path

About 10 days after the virus enters the body symptoms of a high fever (up to 105°F) and general sick feeling occur. This is followed the next day by red, sore eyes, a stuffy nose, and cough. On the second day of fever, a rash (Koplik's spots) of tiny white dots on a red base appears inside the mouth. After three or four days, a bright red splotchy rash will begin on the head and neck and spread down to cover the entire body. The spots may be so numerous that they appear together as a large red area.

The rash begins to fade within three days and will disappear by six days.

The fever will begin to drop on the second day of the rash, and the runny nose and sore eyes also diminish as the fever falls. The cough, however, may last for up to two weeks.

Everyone with measles feels uncomfortable, but babies and young children usually fare the worst, feeling much sicker than they would with a COLD, the flu, or CHICKEN POX.

Patients are infectious from just before the fever begins to the fifth day after the rash appears. The most infectious period occurs right before the rash begins. Patients during the infectious stage must remain isolated.

Physicians can diagnose measles from symptoms alone, although blood tests that check for antibodies to the virus are available in large labs.

Treatment Options and Outlook

There is no cure for measles. Symptoms are treated with fluids and acetaminophen. Antibiotics will not eradicate the virus, but may be needed to treat a secondary infection. Patients need to rest in a darkened room because their eyes are sensitive to light.

A physician should be called immediately if any of the following signs appear:

- vomiting
- signs of dehydration
- wheezing or breathing problems (which may be a sign the virus has spread to the lungs, causing measles PNEUMONIA)
- fever for more than four days after the rash appears
- fever that subsides and then returns
- unusual drowsiness, fussiness, stiff neck (signs of measles ENCEPHALITIS) caused by the spread of virus into the brain
- ear pain, pulling at the ear

Infants, older people, and those with serious health problems may become severely ill with measles and die. It is a common cause of death and blindness in developing countries.

Infants are the most likely to get complications including secondary ear and chest infections, which usually occur as the fever returns a few days after the rash appears. There may also be diarrhea, vomiting, and abdominal pain. Measles pneumonia in children may trigger serious breathing problems.

About 1 in every 1,000 patients goes on to develop encephalitis (brain inflammation), with headache, drowsiness, and vomiting beginning seven to 10 days after the rash begins. This may be followed by seizures and coma, leading to mental retardation or death. (However, febrile seizures are common with measles and do not necessarily indicate the presence of encephalitis.) Very rarely (one in a million cases) a progressive brain disorder called subacute sclerosing panencephalitis develops many years after the original illness.

Measles during pregnancy causes fetal death in about one-fifth of cases, but there is no evidence that measles causes birth defects.

Risk Factors and Preventive Measures

In the United States, children are routinely vaccinated first at age 12 months and again at age four or older by an injection usually combined with MUMPS and rubella that produces immunity in 97 percent of patients. Side effects of the vaccine are reported to be mild, including low fever, slight cold, and a rash about a week after the shot. The vaccine was first licensed for use in 1963 and is very effective; only one injection produces long-lasting (probably lifelong) protection.

The vaccine should not be given to infants under age one or to those with a family history of epilepsy or who have had seizures before. In these cases, simultaneous injection of measles-specific immunoglobulin, which contains antibodies against the virus, should be given.

The booster now recommended at four to six years of age or at 10 to 12 years, will protect 95 percent of those who may have failed to become immune after their first vaccine dose.

Pregnant women who have never had measles or been immunized should avoid anyone with measles. If the pregnant patient does come in contact with an infected person, she should be passively immunized against measles with immunoglobulin within five days.

Schools require evidence of measles immunity upon enrollment. Some people need to be reimmunized against measles. Everyone immunized before their first birthday or who received the previously available "killed" measles vaccine (or a vaccine of unknown type) between 1963 and 1967 should be reimmunized. It is safe to be reimmunized even if a person is actually already immune. People born before 1957 are probably immune to measles because of exposure to the disease. Thus, people who are now between the ages of 30 and 40 are those most likely to require reimmunization.

meningitis Any infection or inflammation of the membranes covering the brain and spinal cord, caused by either BACTERIA, FUNGI, or VIRUS. Bacterial meningitis is by far the most serious type of meningitis. Most of the time, however, the infectious agent is a virus.

Regardless of cause, the onset of meningitis is usually sudden, and characterized by a severe headache, neck stiffness, irritability, malaise, and nausea and vomiting.

See also MENINGITIS, BACTERIAL; MENINGITIS, MENINGOCOCCAL; MENINGITIS, PNEUMOCOCCAL; MENINGITIS, VIRAL.

meningitis, bacterial A bacterial infection of the fluid covering of the brain or the fluid in the spinal cord. More than two-thirds of all patients with bacterial meningitis are children.

Until 1992, most of them were infected with HAEMOPHILUS INFLUENZAE TYPE B (called "H. flu" or "Hib"). The illness has nothing to do with influenza, however, despite the name of the bacterium. Because of an effective vaccine, Hib meningitis has practically disappeared among young children.

The fears of bacterial meningitis is based not only on its reputation as a killer, but on the possibility of neurological complications—lingering problems that can be devastating in infants and children who are still developing. These complications can include hearing loss, mental retardation, and recurrent convulsions; they occur in 20 to 30 percent of patients who survive.

The two most common causes of bacterial meningitis today are pneumococcal meningitis (caused by *Streptococcus pneumoniae*) and meningococcal meningitis (caused by *Neisseria meningitidis*). Bacterial meningitis can be spread by coughing or kissing, but none of the bacteria that cause meningitis are as contagious as the common cold or flu viruses. Moreover, these bacteria are not spread by casual contact or by simply breathing the air where a person with meningitis has been.

However, the bacteria that cause meningitis can spread to other people who have had close or prolonged contact with a patient with meningitis caused by *Neisseria meningitidis* (also called meningococcal meningitis) or Hib. People in the same household or day-care center, or anyone with direct contact with a patient's oral secretions, are at higher risk of infection. Close contacts of a person with meningitis caused by *N. meningitidis* should receive antibiotics to prevent the disease. Antibiotics for contacts of a person with Hib meningitis disease are no longer recommended if all contacts four years of age or younger are fully vaccinated against Hib disease.

Symptoms and Diagnostic Path

Classic signs of meningitis include sudden high fever (100–106°F) with chills, vomiting, vision problems, stiff neck intense headache in the front of the head, or a seizure. The neck will hurt if the patient tries to touch the chin to the chest. There may be muscle spasms or leg pains, and bright light may irritate the eyes.

All types of bacterial meningitis can appear suddenly or gradually. The less common gradual type is harder to diagnose because symptoms are similar to other mild childhood illnesses: cold symptoms, fever, lethargy, vomiting, loss of appetite. A sudden attack is easier to diagnose, although it may indicate a more serious case.

Abnormal behavior may also announce the onset of meningitis, including aggressiveness, irritability, agitation, delirium, or screaming. This is followed by lethargy and stupor or coma.

Babies between ages three months and two years may have fever, vomiting, irritability, seizures, and a high-pitched cry. Rigidity may appear. The front soft spot on the baby's head may bulge.

Sometimes the illness is preceded by a cold or an ear infection. Any sudden change in consciousness or any unusual behavior in a young child may be a sign of meningitis.

A spinal tap must be done to diagnose meningitis. Normally clear, the fluid is analyzed for the presence of bacteria and other evidence of infection. Bacteria will grow in the fluid within 48 hours; rapid tests on urine or blood can give results in a few hours and are most helpful in determining what type of bacteria are causing the meningitis.

However, since the disease can progress so quickly, treatment with intravenous antibiotics should be started even before any test results are available.

Treatment Options and Outlook

Without treatment, most patients would die; with antibiotics, 85 percent recover. Current antibiotics used in the treatment of bacterial meningitis include a class of antibiotics called CEPHALOSPORINS, especially cefotaxime and ceftriaxone, and various members of the PENICILLIN family. At least a week of treatment is needed.

Risk Factors and Preventive Measures

Vaccinations are available against Hib, against some serogroups of *N. meningitidis*, and against many types of *Streptococcus pneumoniae*. The vaccines against Hib are very safe and highly effective. There are two vaccines against *N. meningitidis* available in the United States: Meningococcal polysaccharide vaccine (Menomune) has been approved since 1981; meningococcal conjugate vaccine (Menactra) was licensed in 2005. Both vaccines can prevent four types of meningococcal disease, including two of the three types most common in the United States and a type that causes EPIDEMICS in Africa.

Although meningococcal vaccines cannot prevent all types of the disease, they do protect many people who might get sick if they had not had the vaccine.

Menactra is recommended for all children 11 to 12 years of age; for those who have never gotten the vaccine before, a dose is recommended when a student enters high school. Others at increased risk for whom routine vaccination is recommended are college freshmen living in dormitories, microbiologists who are routinely exposed to meningococcal bacteria, U.S. military recruits, anyone with a damaged or missing spleen, anyone with an immune system disorder, anyone traveling to endemic countries, or anyone exposed to meningitis during an outbreak.

Menactra is the preferred vaccine for people 11 to 55 years of age in these risk groups, but Menomune can be used if Menactra is not available. Menomune should be used for children aged two to 10 years old and for at-risk adults over 55.

Epidemics of meningococcal meningitis are not a problem in the United States, but some other countries experience periodic epidemics. Overseas travelers should check to see if meningococcal vaccine is recommended for their destination; if it is, the vaccine should be given at least one week before departure.

See also MENINGITIS, MENINGOCOCCAL; MENINGITIS, PNEUMOCOCCAL; MENINGITIS, VIRAL; MENINGOCOCCUS.

meningitis, meningococcal A severe bacterial infection of the bloodstream and meninges also known popularly as "spinal meningitis." It is one of the more serious types of MENINGITIS, caused by a specific type of bacteria that can be fatal in some cases.

This type of meningitis is one that usually occurs as an isolated event. It affects about 3,000 Americans a year; half are younger than two and two-thirds are younger than 20. Between 10 percent and 13 percent of patients die despite receiving antibiotics. Of those who survive, 10 percent have severe after effects, including hearing loss and mental retardation. The highest rates occur among babies between four months and one year of age, and in young adults living together (as in a college dorm). EPIDEMICS of meningitis have not occurred in the United States or most other industrial countries since World War II. Virulent epidemics still happen in developing countries, however. More than 40,000 cases were diagnosed during a 1989 epidemic in Ethiopia; as many as 3 million cases may have occurred during the 1960s in China.

Before the development of antibiotics, about half of all patients with this type of meningitis died. Today, most recover—except those with massive blood infection caused by the bacteria. Because the bacteria multiply and spread so quickly, it is very difficult to treat and antibiotics cannot destroy enough of the bacteria fast enough. In this group of patients, 10 to 12 percent of victims will die.

The fear of this type of meningitis is based not only on its reputation as a killer but also on the pos-

sibility of neurological complications—lingering problems that can be devastating in infants and children. These complications can include hearing loss, mental retardation, and recurrent convulsions; they may occur to a greater or lesser degree in 20 to 30 percent of patients who survive.

The bacteria that cause meningococcal meningitis is *Neisseria meningitidis* (or MENINGOCOCCUS), divided into nine separate groups (groups B and C are common in North America). The organism is a close relative of the bacterium responsible for GONORRHEA.

Patients can become infected by inhaling the bacteria, by direct mouth to mouth contact, or by indirect contact. Most patients develop only very mild upper-respiratory symptoms. More serious cases occur when the bacteria enter the bloodstream.

Up to 30 percent of any group of healthy people will have this bacteria in their throats at any one time without having symptoms. This type of meningitis is contagious but requires close personal contact to transmit. It is more commonly found in institutions and schools, such as colleges, child care centers, military barracks, and homes for the developmentally delayed.

In North America the disease usually occurs in isolated cases, although there may be a small outbreak of five to 10 cases at a time. It occurs most often in February and March and least often in September. In some parts of the world, meningococcal meningitis has been epidemic; there are also occasional smaller outbreaks. Epidemics are rare in the Western world. In other areas, epidemics last one to three years.

Symptoms and Diagnostic Path

Signs of meningococcal meningitis include sudden high fever (100–106°F) with chills, vomiting, stiff neck, and intense headache in the front of the head, or a seizure. The neck will hurt if the patient tries to touch the chin to the chest. There may be muscle spasms or leg pains, and bright light may irritate the eyes. Abnormal behavior may also announce the onset of meningitis, including aggressiveness, irritability, agitation, delirium, or screaming. This is followed by lethargy and stupor or coma. Sometimes the illness is preceded by a cold or an ear infection. Any sudden change in consciousness or any unusual behavior in a young child may be a sign of meningitis.

Babies between ages three months to two years may have fever, vomiting, irritability, seizures, and a high-pitched cry. Rigidity may appear. The front soft spot on the baby's head may bulge.

A spinal tap must be done to diagnose meningitis; the procedure samples a small amount of fluid from the spinal cord to check for appearance, bacteria, protein, and sugar. Bacteria will grow in the fluid within 48 hours; rapid tests on spinal fluid or blood can give results in a few hours and are most helpful in determining what type of bacteria are causing the meningitis.

Throat cultures are not helpful, since so many people have this bacteria in their throats.

Treatment Options and Outlook

Penicillin G administered intravenously in high doses will cure most patients with this disease. Patients should be carefully nursed with supportive care and maintained in isolation for the first 24 hours.

People diagnosed with this type of meningitis are infectious until they have taken antibiotics for 24 hours. Healthy carriers with the bacteria in nose and throat rarely develop the disease, as the organism is part of the normal bacteria in humans. The carrier state lasts weeks to months. It is the carrier state that predisposes to epidemics.

Signs of the blood infection are fever, unresponsiveness or coma, rapid spreading rash, and shock. If the bacteria penetrate and damage the blood vessel lining, blood seeps out and causes a rash of small flat spots on arms, legs, and trunk. A child with a high fever and this type of rash needs immediate medical attention; in about 10 to 20 percent of patients, the infection quickly overwhelms the body. Called fulminant meningococcemia, it causes large purple bruises all over the skin and leads to fatal shock.

In addition, bacteria in the blood can lead to arthritis, heart problems, and PNEUMONIA. There may be long-term complications due to damaged nerves leading to the brain, such as hearing loss or mental retardation.

Risk Factors and Preventive Measures

There are two vaccines against *N. meningitidis* available in the United States: Meningococcal polysaccharide vaccine (Menomune) approved in 1981, and meningococcal conjugate vaccine (Menactra) was licensed in 2005. Both vaccines can prevent four types of meningococcal disease, including two of the three most common in the United States. Meningococcal vaccines cannot prevent all types of the disease, but they do protect many people who might get sick if they had not had the vaccine.

Menactra is recommended for all children 11 to 12 years of age. Students who were not vaccinated in childhood should have a dose in high school, as should college freshmen living in dormitories, microbiologists routinely exposed to meningococcal bacteria, U.S. military recruits, or anyone with a damaged or missing spleen, an immune system disorder, traveling to endemic countries, or who was exposed to meningitis. Menactra is the preferred vaccine for people 11 to 55 years of age in these risk groups, but Menomune can be used if Menactra is not available. Menomune should be used for children aged two to 10 years old and for at-risk adults over 55.

Epidemics of meningococcal meningitis are not a problem in the United States, but some other countries experience periodic epidemics. If a meningococcal vaccine is recommended for an overseas destination, the traveler should get the vaccine at least one week before departure.

Physicians must report cases of meningococcal meningitis to the health department. When someone is diagnosed with meningococcal meningitis, prophylactic ciprofloxacin or rifampin should be given to household members, close friends at school, and all preschoolers cared for in the same room as soon as possible (within 24 hours) of the diagnosis. "Close contact" would include anyone who has shared glasses, food, or utensils, or who has kissed or had sexual contact with the patient.

Casual contact among people in a classroom, office, or factory setting is not usually significant enough to cause concern.

See also MENINGITIS, BACTERIAL.

meningitis, pneumococcal The second most common cause of bacterial meningitis, this version is fatal in one out of every five cases. It occurs sporadically during the cold and flu season, not in epidemics, and is found more often in males. Highest rates are among children under the age of two, elderly people, and alcoholics.

Pneumococcal meningitis is caused by STREPTO-COCCUS PNEUMONIAE, a circular-shaped bacterium found in pairs, a common cause of EAR INFECTIONS, PNEUMONIA, and SINUSITIS, in addition to meningitis. There are more than 80 types of this bacteria.

Most people have this bacteria in their nose and throat and can spread the infection by sneezing, coughing, or direct contact. However, most people do not get sick; it requires another condition to allow the bacteria to get into the bloodstream, such as a weakened immune system, HIV infection, sickle cell disease, or cancer. The bacteria can also invade the brain if there is injury or weakness in the nose cavity or a fracture line in the skull. Cases have been reported as a result of a violent sneezing attack.

Symptoms and Diagnostic Path

Classic signs of meningitis include sudden high fever (100–106°F) with chills, vomiting, stiff neck and intense headache in the front of the head, or a seizure. The neck will hurt if the patient tries to touch the chin to the chest. There may be muscle spasms or leg pains, and bright light may irritate the eyes.

Sometimes, the symptoms are similar to other mild illnesses: cold symptoms, fever, lethargy, vomiting, loss of appetite. A sudden attack is easier to diagnose, although it may indicate a more serious case.

Abnormal behavior may also announce the onset of meningitis, including aggressiveness, irritability, agitation, delirium, or screaming. This is followed by lethargy and stupor or coma.

Babies between ages three months to two years may have fever, vomiting, irritability, seizures, and a high-pitched cry. Rigidity may appear. The front soft spot on the baby's head may bulge. Adults most often experience a headache, fever, and stiff neck.

Sometimes the illness is preceded by a cold or an ear infection. Any sudden change in consciousness or any unusual behavior in someone ill with a respiratory infection may be a sign of meningitis.

A spinal tap must be done to diagnose meningitis. Normally clear, the fluid is analyzed for the presence of bacteria and other evidence of infec-tion. Bacteria will grow in the fluid within 48 hours; rapid tests on spinal fluid can give results in a few hours and are most helpful in determining the presence of bacteria in the usually sterile spinal fluid.

However, since the disease can progress so quickly, treatment with intravenous antibiotics must be started before any test results are available.

Treatment Options and Outlook

Some types of *S. pneumoniae* are not resistant to PENICILLIN and other common antibiotics. Hospital care and IV drugs will be prescribed. Patients should be kept in darkened, quiet rooms, with painkillers and treatment for fever.

Risk Factors and Preventive Measures

The vaccine to prevent infections including meningitis due to *S. pneumoniae* is not effective in children under two years of age but is recommended for all persons over 65 years of age, younger persons with certain chronic medical problems, and people who do not have a spleen.

See also MENINGITIS, BACTERIAL.

meningitis, viral A form of MENINGITIS (inflammation of the brain's lining) caused by a virus, which is usually less serious than its bacterial form. Viral meningitis is a fairly common and relatively mild illness when compared to its bacterial cousin. It is also called aseptic meningitis because there is no bacteria in the spinal fluid.

Viral meningitis is usually caused by an ENTERO-VIRUS, a type of virus that affects only humans and is spread by the fecal-oral route. Enteroviruses live in human intestines; the two most common are ECHOVIRUSES and COXSACKIE VIRUS.

The virus is spread by direct contact with infected feces or nose or throat secretions. Most children are carriers without symptoms; the virus spreads most easily among young children in a group situation. Viral meningitis usually strikes young children in the summer and early fall; although anyone can get viral meningitis, most people over age 40 are immune.

Scientists do not know why so few children who are exposed to the disease come down with symptoms; those who are well-fed, well-rested, and healthy are less likely to become infected.

Symptoms and Diagnostic Path

Symptoms usually appear quite suddenly, with a high fever, severe headache, vision problems nausea and vomiting, and stiff neck. There may be sensitivity to light and noise, sore throat, or eye infections. There may also be accompanying neurological problems, such as blurred vision.

Most people recover completely within two weeks, although there may be muscle weakness, tiredness, headache, muscle spasms, insomnia, or personality changes (such as an inability to concentrate) for months afterward. These are rarely permanent.

Viral meningitis can be diagnosed by spinal tap.

Treatment Options and Outlook

There is no cure for viral meningitis; eventually the immune system will develop antibodies to destroy the virus. Hospitalization with IV fluids and painkillers may be necessary for the severe headache, dehydration, nausea, and vomiting.

Patients should drink clear fluids, eat a bland diet, and get plenty of rest. Children should be taken for a hearing test several weeks after recovery.

Increased pressure on the brain from a buildup of fluid in the meninges is a serious complication. Some infants who have meningitis early in life have delayed language. Patients with a weakened immune system may have chronic infections with enterovirus.

meningitis, West Nile   An infection of the membrane around the brain and the spinal cord caused by infection with the West Nile virus, a type of virus transmitted by mosquitoes. This infection first appeared in the United States in New York in 1999. Since then, it has spread throughout the country and affected thousands of individuals. However, severe brain involvement after infection with this virus is uncommon; only about 1 percent of all cases of West Nile virus infection go on to involve the brain.

Symptoms and Diagnostic Path

Symptoms of West Nile meningitis include headache, high fever, stiff neck, stupor, sensitivity to light and noise, and nausea and vomiting. The condition is diagnosed by an analysis of symptoms and blood tests, which look for antibodies to the virus. Meningitis is also diagnosed by a spinal tap.

Treatment Options and Outlook

Viral meningitis, such as West Nile virus meningitis, cannot be treated effectively with antibiotics and is typically considered to be less serious than bacterial meningitis. Treatment may include medication for pain, fever, and nausea; severe cases may require hospitalization in a quiet, darkened room with intravenous medication.

Because West Nile virus is an emerging disease, the long-term effects are not fully understood, but some patients experience lingering problems with memory loss, headaches, muscle weakness, and so on.

Risk Factors and Preventive Measures

The risk for severe complications from West Nile virus infection increases with age, chronic illnesses, impaired immunity, and poor health. Infection can be prevented only by avoiding mosquitoes; there is no vaccine.

See also ENCEPHALITIS, WEST NILE; WEST NILE FEVER.

meningococcus   A bacterium of the genus *Neisseria meningitidis,* an organism that can cause MENINGITIS. The bacteria are often found in the nose and throat of healthy carriers. While not highly communicable, crowded conditions (such as in army camps or college dorms) concentrate the number of carriers.

meningoencephalitis   An inflammation of both the brain and the meninges, usually caused by a bacterial infection.

meningoencephalitis, primary amebic (PAM)   A severe infection of the gray matter of the brain caused by a free-living single-cell amoeba that lives in warm freshwater. Most cases have been reported in young boys and teenage boys and girls. PAM is a relatively rare infection in the United States.

The amoeba (*Naegleria fowleri*) found in stagnant or slow-moving water causes amebic meningoencephalitis. It can live in the soil as a cyst that reactivates when placed in water. If water containing the amoeba goes up the nose while swimming, the person will be exposed to the disease. The amoeba can survive in warm inland water, unchlorinated or incorrectly chlorinated water, dams, and ponds but not in sea water or salty estuaries. Flowing streams and rivers with cool water have not been associated with the disease. Most patients got the infection after diving into freshwater swimming holes.

Symptoms and Diagnostic Path

The disease is characterized by fever, headache, vomiting, and ENCEPHALITIS, followed rapidly by coma and death.

Treatment Options and Outlook

Early treatment with amphotericin B can successfully treat the disease.

meningomyelitis   Inflammation of the spinal cord and its surrounding membranes.

methicillin-resistant *Staphylococcus aureus* **(MRSA)**   A virulent type of bacteria resistant to many antibiotics (including potent methicillin) that can turn into a fatal flesh-destroying infection. Once found only in hospitals, the bacteria is now emerging in gyms, jails, schools, and almost anywhere that bacteria thrives. *Staphylococcus aureus* (also called "staph" or "staph A") is a common bacteria found on the skin of healthy people and that can cause infections ranging from boils or pimples to more serious problems such as PNEUMONIA or blood infections. Methicillin is very effective in treating most staph infections, but some staph bacteria have become resistant to methicillin and can no longer be killed by this antibiotic. These resistant bacteria are termed *methicillin-resistant Staphylococcus aureus.*

Now considered to be EPIDEMIC in the United States, it remains virtually unknown by the average citizen, but it is growing at such astonishing speed that it has alarmed infectious disease experts, far surpassing other new and emerging infections. Exact statistics are difficult to find, since staph infec-

tions are not reportable diseases, but one study has estimated that there were 126,000 cases between 1999 and 2000.

Many Americans carry staph bacteria in their nose, on their skin, or in their blood or urine, and a percentage of these bacteria are the methicillin-resistant variety. MRSA is usually spread through physical contact (especially the hands) and not through the air. Health-care workers' hands may become contaminated by contact with patients, surfaces in the workplace, or medical devices that are contaminated with bodily fluids containing MRSA.

MRSA produces the symptoms that would be caused by any other type of *Staphylococcus aureus* bacteria: reddened, inflamed skin at the wound site, fever, lethargy, and headache. MRSA can lead to urinary tract infections, pneumonia, TOXIC SHOCK SYNDROME, and even death.

While MRSA is resistant to many antibiotics and can be difficult to treat, there are a few antibiotics that can cure MRSA infections.

Microban   A colorless, odorless antibacterial product registered and approved by the U.S. Food and Drug Administration that can be embedded in toys, and hospital equipment, textiles, coatings, paper, adhesives, to protect against the growth of mold, fungus, and bacteria (including ESCHERICHIA COLI, SALMONELLA bacteria, *Staphylococcus,* and *Streptococcus*). The product, which cannot be washed off, has been introduced in a line of products for the home. Since 1994, the company's products have undergone extensive testing.

microbes   Life-forms (also called microorganisms) that are too small to be seen by the human eye. Some of them are so small they cannot be seen with even the most powerful microscope. There are hundreds of thousands of different microbe species that come in all different shapes and sizes, including the PROTOZOANS, algae, FUNGI, slime molds, BACTERIA, RICKETTSIAE, and VIRUSES.

Many scientists believe that microbes were probably the first life-forms on Earth, but they were not discovered until about 300 years ago, when Dutch scientist Antonie van Leeuwenhoek first saw the tiny moving creatures with a microscope he had made himself. He called these creatures "animalcules."

Microbes are a necessary and useful part of the environment; no area of the body other than the brain is totally free of bacteria. Human feces are made up of 94 percent microbes. They process digestion and produce most antibiotics, maintain soil and plant environment, and even produce alcoholic beverages by the process of fermentation. All but a few of the millions of microbial life-forms are beneficial. The very few that do cause disease are called pathogens.

Microsporum A genus of dermatophytes of the family Moniliaceae. One type (*M. audouinii*) causes TINEA CAPITIS (RINGWORM) in children. Other types include *M. canis* and *M. gypseum*. The genus was formerly known as *Microsporon*.

Microsporum canis A species of FUNGI that is found most often among dogs and cats but also occurs among humans and causes RINGWORM. *Microsporum canis* has specifically adapted itself to cats, which are often carriers without symptoms. The fungi can live in the environment for up to 18 months. Any building or room in which infected animals have been housed could potentially be a source of infection.

Brushes, bedding, cages, and other items are all potential sources of infection. These fungi have also been cultured from dust, heating vents, and furnace filters. They can be diagnosed by observing the skin with a special light called a Wood's lamp, where about 50 percent of the time affected hairs may glow green.

middle-ear infection See EAR INFECTION.

miliary tuberculosis See TUBERCULOSIS.

molluscum contagiosum A harmless viral infection that causes groups of tiny pearly white lumps on the skin's surface; palms of the hands and soles of the feet are not affected. This virus is a frequent infection in AIDS patients.

The virus is one of two poxviruses that specifically infect humans, causing a skin disease that responds to treatment in most people with healthy immune systems. But in AIDS patients, the virus is often progressive and resists treatment. (Variola, the cause of SMALLPOX, is the other poxvirus specific to humans.) Despite being in the same family, variola and molluscum contagiosum virus have very different ways of infection. Infection with molluscum is easily transmitted by direct skin contact or during intercourse.

The virus is transmitted from person to person by direct or indirect contact and can live in the body for up to three years, although individual lesions persist for only six to eight weeks.

Symptoms and Diagnostic Path
Each pimple looks like a shiny small circle with a central depression. The pimples appear primarily on the genitals, thighs, and face.

Diagnosis is made by direct examination of the skin.

Treatment Options and Outlook
In healthy patients, the infection usually clears up within a few months without treatment. Because they are unattractive, most people want them removed.

moniliasis Another name for *CANDIDA ALBICANS*.

monkeypox A genetic cousin of the SMALLPOX virus, monkeypox is native to monkeys but is occasionally able to infect and kill humans. In 1997, monkeypox among humans broke out in Zaire, where it has been responsible for at least 92 cases of sickness (including three deaths in children under age three). The Zaire outbreak may have originated in tree squirrels native to the rain forest; once it crossed into humans, it spread through 12 villages in central Zaire.

For years, experts understood that it was possible for monkeys to infect humans with monkeypox. But now, according to the Centers for Disease Control, it appears that for the first time humans have infected other humans. Researchers were evacuated from politically troubled Zaire before they were able to pinpoint how the disease is transmitted from animals or between people. So far, the virus has remained in Zaire and is not likely to reach the United States.

Symptoms and Diagnostic Path

Symptoms include a disfiguring rash similar to smallpox, featuring head to toe blisters, with a high fever and respiratory problems.

Treatment Options and Outlook

Viral medication as for smallpox may be used.

Risk Factors and Preventive Measures

Vaccinia vaccine, which prevents smallpox, also protects against monkeypox. But because vaccination was stopped once smallpox was eradicated from the Earth, the generation born after 1980 may be vulnerable to the new disease.

mononucleosis, infectious An acute HERPES virus infection caused by the EPSTEIN-BARR VIRUS and characterized by sore throat, fever, swollen lymph glands, and bruising. Known as the "kissing disease" because it is transmitted in saliva, young people are most often infected. In childhood the disease is most often mild. The older the patient, however, the more severe the symptoms are likely to be. Infection confers permanent immunity.

The disease is usually transmitted by droplet EBV virus but is not highly contagious. CYTOMEGALOVIRUS (CMV) can cause a similar infection; both EBV and CMV are members of the HERPES family of viruses.

Symptoms and Diagnostic Path

Between four to six weeks after infection, the disease begins gradually with symptoms of sore throat, fatigue, swollen lymph glands, and occasional bruising. Although the symptoms usually disappear in four to six weeks, the virus remains dormant in the throat and blood for the rest of the patient's life. Periodically the virus can reactivate and be found in the patient's saliva, although it does not usually cause symptoms.

Mono may also start abruptly with high fever and severe, swollen sore throat similar to strep throat.

Rarely, about 10 percent of patients have a third type, with a low persistent fever, nausea and vomiting, and stomach problems.

About half of all patients have an enlarged spleen and a few have an enlarged liver or mild jaundice.

Symptoms of fever, sore throat, and swollen glands, are used to diagnose the disease. Blood tests and blood counts are needed for confirmation. The mono spot is a rapid antibody test that looks for a specific reaction in the blood of infected patients. Liver function tests will reveal abnormal liver function—so-called mono-hepatitis that may occur.

Treatment Options and Outlook

There is no specific treatment for the disease other than symptom management. No antiviral or antibiotic drugs are available. Some doctors prescribe steroids to reduce the tonsil inflammation because the patient cannot swallow. Enforced bed rest may prevent injury to the swollen spleen. Painkillers and saline gargles may help the sore throat.

There may be a swollen spleen or liver inflammation; heart problems or involvement of the central nervous system may rarely occur (mono-meningitis), but this disease is almost never fatal. If the spleen ruptures, immediate surgery and blood transfusions will be necessary.

About half the time, the patient will also have a strep throat, which does require antibiotic treatment. Occasionally, patients will have such intense swelling of the lymphatic system of their throat that they require hospitalization for IV fluids to prevent dehydration.

Risk Factors and Preventive Measures

Most people exposed to patients have already been infected with EBV and are not at risk for developing disease themselves, since 95 percent of adults over age 35 have antibodies to the virus. Transmission routes are not fully understood, although doctors suspect it is transmitted via saliva.

Morbidity and Mortality Weekly Report A weekly epidemiologic report on the incidence of communicable diseases and deaths in 120 urban areas of the

United States. It is published by the U.S. CENTERS FOR DISEASE CONTROL AND PREVENTION in Atlanta, Georgia. The publication also includes information on accident rates and important international health data.

morbidity rate The number of cases of a particular disease occurring in a single year per specified population unit. It may be calculated on the basis of age groups, gender, occupation, or other population group.

morbilli See MEASLES.

morbillivirus, equine See EQUINE MORBILLIVIRUS.

mosquito bites Mosquitoes are found throughout the world; the females bite in order to obtain blood to produce their eggs. Because their eggs are laid and hatched in stagnant water, they are most commonly found in areas near marshes, ponds, reservoirs, and water tanks.

Symptoms and Diagnostic Path
Mosquito bites may cause swelling and itching for several days; the main problem of these bites is the infections that may be transmitted in the insect's saliva.

Treatment Options and Outlook
Because mosquitoes can spread disease, mosquito bites should be washed with soap and water followed by an antiseptic. To control itching, a nonprescription antihistamine, calamine lotion, anesthetic gels, or ice pack may help. Alternatively, a paste of salt and water or baking soda and water can be applied to the bite.

Risk Factors and Preventive Measures
Insect repellents can repel mosquitoes, such as

- *DEET* (N1N-diethyl-m-toluamide): By far the best repellant that can be applied on all exposed skin. It comes in various strengths, but the more

concentrated is more effective; children should use milder versions because there have been a few cases of toxicity with small children.
- *bath oil:* Although many consumers believe Avon's Skin-so-Soft is an effective repellent recent research by the military (and the Avon company) demonstrate that it is not nearly as effective as DEET.
- *zinc:* Some experts recommend daily doses (at least 60 milligrams), although they warn it can take up to four weeks to work; extra supplements should be taken only with approval of physician.

Because mosquitoes spread so much disease, scientists are continually working to develop new methods to eradicate them. Among the new possibilities include a protozoan, a fungus, and an Argentian nematode that may attack mosquitoes. Some scientists are developing poisoning bacteria and blue-green algae; others are developing new types of repellents.

The problem with eradicating mosquitoes is that they continually become resistant to almost any poison that scientists can develop; in any population of insects, some are likely to have a genetic resistance to any insecticide. Those few survive and reproduce, passing on their genes to offspring; eventually most of the insects in later generations have inherited the ability to survive the insecticide.

mud fever See LEPTOSPIROSIS.

Muerta Canyon virus See SIN NOMBRE VIRUS.

mumps An acute viral illness that was at one time a common childhood disease, featuring swollen and inflamed salivary glands on one or both sides of the face or under the jaw. In 1968, there were 152,000 mumps cases; today, there are fewer than 300 cases a year.

Before the mumps vaccine was available, almost every child got mumps sometime in childhood. While the incidence of the disease is much lower today, an unimmunized child remains at high risk for getting mumps. The disease is still widely found in developing countries, which is why anyone over one year of age should have a vaccine when traveling abroad.

Mumps is spread by airborne droplets of the mumps virus that are expelled by a patient with mumps who is coughing, sneezing, or talking. The virus invades and multiplies in the parotid gland, but it is attracted to all the glands.

Symptoms and Diagnostic Path

The disease will appear two to three weeks after exposure, beginning with mild discomfort in the area just inside the angle of the jaw. Many infected children have no symptoms. In more serious cases, however, the child complains of pain and has difficulty chewing; the glands on one or both sides become painful and tender. Fever, headache, and swallowing problems may follow, but the fever falls after two to three days and the swelling fades within 10 days. When only one side is affected, the second gland often swells as the first one subsides.

Mumps is usually diagnosed from symptoms; it can be confirmed by culturing the virus from saliva or urine, or by measuring antibodies to mumps virus in the blood.

The skin test for mumps—considered unreliable—is no longer available.

Treatment Options and Outlook

There is no specific treatment, but a patient may be given painkillers and plenty of fluids. In moderate to severe cases the child may need to stay in bed. Males with testicular involvement may be given a stronger painkiller; corticosteroid drugs may be needed to reduce inflammation.

While mumps is normally considered to be a mild disease, sometimes it can be more serious, causing a mild inflammation of the coverings of the brain and spinal cord (MENINGITIS) in about one in every 10 children with mumps. More rarely, it can cause an inflammation of the brain itself (ENCEPHALITIS), which usually improves by itself without permanent brain damage.

While serious complications are not common, one out of every teenage and adult males with the disease will have an inflammation and swelling in one or both testes. In extremely rare cases, this can lead to sterility. Mumps can also cause inflammation of the ovaries in older girls and women, inflammation of the pancreas or heart muscle, or auditory nerve damage resulting in deafness.

There is no evidence that mumps in pregnancy has any effect on the fetus.

Risk Factors and Preventive Measures

All healthy children who have never had mumps should be immunized on or before their first birthday. If in doubt, it is safe to be immunized or reimmunized against mumps.

The vaccine is available by itself, or in combination with measles and rubella (MMR), or with rubella (MR). Typically, the combination MMR vaccine is given at 15 months of age because it includes a measles vaccine; it protects the child against all three diseases. The vaccination, which has been used since 1967, can also be given to older children and adults. It is highly effective and one injection produces long-lasting (probably lifelong) immunity.

According to the U.S. CENTERS FOR DISEASE CONTROL AND PREVENTION, in very rare instances the mumps vaccine produces a mild, brief fever. This fever may occur one to two weeks after receiving the vaccine. Occasionally there is some slight swelling of the throat glands. Serious reactions are extremely rare.

Males who have already gone through puberty who have never been immunized against mumps or had the infection should avoid contact with any infected person. If symptoms do develop, passive immunization with antimumps immunoglobulin can provide some protection against the development of swelling in the testes.

Anyone who has a severely impaired immune system, a severe allergy to eggs, or anyone with a high fever or who has received blood products or immune globulin in the past three months should not receive the mumps virus vaccine.

mycetoma   A rare tropical skin and bone infection that can be extremely disfiguring. Mycetoma occurs primarily in tropical or subtropical areas, including the southern United States.

Mycetoma is caused by FUNGI or a type of bacteria called actinomycetes that enter the body through cuts or wounds on bare feet, legs, and arms, or on the backs of workers carrying contaminated vegetation. Men aged 20 to 40 are most often affected, probably because of injuries incurred during work outdoors.

Symptoms and Diagnostic Path

The infection forms multiple draining sinuses. The lesions can be disfiguring, producing a hard swelling covered by the openings of multiple drainage channels that discharge pus.

Treatment Options and Outlook

Sulfonamides and other antibacterial drugs, sometimes in combination, are used to treat mycetoma. The organisms may respond at least partially to amphotericin B or to itraconazole or ketoconazole, but many are resistant to all available antifungal drugs. Relapses occur after antifungal therapy in most cases, and many cases do not improve or worsen during treatment. Surgical debridement is necessary, and limb amputation may be needed to prevent potentially fatal severe secondary bacterial infections.

Infection progresses slowly over months or even years, gradually destroying nearby muscles, tendons, and bones. Eventually, muscle wasting, deformity, and tissue destruction prevent use of affected arms or legs. In advanced infections, the arms or legs appear grotesquely swollen. The infection may last longer than 10 years, ending in death from neglected bacterial superinfection and blood infection.

Mycobacterium A genus of rod-shaped bacteria with several significant species. *Mycobacterium leprae* causes LEPROSY; *M. tuberculosis* causes TUBERCULOSIS; *M. avium intracellulare* causes *MYCOBACTERIUM AVIUM COMPLEX* (MAC), a significant cause of death in AIDS patients. Currently, more than 60 species of mycobacteria have been well defined.

Mycobacterium avium complex (MAC) The most common bacterial opportunistic infection in people with HIV, it consists of two similar organisms— *Mycobacterium avium* and *M. intracellulare*. In one study, 43 percent of people with AIDS surviving two years after diagnosis tested positive for MAC,

suggesting that the infection may be an almost inevitable complication of HIV infection. MAC is also sometimes called *Mycobacterium avium intracellulare* (MAI). Some studies have shown that MAC occurs more often in Caucasians than in Latinos and African Americans; homosexual and bisexual men may have a higher incidence of infection than those in other risk groups.

The MAC organisms are found commonly in water, water mists or vapors, dust, soil, and bird droppings. They usually enter the body via contaminated food and water, although they also can be inhaled into the lungs. Once inside the body, the organisms colonize and grow in the gastrointestinal tract or the lungs, where they do not usually cause any symptoms at first. Eventually, since they are not stopped by the body's normal response to infection, they attack the tissue lining the gut and reproduce tremendously. After a local infection, the MAC organisms usually enter the bloodstream and spread throughout the body.

Symptoms and Diagnostic Path

The most common symptoms include fevers, night sweats, weight loss, loss of appetite, fatigue, or progressively severe diarrhea. Other symptoms include abdominal pain, nausea, and vomiting. Respiratory symptoms (cough and breathing problems) are fairly uncommon. However, painful joints, bone, brain, and skin infections can result when MAC bacteria spreads to other parts of the body.

Treatment Options and Outlook

Since MAC bacteria are closely related to the organism that causes tuberculosis, some of the drugs used to treat TB are also used against MAC. While it is not clear if treating MAC prolongs survival, treatment definitely reduces symptoms and improves the quality of life. A dozen or more drugs are available to treat MAC; most experts agree that treating an advanced MAC infection requires several drugs because no drug is effective alone. MAC bacteria can quickly become resistant to a particular drug.

Risk Factors and Preventive Measures

Research has shown that rifabutin (Mycobutin) can almost cut in half the rate at which people develop

MAC and also reduce the risk of dying by 14 percent. The drug is approved for preventing MAC, and recent information from studies of rifabutin show that the drug may also help people live longer.

The most serious side effects of rifabutin are low white blood cell counts and elevated liver enzymes. Very few people in trials had to discontinue the drug because of toxicity.

Clarithromycin (Biaxin) is the second drug to be approved for the prevention of MAC, cutting the number of MAC infections by 69 percent (more than two-thirds).

A third drug (azithromycin) taken once a week also has been approved for preventing MAC. A recent study found that azithromycin was better at preventing MAC than rifabutin. Still, azithromycin has not been directly compared to clarithromycin for preventing MAC.

A recent study comparing rifabutin, clarithromycin, and a combination of the two drugs found clarithromycin to be clearly superior to rifabutin for the prevention of MAC. Since MAC organisms have been found in most city water systems, as well as hospital water supplies and bottled water, boiling drinking water is suggested. AIDS patients should not eat raw foods (especially salads, root vegetables, and unpasteurized milk or cheese). Conventional cooking (baking, boiling, or steaming) destroys MAC bacteria, which are killed at 176°F. Fruits and vegetables should be peeled and rinsed thoroughly.

Patients should avoid animal contact (especially birds and bird droppings). Pigeons, in particular, can transmit not just MAC but also the organism that causes CRYPTOCOCCOSIS, another opportunistic infection found in people with HIV infection.

HIV patients should avoid or reduce alcohol consumption, since regularly drinking alcohol can hasten the development of MAC infection in those with HIV.

Mycobacterium avium intracellulare See MYCO-BACTERIUM AVIUM COMPLEX.

Mycobacterium leprae Also called Hansen's bacillus, this organism causes LEPROSY. The rod-shaped bacterium was identified in 1874 by a Norwegian Armauer Hansen; as a result, both the microbe and the disease were named for him.

Mycobacterium nebraskense A newly discovered bacterium species that causes life-threatening lung infections. It is in the family Mycobacterium, which includes diseases such as TUBERCULOSIS and LEPROSY. Nebraskense, commonly found in soil and water, grows slowly and causes chronic lung infection, including PNEUMONIA. The discovery of nebraskense will be of special interest to those treating patients with weak immune systems.

Mycobacterium tuberculosis Also known as Koch's bacillus, this slow-growing organism is the cause of TUBERCULOSIS. (TB) Often shortened to *M. Tb*, the bacterium was discovered in 1882 by German physician Robert Koch, the father of modern bacteriology and discoverer of the organisms that cause ANTHRAX and CHOLERA.

This bacillus (rod-shaped bacterium) belongs to the family Mycobacterium. Most members of this family live in water or soil and do not infect humans, although *M. bovis* infects cows and can cause TB in those who drink unpasteurized milk from infected cows.

A single bacterium is called a tubercule bacillus. An extremely tough type of bacteria, the TB bug can live for weeks in the dark, where it forms spores. It cannot survive in a clean, well-ventilated sunny environment. It is most often transmitted by respiratory secretions from coughing. The organism can remain airborne and alive in these secretions and on surfaces for days.

mycology The study of FUNGI and fungoid diseases.

mycoplasma A type of free-living bacteria that lack a cell wall, which means that the bacteria are resistant to antibiotics such as PENICILLIN, which work by attacking cell walls.

Mycoplasmas are found everywhere in nature, some living on decaying matter or occupying harmless places within other organisms. But many others are disease-causing bacteria of vertebrates, insects, and plants.

Only a limited number of mycoplasma species infect humans; the most important of these is MYCO-PLASMA PNEUMONIAE, a common cause of respiratory infection (including PNEUMONIA). It is also possible that mycoplasmas could be involved in the progression of AIDS.

Mycoplasmas were first isolated in 1898 in France, as the source of a cattle disease called pleuropneumonia. When similar microbes were found to cause other infections (including a particular form of human pneumonia) they were called pleuropneumonia-like organisms or PPLOs. They were later correctly reclassified as mycoplasmas, and M. pneumoniae was identified in the early 1960s.

The term mycoplasma is used as a general designation for any member of the class, or as Mycoplasma, the name of a particular genus within that class.

These organisms are halfway between bacteria and viruses, with characteristics of both. Much smaller than bacteria, they reproduce slowly—but unlike viruses, they can be killed by some antibiotics.

Mycoplasma infections, which cannot be detected by standard bacterial cultures, are often misdiagnosed, so that these infections often are treated inappropriately or not at all. A DNA analysis technique is required to detect the presence of the mycoplasm in patients' blood.

One recent study found that people with chronic illnesses were more than seven times more likely to have mycoplasmal infections compared to healthy subjects. In one test group of 203 patients diagnosed with chronic fatigue syndrome, a full 70 percent showed signs of mycoplasma DNA in the blood compared with an infection rate of only 9 percent of healthy subjects. Another group of 200 GULF WAR SYNDROME patients showed 45 percent positive for mycoplasm, while the control group of healthy subjects tested at the rate of less than 6 percent.

In yet another study, mycoplasma bacteria has been linked to the triggering or exacerbation of rheumatoid arthritis. In this study, researchers found that fluids from the inflamed joints of many patients contained the specific DNA of Mycoplasma fermetans, a well-known bacterium of the mycoplasma family commonly found in the throat.

Because mycoplasmas definitely cause arthritis in animals, doctors since the early 1950s have suspected a mycoplasma in humans might be involved in human arthritis. Scientists suspect that mycoplasmas in the joint may stimulate the immune system to produce antibodies which provoke local inflammation and tissue damage.

See also MYCOPLASMA PNEUMONIA.

mycoplasma pneumonia   A contagious disease of children and young adults caused by MYCOPLASMA PNEUMONIAE, affecting about 2 million Americans a year. The disease is also called Eaton-agent pneumonia, primary atypical pneumonia, or walking pneumonia.

Anyone can get the disease, but it occurs most often in older children and young adults. The infections occur sporadically throughout the year, but they are most common in late summer and in fall; widespread community outbreaks may occur every four to eight years.

Mycoplasma pneumonia is caused by M. pneumoniae, a microscopic organism related to bacteria. It is spread through contact with droplets from the nose and throat of infected people when they cough or sneeze. Scientists believe transmission requires close contact with an infected person. The contagious period is probably less than 10 days.

Symptoms and Diagnostic Path

After an incubation period of between nine to 25 days, symptoms of dry cough, fever, sore throat, headache, and malaise appear. Ear infections may also occur. Symptoms may last from a few days to a month or more.

The disease can be diagnosed based on the symptoms; a nonspecific blood test may help in the diagnosis.

Treatment Options and Outlook

Antibiotics including erythromycin or tetracycline are effective.

Risk Factors and Preventive Measures

There are no vaccines to prevent the spread of mycoplasma infection, and there are no reliable methods for control.

Mycoplasma pneumoniae The organism that causes the contagious disease MYCOPLASMA PNEUMONIA. While classified as a bacterium, it does not have a cell wall and cannot be seen on routine smears or grown on routine culture plates. It does not usually cause any disease other than a respiratory condition.

mycosis Any disease caused by a fungus.

mycotic infections, systemic See FUNGAL INFECTION.

mycotoxicosis A type of fungus-derived metabolite found on certain kinds of food capable of causing one type of food poisoning. Ever since the Middle Ages, thousands of people have died from various types of mycotoxins—most notably, ergot poisoning. But it was a 1960 turkey EPIDEMIC in England that spurred a worldwide research effort to track down the vast number of toxic compounds derived from fungus that cause these poisonings. While most of the deaths from mycotoxicosis have been among animals eating tainted food, symptoms are still found frequently among humans.

One of the most widespread of these toxins are aflatoxins found in a wide variety of food, including grains, peanuts, tree nuts, and cottonseed meal; meat, eggs, milk, and other products from animals that consume aflatoxin-contaminated feed are additional sources of potential exposure.

Peanuts can develop a toxic mold when not properly stored, which is why consumers should never eat moldy or shriveled food (especially grains or peanuts) and should be cautious about eating unroasted peanuts sold in bulk.

Aflatoxin is a cancer-causing byproduct of the *Aspergillus flavus* mold found in peanuts, corn, wheat, rice, cottonseeds, barley, soybeans, Brazil nuts, and pistachios. The molds that produce aflatoxin grow in warm, humid climates in the southeastern United States, but the mold can also be produced in the field when rain falls on corn and wheat left in the field to dry. Aflatoxin-producing mold can even grow on plants damaged by insects or drought, poor nutrition, or unseasonable temperatures.

Aflatoxin has been called the most potent natural carcinogen known to humans; poor diet also seems to predispose animals to cancer in the wake of aflatoxin ingestion.

Still, scientists know very little about why or how the aflatoxins are produced by the mold, and because it is sometimes difficult to see, all susceptible crops are subject to routine testing in the United States. Unfortunately, it is not possible to detect the mold with 100 percent accuracy.

While the way agricultural products are stored can affect the mold's growth, the length of time of such storage is also important; the longer agricultural products are stored in bins, the greater the chance that environmental conditions favorable to aflatoxin production will be created. Stored nuts or seeds might accidentally get wet or the storage bin might not facilitate drying quickly enough to stop the mold from growing.

Aflatoxins are more common in poor-quality cereals and nuts; while most of these low-grade products do not enter the human food market, they are sold as animal feed, which can go on to contaminate animal products (such as meat and milk). For this reason, cottonseed meal (a product often contaminated with high levels of aflatoxin) is banned for use as an animal feed. Cottonseed oil, however, rarely contains aflatoxin, since the toxin sticks to the hulls of the seed.

Milk is commonly contaminated with aflatoxin, and powdered nonfat milk can contain eight times more than the original liquid product since the aflatoxin adheres to the milk's proteins. In addition, measurable levels of aflatoxin can be found in some baby foods that use dry milk to boost the protein content of the product.

Symptoms and Diagnostic Path

In humans, aflatoxin is believed to cause liver cancer, according to some East African studies, which seem to show a correlation between the two. Epidemiological evidence also suggests men are more susceptible than women; many scientists believe a poor diet and liver disease also increase susceptibility to liver cancer as a result of aflatoxin exposure. Data from the African studies were strong enough to prompt the U.S. Food and Drug Administration and the Environmental Protection Agency to develop strict regulations to control levels in food and animal food sold in the United States.

Aflatoxin can also cause acute poisoning; severe liver disease has been detected in those who ingest highly contaminated food, and children around the world exhibit symptoms similar to Reyes syndrome (fever, vomiting, coma, and convulsions) after exposure.

Risk Factors and Preventive Measures

Pasteurization, sterilization, and dry processing techniques can substantially reduce aflatoxin contamination of dried milk. Meat products are less often contaminated because little aflatoxin is carried over into the meat, except for pig liver and kidneys. Chicken may become contaminated with aflatoxin when the bird appears to be only mildly sick.

myiasis, cutaneous   A fly larvae infestation of the skin usually found only in the Tropics. When the African tumbu fly lays eggs on clothing, the larvae from the eggs penetrate the skin, eventually causing a swelling that looks like a boil. Various other types of flies may lay eggs in open wounds, on the skin, or in the ears or nose.

Treatment Options and Outlook

Oil drops over the swelling suffocates the larvae, which then migrate to the surface where they can be removed with a needle.

Risk Factors and Preventive Measures

Infestation can be avoided by covering open wounds and (in Africa) by thoroughly ironing clothes that have been drying outside.

myocarditis   An acute inflammatory condition of the heart muscle (myocardium) caused by viral, bacterial, or fungal infection. Myocarditis may also be produced as a result of RHEUMATIC FEVER.

After a bout of myocarditis, patients usually experience some residual heart enlargement. People with a virus infection that affects the lungs may have a mild myocarditis that may be detected with an electrocardiogram (ECG).

The most common cause of myocarditis in Central and South America is the parasitic infection called CHAGAS DISEASE. Many years after the initial infection, these patients can develop extensive fatal damage to the heart muscle.

Symptoms and Diagnostic Path

The symptoms depend on the type of infection that causes the inflammation, the degree of damage, and the capacity of the heart muscle to recover. Symptoms may be mild or nonexistent; if they do occur, they may include fatigue, pain, fever, and rapid heartbeat. Rarely, the inflammation can lead to chest pain and heart failure, followed by cardiac arrest and death. Acute inflammation of the outer lining of the heart (pericarditis) often accompanies myocarditis.

Treatment Options and Outlook

Most cases clear up without treatment, although corticosteroid drugs are occasionally prescribed to reduce inflammation. Treatment of the cause of the inflammation together with painkillers, oxygen, and rest are helpful. Most physicians believe that exercise is not helpful for people with myocarditis; they recommend that patients not engage in strenuous exercise until their ECG returns to normal.

myxovirus   Any of a group of medium-sized viruses that include those that cause INFLUENZA, MUMPS, and PARAINFLUENZA.

nairovirus Tick-borne viruses that are subdivided into several serogroups. Crimean-Congo hemorrhagic fever virus is the most medically significant member of this genus.

nanobacteria (NB) A novel self-replicating mineralizing agent discovered in the 1990s that has been found in the calcium phosphate centers of kidney stones. This agent has also been detected in related conditions, including Alzheimer's disease, heart disease, prostatitis, and some cancers. In addition, it has been identified by NASA scientists as a potential culprit in kidney stone formation among astronauts. During studies at NASA, scientists discovered that, in a microgravity environment, NB multiplied five times faster than when in normal gravity, supporting earlier discoveries that germs behave quite differently in weightless environments. NB is also an infectious risk for crew members living in close quarters.

However, the idea that nanobacteria are living organisms is still controversial. Further testing for the presence of NB in humans can help reduce the risk for kidney stone formation in astronauts and would also be of benefit to the nearly 1 million Americans who are treated for kidney stones each year.

nanophyetiasis The name for a human disease caused by infection with parasitic flatworms (flukes); it is also called "fish flu."

There have been no reported massive outbreaks of the disease in North America; the only scientific reports are of 20 individuals in one Oregon clinic. The disease is endemic in Russia, where the infection rate is reported to be more than 90 percent and growing.

The disease is caused by the *Nanophyetus salmincola* or *N. schikhobalowi,* the North American and Russian troglotrematoid trematodes (respectively). It is transmitted by the larval stage of a worm that embeds itself in the flesh of freshwater fish; North American cases were all associated with salmon. Raw, underprocessed, and smoked salmon and steelhead were implicated.

Symptoms and Diagnostic Path
The first reported U.S. cases were characterized by diarrhea, usually accompanied by abdominal discomfort and nausea. A few patients reported weight loss and fatigue.

The disease is diagnosed by finding the eggs in feces. However, it is hard to tell the difference between these eggs and those of another parasite, *Diphyllobothrium latum.*

Treatment Options and Outlook
Treatment with bithionol or niclosamide appears to resolve the problem.

National Childhood Vaccine Injury Act of 1986 A vaccine safety and compensation system established by Congress in 1986 to create a no-fault compensation alternative to suing vaccine manufacturers and providers for citizens injured or killed by vaccines. The act also created safety provisions to help educate the public about vaccine benefits and risks, and to require doctors to report adverse events after vaccination as well as keep records on vaccines administered and health problems which occur following vaccination. Finally, the act also created incentives for the production of safer vaccines.

Compensation is divided into two parts. For any injuries or deaths before October 1, 1988 (no matter how long ago the injury occurred), a citizen:

- may choose to pursue a lawsuit unrestricted
- could have filed a claim in the compensation system by January 31, 1991. If the claim was not filed by January 31, 1991, the statute of limitations has run out.

For any injuries or deaths occurring after October 1, 1988, a citizen is required to apply for federal compensation before pursuing a lawsuit. The government will offer to pay up to $250,000 for a vaccine-associated death, or will offer to pay for all past and future unreimbursed medical expenses, custodial and nursing care, up to $250,000 for pain and suffering; and loss of earned income. If a citizen rejects the award or is turned down, a lawsuit may be filed.

Claims must be filed within 24 months of a death and 36 months of an injury. Restrictions apply to lawsuits, if compensation is denied or rejected by the parent. The system is funded by a surcharge on each dose of vaccine sold.

See also VACCINE ADVERSE EVENTS REPORTING SYSTEM.

National Nosocomial Infections Surveillance (NNIS) System   A cooperative effort that began in 1970 between the U.S. CENTERS FOR DISEASE CONTROL AND PREVENTION (CDC) and participating hospitals to create a national nosocomial (hospital-acquired) infections database. The database is used to describe the origin of nosocomial infections and antimicrobial resistance trends, and develop nosocomial infection rates.

Participation in the NNIS System is voluntary and involves only acute care general hospitals in the United States. Long-term facilities such as rehabilitation, mental health, and nursing homes are not included in the NNIS System. About 300 hospitals participated in the NNIS System. Data from the NNIS System are reported annually in the NNIS Report located on the NNIS website (http://www.cdc.gov/ncidod/dhqp/NNIS_pubs.html) and in the November–December issue of the *American Journal of Infection Control.*

necrotizing fasciitis   See FLESH-EATING BACTERIA.

Neisseria gonorrhoeae   A gram-negative bacterium that causes GONORRHEA, also called GONOCOCCUS or diplococcus. This circular bacterium was identified in 1879 by the German dermatologist Albert L. S. Neisser. It was not until 1937 that scientists discovered sulfa drugs could kill the microorganism. Unfortunately, today there are PENICILLIN-resistant strains (known as PPNG, for penicillinase-producing *Neisseria gonorrhoea*), coming primarily from the Philippines. Other strains are resistant to tetracycline.

Neisseria meningitidis   See MENINGOCOCCUS.

nematodes   See ROUNDWORMS.

neonatal infections   Newborns are especially vulnerable to a number of infections because their immature immune systems are not well enough developed to fight off bacteria, viruses, and parasites. As a result, when newborns are diagnosed with one of these illnesses, they may need to spend time in a hospital or neonatal intensive care unit to recover. Common neonatal infections include CANDIDIASIS, *E. coli* infection, group B Strep disease (GBS); LISTERIOSIS, pinkeye, MENINGITIS, SEPSIS, and CONGENITAL INFECTIOUS DISEASES.

Candidiasis   An overgrowth of the common fungus *Candida,* a common fungus that most healthy people carry, can lead to candidiasis in a newborn, typically heralded as diaper rash. However, infants also can develop candidiasis in the mouth and throat (called THRUSH), characterized by cracks in the corners of the mouth and white patches on the tongue, palate, lips, and insides of the cheeks. Newborns who get thrush usually are infected during birth from fungus in the mother's vagina. Thrush can be treated with antifungal medicine in liquid form.

E. coli infection   *Escherichia coli* is a common bacterial infection in newborns. Because *E. coli* is common in almost everyone, babies can become infected during birth or by touching something in the hospital or home. Most newborns who get sick from *E. coli* infection have an especailly fragile immune system. Typical symptoms include fever, fussiness, listlessness, or lack of interest in eating.

Doctors can diagnose *E. coli* infection by lab tests of blood, urine, or cerebral spinal fluid and treat the infection with antibiotics.

Group B streptococcal disease (GBS) Strep bacteria can cause many different newborn infections, including sepsis, PNEUMONIA, and meningitis. Babies usually become infected during birth, since one in four or five pregnant women carries this common germ in the rectum or vagina, where it can easily pass to the newborn if the mother has not been given preventive antibiotics. Babies with GBS often develop symptoms within the first week of life, although some cases do not appear until several weeks or even months after birth. Depending on the infection that the bacterium causes (such as sepsis or pneumonia), the infant might experience breathing problems, poor appetite, a fever, listlessness, or fussiness. GBS is diagnosed from blood tests and cultures. Infections caused by GBS are treated with antibiotics as well as careful care and monitoring in the hospital.

Listeriosis Infection with *Listeria monocytogenes* can cause pneumonia, sepsis, and meningitis. The bacterium, found in soil and water, can contaminate poorly cleaned, cooked or pasteurized fruits and vegetables, meat, and dairy products. Infants can become infected if their mothers develop listeriosis while pregnant. In severe cases, listeriosis may lead to premature delivery or even stillbirth. Babies born with listeriosis may show signs of infection that are similar to those of GBS. A blood or spinal fluid culture can reveal the presence of the bacterium, and infected infants are given antibiotics in the hospital.

Meningitis An inflammation of the membranes surrounding the brain and spinal cord, meningitis can be caused by viruses, fungi, and bacteria, including listeriosis, GBS, and *E. coli,* that a baby can contract during birth or from surroundings. Symptoms of the infection in newborns include persistent crying, irritability, sleepineess, lethargy, poor appetite, low or unstable body temperature, jaundice, pallor, breathing problems, rashes, vomiting, or diarrhea. As the disease worsens, the soft spot at the top of the head may begin to bulge. Bacterial meningitis is a much more serious infection in newborns than is viral meningitis. Meningitis is diagnosed with a spinal tap to check a sample of cerebrospinal fluid. Bacterial and fungal meningitis are treated with antibiotics; viral meningitis may be treated with antiviral medication. All infants with meningitis are typically hospitalized and given intense supportive care.

Pinkeye (CONJUNCTIVITIS) Some newborns develop an inflammation of the eye's membranes that causes redness, swelling, and discharge. Both bacterial and viral infections can cause pinkeye in newborns, which is treated with antibiotics, eye drops, or ointments. The infection can be very contagious, so other children in the family should avoid contact with the baby. More serious types of conjunctivitis require hospitalization.

Sepsis Sepsis is a serious infection in which germs spread throughout the body. Sepsis is caused by viruses, FUNGI, parasites, or bacteria acquired during birth or picked up from the environment. Symptoms of sepsis may vary from child to child and include a slower heart rate, breathing problems, jaundice, lack of interest in eating, low or unstable body temperature, lethargy, and fussiness. Sepsis is treated with antibiotics in the hospital.

Congenital infections Many infections that affect newborns are transmitted from the mother during pregnancy or birth, and the baby is born with the disease. Congenital infections are often caused by viruses, but bacteria, fungi, and parasites also may cause disease in infants at birth. Congenital infections include HIV, rubella (GERMAN MEASLES), CHICKEN POX (varicella zoster), SYPHILIS, TOXOPLASMOSIS, and CYTOMEGALOVIRUS—the most common congenital infection and the leading cause of congenital hearing loss.

Some infections (such as GBS infection or listeriosis) can be transmitted either before birth or later, as a result of a contaminated environment.

A baby is more likely to be born with an infection if its mother became infected for the first time with a germ during pregnancy. Luckily, not all babies born to infected mothers develop disease; others may not show symptoms at first, but then later develop symptoms.

The seriousness of the infection often depends on when the infant's mother was exposed to the germ. For many infections, such as rubella and toxoplasmosis, the risk to the infant is highest during the first three months of pregnancy and can lead to heart disease, brain damage, deafness, visual problems, and miscarriage. Infection later in the pregnancy may cause less severe effects with the infant, although these infections may still interfere with the baby's development.

Early signs of a possible congenital infection include an unusually sized head (either too large or small), small body size, seizures, eye problems, skin rashes, jaundice, enlarged abdominal organs, and a heart murmur. To diagnose a congenital infection, the doctor will order blood tests and cultures of other fluids from the infant and sometimes the mother.

Treatment typically includes the same antiviral or antibiotic medications used to treat the same diseases in older patients, as well as intensive care while the baby is in the hospital. The baby should be closely watched to identify any futher symptoms or lingering problems as the infant grows.

Complications of Neonatal Infections

Neonatal infections can have serious consequences if they are not promptly treated. Because an infant's body and organs are rapidly growing, any infection can lead to complications, including problems with growth, development, the brain, heart, breathing, or senses. In some severe cases, these infections can be fatal.

With their brand-new immune systems, babies cannot deal well with overwhelming infection; babies born too soon have an even higher risk of developing a severe disease from a bacterium or virus that might cause a simple illness in an older child. This is why early diagnosis, swift treatment, and close monitoring and care are so vital to infected neonates.

Risk Factors and Preventive Measures

If a pregnant woman is diagnosed with an infection or if she is considered at risk of infection, preventive measures can lower the risk that she will pass it to her baby. Many infections can be treated with medicine given to the mother while she is pregnant.

In many cases, a quick blood or fluid test can determine if a pregnant woman should receive treatment. Antibiotics can prevent transmission of listeriosis to an unborn baby, and antiretroviral medication taken during pregnancy by an HIV-infected mother can lower the risk that her baby will contract the infection.

Other neonatal infections are best prevented by keeping the expectant mother from developing the infection in the first place. Women should be immunized against rubella and chicken pox infection (if they have not already had the infection) before trying to become pregnant. Pregnant women should thoroughly wash and cook food; regularly wash hands before and after preparing food, after using the toilet, and after coming into contact with bodily fluids and waste; and avoid all contact with cat and other animal feces to lower the risk of contracting bacteria and parasites that lead to infections such as listeriosis and toxoplasmosis. Pregnant women also should practice safe sex to avoid sexually transmitted diseases that can lead to congenital infections.

Some preventive measures are routine parts of pregnancy and delivery. A simple swab test late in pregnancy can identify whether a pregnant woman is carrying GBS; if she is, intravenous antibiotics during delivery can lower the risk of transmitting the bacteria to her baby. Doctors also routinely put antibiotic drops or ointment in newborns' eyes to prevent pinkeye caused by GONORRHEA bacteria.

Medical help should be obtained if a new baby does not eat well, has trouble breathing, is listless, has a low or high fever or skin rash, cries persistently, or is unusually fussy. A marked change in a baby's behavior, such as suddenly sleeping all the time or not sleeping at all, may indicate that something is wrong. These signs are especially serious if the infant is less than two months old.

neurocysticercosis   See TAPEWORM.

neurotoxic shellfish poisoning   See SHELLFISH POISONING, NEUROTOXIC.

Nipah virus   A virus that belongs to the family Paramyxoviridae and that is related but not identical to the HENDRA VIRUS. The Nipah virus was first isolated in 1999 after examining samples from an outbreak of ENCEPHALITIS and respiratory illness among Malaysian and Singaporean men. Scientists suspect that bats of the genus *Pteropus* are the reservoirs for Nipah virus in Malaysia. Nipah virus caused a relatively mild disease in pigs in Malaysia and Singapore, which was then transmitted to humans, cats, and dogs.

Symptoms and Diagnostic Path
Illness with Nipah virus begins with three to 14 days of fever and headache followed by drowsiness and disorientation and sometimes a respiratory infection. These symptoms can lead to coma within 24 to 48 hours.

Serious nervous disease with Nipah virus encephalitis has included persistent convulsions and personality changes. During a Nipah virus disease outbreak in 1998–99, almost half the patients with serious nervous disease died from the illness.

Treatment Options and Outlook
The drug ribavirin has been shown to be effective against the viruses, but the usefulness of this drug in patient populations is uncertain.

Risk Factors and Preventive Measures
Nipah virus infection can be prevented by avoiding infected animals and using personal protective equipment when in contact with potentially infected animals.

nitric oxide A simple molecule with one atom of oxygen and one of nitrogen that may be used by the immune system to fight a wide variety of infections.

It was best known as a toxic gas and an ingredient in air pollution until 1987, when scientists discovered it was produced by cells throughout the body. Since then, it was identified as a player in a vast number of body activities. In addition to its ability to fight infections, it boosts cell communication, regulates blood pressure, causes penile erections, transmits messages between nerve cells, kills certain parasites, and may play a part in learning and memory.

Scientists have known for some time that nitric oxide disables or kills certain protozoans, worms, FUNGI, and bacteria. Now, new research suggests that nitric oxide is a potent antiviral that attacks both poxviruses and HERPES simplex, type 1 (HSV1), which causes COLD SORES in humans. It appears to be triggered by cytokines such as INTERFERON (proteins secreted by immune system cells).

Nitric oxide appears to have potential as a broad-spectrum antiviral because it affects many different kinds of viruses. Scientists believe if they can design ways to deliver the right amount of nitric oxide to the site of infection without causing side effects, they could produce a new approach to antiviral therapy.

Other recent studies suggest that nitric oxide may help the body defend itself against diseases such as MALARIA. Nitric oxide may play a key role in determining whether a child develops the most dangerous complication of the disease, cerebral malaria, which causes fatal convulsions and coma. Scientists do not know why only some people develop the complication, but they found that those who do had the lowest levels of nitric oxide.

nocardiosis An infection by a fungus-like bacterium found throughout the world. This infection is not normally found in healthy patients, but it occurs in those with a compromised immune system, beginning in the lungs and spreading to tissues under the skin.

The disease is caused by infection with *Nocardia asteroides,* an aerobic species of actinomycetes. The organism enters the respiratory tract and spreads throughout the bloodstream.

Symptoms and Diagnostic Path
Symptoms include fever and cough similar to pneumonia, with lung damage and BRAIN ABSCESSES. Occasionally, this bacterium causes skin abscesses only (especially in gardeners).

Treatment Options and Outlook
Sulfonamide drugs for 12 to 18 months, sometimes in conjunction with other antibiotics, together with surgical drainage of abscesses, cures between 50 percent and 60 percent of cases. Symptoms do not respond to short-term antibiotics.

noroviruses A group of viruses that cause stomach flu (GASTROENTERITIS) in humans. The term *norovirus* was approved in 2005 as the official name for this group of viruses, replacing earlier names for noroviruses including Norwalk-like viruses (NLVs), caliciviruses (because they belong to the virus family Caliciviridae), and "small round structured viruses." There are many different strains of norovirus, which makes it hard for a person's body to develop long-lasting immunity. Therefore, norovirus illness can recur throughout one's life.

This virus is very contagious and can spread rapidly, although it is usually not serious. People infected with norovirus are contagious from the moment they begin feeling ill to at least three days to two weeks after recovery. Therefore, it is particularly important for people to use good handwashing and other hygienic practices after they have recently recovered from norovirus illness.

Noroviruses are found in the stool or vomit of infected people. The virus can be passed on by

- eating or drinking anything contaminated with norovirus
- touching anything contaminated with norovirus and then putting hands in the mouth
- having direct contact with another infected person (such as taking care of someone with norovirus or sharing foods or eating utensils with a patient)
- working in day-care centers or nursing homes

Symptoms and Diagnostic Path

The symptoms appear between 12 and 48 hours after infection and include nausea, constant vomiting, diarrhea, and stomach cramps. Other symptoms may include a low-grade fever, chills, headache, muscle aches, and a general sense of fatigue. The illness often begins suddenly, and the infected person may feel very sick, but the illness lasts only about one or two days. Children typically experience more vomiting than adults.

Treatment Options and Outlook

No antiviral medication is effective against norovirus. Patients with vomiting and diarrhea should drink plenty of fluids to prevent dehydration. By drinking rehydration fluids such as juice or water, people can reduce their chances of becoming dehydrated. (Sports drinks do not replace the nutrients and minerals lost during this illness.)

Most people have no long-term health effects related to their illness, although dehydration may be a problem if patients cannot drink enough liquids to replace those lost by vomiting and diarrhea. Dehydration is usually only seen among the very young, the elderly, and patients with weakened immune systems. There is no evidence to suggest that an infected person can become a long-term carrier of norovirus.

Risk Factors and Preventive Measures

There is no vaccine to prevent this infection. People can lessen the chance of being infected by noroviruses by frequently washing their hands, especially after going to the bathroom, changing diapers, and before eating or preparing food.

Fruits and vegetables should be washed carefully, and raw oysters should be avoided. Contaminated surfaces should be thoroughly disinfected right after illness with a bleach-based household cleaner. Clothing or linens that may be contaminated with virus should be washed with hot water and soap right after an episode of illness. Vomitus or stool in the toilet should be flushed immediately, and the surrounding area kept clean.

Recovering patients should not prepare food while they have symptoms or for three days after they recover from their illness. Food that may have been contaminated by a patient should be thrown away.

Norwalk-like virus   The former name for norovirus.

Norwalk virus infection   Common infection by a family of several small viruses that can cause viral GASTROENTERITIS featuring a mild diarrhea. The virus was first identified in 1972 after an outbreak of gastrointestinal illness in Norwalk, Ohio. Later, other viruses with similar features were described and called Norwalk-like viruses; these have since been reclassified as NOROVIRUS. Although viral gastroenteritis may be caused by a number of viruses, the Norwalk family are responsible for about one-third of all cases not involving young infants. Studies show that more than 60 percent of adults develop antibodies to Norwalk agent infection by the time they reach age 50.

Norwalk virus also is the most common cause of viral contamination in shellfish. The specific agent is named for the area where the outbreak of the virus first occurs, such as Norwalk, Hawaii, or Marin agent.

During the Gulf War of 1991, more than 10 percent of the troops were infected by the Norwalk virus when they ate local unwashed fruits and vegetables. Other outbreaks commonly occur in nursing homes, schools, camps, or hospitals. Outbreaks are particularly common in tropical countries with inadequately treated water.

Norwalk virus and noroviruses are being recognized more frequently as important causes of food-borne disease in the United States. However, since no routine diagnostic test is available, the true prevalence is not known. These viruses have been linked to outbreaks of intestinal illness on cruise ships and in communities, camps, schools, institutions, and families.

Many oyster-related outbreaks of intestinal illness linked to Norwalk-like viruses have been reported in Louisiana, Florida, Maryland, and other states where oyster harvesting is common. During 1998, a number of soldiers in El Paso, Texas, were hospitalized with Norwalk virus.

Norwalk gastroenteritis can be transmitted by ingesting contaminated food or water. In addition, the infection can be transferred from person to person. Water is the most common source of outbreaks and may include water from city supplies, wells, recreational lakes, swimming pools, and water stores in cruise ships.

Shellfish and salad ingredients are foods most often implicated in Norwalk outbreaks. Eating raw or insufficiently steamed clams and oysters poses a high risk for infection with Norwalk virus. Foods other than shellfish may be contaminated by food handlers who have the virus.

Everyone who ingests the virus and who has not recently had an infection with the same strain is susceptible to infection and can develop symptoms. Infection is most common in adults and older children.

Symptoms and Diagnostic Path
Within two to three days of infection, symptoms of vomiting, abdominal cramps, mild diarrhea, fatigue, and muscle aches appear. Most people experience only a mild illness and recover within 48 hours.

For about three months following an infection, patients will develop a short-term immunity. After this period of time, however, it is possible to become reinfected. Severe illness or hospitalization is very rare.

Research labs can look for virus in stool specimens; a blood test can uncover antibodies to the virus. Specific diagnosis of the disease can be made only by a few labs that possess reagents from human volunteer studies. Identification of the virus can be made on early stool specimens using immune electron microscopes. However, this disease is usually diagnosed by the characteristics of the illness itself, without tests.

Treatment Options and Outlook
Because the diarrhea is caused by a virus, there is no cure. When a person becomes infected, the body develops antibodies that destroy the virus. Rest, clear fluids, and acetaminophen for headaches and body aches will help. Patients who do not experience vomiting can continue to eat solids.

Risk Factors and Preventive Measures
There are no specific preventive measures, since scientists do not know enough about how the virus is transmitted. Consumers should follow guidelines for avoiding other food-borne illnesses, and follow precautions for food and beverage safety when traveling to tropical countries.

nosocomial infection An infection acquired in a hospital. See HOSPITAL-ACQUIRED INFECTIONS.

notifiable disease See REPORTABLE DISEASE.

onchocerciasis A chronic tropical disease (also called river blindness) that is a parasitic disease transmitted by small black flies that breed in rivers and streams. It is the second-leading infectious cause of blindness in the world. The disease is a type of FILARIASIS. The World Health Organization estimates that 17.7 million people are infected, 500,000 have vision problems, and another 270,000 are blind in 37 endemic countries (especially Nigeria). About 123 million people live in endemic areas worldwide and are at risk of infection; more than 99 percent of those infected reside in Africa.

American travelers appear to be at low risk for infection; the risk only rises for those who stay in an area for a long time, such as missionaries, field scientists, and Peace Corps workers. Eye lesions are more common among people of the African savannah, whereas skin lesions are more often seen among rain forest inhabitants.

The disease is caused by the parasite *Onchocerca volvulus* transmitted by the bite of the blood-sucking female *Simulium* black fly.

The black fly deposits infected larvae beneath the skin of humans; the larvae penetrate the human tissue and develop into an adult worm after about a year. The female adult, which can live for 15 years, produces large numbers of microfilariae that migrate throughout the body.

Symptoms and Diagnostic Path
About a year after the black fly bite, symptoms appear and may include severe localized or generalized itching of the skin. The patient may scratch so hard that the skin is broken; hard lumps then appear in the skin. Other symptoms may include fever, headache, and tiredness. Eye inflammation can lead to blindness. In the Americas, lesions are seen usually on the scalp; in Africa, they are found mostly around the pelvis and on the trunk. The development of blindness depends on the number of larvae around the eye.

Treatment Options and Outlook
In some cases, treatment may include surgical removal of the nodules, together with medication. Ivermectin kills the parasite at the stage where it causes symptoms. Merck, Sharp & Dohme provides this drug free to countries where river blindness is common. It is available in the United States from the U.S. CENTERS FOR DISEASE CONTROL AND PREVENTION under an agreement with the U.S. Food and Drug Administration (FDA). Ivermectin and other drugs for tropical diseases available through the drug service are not approved in the United States but are provided under investigational drug exemptions granted by the FDA. They are provided free to other countries as a public health service. The drugs must be given carefully because of the severe reaction caused by worms dying from the drug.

Researchers are studying a possible vaccine for river blindness using antibodies produced by the few individuals who appear to be resistant to river blindness. (Nearly everyone else who is exposed to the parasites becomes infected.)

o'nyong-nyong An alphavirus that causes disease similar to DENGUE FEVER and CHIKUNGUNYA FEVER in Africa and Asia. The name, which means "weakening of the joints" or "joint breaker" in a Uganda dialect, first appeared in that country in 1959, when it infected millions of Africans over the ensuing two years. Researchers first thought the virus was related to dengue fever or chikungunya, but eventually isolated the virus and recognized it as something new. The EPIDEMIC started in northern Uganda and spread south and eastward into Kenya, Tanzania, and Zambia, and then northward from Tanzania into southwestern Uganda, where it subsided.

Suddenly, the virus reappeared after 35 years, in mid-1996 in Uganda and Kenya. The disease spread into the neighboring Mbarara and Masaka districts of Uganda and in the bordering Bukoba district of northern Tanzania. By October, 1997, the virus appeared to be moving slowly northward within Uganda, following valleys and swampy areas, apparently helped by the current rains.

Symptoms and Diagnostic Path

The initial symptoms of o'nyong-nyong fever are high fever and generalized skin rash with crippling arthritis, primarily in the big joints. Other symptoms include headache, eye pain and reddening with no discharge, chest pain, and general malaise. Patients recover within about two weeks, though occasionally continued joint pain can occur. All age groups and both sexes are equally affected.

In areas where the disease is epidemic, up to 80 percent of the people are infected, many of which cluster in affected households.

The virus is carried by two mosquitoes—*Anopheles funestus* and *Anopheles gambiae*, which also carry MALARIA.

Treatment Options and Outlook

There is no cure. Treatment of symptoms can ease discomfort. No deaths have been reported, but two miscarriages have been associated with infection.

opportunistic infections   An infection caused by normally harmless organisms that do not usually produce disease in healthy people. These infections usually occur among patients whose resistance has been impaired by such disorders as diabetes, AIDS, or cancer; by a surgical procedure such as a urinary tract catheterization; or by immunosuppressive drugs.

Long-term use of antibiotics or other drugs also may interfere with the normal function of the immune system, creating a chance for normally harmless organisms to become harmful.

Most AIDS patients die not of their disease but of the accompanying opportunistic infections (especially *Pneumocystis pneumonia*). Other infections often contracted by AIDS patients include fungal infections (such as CRYPTOCOCCOSIS and CANDIDIASIS) and some viral infections (such as CYTOMEGALOVIRUS and HERPES). Because of the underlying immune system problems of AIDS patients, opportunistic infections are often unavoidable. However, they can be prevented to some extent with prophylactic antimicrobial drugs.

oral polio vaccine   See POLIOMYELITIS.

orbital cellulitis   See CELLULITIS.

ornithosis   Also known as psittacosis or parrot fever, this serious bacterial disease is caught from infected exotic imported birds. It is not possible to catch the disease from another human. The disease is found throughout the world and occurs all year long. Adults are more likely to be infected than children.

Cases must be reported to the local health department so the source of the infection can be traced. Infected birds that cannot be treated with tetracycline must be killed to prevent spread of the disease. The cage of an infected bird must be cleaned, disinfected, and thoroughly aired, since the droppings contain the bacteria. When purchasing a pet bird, consumers should always ask whether the bird has been checked for parrot fever.

Parrot fever is caused by the bacteria CHLAMYDIA PSITTACI, carried by parakeets, parrots, pigeons, turkeys, ducks, geese, and canaries. Rarely, the snowy egret or seagulls carry the disease. The bacteria is shed in droppings and feathers, which are infectious for months; the more stressed the infected bird, the higher percentage of virus shed. A human can become ill by inhaling dust containing the bacteria or by being bitten by an infected bird. Pet birds kept indoors or in an enclosed area (such as a pet shop) are at higher risk for the disease.

Symptoms and Diagnostic Path

Symptoms appear within four to 15 days after infection, and include headache, loss of appetite, muscle aches, chills, sore throat, congestion, chest pain, and sometimes pneumonia. As the fever rises, a dry cough develops. Chest X-rays will show PNEUMONIA. The fever may last for up to three weeks, only gradually falling back to normal. Patients with a particularly bad case (and older people usually are sickest) may not feel completely well for a long time.

Because parrot fever is similar to other pneumonias, a physician will reach a diagnosis in part if there is a history of proximity to birds, since it is not easy to isolate the bacteria. A blood sample taken during the illness can be compared with another sample taken three weeks later; an increase in antibodies to the bacteria confirms the diagnosis.

Treatment Options and Outlook

Tetracycline will cure parrot fever. Acetaminophen can bring down fever above 101°F, and bed rest and fluids will help ease symptoms. Codeine or other cough suppressants may be prescribed for an especially bad cough.

Rarely, parrot fever can lead to infections of the brain and heart. About 30 percent of untreated victims will die.

osteomyelitis   A local or generalized infection of bone and bone marrow, most commonly affecting the long bones in children and the vertebrae in adults. A chronic form of the disease may persist for years, with periodic flareups, despite treatment.

Osteomyelitis is usually caused by bacteria (usually staphylococci) introduced into the bone directly during surgery or trauma, from a nearby infection or from the bloodstream.

Symptoms and Diagnostic Path

Symptoms include persistent, severe, and increasing bone pain; tenderness; regional muscle spasm; and fever. During the early stages of the disease, pain is severe.

Treatment Options and Outlook

Bed rest, antibiotics for months. Surgery may be necessary to remove bone and tissue and to stabilize affected bone. Absolute rest of the affected part may be necessary, with careful positioning using pillows and sandbags.

otitis externa   Also known as "swimmer's ear," this is an inflammation of the outer ear caused by infection or because of a generalized skin disorder (such as atopic eczema or seborrheic dermatitis). It is most common in people with dry or waxy ears.

A generalized infection of the ear that may be caused by BACTERIA, VIRUSES, FUNGI, or trauma. It may affect the entire ear canal and sometimes also the external ear, producing a persistent inflammation called otomycosis. STAPHYLOCOCCUS AUREUS, PSEUDOMONAS AERUGINOSA, and Streptococcus pyogenes are common bacterial causes. HERPES simplex and herpes zoster viruses may be involved.

Malignant otitis externa is a rare (and sometimes fatal) form of the disease caused by the bacterium Pseudomonas aeruginosa. This type of otitis sometimes spreads into surrounding bones and soft tissue and usually affects elderly diabetics with a lowered resistance to disease.

Treatment Options and Outlook

Usually the only required treatment is a thorough cleaning and drying of the ear together with local antibiotic, antifungal, or antiinflammatory drugs. Patients should avoid getting the ear wet until the condition is completely healed; ear canals that are badly swollen may need to use a wick to instill drops into the ear. Nonprescription painkillers may ease pain. Consult a doctor if there is blood, pus, or serum flowing from the ear, or if the ear is red and tender to touch.

Risk Factors and Preventive Measures

People should avoid swimming in dirty water and dry ears after swimming with a blow dryer.

otitis media   See EAR INFECTION.

otomycosis   A fungal ear infection also known as mycotic OTITIS EXTERNA.

Otomycosis is caused by a fungus infection of the outer ear canal, including either *Aspergillus fumigatus, A. niger, Candida albicans,* or *C. tropicalis.* Secondary bacterial infections are common.

Symptoms and Diagnostic Path

Symptoms include inflammation, itching, scaling, and severe discomfort.

Treatment Options and Outlook

This can become a chronic, recurring infection; it is treated with Burow's solution or 5 percent aluminum acetate solution to reduce swelling. Debris is removed in the physician's office. Antifungal drops are often helpful.

pandemic A widespread epidemic occurring throughout the population of a country or the world.

papillomavirus, human (HPV) A group of more than 70 viruses that cause WARTS, including genital warts, PLANTAR WARTS, and a host of other types that cause warts on the hands or feet. There is no cure for the HPV virus.

See WARTS, GENITAL.

paragonimiasis A disease caused by a lung fluke (parasitic flatworm) that is found throughout the Far East, West Africa, South Asia, Indonesia, New Guinea, Central America, and northern South America. It is not likely that casual travelers would come in contact with this disease because it is not found in areas frequented by tourists.

The disease is caused by a type of flatworm that infects humans who eat raw crabs or crayfish. The infectious cycle begins when the eggs of the infective lung fluke reach water through sputum or feces and hatch in three to six weeks. These first develop in the freshwater snail, then enter crayfish and freshwater crabs, where they develop tissue cysts. Humans become infected when they handle or eat the raw or pickled crabs and crayfish; the immature flukes are then released and penetrate the peritoneal cavity in the stomach area and travel to other tissues (such as the lungs).

Symptoms and Diagnostic Path

Some people with mild infection have no symptoms. In others, the worms develop in tissue and start to reproduce about six weeks after ingestion. The most common symptoms of a lung infestation begins with a low fever and dry cough followed by a productive cough that may be bloody. The infection progresses slowly, eventually causing fatigue, weight loss, shortness of breath, and weakness. Other symptoms may depend on the area of the body that is involved, such as the abdomen or central nervous system.

Treatment Options and Outlook

Praziquantel is the drug treatment of choice. Bithionol is an alternative choice. Surgery may be needed to remove the cysts.

Risk Factors and Preventive Measures

The best way to avoid this disease is not to eat raw, undercooked, or pickled crabs, crayfish, or other crustaceans.

parainfluenza A common virus that causes respiratory infections in infants and young children and more rarely, in adults. Types I and II may cause CROUP; type III is also a cause of croup, BRONCHIOLITIS, and bronchopneumonia in children; types I, III, and IV are associated with sore throats and the COMMON COLD.

The parainfluenza virus are included in the paramyxovirus group (a group of RNA-containing viruses) that includes the RESPIRATORY SYNCYTIAL VIRUS and the agents causing MEASLES and MUMPS.

Between 90 percent and 100 percent of children over age five have antibodies to type-III, and about 75 percent have antibodies to type-I and -II. The different types occur at different times of the year and have different symptoms. Type-I causes biennial outbreaks of croup in the fall during odd numbered years. Type-II causes annual or biennial fall outbreaks, while type-III occurs mostly during the spring and early summer months each year, although the virus can be found throughout the year.

Symptoms and Diagnostic Path

Symptoms vary depending on the type of infection. A runny nose and mild cough are common. Life-threatening respiratory symptoms may occur in young infants with bronchiolitis.

Treatment Options and Outlook

Most infections in adults and older children are mild and do not require treatment. Treatment may be necessary if breathing difficulties or respiratory distress develop.

Secondary bacterial infections are the most common complication. Airway obstruction in croup and bronchiolitis can be severe and potentially life-threatening.

Risk Factors and Preventive Measures

No vaccine is currently available to protect against infection; however, researchers are developing vaccines against type-I and -III infection. Passively acquired maternal antibodies may play a role in protection from types-I and -II in the first few months of life.

Frequent handwashing and using separate cups, glasses, and utensils should decrease the spread of virus. Excluding children with colds or other respiratory illnesses (without fever) who are well enough to attend child care or school settings will probably not decrease the spread of the parainfluenzas, because the viruses are often spread in the early stages of illness.

parasites Any living thing that dwells in or on another living organism. The parasite, which may spend part or all of its time on the host, gets food and shelter from the host and contributes nothing to its welfare. It satisfies its nutritional requirements from the host's blood or tissues, or from the host's diet, which allows the parasite to multiply.

Some parasites carry disease, irritate tissue, and interfere with bodily functions. Others release toxins into the body's tissue. Human parasites include FUNGUS, BACTERIA, VIRUSES, PROTOZOA, and WORMS.

parasiticide An agent that destroys PARASITES (excluding bacteria and fungi).

paratyphoid fever A serious bacterial infection sometimes called Salmonella paratyphi infection or SALMONELLOSIS. It is also grouped together with TYPHOID FEVER under the name "enteric fever."

In the past, medical workers found that some instances of what appeared to be a milder version of typhoid fever were not caused by the same bacterium that produces typhoid, so they named the infection paratyphoid fever. Because bacteria in the same family as that which produces typhoid are the cause, the disease is known popularly as Salmonella (the name of the bacterial genus). Thus the disease today is more often called salmonella, salmonella poisoning, or salmonellosis than paratyphoid fever.

There are about 2,200 species of Salmonella bacteria and a few of these species infect as many as 2 to 4 million persons in the United States each year. It is considered to be a food-borne illness.

Paratyphoid fever is caused by infection of any of four different species of Salmonella bacteria: *Salmonella typhi* and *S. paratyphi A, B,* and *C.* The virus can be transmitted from animals or animal products to humans, or from person to person. It is often transmitted by consuming contaminated water and food, especially contaminated shellfish, raw fruits and vegetables, and raw milk.

Symptoms and Diagnostic Path

Symptoms appear slowly in adults, but are often sudden in children. Paratyphoid fever has three stages: a high fever heralds the first stage, together with headache and loss of appetite. The patient typically develops an enlarged spleen. About 30 percent of patients have rose spots on the front of the chest during the first week of illness. The rose spots develop into small hemorrhages that may be hard to see in African or Native Americans.

This is followed by a toxic stage with abdominal pain and intestinal symptoms of constipation or diarrhea. At this point, symptoms may resemble appendicitis, with intense cramping pain and tenderness in the right lower quadrant of the abdomen. During this stage, there is a one percent to 10 percent chance of intestinal perforation or hemorrhage.

The third stage involves a prolonged recovery period.

In adults, these three phases may last from four to six weeks, but illness in children may cover 10 days to two weeks. The incubation period is one to two weeks but is often shorter in children.

Since symptoms are similar to those of viral gastroenteritis, a physician needs to make a positive identification of bacteria using a culture of a stool sample so that an appropriate antibiotic can be prescribed. If the symptoms are caused by a virus, an antibiotic is ineffective.

Treatment Options and Outlook

Paratyphoid fever is treated over a two- to three-week period with trimethoprim-sulfamethoxazole, amoxicillin, and ampicillin. Third-generation cephalosporins or chloramphenicol may be given if the specific strain is resistant to other antibiotics. Patients with intestinal perforation or hemorrhage may need surgery if the infection cannot be controlled by antibiotics.

Most patients with paratyphoid fever recover completely, although intestinal complications can be fatal. With early treatment, the mortality rate is less than 1 percent.

paronychia   An infection of the skin at the base of the nail usually caused by the yeast CANDIDA ALBICANS, although bacteria are sometimes at fault. The condition is most often found among women with poor circulation or who must wash their hands often.

Symptoms and Diagnostic Path

Symptoms include a painful lesion at the base of the nail at the cuticle, with redness and swelling. There may be pus-filled blisters. Paronychia can be diagnosed by the appearance of the lesion.

Treatment Options and Outlook

Antifungal or antibiotic drugs will cure this problem. The hands must be kept dry; any abscess must be surgically drained.

parrot fever   See ORNITHOSIS.

parvovirus B19   The virus that causes FIFTH DISEASE (erythema infectiosum), a mild and common childhood illness. Fifth disease got its name in 1899 because it was the fifth of six common childhood illnesses discovered that caused a rash.

The virus was discovered in 1975 by English scientists, who did not know what disease it caused. Six years later; researchers were able to link parvovirus with a plastic crisis (a serious complication that affects people with sickle-cell disease when exposed to the virus). In 1983 scientists finally discovered that it caused fifth disease. The virus is present in blood and mouth or nose secretions.

Pasteurella   A genus of bacilli, including species that cause disease in both humans and animals. Pasteurella infections may be transmitted to humans via animal bites. The plague bacillus Pasteurella pestis is now called YERSINIA (PASTEURELLA) PESTIS; P. tularensis (which causes TULAREMIA) has been reclassified as FRANCISELLA TULARENSIS.

Pasteurella multocida   A species of gram-negative bacteria that usually infects animals but can be transmitted to humans through a bite or scratch. It causes wound and skin infections and occasionally blood poisoning. The bacteria live in the mouths and throats of 90 percent of cats and up to 60 percent of dogs.

See also PASTEURELLOSIS.

Pasteurella pestis   The PLAGUE bacillus that is now known as YERSINIA (PASTEURELLA) PESTIS.

Pasteurella tularensis   A type of bacillus that causes TULAREMIA and has been reclassified as FRANCISELLA TULARENSIS.

pasteurellosis   A bacterial disease transmitted by cats or dogs, who harbor the bacteria PASTEURELLA MULTOCIDA in their mouths and throats. About 90 percent of cats, and about half of all dogs, are colonized.

The disease is usually transmitted by the bite or scratch of an infected cat; dog bites are much less likely to cause an infection. About half of the people who are bitten by cats develop the infection. It is also possible (although very unlikely) to pick up this infection simply by breathing in the bacteria, if the patient lives in close proximity with a pet.

Wild animals also carry this bacteria.

Symptoms and Diagnostic Path

One to two days after being bitten or scratched, symptoms of pain, heat, redness, or swelling will appear. The area of the bite may begin to drain (either clear or puslike), and there may be fever or chills. The glands nearest the wound may swell.

If the infection was transmitted by breathing in bacteria, symptoms may include cough, fever, chills, and ear or chest pain.

A lab can easily identify the bacteria found in drainage from the wound by culturing the organism.

Treatment Options and Outlook

Augmentin (amoxicillin-clavulante) will cure the infection; those who are allergic to PENICILLIN can take tetracycline. Wounds that swell and fill with pus must be drained.

Risk Factors and Preventive Measures

All bites and scratches should be washed immediately with soap and water. A serious infection can be prevented by prompt antibiotic treatment, so patients should seek medical treatment if the bite wound is significant.

There are no vaccines for animal to protect cats and dogs against pasturella.

pasteurization The process of applying heat for a certain amount of time in order to kill bacteria. By law, milk pasteurization requires a temperature of 145°F to 150°F for not less than 30 minutes, followed by a temperature of 161°F for 15 seconds, followed by immediate cooling.

The process was developed by French chemist Louis Pasteur (1822–95), who established the germ theory of infection and masterminded the development of several types of vaccines.

pea pickers' disease See LEPTOSPIROSIS.

pediculosis An inflammation of the hairy parts of the body or clothing with LICE—head lice, body lice, or pubic lice. Head lice are usually found on the scalp; crab lice in the pubic area; and body lice, along seams of clothing.

The crawling stages of lice feed on human blood. Anyone can become louse-infested under suitable conditions; lice are easily transmitted from person to person during direct contact. Head lice infestations are often found in schools or institutions, where children share hats or combs. Crab lice can be found among sexually active individuals. Body lice can be found among people living in crowded, dirty conditions where clothing is not often changed or washed. The lice can be spread as long as lice or eggs remain alive on the body or clothing.

Symptoms and Diagnostic Path

It may take up to two or three weeks between infestation and the onset of intense itching. The first indication of lice infestation is usually itching or scratching in an area of the body where the lice feed. Head lice often cause itching around the back of the head or around the ears. Itching in the genital area may be caused by pubic lice, and can be so severe that it leads to a secondary bacterial infection.

Treatment Options and Outlook

Medicated shampoos or cream rinses containing pyrethrins are used to kill lice, and are available without prescription. While products containing lindane are still available through prescription, lindane is no longer the recommended drug of choice because of concerns about side effects. Retreatment after seven to 10 days is recommended to assure no eggs have survived. Nit combs are available to help remove nits from the hair.

Risk Factors and Preventive Measures

Physical contact with infected individuals and their belongings (especially clothing, headgear, and bedding) should be avoided. Bedding and clothing should be washed in hot water (140°F for 20 minutes) or dry cleaned to kill the lice and eggs.

Pediculus humanus capitis A species of LICE that lives only on the human scalp, where it feeds by sucking blood.

Pediculus humanus corporis A species of body LICE.

Pediculus humanus pubis The medical term for crab LICE (crabs).

pelvic abscess A pelvic infection that contains pus.

pelvic inflammatory disease (PID) Infection of the ovaries, uterus, or fallopian tubes that can lead to infertility, ectopic pregnancy, chronic pelvic pain, ABSCESSES, and other serious problems. PID is the most common preventable cause of infertility in the United States, and more than 1 million American women are treated for this condition every year. However, an equal number of women may have PID and not know it. PID is more common among teenagers than adults and more common among African-American and Hispanic women than Caucasians. Every year, more than 100,000 women become infertile and more than a 100 women die from PID or its complications.

PID is second only to AIDS as the most serious complication of sexually transmitted diseases.

While it may not have an obvious cause, PID often is linked to an untreated sexually transmitted disease such as GONORRHEA or CHLAMYDIAL INFECTION. It also may occur after childbirth, abortion, or miscarriage. Young, sexually active women and those who use an intrauterine device are at higher risk.

The bacteria travel from the cervix to the fallopian tubes and ovaries, leading to permanent scarring of the tubes. The more times a woman contracts PID, the greater the likelihood she will be sterile because of scarring. Younger women are more at risk for the disease because their reproductive organs are not as good at fighting off infection.

Symptoms and Diagnostic Path
Most women have no symptoms in the early stages. As the disease progresses, symptoms may include fever, painful urination or intercourse, pelvic pain, heavy menstrual flow with severe cramps, bleeding between periods, vaginal discharge, low backache, nausea, and vomiting. The cervix is tender if palpated during physical exam. Youngest women tend to have the most severe symptoms.

A sample from the cervix can be cultured, and blood counts will help reveal the infection. If the diagnosis is still unclear, a physician can examine the fallopian tubes with a laparoscope in the hospital to assess the condition of the tubes.

Treatment Options and Outlook
Antibiotics will kill the bacteria that cause the disease; because PID may be caused by many different types of bacteria, several different types of antibiotics effective against a wide range of bacteria (including those causing chlamydia and gonorrhea) will be prescribed.

Patients may require hospitalization if they are severely ill, are pregnant, do not respond to or cannot take oral medicine, need IV antibiotics, or have an abscess in the fallopian tube or ovary. If symptoms continue or the abscess does not improve, surgery may be required. Complications of PID, such as chronic pelvic pain and scarring, are difficult to treat, but sometimes improve with surgery.

A woman's sex partner may be infected with bacteria that can cause PID even without symptoms. To protect herself from being re-infected with bacteria that cause PID, a woman's sex partners should be treated even if they do not have symptoms. Women should not have sex with partners who have not been treated.

Risk Factors and Preventive Measures
Women who have the highest risk for developing PID include those at risk for sexually transmitted infections and those with a prior episode of PID. Sexually active women under age 25 also are at risk

because the cervix of a teen or a young woman is more susceptible to a sexually transmitted infection. Other potential risk factors include frequent douching. Some women who use an intrauterine device as a birth control method also develop PID. Rarely, PID results from gynecological procedures or surgeries.

PID can be prevented by avoiding exposure to sexually transmitted diseases. Any unusual discharge or pelvic pain should be checked out by a physician.

Because PID is a very serious disease that can permanently damage the reproductive organs, it is important for patients who engage in unprotected sex or who have many partners to have regular checkups.

penicillin The first antibiotic prescribed for general use, it was developed from a type of mold first discovered by Scottish scientist Alexander Fleming. His discovery led to the development of a wide range of antibiotics, one of the most powerful weapons in the war against bacterial infection.

Although penicillins are still used, their value has been lessened by the widespread development of resistance among bacteria, and also by some people's allergic reactions to penicillin.

The biggest difference between bacterial and normal cells is the thick cell wall that protects the bacterial cell membrane. Normal human cells do not have this cell wall, and so any substance that interferes only with cell wall formation could not damage a human host. Penicillins and related antibiotics work by interfering with the synthesis of the bacterial cell wall. This is why they are among the safest of drugs—they cannot harm healthy cells.

Fleming first reported his findings in the British medical journal *Lancet* in 1941, together with Ernst Chain, Howard Florey, and other Oxford University scientists. Four years later, Fleming shared the Nobel Prize in medicine with Chain and Florey.

It is difficult today to fully comprehend the profound danger of bacterial infection prior to the late 1930s. Even in young and strong patients, PNEUMONIA was a common cause of death. Each year, many women died from "childbed fever"—strep infection of the uterus (puerperal septicemia), and infections

caused 40 percent of all children's deaths in the United States.

The story of penicillin's discovery began in 1928, when Fleming noticed mold had contaminated a dish in which he had been growing staphylococci bacteria. Oddly enough, the bacteria had almost completely disappeared in areas where the mold was growing, destroyed by some substance the mold had produced. Because the particular mold was called *Penicillium notatum,* Fleming named the substance penicillin.

It was not until 1938 that Ernst Chain, a refugee from Nazi Germany, came across Fleming's work; he and Howard Florey obtained a grant from the Rockefeller Foundation for further research. By 1940 the two had recorded incredible results from their experiments. In 1941, *Lancet* reported their amazing findings, in which penicillin had been prescribed for "hopeless" cases. A year later, a Russian-American microbiologist coined the term *antibiotic* for this new type of drug.

It was very difficult to produce enough penicillin, especially since Britain's chemical industry was dedicated to meeting wartime needs. As a result, Oxford scientists grew penicillin-producing cultures in bedpans and cookie tins, and doctors recovered penicillin from the urine of treated patients. Not until the end of World War II was there enough penicillin available for general use outside the military. It was still so hard to find that in liberated Europe in 1945, there was a substantial black market for penicillin.

Penicillin had a significant impact on war casualties, dramatically improving the survival rate of soldiers with infected wounds. At the time, the only antimicrobial drugs available were quinine, quinacrine, the arsenicals, and the SULFONAMIDES. Of these, only the sulfa drugs fought bacterial infections, and they had only limited use because of their toxicity.

Once scientists understood the structure of the original penicillin molecule, they began to modify it, leading to semisynthetic penicillins.

There are at least 20 different kinds of penicillin (see box) divided into four different types:

- *narrow-spectrum penicillin-G types:* These are effective against gram-positive strains of streptococci, staphylococci, enterococci, and meningococci and are used to treat such diseases as SYPHILIS, GONOR-RHEA, MENINGITIS, ANTHRAX, and YAWS. The related penicillin V is used for respiratory infections.

- *ampicillin and its relatives:* Ampicillin and amoxy-cillin have a range of effectiveness similar to that of penicillin-G types, with a slightly broader spec-trum, including gram-negative bacteria. Ampicill-in and its relatives are effective against TYPHOID FEVER, BRONCHITIS, URINARY TRACT INFECTIONS, PNEUMONIA, meningitis, and BACTEREMIA.
- *penicillinase-resistants:* These penicillins combat bacteria that have developed resistance to peni-cillin G.
- *antipseudomonal penicillins:* The aminoglycosides are penicillins that fight infections caused by gram-negative Pseudomonas bacteria, a particu-lar problem in hospitals. These penicillins are administered as a preventive to patients with impaired immune systems who are at risk from gram-negative infections.

PENICILLINS
amdinocillin
amoxicillin
amoxicillin and clavulanate
ampicillin
ampicillin and sulbactam
azlocillin
bacampicillin
carbenicillin
cloxacillin
cyclacillin
dicloxacillin
methicillin
mezlocillin
nafcillin
oxacillin
penicillin G
penicillin V
piperacillin
ticarcillin
ticarcillin and clavulanate

Today, 25,000 metric tons of penicillin are pro-duced each year, most of which are used to help produce other antibiotics.

Unfortunately, scientists are faced with a growing problem of bacterial resistance to many of the peni-cillins. Bacteria are broadly classified into two types, gram-negative and gram-positive, depending on how they respond to a particular staining technique. The gram-negative bacteria (such as *ESCHERICHIA COLI, Proteus,* and *Pseudomonas*) are far less susceptible to the penicillin family than are the gram-positive bac-teria, such as *STREPTOCOCCUS.* Later antibiotics (includ-ing newer forms of penicillin) are much more effective against the gram-negative organisms.

Still, the bacterial ability to adapt to antibiotics seem almost limitless. As antibiotic use became common, the incidence of bacterial resistance increased to the point where some scientists con-sider it an overwhelming problem. Sometimes, the extensive use of an antibiotic eliminates sensitive bacterial strains and favors the development of strains that possess natural resistance. This occurred with the proliferation of penicillin-resistant staphy-lococci. This resistance can be transferred from resistant bacteria to nonresistance forms because

genetic material tends to be shared and traded among bacteria.

In addition, using inadequate doses of antibiotics encourages resistance because instead of killing them, it allows bacteria to adapt. Using antibiotics inappropriately has also played a significant role. Physicians who prescribe certain types of broad spectrum antibiotics instead of reserving them for resistant infections curtail the drugs' useful life.

pertussis   See WHOOPING COUGH.

pets and infectious disease   Pet owners can point to a plethora of benefits from their cats and dogs, including reduced stress, higher survival rates, increased self-confidence, and improved self-esteem among children. But pets also can carry very real health risks:

Cats, dogs, birds, reptiles, and other small ani-mals can transmit diseases to humans.

The realization that pets can carry disease is not a new one. Ancient Greeks knew exactly where RABIES came from—the bite of a rabid dog. And the bubonic PLAGUE that wiped out half of the population of 15th-century Europe was understood to move from rodents to animals by way of fleas.

The list of animal-transmitted conditions is constantly lengthening. Fortunately, most of these diseases are rare and almost all can be treated. They include

BIRD FLU Bird flu is an emerging infection now spreading around the world caused by avian influenza viruses that occur naturally among birds. Wild birds worldwide carry the viruses in their intestines and have begun fatally infecting domesticated birds including chickens, ducks, and turkeys.

As infected birds shed the virus in their saliva, nasal secretions, and feces, other birds become infected from contaminated secretions or excretions. If humans come into contacted with the infected birds, they may contract an often-fatal case of bird flu. A particularly virulent strain of bird flu (H5N1 strain) has been found throughout Asia and parts of Europe, Iran, and India. At the moment, bird flu is not transmitted by eating poultry, but by very intimate, close contact between humans and infected poultry.

CAT-SCRATCH DISEASE This infection is caused by a cat bite or scratch. The bite wound is slow to heal and may cause other mild symptoms. The disease is rarely serious, but antibiotics can help treat it if necessary.

LYME DISEASE This disease is not in itself caused by animals, but by a tick to on a cat or dog. Lyme disease has many symptoms including rashes and arthritis. Antibiotic treatment is imperative to prevent the disease from progressing. There is now a vaccine for dogs who live in high-risk areas, but its effectiveness is as yet uncertain.

PSITTACOSIS "Parrot fever" is a bacterial disease infecting 130 species of domestic and wild birds, most commonly ducks, turkeys, chickens, parrots, and pigeons. Humans get the disease from parrots or parakeets by contact with feces and feather dust, experiencing cough, fever, chills, and vomiting. Bird symptoms may include poor eating habits or droopy feathers. Wearing a surgical or dust mask and rubber gloves while cleaning a bird's cage will help protect against this disease. A blood test can confirm the diagnosis and antibiotics will treat the disease in both bird and human.

RABIES Currently epidemic among certain wild animals in the northeast, rabies can be transmitted to humans by a bite from a rabid animal. In the Northeast, canine rabies is controlled and the main source of infection is from bats, although unvaccinated cats and other wildlife are also sources. Vaccination of pet dogs and cats is imperative to stop the spread of this deadly disease. In humans bitten by an infected animal, the disease can be prevented if treatment with rabies shots is begun immediately.

ROCKY MOUNTAIN SPOTTED FEVER This tick-borne disease is found throughout the United States; early antibiotic treatment can head off serious complications, including a sometimes-fatal inflammation of lungs, liver, and heart.

RINGWORM Cats (especially long-haired kittens), dogs, horses, and cows can all pass on this fungal skin disease that has nothing to do with worms. Pets are the usual carriers. The fungus infects cat hair, which is passed on to humans who pet a cat. It causes an inflamed lesion on the skin or in the scalp. Antifungal drugs and iodine-based soap cure the problem in humans.

ROUNDWORM This parasite is carried most often by nursing dogs and their puppies, and less often by cats. Virtually all puppies have roundworm, and because children play in the dirt they are most likely to pick up the parasite. The disease is transmitted through contact with the dog's feces or contaminated soil. So common is the presence of the dog roundworm that worm-free pups can only be produced by raising several generations in isolation, or giving high doses of worm medication to the pregnant mother. Both pups and humans can be treated with worm medication (ANTI-HELMINTIC DRUGS).

SALMONELLOSIS Infections with the *Salmonella* bacteria can cause GASTROENTERITIS. The bacteria are carried by birds and dogs, although turtles present the largest risk. The sale of pet-sized turtles (less than 4 inches) was banned in 1975. Since a wild turtle is just as likely to have *Salmonella*, it should not be considered as a pet either.

HOW TO PROTECT PETS AND FAMILY

- Cages/pens should be scrupulously clean and free from droppings.
- Solid waste should be removed from cat litter box daily.
- Pets should be clean and free from ticks, fleas, and mites.
- Pets should not eat raw meat.
- Children should not handle unfamiliar pets.
- Children should not handle a sick animal.
- Children should wash hands after handling an animal.
- Wild animals should not be adopted as pets if they are injured;
- Dogs should not be walked in tick-infested areas in summer.
- Pet waste should not be used as fertilizer; this material has little value and can spread disease.
- Sandboxes should be covered when not in use.
- Pets should be checked daily for ticks.

STREP THROAT Unknown to many people, the streptococcal bacteria that cause strep throat can be carried in a dog's throat and can cause repeated infections in its human family. In cases of repeated infection in a family, the dog's throat should be checked as a possible source of infection.

TOXOPLASMOSIS This disease is transmitted to humans most often by a parasite in cat feces or contaminated dirt. All cat breeds can become infected with the parasite. Cats become infected by killing and eating small rodents. Most people contract the disease not from cats, however, but from raw meat. The meat becomes infected because sheep and cattle graze in pastures contaminated with toxoplasmosis. The disease, which causes few symptoms, except in AIDS patients, when it can be lethal, can be treated with antibacterial drugs. Expectant mothers can suffer miscarriage, premature birth, or birth defects if they are infected during the first three months of pregnancy.

Pfiesteria piscicida A member of a 450-million-year-old family of one-celled marine organisms that live in warm brackish waters of tidal estuaries and cause huge fish kills from Delaware to North Carolina similar to RED TIDE. It also has been blamed on some human health problems. The microscopic toxic dinoflagellate sometimes behaves like a plant and sometimes like an animal.

Discovered in 1988 by researchers at North Carolina State University, *Pfiesteria piscicida* is now known to have a highly complex life cycle with 24 reported forms, a few of which can produce toxins. However, *Pfiesteria* is not an infectious agent such as BACTERIA, VIRUSES, and FUNGI.

Pfiesteria normally exists in nontoxic forms, feeding on algae and bacteria in the water and in sediments of tidal rivers and estuaries. Scientists believe it only becomes toxic in the presence of schooling fish such as Atlantic menhaden, triggered by their secretions or excrement in the water. At that point, *Pfiesteria* cells begin emitting a powerful toxin that stuns the fish. Other toxins are believed to break down fish skin tissue, opening bleeding sores or lesions.

The toxins or lesions are frequently fatal to the fish. Fish also may die without developing lesions. As fish are incapacitated, the *Pfiesteria* cells feed on their tissues and blood.

Toxic outbreaks of *Pfiesteria* typically last a few hours, and the subsequent toxins in the water break down within a few hours. However, once fish are weakened by the toxins, *Pfiesteria*-related lesions or fish kills may persist for days or weeks.

P. piscicida is known to occur in brackish coastal waters from the Delaware Bay to North Carolina. Other *Pfiesteria*-like organisms occur along the southeast coast from Delaware to the Gulf of Mexico. *P. piscicida* has been implicated as a cause of major fish kills at many sites along the North Carolina coast; millions of fish have died from *Pfiesteria* in North Carolina. In 1997, *Pfiesteria* or *Pfiesteria*-like organisms killed thousands of fish in several Eastern Shore tributaries of the Chesapeake Bay.

Pfiesteria is not contagious or infectious. There is no evidence that *Pfiesteria*-related illnesses are associated with eating finfish, shellfish, or crustaceans. Human health problems associated with the microbe stem from the release of toxins into river and estuarine waters. Preliminary evidence suggests that exposure to waters where toxic forms of

Pfiesteria are active may cause memory loss, confusion, and a variety of other symptoms including respiratory, skin, and stomach problems. Similar human health effects can be caused by exposure to *Pfiesteria* toxins in a laboratory setting.

The U.S. CENTERS FOR DISEASE CONTROL AND PREVENTION, together with state health departments in Delaware, Florida, Georgia, Maryland, North Carolina, South Carolina, and Virginia, have established a surveillance system to collect reports of human illness thought to be related to exposure to *Pfiesteria* and *Pfiesteria*-like organisms.

There has never been a case of illness caused by eating fish or shellfish exposed to *Pfiesteria,* and there is no evidence of *Pfiesteria*-contaminated fish or shellfish on the market.

Scientists do not understand the exact conditions that cause toxic outbreaks of *Pfiesteria* to develop, although it is believed that a high density of fish must be present to trigger the shift of *Pfiesteria* cells into toxic forms. However, other factors may contribute to toxic *Pfiesteria* outbreaks by promoting the growth of *Pfiesteria* populations in coastal waters. These factors include warm, brackish waters and high levels of nutrients such as nitrogen and phosphorus. Some evidence suggests that nutrients may also directly stimulate the growth of Pfiesteria.

The precise role that nutrients and other factors may play in promoting toxic outbreaks of *Pfiesteria* is not clear. Excess nutrients are common pollutants in coastal waters. Chief sources of nutrient pollution in coastal areas are sewage treatment plants, septic tanks, polluted runoff from suburban landscape practices and agricultural operations, and air pollutants that settle on the land and water.

pharyngitis Acute inflammation of the pharynx (the part of the throat between the tonsils and the larynx). The chief symptom is a sore throat.

The illness is most often caused by a viral infection, although it also may be due to a bacterial infection such as *STREPTOCOCCUS*, MYCOPLASMA, or CHLAMYDIAL INFECTION. It is a common symptom of a COLD or INFLUENZA, of MONONUCLEOSIS or SCARLET FEVER. DIPHTHERIA is a rare cause of pharyngitis.

Symptoms and Diagnostic Path
In addition to the sore throat, there may be pain when swallowing, with a slight fever, earache, and tender, swollen lymph nodes in the neck. In very severe cases the fever may be quite high and the soft palate and throat may swell so that breathing becomes difficult. Extensive swelling and fluid buildup in the larynx can be life threatening.

Treatment Options and Outlook
Warm saltwater gargles and treatment may help, depending on the cause. Bacteria infections can be treated with antibiotics.

Especially severe or prolonged sore throats should be reported to a physician, who may take a THROAT CULTURE and prescribe antibiotics.

phlebovirus A genus including more than 50 viruses that are transmitted by mosquitoes or phlebotomine flies. RIFT VALLEY FEVER virus and SANDFLY FEVER virus are the most medically important of these viruses.

Phthirus Genus of lice that includes the species *Phthirus pubis*, the pubic louse (or crab).

pian See YAWS.

picornavirus A group of very small, single-strand RNA viruses that cause many different diseases, including colds, CONJUNCTIVITIS (pinkeye), herpangina, muscle infection, heart infection, and hepatitis. Probably no other family of viruses causes so many very types of different illnesses. The POLIOMYELITIS virus was one of the first recorded infections by a virus in this family. Another member of the picornaviruses is the HAND, FOOT, AND MOUTH DISEASE virus. (Foot-and-mouth disease in cows is caused by a separate bovine picornavirus).

The picornaviruses are divided into nine genra, including the ENTEROVIRUS (containing poliovirus, enterovirus, COXSACKIE VIRUS, ECHOVIRUS), RHI-

NOVIRUS (with about 105 serotypes), and HEPATOVI-RUS (hepatitis A virus), plus six other genera.

See also COLD, COMMON.

PID   See PELVIC INFLAMMATORY DISEASE.

pinkeye   See CONJUNCTIVITIS.

pinta   A rare skin infection found in some remote tropical South and Central American villages, caused by the organism *Treponema carateum*, a close relative of the bacterium *Treponema pallidum* that causes SYPHILIS. Pinta is also called azula, carate or mal del pinto.

The bacterium enters the body through a break in the skin; prolonged exposure and close contact seem to be required for transmission.

Symptoms and Diagnostic Path
The infection begins with a large flat spot surrounded by smaller reddened areas on the face, neck, buttocks, hands, or feet; up to a year later these spots are followed by red skin patches that turn blue, brown, and then white. Lymph nodes are also swollen.

Because the bacteria causing the treponematoses and syphilis are so similar, a person with one of these infections tests positive for syphilis. Standard tests cannot tell the difference between treponematoses and syphilis.

Treatment Options and Outlook
PENICILLIN G or tetracycline will cure the disease, but patients may be permanently disfigured.

pinworm infestation   The most common parasitic infection in the United States known medically as ENTEROBIASIS. The human pinworm *(ENTEROBIUS VERMICULARIS)* lives only in the intestine. While it is not technically a worm, it does look like one. The species may sometimes be called "threadworm" or "seat worm." Pinworm infections affect about 200 million people across the world, including about one-third of the U.S. population. Schoolchildren are most at risk for pinworm infections.

The female pinworm is white, about a third of an inch long. Pinworms lay eggs in the skin around the anus. When a child scratches the area, the eggs are transferred directly by the fingers to the mouth to cause reinfestation. The eggs may also be carried on toys or blankets to other children. Once swallowed, the eggs hatch in the intestine, where they grow and reach maturity in about six weeks. Animal pinworm does not infect humans.

People become infected by unknowingly ingesting microscopic pinworm eggs found on a wide variety of objects, including bed linens and towels, underwear and pajamas, toilets and bathroom fixtures, food, glasses and silverware, kitchen counters, toys, school desks or lunch tables, and sandboxes.

Symptoms and Diagnostic Path
Pinworms cause tickling or itching in the anal region at night. Despite common folklore, neither teeth grinding, bed wetting, stomach aches, weight loss, poor appetite, nor appendicitis are caused by pinworms. Pinworms actually cause very little harm, but they do itch quite a lot.

The eggs can be picked up from the patient's anal area via sticky tape; they can then be identified under a microscope.

Treatment Options and Outlook
Ointment or carbolated petroleum jelly can relieve the itch, as can a sitz bath followed by cleaning with witch hazel around the anal area. One dose of a deworming drug (pyrantel pamoate) will kill the infestation; mebendazole is the alternative for children over age two. In order to kill the newly hatched adults, it is best to repeat the treatment in two weeks. All members of the household should be treated, whether or not they have symptoms. Bed linens of the affected patients should be changed daily without shaking the eggs into the air.

In rare cases, pinworms migrate into the vagina or bladder, leading to CYSTITIS or infection of the fallopian tubes. Severe infestations can interfere with sleep or cause secondary bacterial infections because of constant scratching.

Risk Factors and Preventive Measures
In order to prevent reinfection, all family members should be treated and bathe frequently. Everyone should wear pajamas to limit the number of eggs on

the bed sheets, and all bed linens and clothing should be washed in hot water to kill the eggs. All sleeping areas should be vacuumed daily for one week after treatment.

plague The scourge of early history, plague is a serious infectious disease transmitted by the bites of rat fleas. There are three major forms of the disease: bubonic, septicemic, and pneumonic, each of which can occur alone or together, as the disease moves throughout the body. *Bubonic plague* is centered in the lymphatic system, creating swelling lymph nodes (buboes), from which it gets its name. *Septicemic plague* affects the bloodstream. *Pneumonic plague* occurs when the bacteria enters the lungs.

Plague has been responsible for three great PANDEMICS, which caused millions of deaths around the world and significantly affected the course of history. Although the cause of the plague was not identified until the third pandemic in 1894, scientists are virtually certain that the first two pandemics were plague because a number of the survivors wrote about their experiences and described the symptoms, including the appearance of buboes.

The first great pandemic began in 542 C.E. during the reign of Emperor Justinian, and lasted for about 60 years. Plague affected parts of the Mediterranean region most heavily, and an estimated tens of millions of citizens died.

The second pandemic during the 14th century was nicknamed the "black death" because its primary symptom was black patches on the skin caused by bleeding around the buboes (swollen lymph glands). This was the most severe and historically significant pandemic of the three; it began in the mid-1300s in central Asia, and some historians believe it lasted for more than 400 years. About one-fourth of the entire population of Europe died within a few years after plague was first introduced into the continent in 1347. The Middle and Far East also suffered during this time.

The final pandemic (or Modern Pandemic) began in northern China, reaching Canton and Hong Kong in 1894. From here, plague quickly spread to all of the continents, killing millions. The bacteria also became established during this pandemic in wild rodent flea populations in areas that previously were plague-free, including some parts of North and South America and southern Africa.

Each of the great pandemics eventually came to an end, probably due to a number of factors. Seasonal or weather changes can adversely affect the survival of rodent hosts and fleas, together with control measures aimed at controlling rodents and fleas, sanitation measures, and use of antibiotics to prevent disease.

Recent outbreaks among humans have occurred in Africa, South America, and Southeast Asia. Plague is also found among ground squirrels, prairie dogs, and marmots in parts of Arizona, New Mexico, California, Colorado, and Nevada. Between 10 and 50 Americans each year contract plague during the spring and summer months. The last rat-borne epidemic in the United States occurred in Los Angeles in 1924–25; since then, all plague cases in the United States have been sporadic, acquired from wild rodents or their fleas.

Rock squirrels and their fleas are the most frequent sources of human infection in the southwestern states. In the Pacific states, the California ground squirrel and its fleas are the most common source. Many other rodents (prairie dogs, deer mice, wood rats, chipmunks, and other squirrels) suffer plague outbreaks that sometimes can infect humans.

The great pandemics of the past occurred when wild rodents spread the disease to rats in cities and then to humans when the rats died. A bite from an infected flea leads to bubonic plague; pneumonic plague is a complication of bubonic plague but is also spread via infected droplets during coughing.

In the United States during the 1980s, there were about 18 cases a year, usually in people under age 20.

Major epidemics are most likely to occur when rats live closely with humans in poverty-stricken areas with poor sanitation, and when humans share habitat with wild rodents infected with plague bacteria. Major outbreaks of primary pneumonic plague are most likely to occur under crowded conditions.

Recently, an outbreak of pneumonic plague struck the western Indian city of Surat. In addition, at least 41 cases of bubonic plague also had been reported in the city.

There are 1,000 to 2,000 cases of plague around the world each year. At present, there is no plague in Australia or in western Europe. In Asia and eastern Europe, plague is distributed from the Caucasus Mountains through much of the Middle East, eastward through China, southward to Asia. Plague also occurs in Africa, North America, and South America.

Fleas found on rodents can carry the plague bacterium YERSINIA PESTIS (formerly *Bacillus pestis* or *Pasteurella pestis*). More than 100 species of fleas have been reported to be naturally infected with plague.

Since 1924, there has been no documented case of human-to-human transmission of plague from droplets in the United States. All but one of the few pneumonic cases have been associated with handling infected cats. Dogs and cats can become infected after capturing or eating infected rodents. Dogs rarely exhibit signs of illness and are not known to transmit the disease to humans. However, plague *has* been transmitted from infected coyotes to humans. Cats often survive severe disease, and can pass their infections to humans via direct contact or the inhalation of infectious droplets from cats with plague pneumonia.

Person-to-person transmission without symptoms is very unlikely, but close contacts with pneumonic plague patients could transmit the disease through exposure to infected droplets.

Most experts believe that Swiss bacteriologist Alexandre Yersin first identified the bacterium that causes plague in 1894, while studying a plague outbreak in Hong Kong. The bacterium was later renamed in his honor.

Three different types of plague bacteria have been associated with the three pandemics. The first pandemic (Justinian's Plague) was caused by the "antiqua" type, the Black Death was related to the "mediavalis" type, and the Modern Pandemic to the "orientalis" strain.

Symptoms and Diagnostic Path

Two to five days after infection, patients experience sudden fever, shivering, seizures, and severe headaches followed by buboes—smooth, oval, reddened, and very painful swellings in the armpits, groin, or neck.

Pneumonic plague causes severe, overwhelming pneumonia, with shortness of breath, high fever, and blood in the phlegm. (Onset of these symptoms begins only one to three days after exposure.) If untreated, half the patients will die; if blood poisoning occurs as an early complication, patients may die before the buboes appear.

The most commonly affected sites are the lymph nodes nearest the site of first infection. As the bacteria multiply in the lymph nodes, they become swollen; as they collect fluid, they become extremely tender. If the bacteria invade the bloodstream, they can spread to other sites, including liver, kidneys, spleen, lungs, and sometimes the meninges and eyes. Occasionally, the bacteria will cause an ulcer at the point of first infection.

Discovery of a painful bubo, together with fever, exhaustion, and a history of possible exposure to rodents, rabbits, or fleas in the western United States, leads to a suspicion of plague. As soon as a diagnosis is suspected, the patient should be isolated, and local and state health departments should be notified. Blood cultures and examination of lymph node specimens can help diagnose the disease.

Treatment Options and Outlook

Plague can be treated successfully if it is caught early. Untreated pneumonic plague is almost always fatal, and the chances of survival are very low unless specific antibiotic treatment is started within 15 to 18 hours after symptoms appear.

Administration of streptomycin as soon as possible is the preferred treatment; alternatives include gentamicin, chloramphenicol, tetracycline, and trimethoprim/sulfamethoxazole. Chloramphenicol is specifically indicated in treating plague meningitis. Drug treatment reduces the risk of death to less than 5 percent.

Contacts of anyone with pneumonic plague are given antibiotics as a preventive measure at the first sign of disease.

Risk Factors and Preventive Measures

Untreated pneumonic plague patients can pass on their illness to close contacts throughout the course of the illness. All plague patients should be isolated for 48 hours after antibiotic treatment begins. Pneumonic plague patients should be completely isolated until sputum cultures are negative.

Residents of areas where plague occurs in the wild animals should make sure their home is rodent-proof. Anyone working in a rodent-infested area should use insect repellent on skin and clothing; pets should be treated with insecticidal dust and kept indoors. Handling sick or dead animals (especially rodents, rabbits, and cats) should be avoided.

Plague vaccines have been used since the late 19th century, but their effectiveness has not been proven. Field experience indicates that vaccination lowers the incidence and severity of disease caused by the bites of infected fleas. But the degree of protection against primary pneumonic infection is not known.

In the United States, plague vaccine comes in an injectable form, but it is not required by any country as a condition of entry. Because immunization requires multiple doses over a six to 10 month period, plague vaccine is not recommended for immediate protection during outbreaks. Its unpleasant side effects mean that it should not be considered unless the long-term risk of infection is substantial. Ordinary travelers do not need this vaccine.

Even those who receive the vaccine may not be completely protected; this is why it is still important to take precautionary measures against rodents, fleas, and people or animals with plague. For significant risk, antibiotic preventive treatment may boost immunity.

Those who should receive the plague vaccine include the following:

- those in direct contact with wild or domestic rodents or other animals where an epidemic is occurring among animals
- those who reside or work in plague-infested areas where it is hard to avoid rodents and fleas, especially in developing countries
- lab personnel or vets who work regularly with *Yersinia pestis* organisms or potentially plague-infected animals in risk areas
- military personnel deployed in plague-risk areas

However, the safety of the vaccine for those under age 18 or older than 61 has not been established. Anyone with a moderate or severe illness should delay receiving the vaccine. Pregnant women should not be vaccinated unless the need for protection surpasses the risk to the unborn child. Since beef protein, soy, casein, sulfite, phenol, and formaldehyde are all components of the vaccine, anyone with an allergy to any of these substances should inform the physician providing the vaccine. Anyone with a severe bleeding disorder should discuss the options, since the vaccine is given intramuscularly.

Side effects of the vaccine include tenderness at the site; a small percentage experience sore, swollen lymph glands, headache, and malaise. In rare cases, some people have nausea and vomiting or joint pain. There is a rare chance that other serious problems and even death may occur after getting the vaccine. Travelers should allow at least six months before departure for the three-dose primary vaccination schedule.

Plague is one of three diseases still subject to the International Health Regulations, which require that all confirmed cases be reported to the World Health Organization within 24 hours. The rules also state that all human cases be investigated to make sure the disease is not spread, and that passengers arriving on an infected (or one suspected of infection) ship or aircraft may be treated with insecticides and held for a period of up to six days after arrival. Health authorities also can require disinfection of baggage and any portion of the ship or aircraft.

According to the regulations, passengers on an international voyage who have been to an area where there is an epidemic or pneumonic plague must be placed in isolation for six days before being allowed to leave.

plane wart See WARTS.

plantar warts A hard, rough and painful WART found on the sole of the foot that may appear alone or in clusters. This type of wart is usually spread when infected people walk on a communal shower floor, contaminating it with the common wart virus PAPILLOMAVIRUS.

Symptoms and Diagnostic Path

Plantar warts are soft with a central core surrounded by a firm ring, much like a callus. Because of the constant pressure from the body, the wart is compressed, flattened, and forced into the sole of the foot. The wart usually has tiny black spots on the surface that are actually bits of coagulated blood.

Treatment Options and Outlook

Like many warts, plantar warts may disappear without treatment; some may come and go; and others may persist for years. A foam shoe pad may relieve discomfort. Alternatively, the warts may be removed by burning or cutting with laser treatment, or by salicylic acid plasters.

Plasmodium A genus of protozoa, four species of which cause MALARIA, transmitted to humans through the bite of an infected *Anopheles* mosquito. The two most important malaria-causing protozoa are *P. vivax*, and *P. falciparum*, which causes falciparum malaria (the most severe form of the disease). *P. malariae* and *P. ovale* are not as common, but are endemic to the Tropics.

Plesiomonas shigelloides A gram-negative rod-shaped bacterium found in freshwater, freshwater fish, shellfish and many animals, which may cause one type of gastroenteritis.

Most infections occur during the summer in tropical or subtropical areas in places with polluted freshwater, when a person ingests contaminated water or raw shellfish. Because most infections are so mild people do not seek medical treatment, the occurrence rate in the United States is not known. Infection with this bacterium may be included in the group of diarrheal disease of "unknown origin," which are treated with and respond to broad spectrum antibiotics.

Moreover, most cases that are reported in the United States involve individuals with preexisting health problems or very young patients. A cluster of cases occurred in New York in the summer of 1996, when 30 people got sick with diarrhea after a party. Water contaminated with *P. Shigelloides* was implicated as the cause.

Most human *P. shigelloides* infections seem to be connected with tainted water; the organism is found in unsanitary water used for swimming, drinking, or rinsing foods that are eaten raw. The dose required for infection is believed to be very high (at least more than 1 million organisms).

Symptoms and Diagnostic Path

P. shigelloides gastroenteritis is usually a self-limiting disease with fever, chills, abdominal pain, nausea, watery diarrhea, or vomiting. Symptoms usually begin about a day after eating contaminated food or water. In severe cases, diarrhea may be foamy, green-yellow, and tinged with blood.

Diarrhea is usually mild, but in infants and children under age 15 there may be high fever and chills. Patients with impaired immune systems or who are seriously ill with cancer or blood disorders can develop fatal blood poisoning.

This infection can be identified through bacteriological analysis.

See also GASTROENTERITIS, BACTERIAL.

pneumococcal vaccine An effective vaccine that has been available for a number of years to prevent pneumococcal PNEUMONIA in adults. Although it is safe and inexpensive, it has been underutilized. Doctors recommend the vaccine for high-risk patients, including those who

- are over age 50
- have no spleen
- have chronic lung problems
- have heart or kidney disease
- are diabetic or alcoholic
- live in an institution

A vaccine was approved in 2000 to prevent invasive pneumococcal diseases in infants and toddlers— diseases which can cause brain damage and, in rare cases, death. This vaccine (pneumococcal conjugate vaccine or PCV) is not indicated for use in adults or as a substitute for other approved pneumococcal polysaccharide vaccines approved for high-risk children over the age of two. The previous pneumococcal vaccine, called PPV, was not recommended for use in children under age two, who contract the most serious infections from this bacteria.

The PCV vaccine (Prevnar) protects against the organism *Streptococcus pneumoniae* (also known as PNEUMOCOCCUS), the leading cause of pneumonia, SINUSITIS, and MENINGITIS. It has been added to the recommended schedule of childhood immunizations. It is given to infants as a series of four inoculations administered at two, four, six, and 12 to 15 months of age. If a child cannot begin the vaccine at two months, parents should discuss alternative schedules with their doctor.

Prevnar is the first pneumococcal vaccine for children under the age of two that targets the most common seven strains of pneumococcus causing 80 percent of invasive disease in infants. For the first time, doctors have a highly effective way to prevent a major cause of meningitis and serious blood infections in the most susceptible children.

It is estimated that each year in the United States there are about 16,000 cases of pneumococcal bacteremia and 1,400 cases of pneumococcal meningitis among children under age five. In up to half the cases of meningitis, brain damage and hearing loss occurs and about 10 percent die. There are different types of bacterial meningitis. Before the approval of the first Haemophilus influenza type b (HIB) conjugate vaccine in 1990 for infants, Hib was the leading cause of bacterial meningitis, but today *Streptococcus pneumoniae* is one of the leading causes of bacterial meningitis.

Side Effects

Side effects are generally mild and include local reactions, irritability, drowsiness, and decreased appetite. Fewer than one-fourth of children have fevers over 100.3°F.

pneumococcus   A type of bacteria that causes PNEUMONIA, MENINGITIS, acute EAR INFECTION, or a bloodstream infection (BACTEREMIA).

Pneumocystis carinii   A species in the genus of protozoans *Pneumocystis* that causes *Pneumocystis carinii* PNEUMONIA.

See *PNEUMOCYSTIS CARINII.*

pneumonia   An infection of the lungs considered to be the most common infectious cause of death in the United States. About 48 million Americans develop pneumonia each year, and almost 65,000 die. It is a frequent complication of INFLUENZA.

There are many different types of pneumonia, classified by the type of germ causing the infection: bacteria, virus, fungus, parasites, or mycoplasmia. Pneumonias associated with mycoplasmas, fungus, Q FEVER, LEGIONNAIRES' DISEASE, psittacosis, and viruses are included in a category known as atypical pneumonia syndromes.

If a large portion of one or more lobes of the lung is involved, the disease is called a lobar pneumonia. Bronchopneumonia, more common than lobar, implies that the disease process is distributed in different places in the lungs, originating in a localized area within the bronchi and extending to the adjacent surrounding lung area.

There are a number of risk factors that can predispose a patient to develop pneumonia. Any condition that produces mucus or an obstruction (such as cancer or chronic lung disease) can make the patient more susceptible to pneumonia. Also at risk are people with an impaired immune system, smokers, people confined to bed, alcoholics, or the very old.

Patients with cystic fibrosis are prone to respiratory infection with *Pseudomonas* and *Staphylococcus*; *Pneumocystis carinii* pneumonia has been associated with AIDS patients. Anyone with congestive heart failure, diabetes, or chronic lung disease is also more susceptible.

Pneumonia in the elderly may occur spontaneously or as a complication of another disease. These pulmonary infections are often difficult to treat and are more often fatal than similar infections in younger patients. The onset of pneumonia in the elderly may begin with a general deterioration, confusion, and rapid heartbeat and breathing. To reduce the serious consequences of pneumonia in this group, vaccination against pneumococcus and influenza viral infections is recommended.

Pneumonia is usually caused by inhaling a microorganism, although the germ can occasionally pass to the lungs from the bloodstream.

Symptoms and Diagnostic Path

Shaking chills are very common, and coughing becomes frequent and may produce a colored discharge. The fever is high and may reach 105°F. Pain in the chest may occur as the lungs become more inflamed. During the most serious phase of pneumonia, the body loses fluids, which must be replaced in order to prevent shock; pus in the lungs cause severe respiratory distress.

Treatment Options and Outlook

Bacterial pneumonia is treated with antibiotics. When given early enough in the course of the disease, antibiotics are very effective.

See also ORNITHOSIS.

pneumonia, bacterial   Pneumonia (lung inflammation) caused by bacterial infection. *Streptococcus pneumoniae* is the most common bacterial cause and occurs most often in winter and spring, when upper respiratory tract infections are most frequent. *S. pneumoniae* is commonly referred to as the *pneumococcus*.

In addition to *S. pneumoniae*, other bacteria that can cause pneumonia include *Staphylococcus aureus*, *Klebsiella pneumoniae*, *Pseudomonas aeruginosa*, *Haemophilius influenzae*, *Legionella pneumophila*, and *Mycoplasma pneumoniae*.

Symptoms and Diagnostic Path

Classic bacterial pneumonia usually begins with a sudden onset of shaking chills, a rapid rising fever (101–105°F), and a stabbing chest pain made worse by breathing and coughing. The patient is severely ill and breathes with grunting and flared nostrils, leaning forward in an effort to breathe without coughing.

History (especially of a recent respiratory tract infection), physical exam, chest X-rays, blood culture (because BACTEREMIA occurs often), and sputum exam will diagnose the condition.

Treatment Options and Outlook

The treatment of bacterial pneumonia involves antibiotics; PENICILLIN G is the antibiotic of choice for infection with *S. pneumoniae*. Other effective drugs include erythromycin, clindamycin, the cephalosporins, other penicillins, and trimethoprim-sulfamethoxazole (Bactrim). Bed rest is required until the infection clears. Oxygen may need to be given.

pneumonia, chlamydial   This type of PNEUMONIA is caused by a newly recognized strain of CHLAMYDIAL INFECTION. Chlamydial pneumonia was formerly known as Taiwan Acute Respiratory agent pneumonia (or TWAR agent pneumonia) because it was first diagnosed in Taiwan. Today, cases have been reported all over the world, including Europe, Canada, the United States, Australia, and Japan.

Chlamydial pneumonia among people aged five to 35 is the second leading cause of pneumonia after mycoplasma pneumonia. Between 5 and 10 percent of older people admitted to the hospital with pneumonia have this condition.

Patients are infectious as long as they cough, and antibiotics do not reduce the infectious period. Some people may be infectious for weeks; epidemics in military locations have persisted for up to eight months. It appears that healthy carriers may transmit this disease to others.

While one attack conveys a short-term immunity, it is possible to get chlamydial infection more than once.

Chlamydial pneumonia is caused by a tiny organism (*Chlamydia pneumoniae*) similar to both viruses and bacteria that live inside human cells. But because it responds to antibiotics, it is classified as a bacterium. It is related to *Chlamydia psittaci* (transmitted by birds) and *Chlamydia trachomatis* (which causes the sexually transmitted disease chlamydia).

It is transmitted much the same way as any other bacterial pneumonia; by direct contact with infected individuals or by breathing in the bacteria when an infected person coughs or sneezes nearby. The disease may be passed by handling a coughing infected person's towels or sheets.

Symptoms and Diagnostic Path

Symptoms are similar to mycoplasma pneumonia, beginning with fatigue and weakness, sore throat, hoarseness, low fever, and cough. Some sputum may be coughed up. Older patients have fever with severe lung congestion and rapid, difficult breathing.

The incubation period after exposure varies but is usually between one and four weeks.

An antibody test is the best way to diagnose the disease, but many doctors diagnose the disease on the basis of symptoms and on tests that rule out other types of bacterial pneumonias. Chest X-ray may reveal a pneumonia in the lower lobe of one lung. Throat or sputum cultures will reveal the disease, but many labs are unable to culture this.

Treatment Options and Outlook

Erythromycin or tetracycline for 10 to 21 days will cure the disease. Adults should try to rest and return to normal activities slowly. Children should be given humidified air from a cool-mist vaporizer, clear fluids, chest raised while sleeping, and acetaminophen for fevers over 101°F.

Most infections in young adults are mild and recovery is slow but complete; the cough may last two or more weeks. However, between 5 and 10 percent of elderly patients may die.

Those elderly people who recover may experience chronic BRONCHITIS or SINUSITIS.

pneumonia, fungal   PNEUMONIA caused by fungus that typically causes only mild symptoms, although some people become gravely ill. There are three types of fungi that typically cause pneumonia:

- *Histoplasma capsulatum,* which causes HISTOPLASMOSIS

- *Coccidioides immitis,* which causes COCCIDIOIDOMYCOSIS

- *Blastomyces dermatitidis,* which causes BLASTOMYCOSIS

Histoplasmosis   This condition is found throughout the world; in the United States, it occurs most often in the Mississippi and Ohio River valleys and in the eastern river valleys. The infection may cause acute pneumonia, or it may develop into chronic pneumonia with symptoms that persist for months. Rarely, the infection spreads to other areas of the body, especially the bone marrow, liver, spleen, and digestive tract. This form tends to occur in people who have AIDS or other immune system disorders.

Coccidioidomycosis   Also called valley fever, this condition occurs primarily in semiarid climates, especially the southwestern United States. After being inhaled, the fungus may cause no symptoms, or it may cause acute or chronic pneumonia. In some cases, the infection spreads beyond the respiratory system to the skin, bones, joints, and tissues covering the brain. This complication is more common in men, especially Filipinos and blacks, and in people who have AIDS or other immune system disorders.

Blastomycosis   This infection occurs primarily in the southeastern, south-central, and midwestern United States and in areas around the Great Lakes. After being inhaled, the fungus causes infection in the lungs that may linger for months. The disease may spread to other parts of the body, especially the skin, bones, joints, and prostate gland.

Other fungal infections may lead to pneumonia, including CRYPTOCOCCOSIS (caused by *Cryptococcus neoformans*), ASPERGILLOSIS (caused by *ASPERGILLUS*) and mucormycosis (caused by Mucorales fungi).

Symptoms and Diagnostic Path

Symptoms may differ depending on the specific type of fungus (see above). The diagnosis is made by identifying the fungus in a sample of sputum or from a blood test that identifies certain antibodies.

Treatment Options and Outlook

Typically, treatment of fungal pneumonia involves an antifungal drug, such as itraconazole or amphotericin B.

pneumonia, gram-negative bacterial   A type of very serious PNEUMONIA caused by gram-negative bacteria, such as *KLEBSIELLA* (Friedländer's pneumonia), *PSEUDOMONAS*, *Enterobacter*, *Proteus*, *Serratia*, or *ACINETOBACTER*. These types of bacterial pneumonias almost always occur only in hospitalized patients or those who live in nursing homes and rarely affect healthy adults.

Symptoms and Diagnostic Path

The symptoms of gram-negative bacterial pneumonia are the same as for gram-positive pneumonia, except people tend to be sicker and worsen more quickly with gram-negative infections. Common symptoms include fever, coughing, and shortness of breath, with thick, red sputum.

Treatment Options and Outlook

A patient with this type of pneumonia should be treated in a hospital with antibiotics, supplemental oxygen, and intravenous fluids; a ventilator is sometimes needed. Even with the best of treatment, between one-quarter to one-half of all patients with gram-negative pneumonia die.

Risk Factors and Preventive Measures

Gram-negative bacteria are particularly common causes of pneumonia in people who use ventilators. Other people at risk are infants, older people, alcoholics, and people with chronic diseases, especially immune system disorders.

pneumonia, mycoplasma A very common and highly contagious type of PNEUMONIA (often called "walking" pneumonia) caused by the germ MYCO-PLASMA PNEUMONIAE, which is spread primarily by coughing. Most people who contract mycoplasma pneumonia are teens and young adults, although the illness can occur in a patient of any age. *Walking pneumonia* is so termed because its symptoms are not severe enough to require bed rest or hospitalization.

Mycoplasma pneumonia occurs most often in late summer or fall and can affect organs other than the lungs.

Symptoms and Diagnostic Path

Symptoms of mycoplasma pneumonia are typically milder than for other types of pneumonia and appear more slowly; they include fever, cough, headache, weakness, and fatigue.

Treatment Options and Outlook

When needed, treatment may include antibiotics. Although the infection can make patients feel quite sick, most people recover without lasting complications.

pneumonia, pneumococcal One of several types of PNEUMONIA (serious inflammation of the lungs) caused by bacterial infection; it kills about 40,000 Americans each year.

Adults over age 50 are most at risk; 85 percent of the deaths occur in this group. Others at risk include those with no spleen or with disorders of the spleen; those with impaired immune systems; those with chronic lung disease, heart disease, kidney disorders, diabetes, or alcoholism; adult residents of institutions.

Pneumococcal pneumonia is an infection caused by a type of bacteria called *Streptococcus pneumoniae* (also called PNEUMOCOCCUS). It is spread by airborne or direct exposure to respiratory drops from a person who is infected.

Symptoms and Diagnostic Path

Within one to three days after infection, symptoms of fever, chills, headache, cough, chest pain, shortness of breath, and sometimes a stiff neck may appear. Infections occur most often during the winter and early spring, and less often during the summer.

Doctors can diagnose the disease based on the type of symptoms and specific cultures of sputum, blood, or spinal fluid.

Treatment Options and Outlook

In most cases, this disease is treatable with antibiotics.

Risk Factors and Preventive Measures

A reasonably effective, safe vaccine that protects against many forms of pneumococcus has been available for adults for years, although many high-risk patients have still not been vaccinated.

A pneumococcal vaccine (Prevnar) for children under age two (PCV) was approved in 2000 that is designed to prevent invasive pneumococcal diseases in infants and toddlers—diseases which can cause brain damage and death. (This vaccine is not indicated for use in adults or as a substitute for other approved pneumococcal polysaccharide vaccines approved for high-risk children over the age of two.) Prevnar is the first pneumococcal vaccine for children under the age of two that targets the most common seven strains of pneumococcus causing 80 percent of invasive disease in infants. For the first time, doctors have a highly effective way to prevent a major cause of meningitis and serious blood infections in the most susceptible children.

Prevnar prevents invasive diseases caused by the organism *Streptococcus pneumoniae* (also known as PNEUMOCOCCUS), including infection of the bloodstream and MENINGITIS. The vaccine is given to infants as a series of four inoculations administered at two, four, six, and 12 to 15 months of age.

It is estimated that each year in the United States there are about 16,000 cases of pneumococcal bacteremia and 1,400 cases of pneumococcal meningitis among children under age five. Children under the age of two are at highest risk for infection. In up to half the cases of meningitis, brain damage and hearing loss occurs and about 10 percent die. There are different types of bacterial meningitis. Before the approval of the first Haemophilus influenza type b (HIB) conjugate vaccine in 1990 for infants, Hib was the leading cause of bacterial meningitis, but today *Streptococcus pneumoniae* is one of the leading causes of bacterial meningitis.

Side effects are generally mild and include local injection site reactions, irritability, drowsiness and decreased appetite. Approximately 21 percent of the children have fevers over 100.3°F.

See also PNEUMONIA, PNEUMOCOCCAL.

pneumonia, *Pneumocystis carinii* A type of pneumonia (PCP), also known as aids pneumonia, that is the most common AIDS lung infection. Most people who get PCP have a weakened immune system. PCP is an OPPORTUNISTIC INFECTION dangerous only to those patients with immune system impairment, such as patients with AIDS or leukemia. It is a major cause of death among AIDS patients.

PCP is caused by the species *Pneumocystis carinii,* spread in the air from person to person by breathing or coughing. Healthy people will not be affected by these germs, but anyone with an impaired immune system may be vulnerable.

Symptoms and Diagnostic Path

Early signs include breathing problems, fever, or a dry, hacking cough. Lips and nailbeds may turn blue if there are severe breathing problems. Symptoms may last from a few weeks to a few months.

A physician can diagnose the disease by examining the sputum (phlegm) or a lung biopsy.

Treatment Options and Outlook

The infection is fatal if untreated, but it can be cured with high doses of cotrimoxazole or other antibiot-

ics. Mild cases may be treated at home, but more serious infections require hospitalization.

pneumonia, walking The common name for MYCOPLASMA PNEUMONIA.

pneumonic plague See PLAGUE.

poliomyelitis A contagious viral disease that in its severe form can cause permanent paralysis and sometimes death. This extremely dangerous disease causes mild disabilities in about half of all patients; the rest may suffer permanent paralysis. However, due to modern vaccination practices, the disease has all but been wiped out in the United States. The last cases of indigenously acquired polio in the United States occurred in 1979.

Although a polio eradication program eliminated polio in the Western Hemisphere (the last case associated with wild poliovirus was detected in 1991), outbreaks of vaccine-derived poliovirus type 1 occurred in the Dominican Republic, Haiti, and Philippines in 2001, and a type 2 outbreak occurred in Madagascar in 2002. During 2003 and 2004, poliomyelitis outbreaks occurred in a number of countries in west and central Africa, after importation of wild polioviruses types 1 and 3 from Nigeria.

The number of reported polio cases has dropped by more than 99 percent as a result of the global polio eradication initiative since the mid–1980s, and experts believe that worldwide eradication of the disease is possible. As of September 2004, poliovirus remains endemic in Afghanistan, India, Pakistan, Nigeria, Niger, and Egypt.

The Americas were declared polio-free in 1994, and the disease has been eliminated in Europe.

Most American doctors have never seen an active case of polio, but in the first half of this century polio was called the last of the great childhood plagues.

Polio was known for hundreds of years, but the disease was not much discussed in ancient medical literature and did not occur in large epidemics until modern times. In fact, it was only in the late 18th century that the disease was first identified as polio.

In ancient times, sanitation was so appallingly poor that there was plenty of opportunity for people to contract polio, carried as it is in feces. The viruses infected each new generation of infants, who were protected in part by antibodies passed from their mothers. These early infections were usually mild, and were rarely diagnosed as polio.

But when improved public sanitation and other health measures arrived (such as water purification and milk pasteurization), there was less chance for babies and young children to contract the mild form of the disease and become immune. When the disease struck older children and adults, it was more likely to paralyze. In northern Europe and the United States, small EPIDEMICS began to appear in the late 19th and early 20th centuries. But it was not until the summer of 1917 when 27,000 U.S. citizens were paralyzed and 6,000 died that the real threat emerged. The Northeast was especially hard hit; in New York City and its suburbs, more than 9,000 cases were reported and 2,448 people died. The 1917 epidemic set off a panic as thousands fled the city to mountain resorts. Movie theaters were closed, meetings were canceled. Because no one know what spread the disease, public gatherings were shunned. Doctors stopped performing tonsillectomies until fall, and warned youngsters not to drink from public water fountains, not to take rides in amusement parks, or swim in public beaches.

In some towns, New York City natives who came to visit were turned away by armed citizens who feared the spread of the disease. Yet despite these precautions, an epidemic appeared each summer after that, with the most serious outbreaks in the 1940s and 1950s. It was the 1952 epidemic that was the worst, with nearly 58,000 reported cases and 3,145 deaths.

And then came the vaccine developed by Dr. Jonas Salk. The 1954 field trial, sponsored by the National Foundation for Infantile Paralysis, tested 1.8 million children, proving that Salk's killed virus vaccine was very effective in preventing polio. Dr. Salk became a national hero.

After the licensing of the vaccine in 1955, an intense public health campaign was mounted to inoculate every American child in the country. Similar scenes were repeated in 1961, when the attenuated live virus vaccine developed by Dr. Albert Sabin was licensed. This time, the vaccine was given in a sugar cube soaked in liquid vaccine. In a few short years, polio was virtually eliminated in this country, since both vaccines contain all three polio strains and prevent the disease.

The last U.S. epidemic occurred in 1979, when 10 Amish children whose parents had refused to have them vaccinated on religious grounds came down with the disease.

Polio is caused by a virus with three distinct strains (types I, II, and III) that lives in the nose, throat, and especially the intestinal tract of an infected person. Many people are carriers (that is, they are infected but show no symptoms)—but they can still spread the infection to others. The virus is excreted in large amounts in the feces of a carrier, and is probably spread through hand-to-hand or hand-to-mouth contact. Once in the body, the virus multiplies in the throat and intestinal tract. In more serious cases, the virus may attack the nervous system (the brain and spinal cord), where it may kill or injure motor nerve cells. This may lead to extensive paralysis, including paralysis of the muscles involved in breathing, or it may be fatal. Immunity to one type of polio does not confer immunity to the other two.

Symptoms and Diagnostic Path
The mild forms of polio usually begin abruptly and last just a few days. Symptoms (if they appear at all) include fever, sore throat, nausea, headache, and stomach ache. Sometimes there will be pain and stiffness in the neck, back, and legs.

The more serious form—paralytic polio—is the form that causes most epidemics; it begins with the same symptoms, but severe muscle pain is usually present. If paralysis occurs, it begins within the first week. Paralysis may affect only a small group of muscles, or it may be widespread. The legs are more often affected than the arms, but the virus may partially or completely paralyze a single limb, half of the body, or all four extremities.

Those most at risk for serious neurological damage during epidemics due to lowered immunity included patients who had recently been inoculated or operated on (especially those who underwent tonsillectomies and adenoidectomies) and pregnant women.

Treatment Options and Outlook

There is no specific treatment for polio. The degree of recovery varies from one patient to the next.

Post-polio syndrome Patients who had polio in childhood have a one in five chance of experiencing new health problems decades later. Called post-polio syndrome, the symptoms include joint and muscle pain, tiredness, and weakness. While experts are not sure what causes the problem, they do not think it represents a reactivation of the old virus. Some experts suspect the syndrome may be related to chronic overuse of muscles and joints that had appeared to be undamaged by the initial infection.

There is no known cure and no universal treatment for post-polio syndrome. Treatments may include nonstrenuous exercise, physical therapy, electrical stimulation, occupational therapy, and nonsteroidal anti-inflammatory drugs or aspirin.

Risk Factors and Preventive Measures

Mass childhood immunizations with the polio vaccine has virtually eliminated the once-dreaded paralytic disease in this country. It is an essential part of every young child's preventive care. While there are no wild polio cases in the United States, there are thousands in the rest of the world. There is therefore a risk of polio being reestablished in the United States if children are not immunized.

Because the live vaccine carries an extremely small risk of giving polio to the person being vaccinated, especially if that person has an impaired immune system, the killed virus vaccine (IPV) is currently recommended for almost all children in the United States today. Until recently, the live oral polio vaccine (OPV) was recommended for most children. While both vaccines provide immunity to polio, OPV was better at keeping the disease from spreading to other people.

However, for a few people (about one in 2.4 million), OPV actually caused polio. Since the risk of getting polio in the United States is now extremely low, experts believe that using oral polio vaccine is no longer worth the slight risk.

Therefore, as of January 1, 2000, OPV was no longer recommended for routine immunization in the United States, and it is no longer available in this country, although it continues to be used in the majority of countries and for global polio eradication activities.

The killed virus polio shot (IPV) never causes polio nor is it known to produce any side effects other than minor local pain and redness.

The new guidelines were developed following complaints of parents of children who contracted polio from the live vaccine; they contended that even five to 15 cases of polio is too many considering there have been few cases of "wild" polio in the United States.

Pontiac fever See LEGIONNAIRES' DISEASE.

pork and infectious disease Undercooked pork can cause a variety of infectious diseases, including LISTERIOSIS, TRICHINOSIS, and YERSINIOSIS, pork TAPEWORM (taeniasis).

CORRECT COOKING METHODS FOR SAFE PORK PRODUCTS

- All pork should be cooked until internal temperatures reach 171°F or until the meat changes from pink to gray.
- Raw garbage should not be fed to swine; swine must not have access to human feces.
- Freezing pork kills pork tapeworm and roundworm; meat should be kept at 5°F for 30 days to kill roundworm cysts; for four days to kill tapeworm cysts.
- Raw or undercooked pork should not be eaten.

---

pork tapeworm See TAPEWORM.

poultry and infectious disease Undercooked poultry can cause a variety of infectious diseases, including SALMONELLOSIS and YERSINIOSIS. Poultry should be cooked to an internal temperature of at least 180°F or until juices run clear. Poultry should not be thawed at room temperature, and frozen prestuffed turkeys should not be thawed at all, but cooked frozen. After handling raw poultry, wash hands, surfaces, and cutting boards well. Leftover poultry should be divided into small containers and refrigerated for no more than three or four days.

See also AVIAN FLU FOOD POISONING; KITCHEN INFECTIONS.

Powassan (POW) virus   A rare tick-borne virus that causes a sometimes-fatal infection and inflammation of the brain. The virus gets its name from the town of Powassan, Ontario, where the disease was first recognized in 1958 after a fatal pediatric case; the first U.S. case occurred in 1979 in New Jersey. POW is a flavivirus, in the same family as St. Louis encephalitis (see ENCEPHALITIS, ST. LOUIS) virus and WEST NILE VIRUS, although it is very different. In North America, POW virus has been isolated from four tick species: *Ixodes cookei, Ixodes marxi, Ixodes spinipalpis,* and *Dermacentor andersoni.* Evidence of POW virus infection has been found in 38 mammals (primarily groundhogs). The virus has been found in the United States from coast to coast and is widespread throughout Canada, but human disease is rare. In Canada, 12 cases were identified between 1958 and 1999; seven were in children younger than 10. At least four cases were fatal either during the disease or afterward, as a result of chronic debilitation. Four of the eight surviving patients experienced some form of persistent debility.

From September 1999, to July 2001, four residents of Maine and Vermont were infected with the virus and developed encephalitis—the first cases identified in the United States since 1994.

According to experts at the CDC's National Center for Infectious Diseases, the viral infections are probably more widespread than the four cases indicate. These cases were identified because the four patients were tested for West Nile virus, and the results were negative.

Symptoms and Diagnostic Path

POW virus may cause no symptoms or only mild illness, unless it penetrates the central nervous system; at that point, it can cause ENCEPHALITIS. Symptoms usually begin suddenly, between one and two weeks after infection, and include headache, fever, nausea and vomiting, stiff neck, and sleepiness. As the disease progresses, more severe symptoms develop, such as breathing problems, tremors, confusion, seizures, coma, paralysis, and sometimes death. POW encephalitis is often associated with significant long-term illness.

Lab tests are necessary to confirm a diagnosis, which can be performed at the CENTERS FOR DISEASE CONTROL AND PREVENTION (CDC) when requested through state public health laboratories. Blood tests that detect antibodies to POW virus are most often used.

Treatment Options and Outlook

There is no specific treatment for this disease other than to treat symptoms, administer intravenous fluids, and offer breathing help, if needed. It is also important to prevent secondary infections, such as PNEUMONIA and URINARY TRACT INFECTIONS. Corticosteroids may sometimes be used to reduce swelling in the brain. POW encephalitis has a fatality rate of 10 to 15 percent. Of those patients who survive, many suffer permanent brain damage.

Risk Factors and Preventive Measures

There is no vaccine to prevent this disease. Occasionally, POW virus may also be isolated from blood, cerebrospinal fluid, or other tissue. The virus may be prevented by avoiding contact with ticks.

POW virus infections are most common from June to September, when the ticks are most active. One of the four types of ticks that carries the virus is often found on woodchucks and skunks, which suggests that these animals may be the main carriers of the POW virus. For this reason, people should keep areas near their home clear of brush, weeds, trash, and other materials that could harbor small and medium-sized mammals.

pregnancy and infectious disease   There are many infectious diseases that, when contracted by a pregnant woman, can cause serious harm to her unborn child. They include the following:

AIDS If a mother is infected with HIV or AIDS, medication during pregnancy can offer significant protection to an unborn baby. Babies born to infected mothers must be carefully followed and checked for infection at birth.

CHICKEN POX While many pregnant women are immune to chicken pox, those who contract the disease during the first three or four months of pregnancy have a 5 percent risk of damaging the fetus, producing small, poorly formed or scarred arms and legs, brain abnormalities, and premature birth. The earlier in the pregnancy a mother gets chicken pox, the higher the risk of fetal damage. However, chicken pox after 14 weeks of pregnancy is very unlikely to affect the unborn baby. Any pregnant woman who has never had chicken pox and who is exposed to the virus during the first trimester should discuss preventive treatment with her doctor.

CHLAMYDIAL INFECTIONS Some studies—but not all—have linked this infection to a higher risk for premature birth, low birth weight, or premature ruptured membranes.

CYTOMEGALOVIRUS In most women this does not produce many symptoms, but an infection during pregnancy can be devastating to an unborn child. Almost all babies infected before birth are born perfectly normal; only about 10 percent are born sick, and of these, 20 to 30 percent may die. Those ill babies who survive may have convulsions, lethargy, a rash, breathing problems, mental retardation, small brain, water on the brain, eye inflammation, hearing loss, poor coordination, learning disabilities, and liver disease. Some long-term studies suggest that a few apparently normal babies who were infected with CMV at birth develop problems later on in life.

FIFTH DISEASE Up to 2.5 percent of pregnant women who contract fifth disease during pregnancy have spontaneous abortions or stillbirths. Most babies born to women infected during pregnancy are normal and healthy. If a woman is pregnant and a blood test confirms active infection, the doctor may advise a serial ultrasound to check on the baby's health, since the virus can cross the placenta and infect the fetus.

GENITAL HERPES An initial episode of genital herpes in a pregnant woman is much more dangerous to an unborn child than are recurrent episodes in a previously infected woman. Women with recurrent infections but no active lesions at delivery can have safe vaginal deliveries. Women with active lesions near delivery but before labor need a culture every three to five days. If the cultures are negative, a vaginal delivery is possible. Women with lesions at the time they go into labor will require a Caesarean section to prevent the baby from being infected as it moves through the birth canal.

GENITAL WARTS Vaginal delivery may be difficult if the genital warts grow very large during pregnancy, which they often do; the doctor may choose to perform a C-section in this case. Occasionally, a mother with genital warts can pass the infection to the baby during delivery, which can lead to recurrent respiratory papillomatosis (RRP), in which warts grow into the baby's throat and interfere with breathing.

GERMAN MEASLES One of the most serious infections a pregnant woman can contract while pregnant is German measles, a disease so profoundly damaging to a fetus that widespread vaccination is practiced as a way to avoid this problem. If a pregnant woman is infected with German measles during the first 12 weeks of pregnancy, as many as 85 percent of women will miscarry. At 14 to 16 weeks the risk drops to between 10 and 24 percent, and after 20 weeks the risk is close to zero. However, infants surviving infection in the womb may be born with defects, including deafness, eye problems (including blindness), heart defects, mental retardation, growth retardation, and bleeding disorders.

GONORRHEA Untreated gonorrhea during pregnancy can cause a uterine infection, premature birth, a smaller-than-normal baby, or an infection in the amniotic fluid. Babies born to infected mothers get gonorrhea conjunctivitis during delivery; an untreated baby will become blind. This is why drops are placed in every newborn's eyes at birth to prevent both gonorrhea and chlamydia conjunctivitis.

GROUP B STREP This form of strep is a normal part of the healthy intestinal tract, but in up to 40 percent of pregnant women the bacteria migrate to the genital tract, where they live without causing any symptoms. In about half of these cases, the mother will give birth to a child carrying group B strep, but only one out of a hundred babies will have symptoms. The baby can be infected either in the uterus or during delivery. Occasionally, an infant will be infected in the hospital nursery as a result of cross-contamination. If the baby becomes sick with group B strep within 48 hours of birth, symptoms may be severe and can include difficulty in breathing, paleness, lethargy, fever, poor feeding, and low body temperature. After delivery, women who develop infections in the uterus, or wound infections after a Caesarean, are often infected with group B strep.

HEPATITIS B Infected mothers transmit this infection to their infants during the last three months of pregnancy, during delivery, or while breast feeding. There is less risk of infection if a mother is infected early in pregnancy. All pregnant women should be tested for hep B.

JAPANESE ENCEPHALITIS Women who are infected during the first two trimesters may have miscarriages.

LISTERIOSIS Infection with *Listeria* is another very serious infection during pregnancy that is particularly damaging to a fetus or newborn. Babies can be infected via the placenta before birth or during delivery through the birth canal. A pregnant woman with a flulike illness must be tested for this disease if there is a hint that she might have been exposed to *Listeria.* If a baby is infected while in the womb, the infant may be born prematurely, have a low weight, and be very ill with breathing problems, blue skin, and low body temperature at birth. There may be a rash or a sticky eye infection. If the baby survives, the child will be quite ill and may have MENINGITIS or a bloodstream infection. Half of these babies will die, even if promptly treated. Babies who are infected during delivery are born full term with normal birth weight, but may develop meningitis; about 40 percent may die. Some survivors will have permanent brain damage or mental retardation. If listeriosis is suspected during pregnancy, antibiotics given to the mother can prevent disease in the fetus.

LYME DISEASE It is possible for the spirochete to cross the placenta and harm the fetus, although most babies born to women infected during pregnancy are normal. A pregnant woman infected with Lyme disease does have a slightly higher risk of miscarriage or stillbirth or of having a baby born with heart defects or other problems.

MALARIA Pregnant women who become infected with malaria may suffer from miscarriage, premature delivery, or stillbirth.

SHINGLES Sometimes a young, healthy pregnant woman will develop shingles, since pregnancy alters the immune system. Because the virus is not in the bloodstream, however, there is no danger to the fetus from this infection. Babies born to mothers who had chicken pox during pregnancy, and babies who get the disease before age two, often have a mild, short-lasting shingles infection as young children.

SYPHILIS A pregnant woman can pass the infection to her unborn baby at any stage of the disease if she is not treated before 32 weeks of pregnancy, even if she has no symptoms. The bacteria cross the placenta and enter the baby's bloodstream. A baby who is born to a syphilitic mother has congenital syphilis, which can lead to serious illness, birth defects, and death.

TOXOPLASMOSIS This disease is another of the mild infections that can be very serious if contracted by a pregnant woman. If a pregnant woman thinks she has been exposed or has symptoms, blood tests can reveal antibodies; some women with the infection choose to end their pregnancy. There is no way to determine if a fetus has been harmed by the infection, however. Infection is most severe if it occurs during the first three months of pregnancy; complications include miscarriage, premature birth, and poor growth in the womb. Infants who are born apparently normal can develop mental retardation by age 20 and have eye problems.

TRICHOMONIASIS Pregnant women with an untreated infection may experience premature labor or give birth to a low-weight infant.

preseptal cellulitis   See CELLULITIS.

prion   An unusual infectious agent that appears to be neither virus nor bacteria, with no genetic material; a prion consists entirely of protein. Many experts believe prions cause spongiform encephalopathy in animals. It has been implicated in MAD COW DISEASE (bovine spongiform encephalopathy), in sheep (scrapie), in mink (transmissible mink encephalopathy), and in muledeer and elk (chronic wasting disease). Humans are also susceptible to several prion diseases, including CREUTZFELD-JAKOB DISEASE (CJD), variant-CJD, Gerstmann-Straussler-Scheinker syndrome, fatal familial insominia, kuru, and Alpers syndrome.

The prion was first identified in 1982 by Stanley Prusiner of the University of California/San Francisco medical school, who suggested that these prion proteins are structurally similar to proteins that are found naturally in the brains of humans and other animals. But prions differ from these other normal proteins in their three-dimensional shape. Prusiner endured ridicule at first, but his theory has gradually won a strong following. Other scientists still insist that prions must be an unknown form of virus.

Prions seem to be able to cause disease by coming into contact with these normal proteins, stimulating them to change their shape to mimic the prion protein. This shape change appears to set off a chain reaction, with normal proteins metamorphosing into the prions, causing a devastating, ultimately fatal, disease.

Prion diseases are unusual in that they appear to be both infectious and hereditary diseases. They can be acquired from diet or after medical procedures such as surgery, growth hormone injections, or corneal transplants; this implicates prions as an infectious agent. However, these diseases also can be inherited as an autosomal dominant trait. They are also sporadic, which means that sometimes there is no known risk factor, although it seems likely that infection was acquired in one of the two ways listed above.

Symptoms and Diagnostic Path

The human versions of these prion diseases are characterized by loss of motor control, dementia, paralysis, wasting, and eventually death. The prion-related diseases are extremely difficult to diagnose; there is no blood test that reveals the condition.

Treatment Options and Outlook

No treatment has yet been discovered to halt this process. Prions are not destroyed by the usual methods employed to kill infectious agents. They are resistant to everything from boiling temperatures well over 400°F to ionizing radiation.

Continuing research may help determine whether prions consisting of other proteins might play a part in other degenerative conditions, including Alzheimer's disease, Parkinson's disease, and amyotrophic lateral sclerosis.

Proquad A new single-shot vaccine that protects children against MEASLES, MUMPS, rubella (GERMAN MEASLES), and CHICKEN POX, which could mean one less shot and one less doctor visit. The U.S. Food and Drug Administration approved the vaccine, manufactured by Merck, in 2005. The vaccine (a combination of the company's measles, mumps, rubella vaccine and its chicken pox shot) is designed for children from 12 months to 12 years of age.

Proquad is the first and only vaccine approved in the United States to help protect against these four diseases in a single shot. It is also approved for use in children 12 months to 12 years of age if a second dose of measles, mumps, and rubella vaccine is to be given. The approval of this new vaccination combination came after it was tested in more than 5,000 children, according to the drug company.

prostatitis Acute or chronic inflammation of the prostate gland caused by either bacterial, fungal, or mycoplasma infection. It usually affects men between the ages of 30 and 50.

Prostatitis is often caused by an infection that has spread from the urethra. The infection may or may not be sexually transmitted. A urinary catheter increases the risk of prostatitis.

Symptoms and Diagnostic Path

Burning, frequency, and urgency of urination, and sometimes a discharge from the penis or blood in the urine. An acute bacterial infection may produce a sudden fever and chills, with rectal, abdominal, or low back pain. However, some patients may not experience any symptoms.

A careful history, culture of prostate fluid or tissue and sometimes an examination of tissue under a microscope. The physician examines the prostate by inserting a gloved finger into the rectum and assessing tenderness of the gland by palpation.

Treatment Options and Outlook

Administration of antibiotics, sitz baths, bed rest, and fluids. The condition may be slow to clear up and may recur.

protegrin A type of peptide (first discovered in pig white blood cells) that may offer new broad-spectrum microbial treatments for many infectious diseases, including those now resistant to traditional antibiotics.

The peptides seem to be able to kill a wide range of disease-causing organisms quickly, including both gram-positive and gram-negative bacteria. Scientists have evidence that the peptides were able to treat systemic infections by PSEUDOMONAS AERUGINOSA, drug-resistant STAPHYLOCOCCUS AUREUS, and VANCOMY-CIN-RESISTANT ENTEROCOCCUS. In studies, the peptides were also effective against the fungal CANDIDA ALBICANS and HELICOBACTER PYLORI, the bacteria that causes ulcers. Unlike many antibiotics, which only halt the growth of microorganisms, protegrins quickly kill both BACTERIA and FUNGI. They do it while apparently avoiding the normal mechanisms by which bacteria quickly develop resistance to conventional antibiotics. They are not available for clinical use.

protozoa Any of about 30,000 known simple one-celled forms of animal life. Protozoa, which means "first animals," were discovered by the Dutch scientist Antonie van Leeuwenhoek who found them swimming in a rain barrel.

Protozoa include paramecium, a one-celled animal shaped like a shoe, and AMOEBA, another one-celled animal with a constantly changing shape.

Although they consist of only a single cell, they are complete organisms and carry out all necessary life functions, including feeding, moving, excreting wastes, and reproducing. These types of life-forms reproduce very rapidly by cell division. When the cell divides, the nucleus of the cell splits in half; the nucleus of this cell holds the chemical information that the cell needs to function. There may be thousands of new microbes produced in just one day, but most die quickly as well.

Most protozoa are animal-like, obtaining their nutrients from the environment. However, a few contain the pigment chlorophyll and, plantlike, can use the sun's energy to manufacture nutrients in the form of carbohydrates.

Because of this overlap, protozoa have been variously regarded as animals, plants, or as a separate group entirely. Some scientists classify the protozoa as a separate kingdom apart from animals or plants, called the Protista, which also includes single-celled algae.

Protozoa come in many different shapes, but they are usually broadly grouped into three major types related to the way they move: *flagellate, ciliate,* and *amoeboid.* The flagellates move by using a few long, whiplike appendages. Cilia move by short, hair-like appendages. Amoebae move by means of a flowing, shape-changing action.

They may be parasitic and live off hosts, or they may live on their own. They can be found from polar sea ice to tropical rain forests, from the depths of the oceans to the tops of mountains.

Some photosynthetic protozoa (such as species of red-colored dinoflagellates) cause toxic water blooms called RED TIDE.

The parasitic protozoa cause serious disease among humans and animals, especially in tropical climates. This type of protozoa include the malarial trypanosome, a type of organism that invades human red blood cells, causing fatal fever and chills. LEISHMANIA and trypanosome flagellates are found in the tropics, invading body tissue and causing disfigurement and sometimes death. The amoeboid intestinal parasite *Entamoeba histolytica* causes a severe DYSENTERY. Some parasitic species (such as *Pneumocystis carinii*) are more closely related to fungi than protozoa, and are especially harmful to humans with an impaired immune function.

pseudomembranous enterocolitis A sporadic, often fatal type of diarrheal disease that has been linked to hospital-acquired infection with CLOSTRIDIUM DIFFICILE in patients taking antibiotics for another infection. The infection is named for the presence of yellow plaques (or pseudomembranes) scattered over the walls of the colon.

The disease is usually associated with antibiotic therapy (especially Clindamycin) and develops as a result of overgrowth and toxin production by *C. difficile* within the colon, as the normal bacteria is disturbed (usually when the patient takes antibiotics).

Symptoms and Diagnostic Path
There is a wide variety of diarrheal symptoms from mild to severe that begin between four to 10 days

after the patient starts taking antibiotics; they may start as early as the first day of treatment or as late as three weeks after treatment has been discontinued. Diarrhea is always present in this disease and is generally severe, with dehydration, fever, vomiting and cramps, and abdominal distention.

The diagnosis is best made by finding *C. difficile* toxin in the stool.

Treatment Options and Outlook

Once the diagnosis is made, immediate therapy should begin with fluids, electrolyte replacement, and discontinuation of the antibiotic. Many patients respond dramatically once the antibiotic is stopped, within two to three days. The drug of first choice against this disease is oral vancomycin.

Relapses occur in 14 percent of patients between four and 21 days after completing the first course of vancomycin; sometimes, repeated bouts of treatment with vancomycin have been needed. Metronidazole is an alternative to vancomycin.

Pseudomonas aeruginosa A species of gram-negative bacteria that has been isolated from wounds, blood, sputum, burns, and infections of the urinary tract. These bacteria are noted for their resistance to disinfectants and antibiotics. The bacilli cause a range of human diseases, from purulent MENINGITIS to HOSPITAL-ACQUIRED INFECTIONS, and can cause life-threatening lung infections in patients with cystic fibrosis.

See also URINARY TRACT INFECTION.

psittacosis See ORNITHOSIS.

psychiatric disease and infections Because the central nervous system is susceptible to infection, there are a few mental disorders that have been related to certain infectious agents. These include aids dementia, schizophrenia, manic depression, and obsessive-compulsive disorder.

AIDS dementia The HIV virus can cause a wide variety of cognitive and motor problems. The prevalence of dementia among AIDS patients is between 4 and 7 percent; about one third of adults and half of children with AIDS will eventually develop some sort of mental or thinking deficits. HIV infection has also been associated with mood disorders such as manic depression.

Schizophrenia For the past 70 years there have been reports of a link between some cases of schizophrenia-like psychoses and influenza (especially as a result of fetal exposure during the second trimester of pregnancy and subsequent development of schizophrenia in adulthood). In several studies, the risk of schizophrenia was about 88 percent higher among the offspring of women exposed to the flu viruses during the second trimester as compared to those who were not exposed. If exposure to the flu virus does increase the risk for schizophrenia, it is estimated that it is not a major risk factor (perhaps accounting for just about 1 percent of all cases). Some researchers suspect that exposure to the virus during the critical period of fetal central nervous system development could lead to a disruption of brain organization.

Obsessive-compulsive disorder Infection by group A beta-hemolytic strep has been linked to specific neuropsychiatric symptoms, probably due to the production of antibodies that react against neurons. Sudden onset or worsening of obsessive-compulsive disorder or tics has been reported after recent group A beta-hemolytic strep infections in children.

Mood disorders BORNA DISEASE VIRUS (BDV) was first recognized during the 19th century as a cause of severe neurologic disease in animals. Recently, antibodies against BDV has been found in the blood of hospitalized psychiatric patients suffering with major depression, obsessive-compulsive disorder, panic disorder, or organic mood disorder. Researchers suspect that the depressive state may somehow activate a latent infection, but the precise mechanism between the virus and specific mood disorders needs to be determined.

pubic lice See LICE.

pyelonephritis Inflammation of the kidney usually caused by a bacterial infection. This condition may occur as a sudden attack or it may be chronic, in which repeated attacks cause permanent scarring.

The acute version of the disease is more common in women and is more likely to occur during pregnancy.

Acute pyelonephritis is usually caused by an infection of the bladder that spreads into the kidney. The chronic version usually begins in childhood, usually as a result of urine flowing back from the bladder into one of the ureters. Persistent back-flow of urine causes repeated kidney infections that lead to inflammation and scarring. Over a period of years, this can cause kidney damage.

Symptoms and Diagnostic Path

Symptoms include pain in the back, side, and groin; urgent, frequent, painful urination; fever; nausea and vomiting; and pus and blood in the urine. A kidney infection should be treated with an appropriate antibiotic, and abnormalities may need to be surgically repaired.

A urine test can identify bacteria and formations of white blood cells in the kidneys. If an infection cannot be easily cured, X-rays can highlight abnormalities in the kidneys, ureters, and bladder.

Treatment Options and Outlook

Antibiotic drugs may need to be given intravenously in serious cases, is the treatment of choice. SEPTICEMIA (blood poisoning) is a possible complication. An untreated or recurrent kidney infection can lead to a chronic problem involving permanent kidney damage.

See also KIDNEY DISORDERS, INFECTIOUS.

Q fever A little-known respiratory illness of animals, also known as Australian Q fever or query fever, which can be transmitted to humans. The organisms are most plentiful in the uterus and udder of pregnant cattle and sheep.

Q fever is found all over the world and is especially common where cattle are raised and goats and sheep are herded; this includes the western United States and Canada, Africa, England, and the Mediterranean countries. It usually affects veterinarians, dairy workers, and farmers, and those who work in meatpacking plants and animal research.

The disease is caused by a bacterium called *Coxiella burnetii (Rickettsia burnetii)*, which is spread through contact with infected domestic animals, by inhaling the rickettsiae from the hides, drinking contaminated milk, or being bitten by an infected tick. The organism survives for a long time in the environment and is hard to kill with disinfectants.

Animals are usually infected by ticks that carry the bacteria; most animals have no symptoms, although they shed the organisms in urine and feces. It is even possible for the disease to spread from the laundry of infected persons contaminated with animal feces; only small numbers of the organisms can cause human disease, and the organism is able to travel through the air for at least a half mile. Even casual visitors to animal research labs have become infected.

However, the bacteria are not passed directly from one person to the next, which means patients are not infectious to others. After one infection, a person becomes immune to Q fever for life.

Symptoms and Diagnostic Path

Many people have very mild symptoms, but some are very sick. Onset of symptoms is abrupt, with high fever that may last three weeks or more; fever is often misdiagnosed as INFLUENZA or PNEUMONIA. Other symptoms include chills, muscle pain, severe headache, weakness, fatigue, vomiting, diarrhea, confusion, sore throat, and sweats, with chest pain, dry cough, and a mild pneumonia. The fever may rise as high as 104°F.

Some patients can lose weight over a period of time, and between a third to a half of patients with symptoms will develop pneumonia. Most patients also have abnormal liver function tests, and some will develop hepatitis.

More rarely, some patients develop chronic Q fever with a persistent infection for more than six months—a much more serious disease. Patients who have had acute Q fever may develop the chronic form within a year or as long as 20 years after the initial infection. ENDOCARDITIS is a serious complication of chronic Q fever, involving either the aortic or mitral heart valves.

Anyone with flu-like symptoms who is likely to have had contact with infected animals should seek medical advice, stating clearly that contact with the Q fever organism has possibly occurred. A blood test reveals antibodies to the bacteria, which can indicate either a past or current infection.

Confirming a diagnosis of Q fever requires blood tests to detect antibodies to *C. burnetii* antigens. *C. burnetii* also may be identified in infected tissues by using immunohistochemical staining and DNA detection.

Treatment Options and Outlook

Q fever is treated with doxycycline for up to three weeks, which is most effective when started within the first three days. Quinolone antibiotics also may be effective. Chronic infection can be difficult to cure; therapy should be started again if the disease relapses.

Chronic Q fever endocarditis is much more difficult to treat effectively and often requires the use of several drugs. Surgery to remove damaged valves may be required for some cases.

Chronic HEPATITIS and infection in heart valves or lining of the heart are serious but rare complications. There is a high death rate among people who develop the infection in the heart lining or valves.

Risk Factors and Preventive Measures

In the United States, Q fever outbreaks have occurred primarily among veterinarians, meat-processing plant workers, sheep and dairy workers, livestock farmers, and researchers at facilities housing sheep.

Those who work with domestic animals can be vaccinated against Q fever, but the vaccine is not commercially availabe in the United States. A vaccine for animals also has been developed but is not yet available in the United States. Strict hygienic practices must be followed when contaminated hides, wool, straw, or pregnant animals are handled. This involves prevention of inhalation of contaminated dust or fluid droplets, adequate disinfection and disposal of material, and prompt treatment of cuts and abrasions. Placental and other birth material should be burned or buried. Contaminated litter should be burned. All animal milk should be pasteurized or boiled.

query fever See Q FEVER.

rabies An acute viral disease of the central nervous system that is usually transmitted to humans by a bite from an infected warm-blooded animal. Untreated, the disease is a swift, deadly killer, and there is no cure; the only hope lies in a vaccine given immediately after a bite by a rabid animal.

Rabies—the name comes from a Latin word meaning "to rage"—has been deeply feared for centuries. First described in 1800 B.C.E., it was known to the ancient Greeks as *lyssa*, meaning "frenzy," although the Greeks did not think humans could catch the disease. It was the 16th-century Italian physician Girolamo Fracastoro who discovered that rabies was fatal to humans as well as to animals and called it the "incurable wound," but at least some Romans disagreed. It was not until 1885 C.E. that Louis Pasteur created the first rabies vaccine using live rabies virus. Pasteur's early attempts could cause serious (sometimes fatal) reactions—but it was the only hope a person bitten by a rabid animal could have. Only three people who showed clear evidence of rabies have ever been known to survive the illness without treatment, and all of those patients suffered permanent nervous system damage causing physical or psychological problems.

Although most people tend to associate rabies with dogs, in fact rabies today is more likely to be found in cats. Together with dogs and cattle, these animals make up nearly 90 percent of rabies cases in domestic animals, with horses, mules, sheep, goats, swine, and ferrets making up the rest. Among wild animals, the disease occurs most often in skunks and raccoons, but it also appears in bats, foxes, mongeese, groundhogs, and some rodents.

Although rabies in humans is rare in the United States, as many as 18,000 Americans get rabies shots each year because they have been in contact with animals that may be rabid. There were 7,437 cases of rabies reported in (mostly wild) animals in the United States, and one human case was also reported. Rabies occurs in every state except Hawaii, the only state that has not had a single native case of rabies in animals or humans.

The number of human rabies deaths is low in the United States compared with the rest of the world, where each year between 30,000 and 50,000 people die of rabies. These deaths occur because people did not get vaccinations after being bitten by a rabid animal, primarily in Asia, Africa, and Latin America. Millions of people around the world get the anti-rabies shots after an animal bite. Dogs are the primary source of animal bites leading to rabies shots worldwide.

Any wild animal acting unusually tame may have rabies. Because rabies may be contagious before any symptoms appear, a healthy-looking animal can transmit the disease.

Rabies is actually a form of viral ENCEPHALITIS transmitted through infected animal saliva that affects the human's brain and spinal cord. The virus is concentrated in the salivary glands, which is why the disease is usually spread by a bite. The virus also invades and damages muscles involved in drinking and swallowing, causing excruciating pain when swallowing liquids. Although suffering from thirst, animal and human rabies patients can be terrified by the sight of water, hence the other name for the disease—hydrophobia.

Although a bite is the most common way to transmit the disease, rabies also can be transmitted when infected saliva comes in contact with a cut or a skin break. Infected bat droppings may also transmit the disease (at least two people are believed to have been exposed to rabies by breathing the air in caves where rabid bats live). Other unusual causes of transmission include corneal transplants from donors with undiagnosed rabies.

Symptoms and Diagnostic Path

The incubation period in humans may range from 10 days to more than a year, although 30 to 50 days is average. (Animals usually develop symptoms between 20 and 60 days.) The length of the incubation period seems to depend both on the location of the wound (the farther from the brain, the longer the incubation) and the dose of virus received. Without treatment, severe bites on the head or upper body could lead to symptoms sooner than a mild scratch on the ankle.

There are two forms of the disease. "Furious" rabies primarily affects the brain and causes an infected animal to be aggressive, highly sensitive to touch, and vicious—the "mad dog" image of a rabid animal. "Paralytic" (or "dumb") rabies primarily affects the spinal cord, weakening the animal so that it cannot raise its head or make sounds because its throat muscles are paralyzed. In the beginning stage of paralytic rabies, an animal may seem to be choking. In both forms, death occurs a few days after symptoms appear (usually from respiratory failure).

Symptoms in humans begin fairly mildly and worsen over time, starting with an itching or burning at the bite site, followed by malaise, fever, headache, fatigue, and appetite loss. The patient begins to grow restless, excitable, anxious, and irritable, with insomnia or depression. The patient may begin to hallucinate, salivate, and have periods of intense excitement and painful muscle spasms of the throat induced by swallowing. As time goes on, other signs of nervous system damage (such as paralysis, disorientation, and coma) follow. Four or five days later, the patient may then either slip into a months-long coma ending in death or die suddenly from respiratory or cardiac arrest.

There are no tests that can detect rabies in humans at the time of a bite, and by the time symptoms appear it is too late for treatment. The transmission of rabies by a bite can be hard to detect. One four-year-old was exposed to rabies from a bat that flew into her room while she slept. The bat was killed and buried, and the child had no sign of a bite. But when she died of rabies a month later, health officials tested the bat carcass and found both bat and child had the same variant of rabies.

Treatment Options and Outlook

If a person is bitten by a suspected rabid animal, the wound should be *immediately* washed with soap and water; the bite should be allowed to bleed to help wash out the wound. Medical help is needed at once. (If possible, the animal should be trapped and confined, but only if it can be done safely.)

Unlike other immunizations, the rabies vaccine is administered after exposure to the virus. This unusual technique works because unlike other viruses, the rabies virus takes a long time to induce disease. Injections of rabies vaccine should prevent the disease from developing in a person bitten by an infected animal.

There are currently two rabies vaccines licensed in the United States. Both work in the same way, triggering the immune system to produce antibodies to neutralize the virus before it causes disease.

The vaccine is a series of five shots, given after exposure on day zero, three, seven, 14, and 28. On day zero, rabies immune globulin is also given, because the vaccine takes about seven to 14 days to provide an active antibody response. Rabies immune globulin provides a passive immunity until active antibodies are produced from the vaccine.

Over the years, scientists have improved both the effectiveness and safety of human rabies vaccines. Earlier vaccines made from duck embryos required a series of 21 shots, many of which were given in the stomach. (Today, most shots are given in the shoulder muscle.)

The modern vaccines are highly effective and produce few side effects. This vaccine is the only way to treat the disease in humans.

Risk Factors and Preventive Measures

There is a preexposure vaccine series designed for people at high risk for exposure (such as veterinarians, researchers, forest rangers, animal control officers, cave explorers, animal handlers, or those who spend time in countries where rabies is common). The preexposure series for all human rabies vaccines is given in three shots—on day zero, day seven, and day 21 or day 28. How often booster shots are taken depends on how good a person is at producing antibodies. People who have received the preexposure series need only two booster shots if they are later exposed to rabies. People in high-risk jobs are encouraged to have their blood tested at regular intervals so boosters can be given if antibody levels fall below a baseline rate. The average high-risk worker only needed boosters about once every two years.

An individual should seek medical evaluation for any animal bite, but rabies is not common in dogs, cats, and ferrets in the United States; very few bites by any of these animals carry a risk of rabies. If the pet appeared healthy when it bit, it can be confined by its owner for 10 days and observed. No anti-rabies shots are needed during this time. *No person in the United States has ever contracted rabies from a dog, cat, or ferret held in quarantine for 10 days.*

If a dog, cat, or ferret appeared ill at the time it bit a human or became ill during the 10-day quarantine, it should be evaluated by a veterinarian for signs of rabies, and the person who was bitten should seek medical advice about the need for anti-rabies prophylaxis. The quarantine period is a precaution against the remote possibility that an animal may appear healthy, but actually be sick with rabies.

Because of the sharp rise in animal rabies (especially among raccoons), an oral recombinant vaccine was licensed for vaccination of free-range raccoons and is the only effective vaccine for raccoons. The license allows the vaccine to be dropped to wildlife habitats in vaccine-laced bait. The oral vaccine is unique because it was created using genetic engineering.

Although most animal cases involve raccoons, there has never been a reported human rabies death directly or indirectly connected to a raccoon.

Four human deaths in 1995 in the United States were due to bat bites or from animals bitten by rabid bats. Rabid bats have been associated with at least 21 human deaths since 1951 in the United States.

rash in infectious diseases Rashes have many causes, including reactions to drugs, allergic reactions, and insect bites. But many infectious diseases also cause a rash, and these rashes usually have a distinct characteristic that changes as the infection continues. A good history and description of a rash can help a doctor reach a correct diagnosis.

Rash with fever is most likely an infectious disease. Raised, red, and itchy spots that turn into blisters could mean CHICKEN POX. A rash of dull red spots or blotches, together with runny nose, cough, and sore, red eyes could be MEASLES, especially if the rash is on the face or trunk and if the patient has never had the disease. A rash of pink spots with a tender swelling down the back and sides of the neck could be GERMAN MEASLES (rubella), especially if the patient has not been vaccinated or had the disease. A rash of purple spots with headache, vomiting, dislike of light, and a stiff neck could mean MENINGITIS. A widespread red rash that is especially itchy at night, with tiny gray lines or red infected-looking spots between fingers or wrists, could be a parasitic infection (especially SCABIES). One or more red, scaly patches spreading out in a ring could be a fungal infection.

rat-bite fever An infectious disease caused by the bite of a rat, squirrel, weasel, or wild mouse. Rat-bite fever is rare in the United States, but since it is not a notifiable disease, exact numbers of cases are not known. People who work with lab mice have been infected without even being bitten, but just from living and working around the rodents. Some recent cases in the United States have occurred in people with pet rats, but the disease is not transmitted from person to person. Humans only get infected from an infected animal, typically through a bite or scratch. Occasionally, unpasteurized contaminated milk has caused an outbreak; this occurred in 1983 in England, when 208 boarding school children got sick from drinking raw milk. The disease is rare in North America; less than 20 cases have been reported in the last 10 years.

Either of two types of bacteria can cause the disease; the type usually seen in North America is *Streptobacillus moniliformis*. In the Far East, rat-bite fever is usually caused by the bacteria *Spirillum minus*. Rat-bite fever caused by *S. moniliformis* is also called Haverhill fever; infection caused by *S. minus* is also called sodoku.

Symptoms and Diagnostic Path

About 10 days after being bitten, the patient experiences the sudden onset of fever, chills, headache, and muscle pain followed in three days by rash on arms and legs. Within a week, there may be swelling, redness, or pain in the joints. About half of those infected with *Streptobacillus moniliformis* will have joint swelling and pain that comes and goes. Patients with *Spirillum minus* do not experience joint pain but instead notice intermittent fever, swollen glands near the bite site, and a purple-red rash.

The bacteria can be cultured in either blood, drainage from the wound or joint fluid. Blood counts show evidence of a bacterial infection.

Treatment Options and Outlook

PENICILLIN is effective in treating either form of the disease; painkillers can treat fever and pain.

Without treatment, rat-bite fever due to *S. moniliformis* in the United States can cause extremely serious and potentially fatal complications, such as an infection of the heart called ENDOCARDITIS. Up to 10 percent of the patients die.

Risk Factors and Preventive Measures

The most important precaution after any animal bite is to wash the area well with soap and running water and seek medical attention. Rat control is also important.

rats and infectious disease   Rodents live close to humans and in many cities, they actually outnum-

ber people and represent a serious public health threat. Various microorganisms and parasites live in the rat, which can cause illness if spread to people. For example, the organisms responsible for PLAGUE and one sort of TYPHUS are transmitted to humans via the bite of rat fleas. LEPTOSPIROSIS is caused by contact with anything that has come into contact with rat's urine, such as tainted water. The rare bacterial infection RAT-BITE FEVER is transmitted directly by rat bite. The only way to control the spread of these rat-borne infectious diseases is to control the urban rat population.

red measles   See MEASLES.

red tide   Red tides are caused by toxic plankton (called dinoflagellates) that multiply rapidly during the warm summer months; the name "red tide" refers to the plankton's pink or red color. These plankton produce a deadly poison called saxitoxin. Shellfish that eat this plankton become contaminated and can cause disease in anyone who eats them. The toxin is so toxic, even one contaminated shellfish can be fatal if eaten. This is why clams, oysters, and mussels are not sold during the summer months.

Red tides are found in coastal waters in the Pacific from California to Alaska and in the Atlantic from New England to the St. Lawrence. Under good conditions (warm climate, warm water), the plankton may reach 60 million organisms per liter of water. These rapid growths (referred to as a "bloom") discolor the sea and poison fish and marine life. Usually, a person becomes poisoned with the plankton when eating shellfish that have been feeding on them.

Red tides have been known since ancient times; it is believed that the name of the Red Sea was coined by ancient Greeks who were referring to red blooms off the Arabian coasts. In fact, it is believed that the first reference to red tide appears in the Bible: "And all the waters that were in the river were turned to blood. And the fish that was in the river died, and the river stank, and the Egyptians could not drink of the water of the rivers." (Exodus 7:20–21).

Mussels, clams, and oysters are the primary shellfish at risk, and mussels are the most susceptible of all. Healthy bivalve shellfish filter large amounts of toxic plankton, which form the primary ocean food during May through August. During these warm times, the dinoflagellates thrive by photosynthesis and can be so invasive that they kill birds and fish.

The first large epidemic of poisoning caused by red tide–contaminated shellfish occurred in San Francisco in 1927, when 102 people were sickened and six died. Today, largely because of the prohibition against eating certain shellfish during the summer months, such epidemics are rare.

relapsing fever   A comprehensive term for any one of several infectious diseases marked by recurrent fevers, also known as African tick fever, famine fever, recurrent fever, spirillus fever, or tick fever. The disease has occurred in several western states, but is more commonly found in South America, Asia, and Africa.

Relapsing fever is caused by at least 15 different *Borrelia* species, transmitted by both ticks and lice and often seen during wars and famines.

Symptoms and Diagnostic Path

The first episode usually begins with a sudden high fever (104°F to 105°F) with headache, chills, muscle aches, and nausea. A rash may appear over the trunk and arms and legs, and jaundice is common in the later stages. Each attack lasts two or three days and ends in a high fever, profuse sweating, and rising heart and breathing rates. This is followed by an abrupt drop in temperature and a return to normal blood pressure. Typically, patients relapse about seven to 10 days later and eventually recover completely. In louse-borne disease, there is usually only one period of relapse; tick-borne illness causes several relapses, each milder than the last.

The spirochete is identified in a blood smear obtained during an attack.

Treatment Options and Outlook

Long-acting PENICILLIN, tetracycline, or chloramphenicol. However, treatment is withheld during the high-fever stage. Other treatment includes bed rest, sponge baths, and aspirin to alleviate symptoms. Bedding and clothing should be disinfected to destroy any lice or ticks.

reovirus   Any of three viruses (found in the respiratory and alimentary tracts of both healthy and sick people) that have double-stranded RNA. They have been linked in some cases to upper RESPIRATORY TRACT INFECTIONS and infantile gastroenteritis.

reportable disease   Any contagious disease that must be reported by the physician to the public health authorities, who in turn report some of them to the CENTERS FOR DISEASE CONTROL AND PREVENTION.

This notification of certain potentially harmful diseases is important because it helps public health officers take the necessary steps to control the spread of infection. The reporting also provides valuable statistics on the incidence and prevalence of a disease. This information can then be used to help determine health policies (such as immunization programs or sanitary improvements).

Examples of reportable diseases include AIDS, MALARIA, INFLUENZA, POLIOMYELITIS, RELAPSING FEVER, TYPHUS, YELLOW FEVER, SYPHILIS, GONORRHEA, CHOLERA, and bubonic PLAGUE.

respiratory syncytial virus (RSV) infection   The most common respiratory illness in infants and young children. It is caused by a type of virus known as a MYXOVIRUS (an RNA-containing virus that commonly causes upper respiratory infections and the common COLD).

RSV is responsible for more than 125,000 hospitalizations; about 2 percent of these die. Most cases occur in children under age four, with the peak of severe illness under six months of age, especially in infants with preexisting heart or lung conditions. RSV also can cause a serious illness in the elderly and in those with impaired immune systems.

The disease can occur at any time, although epidemics usually take place in fall and winter. The first infection is the worst, but it does not confer immunity; RSV can also cause serious colds in children who have repeat infections.

The highly contagious virus is spread via contact with droplets from the nose and throat of infected patients when they cough and sneeze. RSV can spread through direct respiratory secretions on sheets, towels, and other items. In the winter, this infection is a big problem for hospitalized children who can become seriously ill with PNEUMONIA if they catch RSV.

Air pollution and smoking irritate the lining of the throat and can make it easier to catch RSV; people who live in areas of heavy industrial pollution or live with smokers have more serious and longer RSV infections.

Outbreaks are predictable, occurring in the fall through spring. Studies have found that many children under age one who attend day care centers have been infected.

Symptoms and Diagnostic Path

Symptoms can range from a mild cold to severe pneumonia and include coughing, wheezing, runny nose, and severe fatigue. Fever is unusual in young babies. Pneumonia is most likely among high-risk patients; occasionally, the infection can be fatal to infants. Symptoms occur four to six days after exposure, and may persist for a few days to weeks.

In most cases, babies are not seriously ill; it affects infants under age three months the most severely, since they have a hard time breathing. All babies except those with other medical problems should recover within a week.

Children are infectious from 24 hours before symptoms until two weeks after the cold starts. Adults are infectious for a much shorter time, until about five days before the cold starts.

RSV is usually diagnosed on the basis of symptoms; lab tests may be used in cases of severe illness and in special outbreak investigations. If a child has a bad cold, it is not likely that the pediatrician will test for RSV in an office visit. Children admitted to a hospital with pneumonia or bronchiolitis will be tested for the disease during RSV season.

Treatment Options and Outlook

There is no cure for this virus. Rest, high humidity, and clear fluids can help. The antiviral drug ribavirin will help a child recover if started in the first few days after symptoms appear. Treatment is reserved for the most serious cases because of potential side effects; an expensive medication, it is given in the hospital as a mist treatment. Most hospitalized children with RSV do not need ribavirin.

Because RSV often improves on its own, treatment of mild symptoms is not necessary for most people. Antibiotics are not effective, although in certain patients antibiotics may be used to treat underlying secondary bacterial infections.

RSV can cause BRONCHIOLITIS in infants under age one, pneumonia in babies under age two, or CROUP in children from six months to three years of age. Premature babies who have poorly developed lungs may be quite ill and may survive with permanent lung damage. But it is the babies with heart problems who are most at risk; some of these infants can die from an RSV infection. *Danger signs:* an infant who is not getting enough air into the lungs will have flaring nostrils and dents above and below the breastbone or in between the ribs during breathing.

Risk Factors and Preventive Measures

Palivizumab (Synagis) and RSV immunoglobulin intravenous (RSV-IGIV) helps prevent RSV infection in high-risk children, children younger than 24 months with chronic lung disease, and certain preterm infants. Monthly administration of palivizumab during the RSV season (fall and winter) results in a 45 to 55 percent decrease in the rate of hospitalization attributable to RSV. Because it is easier to administer, monthly palivizumab generally is favored over RSV-IGIV, which requires a four-hour IV infusion.

The treatment does not prevent children from getting the virus, as a vaccine would, but it can help protect high-risk children under age two from the most serious complications. It is given intravenously in five monthly doses beginning each November before the start of RSV season.

No vaccine for RSV currently exists, although some researchers are testing various versions of live attenuated RSV vaccines. Since a baby is most vulnerable during the first three months of life, it is possible to take some steps to protect against RSV: People should not smoke around the baby, crowds should be avoided, and the baby should be isolated from children with obvious colds.

respiratory tract infections Upper respiratory tract infections include the common COLD, PHARYNGITIS, RHINITIS, SINUSITIS, or TONSILLITIS. Lower respiratory tract infections include BRONCHITIS, BRONCHIOLITIS, PNEUMONIA, tracheitis, lung ABSCESS, and TUBERCULOSIS.

retrovirus An RNA virus family that includes HUMAN IMMUNODEFICIENCY VIRUS (HIV), the virus that causes AIDS.

rheumatic fever An inflammatory disease that may appear as a delayed reaction to inadequately treated group A beta-hemolytic streptococcal infection of the upper respiratory tract. Although most symptoms disappear within weeks to months, half the time patients have deformed heart valves. The disorder, which usually appears in young school-age children, also may affect the brain, joints, skin, or other tissues. Once diagnosed, rheumatic fever will tend to recur whenever the patient gets a strep infection.

During the 1950s, the disease was considered to be such a serious threat to the health of young U.S. military recruits that the country set up a special disease lab at Warren Air Force Base in California to handle the problem. When PENICILLIN became available, researchers at the base proved that rheumatic fever could be prevented by an injection of penicillin for everyone with strep throat. By the 1980s, rheumatic fever was considered to be conquered in the United States and other developed countries.

Unfortunately, the disease has not been eradicated; today it causes a much more severe form that leads to heart damage and death in many people, from middle-class suburban families to those in poor, overcrowded conditions. Since 1985, there have been outbreaks in 24 states, especially in Utah, Ohio, and Pennsylvania.

Researchers believe the resurgence can be traced to a reemergence of certain strains of the bacterium group A *beta-hemolytic Streptococcus* (GROUP A STREP). Of the 80 different strains of group A strep, only a few can cause rheumatic fever. This is the same strain of virulent bacteria that killed Muppet creator Jim Henson in 1990.

Rheumatic fever is a delayed complication of group A strep infection, usually either strep throat or SCARLET FEVER. About 1 to 3 percent of untreated people come down with rheumatic fever from 10 days to six weeks after getting over these related illnesses. Scientists are not sure why some people develop rheumatic fever, but it may be a combination of the type of bacteria and the genetics of the infected person. Rheumatic fever occurs because the patient's body creates antibodies to the organism and those antibodies mistakenly attack the person's own tissues. Rheumatic fever usually strikes children from five to 18 years of age.

Symptoms and Diagnostic Path
The onset of the disease is usually sudden, usually about one to five weeks after recovery from scarlet fever or a sore throat. Early symptoms include fever, joint pain, nose bleeds, stomach pain, and vomiting. Other symptoms include palpitations, chest pain, and (in severe cases) heart failure. Sydenham's chorea is usually the only late sign of rheumatic fever and is characterized by an increased awkwardness and a tendency to drop objects. As the chorea progresses, irregular body movements or twitching become severe, sometimes including the tongue and facial muscles.

Rheumatic fever is hard to diagnose because it resembles so many other illnesses; lab studies, throat culture, and EKG can diagnose the condition. Doctors may rely on a variety of criteria, including evidence of previous group A strep infection. A diagnosis of rheumatic fever requires one (and preferably two) of these symptoms:

- joint pain (ankles, knees, elbows, or wrists become painful, red, and swollen)
- clumsy movements that resemble cerebral palsy that last from three to eight months
- inflammation of the heart muscle
- painless swellings under the skin over joints
- flat, painless rash lasting less than a day with fever and fatigue
- fever of at least 100.4°F

Treatment Options and Outlook
Severe restriction of regular activity and painkillers. Penicillin is often given to eliminate any remaining

strep from the old infection, and steroids or salicy-lates may be used, depending on the severity of joint pain.

While bed rest used to be a part of the treatment, it is no longer considered to be helpful.

Rheumatic fever can cause inflammation of the heart muscle in about 50 percent of patients, with heart valve damage that can lead to congestive heart failure. It is one of the most common causes of the need for heart valve replacement.

rhinitis Inflammation of the mucous membrane lining the nose, caused by the common cold virus. This infection can lead to SINUSITIS. It usually causes nasal obstruction, nasal discharge, sneezing, and facial pain.

rhinoscleroma An uncommon bacterial infection caused by *Klebsiella rhinoscleromatis* that is chronic in rural areas throughout the world.

Symptoms and Diagnostic Path
The disease begins with increased nasal secretion and crusting, followed by an enlargement of the nose, upper lip, palate, or neighboring areas. If the infection spreads to the respiratory tract, breathing may become difficult.

Treatment Options and Outlook
This disease is difficult to treat; systemic antibiotics such as gentamicin and tobramycin have been effective. Alternatively, oral administration of cip-rofloxacin may help, although this drug has not been widely studied as a therapy for this condition. The condition may be fatal due to breathing prob-lems or continuing infection.

rhinovirus Any of the more than 200 distinct viruses that cause about 40 percent of all acute respiratory illnesses. Complete recovery is usual.

Symptoms and Diagnostic Path
Infection is characterized by dry, scratchy throat, nasal congestion, malaise, and headache. There is little fever; nasal discharge lasts two or three days.

Children may develop a cough. From onset to end, with or without treatment, the infection lasts two to four weeks.

Treatment Options and Outlook
Symptom-relieving medications such as painkillers, antihistamines, and nasal decongestants. Zinc and vitamin C in large doses have been shown to be somewhat effective at shortening the duration of the illness caused by certain strains of rhinovirus.

See also COLD, COMMON.

Rickettsia akari A type of parasite of insects and insectlike animals such as fleas, lice, ticks, and mites that cause the disease rickettsial pox.

Rickettsia conorii A type of parasite of insects and insectlike animals such as fleas, lice, ticks, and mites that cause TYPHUS.

rickettsial fever See ROCKY MOUNTAIN SPOTTED FEVER.

rickettsial infections Diseases caused by the bite or feces of insects carrying parasitic microorganisms called rickettsia. These diseases include CAT SCRATCH DISEASE, ROCKY MOUNTAIN SPOTTED FEVER, Q FEVER, and various forms of TYPHUS. Rickettsia resemble small bacteria, but they are able to multiply only by invading the cells of another life-form. In this respect, they are more like VIRUSES. The rickettsiae were once classified between bacteria and viruses because they seem to possess the characteristics of both.

Rickettsiae are primarily found in the intestines and saliva of insects and insectlike animals (such as fleas, lice, ticks, and mites). However, these insects can transmit rickettsiae to larger animals (including humans) through their saliva and feces.

They were named for 19th-century American pathologist Howard Taylor Ricketts, who studied them in 1906 when he was at the University of Chicago as part of his studies of Rocky Mountain spotted fever. Ricketts died in Mexico in 1910 from typhus, which he was investigating at the time, and the genus *Rickettsia* was named in his honor.

Rickettsiae that produce disease are usually transmitted by the bite of an infected louse, tick, mite, or flea. The diseases they cause are widespread and are found wherever in the world that humans, rodents, and arthropods live together. The rickettsial human infections are divided into four main groups: the typhus fever group (including classical typhus and rat-borne typhus); spotted fever group (Rocky Mountain spotted fever, South Africa tick fever, boutonneuse fever, and Sao Paulo typhus of Brazil); tsutsugamushi group (TSUTSUGAMUSHI DISEASE of Japan, Malayan scrub typhus, and Sumatran mite typhus); and miscellaneous group (trench fever, Q fever, RICKETTSIAL POX).

Most rickettsial infections are characterized by a fever and a rash, although the fatality rate differs from one variety of illness to the next. It ranges from less than 1 percent for the milder diseases to 70 percent for some outbreaks of typhus and Rocky Mountain spotted fever.

rickettsial pox An urban disease transmitted by the bite of a mite from a house mouse. The responsible microorganism is *RICKETTSIA AKARI*, which belongs to the spotted fever group.

Rickettsia prowazekii A type of parasite of insects and insect-like animals such as fleas, lice, ticks, and mites that causes TYPHUS.

Rickettsia rickettsii A type of intracellular parasitic microorganism that looks like small bacteria but can reproduce only by invading cells of another life-form. These parasites live primarily off insects such as lice, fleas, ticks, and mites; in turn, these insects can transmit the rickettsia to rodents, dogs, or humans through saliva or feces. Human diseases caused by these organisms include ROCKY MOUNTAIN SPOTTED FEVER and various forms of TYPHUS.

Rickettsia tsutsugamushi A type of parasite of insects and insectlike animals such as fleas, lice,

ticks, and mites that cause TYPHUS or TSUTSUGAMUSHI DISEASE.

Rift Valley fever A viral disease uncommon in the United States but found much more often in eastern and southern Africa, most countries of sub-Saharan Africa, and in Madagascar. It is caused by an ARBOVIRUS that affects domestic animals and causes fever in humans.

The virus is transmitted by the *AEDES* and other types of mosquito. It was first discovered in the 1930s as a cause of stillbirth in European cattle in Kenya and a cause of fever in veterinarians who studied the problem and were exposed to blood or viscera. After the Aswan Dam was completed in the 1970s, vast new wetlands were created that boosted the local mosquito population. As a result, an EPIDEMIC of Rift Valley fever swept through the area, killing 598 of the 18,000 patients and wiping out entire livestock herds. Over the next 10 years, other epidemics related to dam construction occurred in Mauritania, Madagascar, and Senegal, followed by a second outbreak in Aswan in 1993. In this latest epidemic, patients were blinded after experiencing fever, headache, and muscle pain.

Humans can get the disease as a result of bites from mosquitoes if they are exposed to the blood or body fluids of infected animals while handling infected animals, or by touching contaminated meat while cooking.

Sleeping outdoors at night in areas where outbreaks occur could be a risk factor. Animal herdsmen, abattoir workers, and others who work with animals in RVF-endemic areas are at higher risk for infection. People in high-risk professions such as veterinarians and slaughterhouse workers have a higher chance of contracting the virus from an infected animal. International travelers may be at risk if they visit RVF-endemic locations during periods when sporadic cases or epidemics are occurring.

Symptoms and Diagnostic Path
People with RVF typically have either no symptoms or a mild illness associated with fever, vision problems, and liver abnormalities. However, in some patients the illness can progress to hemorrhagic fever, ENCEPHALITIS, or diseases affecting the eye.

Symptoms usually begin with fever, generalized weakness, back pain, dizziness, and extreme weight loss. Typically, patients recover within two days to one week after onset of illness. Fatal bleeding can occur in rare cases. Approximately 1 percent of humans who become infected with RVF die of the disease.

Treatment Options and Outlook

Treatment is symptomatic. However, studies in monkeys and other animals have shown promise for the antiviral drug Ribavirin for future use in humans. Additional studies suggest that interferon, immune modulators, and convalescent-phase plasma may also help in the treatment of patients.

The most common complication associated with RVF is inflammation of the retina that may lead to permanent vision loss in up to 10 percent of affected patients.

Risk Factors and Preventive Measures

Avoiding mosquito bites can reduce the risk of infection. People should also avoid exposure to blood or tissues of animals that may potentially be infected. The human live attenuated vaccine MP-12 has demonstrated promising results in laboratory trials in domestic animals, but it is not yet available for humans.

ring rubella   See FIFTH DISEASE.

ringworm   A skin infection caused by a fungus that can affect the scalp, skin, fingers, toenails, or feet. The disease has nothing to do with worms or rings. Scalp ringworm is the most common fungal skin infection in children. While anyone can get ringworm, children are more susceptible to certain varieties.

Patients are infectious for as long as the lesions appear on the body; if untreated, the condition may last for years.

Once thought to be under control in the United States, ringworm now affects up to 15 percent of children between five and 10.

Ringworm is spread by direct skin-to-skin contact with infected people or pets, or with indirect contact with items such as barber clippers, shower stalls, or floors. Children can get it from playing with ringworm-infected dogs or cats or from sharing combs, brushes, headphones, towels, pillows, hats, and sofas.

Symptoms and Diagnostic Path

The infection usually begins as a small pimple that gets larger and larger, leaving scaly patches of temporary baldness; infected hair is brittle and breaks off easily. Sometimes there is a yellow cup-like crusty area. The infection usually is seen 10 to 14 days after contact.

Ringworm of the scalp (TINEA CAPITIS) involves scaly, temporary bald patches with dandruff-like white scales. The hair may be dull, and the infection may affect only one part of the scalp or may spread over the entire head. A severe case may include fever and swollen glands below the hairline.

Ringworm of the nails causes thick, discolored, and brittle or chalky and friable nails.

Ringworm of the body (TINEA CORPORIS) is flat and ring-shaped; the edge is red and may be dry and scaly, or moist and crusted. The center area clears and appears normal. Symptoms occur four to 10 days after contact. The rings can appear on face, legs, arms, or trunk.

Ringworm of the foot appears as a scaling or cracking of the skin, especially between the toes.

Since so many species of fungus can cause ringworm, infection with one species will not make a person immune to future infections from other species.

Microscopic inspection of infected hair or skin scrapings will reveal certain characteristics of the fungus. The doctor may use an ultraviolet light called a Wood's light to diagnose ringworm; when the lamp is shone on an affected area, the fungus may show as a yellowish or brilliant green fluorescence, depending on the type of fungus. (The most common type of scalp fungus will not have this effect.)

Treatment Options and Outlook

Antifungal medication (such as griseofulvin) by mouth or applied to the skin. An antifungal ointment applied directly to the scalp will stop the ringworm from spreading to other areas of the head, and to a child's friends. Any secondary bacterial infection will be treated with antibiotics. Boggy raised areas of the scalp will require a special cream and a cotton cap to cover the scalp until the areas dry. The infected hair will need to be clipped and a special shampoo used.

Body ringworm is easier to treat; a variety of antifungal creams will work. The patient should wash well with soap and water and remove all scabs and crusts. Antifungal cream should then be rubbed into all lesions.

Risk Factors and Preventive Measures

People should not share towels, hats, or clothing of an infected person. Good grooming and hygiene and frequent checks of a child's scalp can prevent the disease.

Once an infection has been diagnosed, all contaminated articles must be cleaned to prevent further infection. Combs, brushes, hats, scarfs, and bedding must be cleaned in hot, soapy water.

risus sardonicus   An unusual grinning expression caused by prolonged contraction of the facial muscles; it is a symptom of TETANUS.

Ritter's disease   The former name for STAPHYLOCOCCAL SCALDED SKIN SYNDROME.

Rocky Mountain spotted fever (RMSF)   An infectious disease characterized by a spotted rash, caused by the organism RICKETTSIA RICKETTSII (similar to bacteria).

In the eastern United States, children are most often infected, whereas in the West disease is highest among men. Although the disease is found most often on the Atlantic coast, it gets its name from its original appearance in the Rocky Mountain states. The incidence of the disease has been rising steadily since 1980; between 500 and 1,000 cases are reported each year, although many likely go unreported.

RMSF is spread by the bite of an infected American dog tick, lone-star tick, or wood tick, or by skin contamination with tick blood or feces. Person-to-person spread of RMSF does not occur.

Symptoms and Diagnostic Path

Symptoms begin with the sudden onset of mild to moderate fever, which can last for two or three weeks. Loss of appetite and a slight headache may develop slowly about a week after a tick bite. Sometimes, however, symptoms appear suddenly, with high fever, prostration, aching, tender muscles, severe headache, nausea, and vomiting. Two to six days after symptoms appear, small pink spots appear on wrists and ankles, spreading over the entire body and darkening, enlarging, and bleeding. The illness subsides after about two weeks. Untreated cases with very high fever may end in death from PNEUMONIA or heart failure.

Diagnosis may be difficult because the disease resembles several other infections. Lab tests on blood and tissues may confirm the disease.

Treatment Options and Outlook

Antibiotic drugs doxycycline or tetracycline usually cure the disease. If patients cannot tolerate these drugs, chloramphenicol may be administered.

Risk Factors and Preventive Measures

People in tick-infested areas should use insect repellent and examine themselves daily for ticks. Local tick populations may be controlled with applications of pesticides to vegetation along trails, and frequent lawn mowing to eliminate areas where small rodents can live.

One attack probably provides permanent immunity.

roseola (exanthem subitum)   A common infectious disease of early childhood that primarily affects youngsters aged six months to two years. Only about a third of children with the infection have any symptoms at all. All children recover completely.

The cause is human HERPES virus-6 and -7. Because scientists recently found the virus in the saliva of healthy children, they have concluded that the virus may be spread through contact with saliva of family members or other children who carry the virus but do not have symptoms.

Research suggests that after an active infection, the virus can become latent and hide in the body, later reappearing to cause other illnesses. Some scientists suggest it may be linked to the development of CHRONIC FATIGUE SYNDROME.

Symptoms and Diagnostic Path

Most cases of roseola occur in spring and summer and are characterized by the abrupt onset of irritability and a fever, which may climb as high as 105°F. By the fourth or fifth day, the fever breaks, suddenly returning to normal. At about the same time, a rash appears on the body, often spreading quickly to the face, neck, and limbs, fading within two days. Other symptoms may include sore throat, enlarged lymph nodes, and occasionally a febrile seizure.

Roseola is usually diagnosed by noting symptoms and ruling out other causes of high fever. Tests have been developed to look for both the virus and its antibodies, but these are available in research labs only.

Treatment Options and Outlook

There are no serious complications, and there is no specific treatment other than acetaminophen or ibuprofen for the fever, rest, and fluids.

Rarely, a child will have seizures due to the high fever, or develop ENCEPHALITIS.

rotavirus   The most common cause of severe diarrhea in children, leading to the hospitalization of about 55,000 children each year in the United States and the death of more than 600,000 children each year around the world. The rotavirus gets its name from its appearance: it looks like a wheel when seen under an electron microscope (rotavirus is derived from the Latin *rota*, meaning "wheel"). The rotavirus is a common name for a family of viruses that share several features.

If an infant or toddler develops diarrhea in the winter, there is a good chance that a rotavirus is the culprit. By age four, most people have been infected and developed antibodies. While the disease is not particularly deadly in the United States among children with healthy immune systems, rotavirus in the developing world is more serious because many infants are malnourished. In the United States, the chance a child will be hospitalized with rotavirus is one in 40. One in every 800

hospitalized will die. The rotavirus season begins in late fall and ends in the spring.

Rotavirus invades the cells of the small bowel so that it cannot absorb liquids, resulting in diarrhea. While the rotavirus also infects animals, scientists do not believe it is passed from pets to humans; the virus is thought to be spread by the fecal-oral route. The virus must be swallowed in order for it to infect the digestive tract. Children infected once can be infected again.

Symptoms and Diagnostic Path

After infection, it takes about two days for symptoms to appear. Most babies begin with vomiting and a low fever, followed by watery diarrhea for three to eight days. Immunity after infection is incomplete, but repeat infections tend to be less severe than the original infection. The child is infectious until the diarrhea stops. As many as 20 vomiting and 20 diarrhea episodes a day are not uncommon.

Physicians can diagnose rotavirus from symptoms alone, noting the age of the child and time of year. A test of stool samples can detect rotavirus in 15 minutes.

Treatment Options and Outlook

There is no cure for rotavirus infection. Nonprescription antidiarrhea medicine should not be given to infants and young children. Infants with severe dehydration and vomiting require IV-fluid replacement.

Risk Factors and Preventive Measures

The newest rotavirus vaccine (RotaTeq, produced by Merck) was approved by the U.S. Food and Drug Administration in February 2006, making it the only rotavirus vaccine sold in the United States. It should be included with all routine immunizations given to infants by mouth at two, four, and six months of age.

A second vaccine, developed by GlaxoSmith-Kline (Rotarix) is also effective, but the company has not yet sought FDA approval. Instead, the vaccine has been approved for use in Mexico and 14 Latin American countries and is expected to be available in Europe in 2006.

There are differences between the two vaccines. Rotarix contains the most common strain of rotavirus and is given in two doses, a month or two apart;

RotaTeq contains five strains and is given in three doses, at two, four, and six months of age. Both are given by mouth.

An earlier vaccine (RotaShield) had been approved in 1998, but it was abruptly withdrawn in 1999 after nine infants developed a bowel obstruction after being vaccinated. Within the first seven days of vaccination, the risk was 14 times higher than normal, and within the first two weeks after vaccination, the risk was 10 times higher. Although the obstruction was considered to be very rare (affecting only one in every 10,000 vaccinated infants), the risk was deemed too great because so few American babies die of rotavirus. However, at the time, many developing countries—where rotavirus is a significant threat—complained that RotaShield could have saved at least 100 of their children's lives for every case of bowel obstruction.

See also DIARRHEA AND INFECTIOUS DISEASE; ANTIDIARRHEAL DRUGS.

roundworms   Also known as nematodes, this class of elongated, cylindrical worms include at least a dozen or so types that are parasites in humans. In temperate climates such as the United States, the only common type of roundworm problem is PINWORM INFESTATION, which primarily affects children. Ascariasis, whipworms, and TRICHINOSIS also are fairly common. TOXOCARIASIS sometimes occurs, caused by the worm *TOXOCARA CANIS* (in dogs) and the *T. cati* (in cats). (Most North American infections are due to *T. canis*.)

In tropical countries, roundworm infestations are much more common and include HOOKWORM DISEASE, STRONGYLOIDIASIS, Guinea worm disease (see DRACUNCULIASIS), and different types of FILARIASIS.

Symptoms and Diagnostic Path
In many cases, adult worms live in the human intestines without causing symptoms unless there are many worms present. Sometimes symptoms occur as worm larvae pass through various parts of the body. The number of worms present is called the "worm burden."

Treatment Options and Outlook
Most infestations are treated relatively easily with ANTIHELMINTIC DRUGS.

rubella   See GERMAN MEASLES.

rubeola   Another name for MEASLES.

Russian flu   See INFLUENZA.

S

St. Anthony's fire   The common name for ERY-
SIPELAS.

St. Louis encephalitis   See ENCEPHALITIS, ST. LOUIS.

Salk vaccine   See POLIOMYELITIS.

Salmonella   A group of more than 2,000 types of
bacteria that cause a type of food poisoning known
as SALMONELLOSIS. Included in this group are *Salmonella enteritidis, S. cubana, S. aertrycke,* and *S. cholerae-
suis.* These bacteria are known for multiplying
rapidly at room temperature and are often found in
raw meat, poultry, eggs, fish, raw milk (and foods
made from them), and in pet turtles. Proper handling and cooking of contaminated food will kill the
Salmonella bacteria.

The most dangerous members of the *Salmonella*
family are *S. typhi,* which causes TYPHOID FEVER. *Salmonella* is also a common cause of OSTEOMYELITIS
(bone infection), especially of the spine. They were
discovered by an American scientist named Salmon,
for whom they were named.

salmonellosis   One of the major types of FOOD POI-
SONING caused by *SALMONELLA* bacteria that multiply
rapidly at room temperatures. Although salmonellosis is fatal in only 1 percent of cases, it is very
dangerous in pregnant women, young children,
the elderly, and those with cancer or AIDS. Each
year about 2 million cases of salmonellosis lead to
between two and 20 deaths in the United States.

Salmonellosis is caused by infection with the *Salmonella* bacteria; even extremely low doses (too low

to be detected by current standards) can cause food
poisoning (see FOOD-BORNE INFECTIONS).

The incidence of salmonellosis appears to be
spreading in EPIDEMIC proportions. Bacteria are now
commonly found in eggs and poultry across the
country; it is estimated that 35 percent of chicken
carcasses in U.S. processing plants harbor the bacteria. *Salmonella* is also present in raw meats, fish, raw
milk, bone meal, fertilizer, and pet foods as well as in
pet turtles and marijuana, and it can also be transferred to food from the excrement of infected animals or people. One type of the bacteria, *S. enteritidis,*
has been found in the eggs of chickens with the disease. The more bacteria ingested, the faster illness
will occur.

Salmonellosis is very common in this country;
bone meal, fertilizer, and pet foods may all be implicated in the spread of the disease. In particular,
recent outbreaks have been linked to chickens and
eggs; it is estimated that 35 percent of chicken carcasses in processing plants harbor the bacteria.

The largest outbreak ever recorded occurred in
1994 and involved more than 200,000 Americans.
In this case, commercially pasteurized ice cream
premix was contaminated by bacteria during transport to a Minnesota ice-cream plant in tanker trail-
ers that had previously carried nonpasteurized
liquid eggs. The outbreak ended after sales of the
ice cream were stopped.

Unfortunately, salmonella resistant to standard
antibiotics used to treat infection in children are
emerging across the nation. Between 1996 and 1998,
13 cases of salmonella infection resistant to the antibiotic ceftriaxone were recorded. Another possible
28 cases occurred in 1999. Because there are several
million salmonella infections each year, researchers
believe this means that several thousand are probably caused by the ceftriaxone-resistant strain.

Symptoms and Diagnostic Path

While tiny amounts of *Salmonella* can be ingested in otherwise healthy people without problem, a minimal number may cause salmonellosis symptoms from 12 to 72 hours after eating tainted food, smoking tainted marijuana, or handling infected turtles. Symptoms vary, depending on the amount of bacteria, but include headache, nausea, vomiting, fever, stomach cramps, and diarrhea. Symptoms usually last two to seven days. Severe cases can lead to shock and can be fatal in infants and the elderly.

Treatment Options and Outlook

As with most types of food poisoning, there is no specific treatment. Patients should eat a bland diet and drink plenty of fluids to combat dehydration. Antibiotic treatment (chloramphenicol, ampicillin, or tetracycline) should be administered only in cases of severe infection or if there is indication of bacteria in the blood.

Risk Factors and Preventive Measures

Fortunately for consumers, proper handling and cooking of contaminated food will kill the *Salmonella* bacteria. Proper refrigeration and cooking methods for meat and eggs must be observed at all times. Eggs should be refrigerated and not used raw (such as in Caesar salad or egg nog). Raw chicken should never touch any other food or utensils during preparation, and cooks should wash their hands after touching raw chicken.

Researchers have developed a bacteria mixture that, when sprayed on newly hatched chicks, blocks the growth of salmonella in their intestines. Industry and health officials hope it will cut down on the amount of salmonella found in raw chicken and lessen the threat of food poisoning from undercooked chicken. The product, called Preempt, is made up of 29 healthy, nonharmful bacteria naturally present in adult birds. Newly hatched chicks sprayed with the mixture peck at their wet feathers and ingest the solution. The culture then grows inside the chicken, preventing salmonella bacteria from attaching to the chicken's intestines.

In tests of 80,000 chickens, 7 percent of the untreated birds developed salmonella—but none of the treated birds became infected. Farmers who use Preempt must not feed their birds preventative antibiotics that could kill the beneficial microbes.

USDA researchers say lab tests show the mixture also looks promising in the fight against other germs that infect chicken, including *Campylobacter*, *Listeria*, and *E. coli*.

See also ANTIDIARRHEAL DRUGS; DIARRHEA AND INFECTIOUS DISEASE; TRAVELER'S DIARRHEA.

sandfly fever A mild viral disease transmitted by the bite of certain mosquitoes, commonly found in hot, dry areas of the world. Although sandfly fever is not lethal, unlike many other BUNYAVIRUSES, it is still an important disease. The sandfly fever virus is transmitted by mosquitos including *Phlebotomus papatasi*, *P. perniciosus*, and *P. perfiliewi*.

Symptoms and Diagnostic Path

After an average incubation period of between two and six days, patients experience a sudden onset of fever, frontal headache, low back pain, generalized myalgia, sensitivity to light and in some cases nausea, vomiting, dizziness, and neck stiffness. Acute neurologic disease can occur in a few people and is marked by fever and headache two to four days before the appearance of more serious symptoms. In some cases, mental confusion and lethargy appear.

Treatment Options and Outlook

Only treatment of the symptoms is possible, since there are no current antiviral drugs that are effective against sandfly fever. There is also no vaccine.

San Joaquin fever Another name for COCCIDIOIDOMYCOSIS.

Sarcoptes scabiei The mite responsible for the skin infestation of SCABIES.

SARS See SEVERE ACUTE RESPIRATORY SYNDROME.

scabies A highly infectious, fairly common skin infestation caused by the mite SARCOPTES SCABIEI, which burrows into the skin and lays its eggs. Scabies infect people from all socioeconomic levels, with no regard to age, sex, race, or standards of personal hygiene. Clusters of outbreaks are sometimes seen in institutions such as child care centers or nursing homes.

Scabies mites are passed by direct skin-to-skin contact; indirect transfer from underwear or sheets can occur only if these have been contaminated by infected people right beforehand. Hatched mites can pass from one individual to another person simply by direct contact, although the mites are usually passed during contact, such as sexual intercourse. A person can continue to spread scabies until the mites and eggs have been destroyed.

Symptoms and Diagnostic Path
The most common symptom is intense itching (especially at night). Tiny gray, itchy swellings appear on the skin, between the fingers, on wrists and genitals, waist, thighs, nipples, breasts, lower buttocks, and in armpits. Reddish lumps may later appear on limbs and trunk.

Symptoms may appear from two to six weeks in people who have not been previously exposed to scabies. Those who have had cases in the past may show symptoms within one to four days after a reexposure.

Treatment Options and Outlook
Insecticide lotion such as prescription permethrin or crotamiton should be applied to all skin below the patient's head, which kills the mites (although itching may continue for up to two weeks later). All members of a family should be treated at the same time.

Itching may persist, but this is not necessarily a failure of treatment or a reinfestation. Those with symptoms should be treated with a second course of lotion seven to 10 days later, followed by a cleansing bath eight hours after application, and a change to clean clothing.

Risk Factors and Preventive Measures
Scabies can be prevented by avoiding physical contact with an infested person or his or her belongings.

scalded skin syndrome See STAPHYLOCOCCAL SCALDED SKIN SYNDROME.

scarlatina Another name for SCARLET FEVER.

scarlet fever An infectious bacterial childhood disease characterized by a skin rash, sore throat, and fever and caused by infection with group A streptococcus. It is less common and dangerous than it was years ago. No longer a reportable disease, experts do not know for sure how many cases occur today in the United States, although it is believed that the disease has been on the increase for the past several years.

With the spread of STREPTOCOCCUS infections around the world has come more cases of scarlet fever. Scarlet fever strains of group A strep produce toxins that are released in the skin, causing a bright red rash.

In the past, the disease was associated with poor living conditions. In 1737, a scarlet fever EPIDEMIC in Boston killed 900 people; another epidemic in New York City in the late 1800s killed 35 percent of children who contracted the disease; that same year, 19 percent of Chicago children who got the disease perished.

Inexplicably, by the 1920s the death rate of the disease dropped to 5 percent for reasons that are still not completely understood. It is believed that the scarlet fever bacteria underwent a natural mutation that made it less lethal. The introduction of PENICILLIN reduced the death rate even more.

Today, most cases are found among residents of middle-class suburbs, not in the inner cities. Because it is possible to get strep and scarlet fever more than once, and because the incidence of all strep infections is rising, prompt medical attention when strep is suspected is important. A patient with a sore throat and skin rash should seek medical care. Anyone can develop scarlet fever, but most cases are found among children aged four to eight.

Scarlet fever bacteria are spread in droplets during coughing or breathing or by sharing food and drink. When bacterial particles are released into the air, they can be picked up by others close by. The hallmark rash is caused by a toxin released by the bacteria.

Symptoms and Diagnostic Path

After an incubation period of two to four days, the first sign of illness is usually a fever of 103°F to 104°F, accompanied by a severe sore throat. The face is flushed and the tongue develops a white coating with red spots, rather like a white strawberry. The child may seem tired and flushed; 12 to 18 hours after the fever, a rash appears as a mass of rapidly spreading tiny red spots on the neck and upper trunk. The scarlet fever rash is unique in that it feels rough, like fine sandpaper, and is quite distinctive.

Other common symptoms include headache, chills and vomiting, tiny white lines around the mouth, as well as fine red striations in the creases of elbows and groin. After a few days, the tongue coating peels off, followed by a drop in fever and a fading rash. Skin on the hands and feet often peel.

Treatment Options and Outlook

A 10-day course of antibiotics (usually PENICILLIN or erythromycin), with rest, liquids, and acetaminophen. Children are contagious for a day or two after they begin treatment, but after that they can return to school.

As with other types of sore throat caused by the streptococci bacteria, untreated infection carries the risk of immunologic disorders, such as RHEUMATIC FEVER or inflammation of the kidneys (glomerulonephritis).

schistosomiasis An infection that occurs worldwide, caused by parasitic worms that live and multiply in freshwater snails. There are two types of human schistosomiasis—cutaneous schistosomiasis (SWIMMER'S ITCH) and visceral schistosomiasis, a serious systemic disorder that occasionally causes minor skin symptoms. The disease is caused by one of three types of worms (called schistosomes) acquired from bathing in infested lakes and rivers.

Visceral schistosomiasis is a parasitic disease (also called bilharziasis) that causes an itchy rash where flukes have penetrated the skin. The disease is found in most tropical countries and affects more than 200 million people around the world.

Fresh water becomes contaminated by worm eggs when infected people urinate or defecate in the water. The eggs hatch, and if certain types of snails are in the water, the parasites grow and develop inside the snails. Eventually the parasite abandons the snail and enters the water, where it can survive for about 48 hours. The parasites can penetrate the skin of anyone wading, swimming, bathing, or washing in contaminated water. Within several weeks, worms grow inside the blood vessels of the body and produce eggs. Some of these eggs travel to the bladder or intestines and are passed into the urine or stool.

Symptoms and Diagnostic Path

Fever, chills, cough, and muscle aches can begin within one or two months of infection, but most people have no symptoms at this early phase of infection.

Eggs travel to the liver or pass into the intestine or bladder. Rarely, eggs are found in the brain or spinal cord and can cause seizures, paralysis, or spinal cord inflammation. For people who are repeatedly infected for many years, the parasite can damage the liver, intestines, lungs, and bladder.

Symptoms of schistosomiasis are caused by the body's reaction to the eggs produced by worms, not by the worms themselves.

Tests of stool or urine samples will reveal the parasite. A blood test has been developed and is available at the U.S. CENTERS FOR DISEASE CONTROL AND PREVENTION. For accurate results, the patient must wait six to eight weeks after the last exposure to contaminated water before the blood sample is taken.

Treatment Options and Outlook

Safe and effective drugs are available for the treatment of schistosomiasis.

Risk Factors and Preventive Measures

Since there is no way to tell infested from noninfested water, travelers should avoid freshwater swimming in rural areas of suspected countries. Accidental exposure to water in suspected areas should be followed by immediate, vigorous towel drying or quick application of alcohol to the exposed areas of skin.

There are no preventive drugs yet available, but scientists have developed a new vaccine that protects against damage caused by the worm. In an animal study, it dramatically reduced the scar tissue. The vaccine did not stop reinfection, but did halt the damage that the organism caused.

scrofula The former term for TUBERCULOSIS of the bones and lymphatic glands (especially in children). The old English name was king's evil, so-called because it was believed that the king's touch could cure the disease.

sepsis See SEPTICEMIA.

septicemia (bacterial sepsis) The medical name for blood poisoning, a potentially lethal blood infection characterized by the rapid multiplication of bacteria and the presence of their toxins that kill almost 215,000 Americans each year. Unlike BACTEREMIA, in which bacteria are present in the blood but do not always cause illness, septicemia is a severe, life-threatening emergency.

Since the 1990s, the reported incidence of sepsis in the United States increased 91.3 percent, according to the Society of Critical Care Medicine. Sepsis, now the 10th leading cause of death in the United States, is more common in men than women and in African Americans than Caucasians.

Sepsis is the body's response to severe infection, mediated through the immune system and involving nearly every system in the body. The condition may produce harmful effects in other organs, leading to very high death rates.

Septicemia can occur when certain forms of bacteria enter the bloodstream. These bacteria give off endotoxins—poisonous substances that remain even after the bacteria disintegrate and that can lead to a dramatic drop in blood pressure (SEPTIC SHOCK), with rapid heartbeat and breathing.

Researchers have discovered a link between sepsis and levels of a substance called protein C. Normally, this protein is converted by the body into activated protein C, which circulates in the body and inhibits inflammation and formation of blood clots. Patients with sepsis tend to have low levels of protein C. Scientists suspect that low levels of protein C leads to small blood clots in vital organs that block blood flow, starving the organ of oxygen and nutrients. Even with good care, up to 45 percent of patients die.

Symptoms and Diagnostic Path

Symptoms include the sudden onset of fever, chills, rapid breathing, headache, nausea or diarrhea, and clouding of consciousness. Skin rashes and jaundice may occur, and the hands may be especially warm. If large amounts of toxins are produced by the bacteria, the patient may pass into a state of septic shock.

Septicemia is diagnosed by a culture of the blood.

Treatment Options and Outlook

The first drug to successful combat sepsis directly was discovered by an international research team in 2001. In studies, patients who took drotrecogin alfa (Xigris) had a 19 percent better chance of survival than those who did not.

Xigris is a laboratory-made version of activated protein C. By replacing the body's levels of the protein, doctors hope to reduce the risk of clot formation and organ damage.

Before this drug was discovered, treatment of symptoms included antibiotics and IV fluids. Approved by the U.S. Food and Drug Administration (FDA), patients with sepsis must have at least one failed organ to qualify for the drug.

Xigris is not indicated for patients with less severe illness who are currently doing well with standard treatment or those whose illness is so severe they are not likely to benefit from it.

Side effects included a small chance of serious bleeding (3.5 percent), and should therefore not be given to patients who are susceptible to bleeding. The drug has not yet been tested in children.

septic shock A type of shock in which there is tissue damage and a dramatic drop in blood pressure as a result of SEPTICEMIA (bacteria causing blood poisoning) and toxemia (the multiplication of bacteria and their toxins in the blood). This type of shock usually follows signs of severe infection (often in the stomach or intestines or in the urinary tract).

Septic shock is especially common in those who have an immune system problem, in people taking drugs for cancer, or in people undergoing prolonged antibiotic treatment.

The toxins released from bacteria into the bloodstream are the primary source of septic shock because they can damage cells and tissues throughout the body. This leads to clotting of blood in the smallest blood vessels, seriously interfering with the normal blood circulation. Damage occurs especially to tissues in the kidneys, heart, and lungs. The toxins may lead to leaking of fluid from blood vessels, interfering with their ability to constrict, which triggers a drop in blood pressure.

Symptoms and Diagnostic Path

Symptoms vary with the extent and type of major tissue damage. In general, the symptoms are the same as those of septicemia, with the additional signs of cold hands and feet; blue coloration; a weak, rapid pulse; and significant drop in blood pressure. Fever, rapid breathing, confusion, or coma are common. There also may be vomiting or diarrhea.

Treatment Options and Outlook

Septic shock must be treated immediately, with rapid fluid replacement and antibiotics; surgery sometimes may be needed. Measures should be taken to boost blood pressure. Despite aggressive treatment, septic shock is a grave condition with a 50 percent mortality rate.

severe acute respiratory syndrome (SARS) A viral respiratory illness that appeared suddenly in 2003, killing a number of patients before fading away. SARS is caused by SARS-associated coronavirus (SARS-CoV), one of a family of viruses that in humans usually causes mild upper respiratory infections such as the common cold. How this new coronavirus evolved or why it turned deadly is not known, though the coronaviruses are known for the ability to evolve. Nor is it clear why some people succumb to the disease and others recover. Although many who died were older adults with other health problems, SARS also killed healthy young adults.

SARS appeared in southern China in November 2002, eventually spreading over the next few months to more than two dozen countries in North America, South America, Europe, and Asia. It was first recognized as a global threat in March 2003, although the outbreak was eventually contained. However, experts worry that person-to-person transmission of the virus might recur.

According to the World Health Organization (WHO), a total of 8,098 people worldwide became sick with SARS during the 2003 outbreak. Of these, 774 died. In the United States, only eight people had laboratory evidence of SARS, and all had traveled to other parts of the world where SARS was endemic. SARS did not spread more widely in the community in the United States.

The rapid and unexpected spread of SARS concerned health officials and the public, and its emergence showed how quickly infection can spread in a highly interconnected world. SARS is particularly troubling because health experts know so little about it, and because its symptoms are similar to those of other respiratory illnesses. Although SARS was contained in the months after its emergence, additional cases later emerged. The sense of concern surrounding SARS remains because as yet there is no known treatment.

SARS appears to spread by close person-to-person contact when an infected person coughs or sneezes. The virus also can spread when a person touches something contaminated with infectious droplets and then touches the nose, mouth, or eye. In addition, it is possible that the SARS virus might be spread through the air or by other ways that are not now known.

Symptoms and Diagnostic Path

Several lab tests can help identify SARS, including a reverse transcription polymerase chain reaction test looking for viral DNA in nose secretions or a blood or stool sample. Blood tests can identify antibodies to SARS-associated coronavirus, and a viral culture also can identify the virus.

The infection begins with a fever above 101°F, which may be associated with chills or other symptoms, including headache, malaise, body aches, and mild breathing problems. Some patients have diarrhea. After two to seven days, patients may develop a dry cough or experience shortness of breath, at which point oxygen levels in the blood may drop. Most patients eventually develop PNEUMONIA.

Treatment Options and Outlook

As a virus, SARS will not respond to antibiotics, and antiviral medications such as ribavirin and oseltamivir, even in combination with steroids, was not always effective. However, a combination of antiviral drugs commonly used to treat AIDS (lopinavir-ritonavir plus ribavirin) has been shown to prevent serious complications and deaths from SARS. Further testing is needed before these drugs are recommended for use in people with SARS.

Even with treatment, between 10 and 20 percent of people with SARS become worse and develop such severe breathing problems that they need a respirator. SARS patients can die from respiratory failure. Other possible complications include heart and liver failure.

Risk Factors and Preventive Measures

People are at greatest risk of SARS if they have had direct, close contact with someone who is infected, such as a roommate or family member. Researchers also have discovered immune system gene variation that may make carriers much more vulnerable to the SARS virus. This genetic variation is common among people of southeastern Asian descent but is rare in others, which may help explain why most SARS cases have occurred in China and Southeast Asia.

As yet, no vaccine has been developed against SARS. To prevent spread of the infection, a patient with SARS should cover the mouth and nose with a tissue when coughing or sneezing and limit activities outside the home. This means avoiding public transportation and staying away from work, school, child care, church, or activities in other public areas. Hands should be washed often and well, especially after blowing the nose. If possible, the patient should wear a surgical mask when around other people in the home, or members of the household should wear a mask when around the patient.

Patients should not share silverware, towels, or bedding with anyone in the home until these items have been washed with soap and hot water. Counters, tabletops, door knobs, bathroom fixtures, and so on, contaminated by body fluids should be cleaned with a household disinfectant. These precautions should be followed for 10 days after the fever and respiratory symptoms have stopped. No one should visit, and other household members should either be relocated or minimize contact with the patient in the home. This is particularly important for persons at risk of serious complications of SARS, such as individuals with underlying heart or lung disease, diabetes mellitus, and older age. Unexposed persons who do not have an essential need to be in the home should not visit.

sexually transmitted disease (STD)   A contagious disease usually transmitted during sexual intercourse or genital contact. In the United States, the most commonly reported infections are sexually transmitted, and the incidence has risen despite improved methods of diagnosis and treatment. Each year, another 19 million infections are diagnosed.

Once known as venereal disease, these conditions are often acquired by people who have many sex partners. Some of the major STDs are also transmitted by blood and can therefore be acquired by drug addicts who share needles, or by people needing transfusions.

STDs affect men and women of all backgrounds and economic levels, and are most common among teenagers and young adults. Nearly two-thirds of all STDs occur in people under age 25.

The incidence of STDs is rising in part because in the last few decades young people have become sexually active earlier but are marrying later. As a result, sexually active people today are more likely to have multiple sex partners.

Venereal diseases include GONORRHEA, SYPHILIS, CHANCROID, GRANULOMA INGUINALE, LYMPHOGRANU-LOMA VENEREUM, SCABIES, HERPES, genital WARTS, pubic LICE, PEDICULOSIS, TRICHOMONIASIS, genital CAN-DIDIASIS, MOLLUSCUM CONTAGIOSUM, HEPATITIS B, nonspecific URETHRITIS, CHLAMYDIAL INFECTIONS, CYTO-MEGALOVIRUS, PELVIC INFLAMMATORY DISEASE and HIV/AIDS.

During World War II, the incidence of STDs rose in the United States, but these declined with the introduction of PENICILLIN and subsequent cure of syphilis and gonorrhea. However, in the 1960s and 1970s the infections began to increase with the introduction of oral contraception. The pill meant that more women were having more sex partners and fewer couples used barrier methods of birth control, which provide some protection against STDs. At the same time, in the early 1980s doctors began to diagnose nonspecific urethritis in about 25 percent of patients who visited STD clinics; most of these people were found to have chlamydial infection. By 2004, chlamydia was the most common of all the reported infectious diseases (929,462 cases). Gonorrhea and AIDS were second and third, according to the CENTERS FOR DISEASE CONTROL AND PREVENTION. Chlamydia was more often reported among women, while gonorrhea and AIDS were reported more often by men.

Symptoms and Diagnostic Path

Most of the time STDs cause no symptoms, especially in women. If symptoms do develop, they may be confused with those of other diseases not transmitted through sexual contact. Even when an STD doesn't cause any symptoms, however, a person who is infected may be able to pass the disease on to a sex partner. That is why many doctors recommend periodic testing or screening for people who have more than one sex partner.

Health problems caused by STDs tend to be more severe and more frequent for women, partly because women may not have symptoms, and therefore do not seek care until serious problems have developed. Some STDs can spread into the uterus and fallopian tubes, causing pelvic inflammatory disease (PID), which in turn is a major cause of both infertility and tubal pregnancy. STDs in women also may be associated with cervical cancer. For example, HUMAN PAPILLOMAVIRUS INFECTION (HPV) causes GENITAL WARTS and cervical and other genital cancers.

In addition, STDs can be passed from a mother to her baby before, during, or immediately after birth; some of these infections of the newborn can be cured easily, but others may cause a baby to be permanently disabled or even die.

STDs are also linked to other problems. Experts believe that having STDs other than AIDS increases the risk for becoming infected with the AIDS virus.

STDs can be diagnosed at special clinics or by specialists in genitourinary medicine and infectious disease.

Treatment Options and Outlook

When diagnosed and treated early, many STDs can be treated effectively, although some infections have become resistant to the drugs used to treat them and now require newer types of antibiotics. When being treated, patients should notify all recent sex partners, complete the full course of medication, and take a follow-up test to ensure the infection has been cured. Patients also should avoid all sexual activity while being treated for an STD.

Once drugs have eased the symptoms, tests are given to make sure the patient is no longer infectious. Treatment is also given to all recent sex partners to prevent transmitting infection. The confidential tracing and treatment of contacts is an essential part of managing STDs.

Risk Factors and Preventive Measures

The best way to prevent STDs is to avoid sexual contact with others. To reduce the risk of developing an STD, people who are sexually active should

- have a monogamous sexual relationship with an uninfected partner.
- correctly and consistently use a condom.
- prevent and control other STDs to decrease susceptibility to HIV infection.
- delay having sex, because the younger a person is when having sex for the first time, the more susceptible to developing an STD. The risk of acquiring an STD also increases with the number of partners over a lifetime.
- have regular checkups for STDs even in the absence of symptoms, and especially if having sex with a new partner. These tests can be done during a routine visit to the doctor's office.
- avoid having sex during menstruation. HIV-infected women are probably more infectious, and HIV-uninfected women are probably more susceptible to becoming infected, during that time.

- avoid anal intercourse, but if practiced, a condom should be used.
- avoid douching, because it removes some of the normal protective bacteria in the vagina and increases the risk of getting some STDs.

shellfish poisoning Consumption of shellfish has been linked to a number of bacterial and viral diseases.

Shellfish are highly susceptible to bacterial and viral contamination, since they live close to the shore where pollution tends to be worse. While shellfish by themselves are not poisonous, they can become contaminated from their environment, passing infection on up the food chain when eaten by humans. Oysters, clams, and mussels are particularly prone to becoming contaminated because of their metabolic system, which pumps water across their gills to isolate plankton; this makes them vulnerable to bacteria, viruses, and contaminants in the water. (Lobsters and other crustacean shellfish only rarely become contaminated.)

Shellfish contamination caused by bacteria and viruses can be prevented by cooking seafood thoroughly, storing it properly, and protecting it from contamination after cooking. However, traditional methods of cooking seafood (such as steaming clams only until they open) may be insufficient to kill all bacteria and viruses inside them.

Most cases of shellfish poisoning have occurred when people ate raw or undercooked shellfish; in fact, raw shellfish have been linked to nearly 1,000 cases of HEPATITIS a year. For this reason, doctors recommend that no one eat raw shellfish.

Good data on the occurrence and severity of shellfish poisoning are largely unavailable, which reflects the inability to measure the true incidence of this disease; cases are often misdiagnosed and infrequently reported.

The shellfish industry and government regulatory agencies try to control the problem of shellfish contamination at the source, by seeing that shellfish are harvested from unpolluted beds not tainted by sewage. Unfortunately, these efforts cannot guarantee that shellfish from unapproved beds do not reach the market.

Viral contamination The most common viral contamination in shellfish is caused by the Norwalk virus, which leads to food poisoning when raw or improperly cooked food has been in contact with water contaminated by human excrement.

It is also possible to contract HEPATITIS A from eating raw shellfish harvested from sewage-contaminated waters. Even though federal regulations and posting of contaminated waters offer some protection, there is still a risk of contracting viruses when eating raw shellfish.

Symptoms begin from two to six weeks after eating and include fever, weakness, anorexia, jaundice; severe cases may damage liver and can be fatal.

Toxins Shellfish also can become tainted by eating toxic plankton (called dinoflagellates) that multiply rapidly during the warm summer months; because the plankton have a pink or red color, this phenomenon has come to be called red tide. Red tides are found in coastal waters in the Pacific from California to Alaska and in the Atlantic from New England to the St. Lawrence. Under good conditions (warm climate, warm water), the plankton may reach 60 million organisms per liter of water. These rapid growths (referred to as a "bloom") discolor the sea and poison fish and marine life. Usually, a person becomes poisoned with the plankton when eating shellfish that have been feeding on them.

The plankton produce a deadly poison called saxitoxin that is so toxic that even one contaminated shellfish can be fatal if eaten. This is why clams, oysters, and mussels are not sold during months without an *R* in them (the summer months).

Mussels, clams, and oysters are the primary shellfish at risk, and mussels are the most susceptible of all. Healthy bivalve shellfish filter large amounts of toxic plankton, which form the primary ocean food during May through August. During these warm times, the dinoflagellates thrive by photosynthesis and can be so invasive that they kill birds and fish.

The first large EPIDEMIC of poisoning caused by red tide–contaminated shellfish occurred in San Francisco in 1927, when 102 people were sickened and six died. Today, largely because of the prohibition against eating certain shellfish during the summer months, such epidemics are rare.

Shellfish poisoning caused by toxic forms of dinoflagellates include paralytic shellfish poisoning, neurologic shellfish poisoning, diarrheic shellfish poisoning, and amnesic shellfish poisoning. Each has different etiology, symptoms, and prognosis for recovery, but of the three, paralytic shellfish poisoning is by far the most serious.

Shellfish containing toxin look and taste normal, and usual cooking methods do not affect the toxin. State shellfish screening programs test shellfish for the presence of these toxins and monitor the safety of shellfish harvest beds.

shellfish poisoning, amnesic This type of SHELL-FISH POISONING first came to the attention of public health officials in 1987, when 156 cases of acute intoxication occurred after people ate cultured blue mussels harvested off Prince Edward Island in eastern Canada. Of those who got sick, 22 were hospitalized and three elderly patients eventually died.

Amnesic shellfish poisoning is the result of an unusual neurotoxic amino acid (domoic acid) that contaminates shellfish. The domoic acid is produced by a phytoplankton called *Nitzschia pungens* f. multiseries. (Phytoplankton are microscopic, photosynthetic, free-floating organisms in the ocean; *N. pungens* is a type of phytoplankton with a particular kind of cell wall.) Many different kinds of phytoplankton exist and only a few of them are toxic.

Symptoms and Diagnostic Path

While everyone is susceptible to shellfish poisoning, elderly people appear to be predisposed to the severe neurological effects of amnesic shellfish poisoning. Within 24 hours of eating contaminated shellfish, the symptoms begin: vomiting and diarrhea, severe headache, abdominal pain, and a host of neurological problems, including confusion, memory loss, disorientation, seizure, and coma.

Diagnosis is based on observing symptoms and recent dietary history.

Treatment Options and Outlook

There is no antidote for this type of shellfish poison. The only treatment is to ease the symptoms. Seizures respond to anti-seizure drugs.

shellfish poisoning, diarrheic This type of SHELL-FISH POISONING is rarely fatal and has not been confirmed in U.S. seafood, although the organisms that produce it are present in U.S. waters. It occurs in Europe in a sporadic, widespread fashion, and an outbreak was recently confirmed in Canada.

It is caused by eating shellfish contaminated by toxin-producing plankton. It is associated in particular with eating mussels, oysters, and scallops.

Symptoms and Diagnostic Path

Symptoms appear between a few minutes to three hours after ingestion, and include gastrointestinal problems accompanied by muscular weakness, chills, headache, and fever. Recovery is rapid and death is rare.

Diagnosis is based on observing symptoms and recent dietary history.

Treatment Options and Outlook

There is no antidote for this type of shellfish poison, but most people recover on their own.

shellfish poisoning, neurotoxic (NSP) A type of SHELLFISH POISONING caused by eating shellfish that have ingested toxin-producing plankton.

While all shellfish are potentially toxic, NSP is generally associated with shellfish harvested along the Florida coast and the Gulf of Mexico. Outbreaks are sporadic and continuous and have been reported along the Gulf coast of Florida and more recently in North Carolina and Texas.

NSP is the result of exposure to a group of toxins called brevetoxins.

Symptoms and Diagnostic Path

Both gastrointestinal and neurological symptoms appear in this type of poisoning within a few minutes to a few hours after eating the shellfish. Symptoms include tingling and numbness of lips, tongue, and throat; muscular aches; dizziness; reversal of the sensation of hot and cold; diarrhea; and vomiting.

Recovery is complete with few aftereffects; no fatalities have been reported.

Diagnosis is based on observing symptoms and recent dietary history.

Treatment Options and Outlook

There is no treatment other than easing symptoms.

shellfish poisoning, paralytic (PSP) The most serious type of SHELLFISH POISONING, PSP is a toxic neurologic condition caused by eating clams, oysters, or mussels that have ingested toxin-producing plankton. The type of toxin is called saxitoxin, among the most potent toxins known and one that is not destroyed by cooking. The saxitoxin comes from algae eaten by filter-feeding shellfish such as clams and mussels; this toxin can be present even when there is no visible discoloration (or RED TIDE) in the ocean water. The shellfish store the toxin from the algae in their tissues and pass the toxin on to anyone who eats them. In recent years, the toxin has been found in snails and in crab viscera as well.

Most victims of this type of poisoning in the United States are individuals who have gathered shellfish for their own use. PSP has generally been considered to be dangerous only in shellfish harvested from cold water, but the incidence of red tides in warmer waters may be increasing. Outbreaks have recently been reported from Central and South America, Asia, and the Pacific.

The 20 toxins responsible for paralytic shellfish poisonings are all derivatives of saxitoxin. PSP is associated with mussels, clams, cockles, and scallops.

Symptoms and Diagnostic Path
Saxitoxin interferes with functions involving the brain, movement, and senses. Soon after eating (sometimes in less than an hour), symptoms appear. At first, there is a tingling or numbness in lips and tongue, often followed by tingling and numbness in the fingertips and toes, nausea, light-headedness, followed by vomiting and diarrhea. This may progress to loss of muscle coordination. This is followed by a gradual paralysis, trembling, headache, and weakness. Death as a result of respiratory paralysis can occur within 12 hours of eating PSP-containing shellfish. Eating as little as 0.5 to 1.0 mg of contaminated shellfish can be fatal, and a person's survival depends on how much has been consumed. If a person survives the first 12 hours, chances of survival are good. However, between 8 and 23 percent of PSP poisonings are fatal. The severity of the illness is less if the water used in cooking is not consumed.

There is no lab test that can determine the presence of PSP in an individual. Diagnosis is made on the basis of recent food consumption, symptoms, and detection of toxin in uneaten shellfish.

Treatment Options and Outlook
There is no known antidote for shellfish poisoning caused by saxitoxin-producing plankton. Administration of prostigmine may be effective, together with artificial respiration and oxygen as needed. It is important that vomiting be induced at the onset of symptoms to help remove remaining toxincontaining shellfish and that medical attention be obtained. Drinking alcohol increases absorption of the toxin.

Risk Factors and Preventive Measures
To prevent outbreaks of PSP, samples of susceptible mollusks are tested for toxin by state health departments during certain times of the year. Affected growing areas are quarantined, and sale of shellfish is stopped. Warning signs posted in shellfish-growing areas, on beaches, and in the news warn the public of the danger.

Because of this constant monitoring, shellfish poisoning in the United States is rare; from 1973 to 1987 only 19 outbreaks were reported, with an average of eight cases per outbreak.

Shigella group A group of four different species of bacteria that lead to the diarrheal disease known as SHIGELLOSIS.

Shigella were discovered more than 100 years ago by Japanese scientist Kiyoshi Shiga. There are several different kinds of *Shigella* bacteria, including *Shigella sonnei* (Group D *Shigella*) that account for more than two-thirds of the shigellosis in the United States. *Shigella flexneri* (group B *Shigella*) accounts for almost all of the rest. Other types are rare in the United States, though they continue to be important causes of disease in the developing world. One especially deadly type found in the developing world is *Shigella dysenteriae* type 1.

shigellosis A bacterial diarrheal disease caused by the bacterium *Shigella*, which includes four different species. The disease is common among the developing countries, where lack of sewage treatment leads to contaminated food and water.

Two-thirds of cases occur in children between six months and 10 years of age, although it is rare in infants under age six months. The highest rates of infection occur in child-care centers, large camps, and institutions.

A person is infectious from the time the diarrhea appears until the bacteria are no longer in the stool, which could take a month. Antibiotics shorten the infectious period to a week.

Shiga toxin is named after Kiyoshi Shiga, who in 1898 first described the bacterial origin of DYSENTERY caused by *Shigella dysenteriae.*

The *Shigella* bacteria are found in milk and dairy products, poultry, and mixed salads, but they can develop in any moist food that is not thoroughly cooked. The bacteria multiply rapidly at or above room temperature. *S. sonnei* is the mildest of the four, and is responsible for most cases around the world. *S. dysenteriae* (also known as bacillary dysentery) is fairly common in rural Africa and India, where it causes illness and many deaths.

A person gets sick after ingesting bacteria; it only takes a few organisms to cause illness. The bacteria may be found in contaminated bodies of water or in food that is left out in the open where flies can contaminate it. Dogs who eat infected human feces can spread the infection to humans (especially children), and the disease can also be spread sexually with anal-oral contact.

Symptoms and Diagnostic Path

Symptoms, which usually appear eight hours to eight days after ingestion, begin with nausea and vomiting, watery or bloody explosive diarrhea and stomach cramps, weakness, vision problems, headache, and difficulty swallowing. Those with weakened immune systems may have more serious diarrhea and may take longer to recover. Young children have more serious symptoms, and those children already malnourished or weak will be much sicker.

Culture of the stool will reveal *Shigella.*

Treatment Options and Outlook

Most people with shigellosis recover on their own. Some may require fluids to prevent dehydration. To shorten severe cases, antibiotics will help stop the diarrhea, although *Shigella* has become resistant

to some drugs. Trimethoprim-sulfamethoxazole, ciprofloxacin, or orofloxacin are usually effective; some strains are susceptible to tetracycline. Those who are infected in a developing country may respond better to nalidixic acid, since the bacteria in those locations are widely resistant.

Antidiarrheal medications should not be taken. Dilute drinks high in sugar and bland foods high in carbohydrates are tolerated best by the patient.

People with diarrhea usually recover completely within several months, but about 3 percent of those infected with *Shigella flexneri* will eventually develop painful joints, irritated eyes, and painful urination. This condition, called Reiter's syndrome, can last for months or years and lead to chronic arthritis that is hard to treat. Reiter's syndrome is caused by a reaction to *Shigella* infection that happens only in people who are genetically predisposed to it.

People who have had shigellosis are not likely to be reinfected with that specific type again for at least several years, although they can still get infected with other types of *Shigella.*

Risk Factors and Preventive Measures

Confirmed *Shigella* cases must be reported to the health department, which will begin an investigation and control measures in order to prevent large-scale outbreaks. Although several vaccines have been tested, none have yet been licensed for use in preventing the disease. The single most important way to prevent the spread of disease is to carefully wash hands after using the toilet, since *Shigella* is passed in feces.

shingles A painful, red blistering viral infection of the nerves that supply certain areas of the skin, caused by reactivation of the VARICELLA-ZOSTER VIRUS (VZV), the same culprit that causes childhood CHICKEN POX.

Shingles is a common illness that strikes one in five Americans. The name comes from the Latin word *cingulum,* meaning "belt" or "girdle." By age 85, people have a 50–50 chance of developing shingles if they have not already had them.

After an episode of chicken pox, the virus lie dormant in sensory nerves along the spine for many years. When the immune system efficiency is weakened, the virus reemerges and migrates along the sensory nerve, breaking out at its receptor ends in the skin. Each year, shingles affects several hundred patients per 100,000 in the United States, usually over age 50.

Scientists suspect that a decline in the activity of white blood cells may allow the virus to reemerge. This idea is bolstered by the fact that shingles also appears in children with leukemia, cancer patients undergoing chemotherapy, and organ transplant patients. The virus often affects a nerve that has had previous trauma.

Symptoms and Diagnostic Path

The first sign is excessive sensitivity in an area of skin, followed by pain; after about five days the rash appears, turning into tense blisters that turn yellow within three more days. The blisters then dry out and crust over, gradually dropping off (leaving small pitted scars behind). Because the nerves have been damaged after the virus attack, after the blisters heal the nerves constantly produce strong pain impulses that may last for months or years.

The older the patient and more severe the rash, the more likely the pain will persist. Shingles often affects a strip of skin over the ribs on one side; sometimes it affects the lower part of the body or the upper half of the face on one side. It can occur in any area of the body.

Treatment Options and Outlook

Prompt use of antiviral drugs such as acyclovir, famciclovir, or valacyclovir can significantly shorten the rash stage and lessen the chance of pain later. Therefore, patients should seek medical help at the first signs of shingles. Acyclovir slows reproduction of the virus and shortens the course of the infection, although it does not prevent the nerve pain following a shingles attack.

Some experts maintain that steroid drugs such as prednisone can prevent this pain. Other treatments include antidepressants and anticonvulsants.

For severe pain from shingles, experts occasionally recommend injecting a nerve block in the appropriate place to block the sympathetic nerves supplying the area of pain. This block typically relieves pain for hours in up to 80 percent of patients.

An over-the-counter product called Zostrix or Valtrex (active ingredient: capsaicin, a red pepper derivative used to make chili powder) may help relieve the post-herpetic shingles pain, once all the blisters have disappeared. Experts believe that capsaicin blocks the production of a chemical necessary for pain impulse transmission between nerve cells. *Zostrix should not be applied to active shingles blisters.* As a counterirritant, Zostrix is designed to be used on unbroken, healed skin with a pain sensation, not for open oozing infections.

Adenosine monophosphate is the newest potential treatment now being studied by researchers.

Almost half of the 600,000 patients who get shingles each year suffer from agonizing pain that may last from days to years. If the pain lasts long after the rash, it is known as postherpetic neuralgia. It can also lead to bizarre sensations that can linger for years, including phantom feelings.

Sufferers complain that a light touch can feel like torture and a drop of water feels like a third-degree burn. Even the softest clothing can be unbearable to these patients.

Postherpetic neuralgia is treated with a variety of medications from amitriptyline to opioids.

Risk Factors and Preventive Measures

In one of the largest adult vaccine clinical trials, researchers found that an experimental stronger version of chicken pox vaccine prevented about half of cases of shingles and dramatically reduced its severity and complications in vaccinated persons who got the disease. The five-year shingles prevention study was carried out in collaboration with the National Institute of Allergy and Infectious Diseases. The results showed that for the first time a vaccine can prevent shingles or lessen the severity of subsequent episodes. The zoster vaccine used in the study (manufactured by Merck) is a new, stronger version of the chicken pox vaccine used to prevent chicken pox in millions of American children. The zoster vaccine was developed specifically for study in older adults. During an average of more than three years of follow-up, there were 642 cases of shingles among the placebo group compared with only 315 in the vaccinated group. Among all vaccine recipients, the total burden of pain and discomfort due to shingles was 61 percent lower, and the zoster vaccine reduced the incidence of pain by two-thirds. The vaccine was well tolerated, with very few serious side effects. The researchers emphasize that the zoster vaccine was tested only as a preventive and not as a treatment for those who already have shingles or postherpetic neuralgia. Merck submitted a license application to the U.S. Food and Drug Administration for the zoster vaccine, which was approved in 2006. The research team estimates the vaccine could prevent 250,000 cases of shingles that occur in the United States each year and significantly reduce the severity of the disease in another 250,000 cases annually.

Sin Nombre virus A strain of HANTAVIRUS (virus carried by rodents) that caused an outbreak of HANTAVIRUS PULMONARY SYNDROME in the Four Corners area of the western United States. The virus first appeared there where it was first called the Muerto Canyon (valley of death) virus, for the spot on a New Mexican Navajo reservation where it was isolated. Because this name offended the Navajo, the virus was renamed Sin Nombre ("no name" in Spanish). It has killed more than 100 patients across the United States (mostly in Arizona, New Mexico, and Colorado). Hantavirus is the third most deadly virus ever found in the United States, after HIV and RABIES.

This American variety appears to be 10 times more deadly than a related hantavirus from Asia, called the Hantaan virus. Scientists suspect the Sin Nombre virus is not at all a new organism but rather one that has been living for eons in deer mice of the southwest, emerging occasionally to infect humans. Navajo legends appear to have mentioned this disease.

Because the virus has been identified as a cause of disease in patients in New York and Virginia, scientists believe that eventually the organism will be found throughout the United States.

There is no vaccine against the Sin Nombre virus. The best defense is proper hygiene and cleanliness. Rodents and their food sources must be eliminated from the home, and all food and water in endemic areas should be stored in a rodent-proof metal containers. Dishes should be washed immediately after use and put away in protected cupboards. Trash, clutter, and spills should be cleaned up immediately, covered in a rodent-proof container, and disposed. Rodent traps should be set within and around the home. Finally, to keep rodents away, all openings into the home should be sealed, and the area around the home should be free from woodpiles and other debris.

sinusitis An inflammation of one or more of the sinuses, often as a complication of an upper respiratory infection or dental infection. (It also may be caused by allergies, air travel, or underwater swimming.) Sinusitis is extremely common and afflicts some people with every bout of the common cold. In many people, once a tendency toward sinusitis develops, the condition recurs with each viral infection.

Sinusitis is often caused by infection spreading from the nose along the narrow passages that drain mucus from the sinuses into the nose. As the nasal mucous membranes swell, the openings from the sinuses to the nose may be blocked. This leads to a buildup of sinus secretions, often teeming with bacteria. The disorder is usually caused by a bacterial infection that develops as a complication of a viral infection (such as the common cold). It is also possible that an infection may occur from an abscess in an upper tooth or from infected water forced into the sinuses while swimming.

Symptoms and Diagnostic Path

Pressure, throbbing headache, fever, and local tenderness, together with a feeling of fullness or tension. It may also cause a stuffy nose and loss of the ability to smell.

X-rays may be taken to determine the location and extent of the disorder, and a culture may be grown from a swab of the sinus to identify the bacteria.

Treatment Options and Outlook

Steam inhalations, nasal decongestants, painkillers, and antibiotics. Surgery to improve drainage may be performed for chronic problems.

Often, sinusitis leads to the formation of pus in the affected sinuses, causing pain and a nasal discharge. Other more rare complications include orbital CELLULITIS, OSTEOMYELITIS, and MENINGITIS.

See also COLD, COMMON.

sixth disease See ROSEOLA.

skin infections Because the skin represents the outer barrier to the world, it is responsible for defending the interior of the body against a wide range of attackers, including BACTERIA, VIRUSES, insect venom, and FUNGI. Skin infections can range from a local superficial problem (such as IMPETIGO) to a widespread and possibly fatal infection.

Examples of skin infections or diseases with skin symptoms include impetigo, ECTHYMA, FOLLICULITIS, BOILS, CARBUNCLES, ERYSIPELAS, SCARLET FEVER, CELLULITIS, ECZEMA, ERYTHEMA TOXICUM, LYME DISEASE, ROCKY MOUNTAIN SPOTTED FEVER, ROSEOLA, TOXIC SHOCK SYNDROME, HERPES SIMPLEX, CHICKEN POX, AND SHINGLES, WARTS, MEASLES, GERMAN MEASLES, FIFTH DISEASE, and AIDS.

sleeping sickness The common name for African TRYPANOSOMIASIS, a serious infectious disease of tropical Africa caused by parasites transmitted by the bite of infected TSETSE FLIES. Between 300,000 and 500,000 people contract this disease each year.

East Africa's version of sleeping sickness is caused by the parasite *Trypanosoma brucei rhodesiense* and is spread mainly to wild animals, only rarely affecting humans. West Africa's chronic *gambiense* variety (caused by the *T. brucei gambiense*) may not cause the "sleeping" part of the illness until years after exposure. This variety is spread primarily from person to person. Within humans, the parasites multiply and spread to the bloodstream, lymph nodes, heart, and brain.

Symptoms and Diagnostic Path
With both versions of sleeping sickness, a painful nodule develops at the site of the fly bite. In the West African version, the disease progresses slowly with bouts of fever and lymph gland enlargement. After a period of months or years, the parasites invade the tiny blood vessels supplying the central nervous system. This causes the legendary drowsiness, lethargy, and sleepiness. The patient may become completely inactive, with drooping eyelids and a vacant expression (hence, the term *sleeping*

sickness). If untreated at this point, the patient may die. The East African form is more virulent; a severe fever develops within a few weeks of infection and effects on the heart may be fatal before the disease gets to the brain.

Microscopic examination of the blood, lymph fluid, or cerebrospinal fluid reveals the presence of the parasites.

Treatment Options and Outlook
The drug suramin can treat both versions of African sleeping sickness. Melarsoprol (a derivative of arsenic) is available from the CDC to treat final stages of both versions. If the patient is known to have the *gambiense* variety, the drug eflornithine (approved by the U.S. Food and Drug Administration [FDA]) is more effective and safer.

Melarsoprol can cause serious or fatal nervous system problems in some patients, according to the FDA. Eflornithine is useful for both early and late stages of *gambiense* sleeping sickness; it is not effective for the *rhodesiense* variety. It works by interfering with the parasite's growth. In most cases, a complete cure is possible, although there may be brain damage if the infection has already spread to the brain.

Risk Factors and Preventive Measures
Eradication of tsetse flies can help prevent spread of this disease. Visitors to rural parts of Africa should take measures to protect against tsetse fly bites.

smallpox A highly infectious serious viral disease causing skin rash and flu-like symptoms that has been totally eradicated throughout the world since 1980. The last naturally acquired case of smallpox occurred in 1977, and the last cases of smallpox (from laboratory exposure) occurred in 1978.

However, after the attacks of September 11, 2001, the government began taking precautions to deal with a bioterrorist attack using smallpox as a weapon. The government has established a detailed nationwide smallpox preparedness program to protect Americans against smallpox as a biological weapon, including the creation of preparedness teams who can respond to a smallpox attack on the

United States. Members of these teams (health-care and public-health workers) have been vaccinated so that they might safely protect others in the event of a smallpox outbreak. As of February 2003, the government has announced that there is enough smallpox vaccine to vaccinate everyone who would need it in the event of an emergency.

Smallpox is classified as a Category A agent by the CENTERS FOR DISEASE CONTROL AND PREVENTION (CDC). Category A agents are believed to pose the highest potential threat for adverse public-health impact and have a moderate-to-high potential for large-scale dissemination. Other Category A agents include ANTHRAX, PLAGUE, BOTULISM, TULAREMIA, and viral hemorrhagic fevers. This is not to say that a smallpox terrorist weapon would be easy to release. The smallpox virus is so fragile that in experiments, 90 percent of smallpox virus released into the air died within 24 hours; in the presence of ultraviolet light, this percentage was even higher.

A common scourge of the 19th century, smallpox was characterized by a rash that spread over the body, turning into pus-filled blisters that crusted and sometimes left deeply pitted scars. Complications included blindness, pneumonia, and kidney damage.

Smallpox was the single most deadly killer during the 18th century. In London alone, fully one-third of the population at the time carried pockmarks from the highly contagious disease.

In the 19th century, English doctor Edward Jenner heard stories that cowpox was not dangerous to humans and caused immunity to small-pox. He began studying ways to inoculate humans with cowpox as a way of preventing the much deadlier disease. Although many people doubted whether vaccination would work, several famous people backed Jenner's theory, including Thomas Jefferson, who had his family and slaves vaccinated.

Although Jenner believed his vaccination would eradicate smallpox in his lifetime, it was not officially wiped out until 1980—157 years after his death in 1823.

Smallpox was eradicated through a cooperative international vaccination program. The disease affects only humans, and its victims are easily recognized and only infectious for a short time.

The last known naturally occurring case of smallpox occurred in Somalia in 1977. In May 1980, the World Health Assembly certified that the world was free of naturally occurring smallpox.

In the United States, vaccination programs and quarantine regulations meant that by the 1960s the risk for importing smallpox had been almost eliminated. As a result, recommendations for routine smallpox vaccination were rescinded in 1971. In 1976, the recommendation for routine smallpox vaccination of health-care workers was also discontinued. In 1982, the only active licensed producer of VACCINIA vaccine in the United States discontinued production for general use, and in 1983, distribution to the civilian population was discontinued. All military personnel continued to be vaccinated, but that practice ceased in 1990.

Since January 1982, smallpox vaccination has not been required for international travelers, and International Certificates of Vaccination forms no longer include a space to record smallpox vaccination.

In the United States, routine vaccination against smallpox ended in 1972. The level of immunity among vaccinated Americans is uncertain, so formerly vaccinated people are assumed to be susceptible. Most estimates suggest immunity from the vaccination lasts only three to five years, which means that nearly the entire U.S. population has only partial immunity at best. Approximately half of the U.S. population has never been vaccinated.

Immunity can be boosted effectively with a single revaccination, and prior infection with the disease grants lifelong immunity. In the absence of a confirmed case of smallpox anywhere in the world, experts had believed there was no need to be vaccinated against smallpox, especially since there can be severe side effects to the smallpox vaccine.

Although smallpox disease had been eradicated, two countries kept smallpox virus (variola) stocks: the WHO Collaborating Centers in Atlanta, and Koltsovo in the Russian Federation.

Most experts now fear that the smallpox store in the Russian lab is no longer secure. Since the terrorist attack against the United States on September 11, 2001, worldwide concerns have focused on the possibility of a bioterrorist attack using smallpox virus. The U.S. CENTERS FOR DISEASE CONTROL AND PREVENTION (CDC) maintains an emergency supply of vaccine that can be released if necessary, since post-exposure vaccination is also effective in preventing the disease.

Symptoms and Diagnostic Path

The incubation period before symptoms appear ranges between seven and 17 days after exposure. Initial symptoms include high fever, fatigue, and head and back aches. A characteristic rash of flat red lesions, most prominent on the face, arms, and legs, follows in two to three days. Lesions become filled with pus after a few days, and then begin to crust early in the second week. Scabs develop, separate, and then fall off after about three to four weeks. Most patients with smallpox recover, but death may occur in up to 30 percent of cases.

In most cases, smallpox is spread from one person to another by infected saliva droplets that expose a susceptible person having face-to-face contact with the ill person. People with smallpox are most infectious during the first week of illness, because that is when the largest amount of virus is present in saliva. However, some risk of transmission lasts until all scabs have fallen off.

Contaminated clothing or bed linen could also spread the virus. Special precautions need to be taken to ensure that all bedding and clothing of patients are cleaned appropriately with bleach and hot water. Disinfectants such as bleach and quaternary ammonia can be used for cleaning contaminated surfaces.

Treatment Options and Outlook

Currently, there is no proven treatment for smallpox, but research to evaluate new antiviral agents is ongoing. Early results from laboratory studies suggest that the drug cidofovir may be effective against the smallpox virus; studies with animals are investigating whether the drug can treat smallpox.

Otherwise, a person with smallpox would need treatment of symptoms and intravenous fluids, plus medicine to control fever or pain and antibiotics for any secondary bacterial infections that may occur.

Risk Factors and Preventive Measures

Smallpox vaccine does not contain smallpox virus, but another live virus called vaccinia virus, which is related to smallpox. Vaccination provides immunity against infection from smallpox virus. If the vaccine is given within four days after exposure to smallpox, it can lessen the severity of illness or even prevent it.

The government has recommended that more than half a million doctors, nurses and other health-care workers should be vaccinated against smallpox just in case of an attack. The Advisory Committee on Immunization Practices, which advises the federal government on vaccination policy, broadened its recommendations for vaccinating those who may have to treat smallpox cases if there were a biological attack against the United States. They include doctors and nurses in intensive care units, emergency room workers, and subspecialists, including doctors specializing in the treatment of infectious diseases. The idea is to make sure key people are protected against the virus so they can help any victims without endangering themselves.

Unfortunately, the vaccine is based on crude 100-year-old technology; it kills one to two people out of every million who receive it, and causes severe, life-threatening disease such as ENCEPHALITIS in 15 people out of every million. In addition, unvaccinated people can catch a related virus from those who have just been immunized. (The vaccine uses a live virus related to smallpox, which is usually—but not always—harmless to people.) Experts predict that between two to six unvaccinated people would contract the virus used in the vaccine for every 100,000 immunized. In infants, people with eczema and those with suppressed immune systems, such as cancer patients and those with AIDS, this other virus could have serious effects such as blisters, a red, raw rash, or blindness.

snail fever See SCHISTOSOMIASIS.

sore throat A scratchy, painful throat often accompanying a cold or other infection and caused by a variety of organisms.

Although a sore throat in itself is not serious, it may indicate a bacterial infection, such as a strep throat, if accompanied by swollen/tender lymph nodes in the neck, fever for more than two days, and pain with swallowing.

southern tick-associated rash illness (STARI) An infection causing a rash similar to that produced by LYME DISEASE that affects residents in southeastern and south central United States. STARI is associated with the bite of the lone star tick (*Amblyomma americanum*).

Amblyomma americanum ticks are found through the southeastern and south central states. Even though spirochetes have been seen in *A. americanum* ticks, attempts to culture it in the laboratory have consistently failed. However, a spirochete has been detected in *A. americanum* by DNA analysis and was given the name *Borrelia lonestari*.

Symptoms and Diagnostic Path

People who live or travel in the South and who develop a red, expanding rash with central clearing after the bite of a lone star tick should see a doctor. The CENTERS FOR DISEASE CONTROL AND PREVENTION is interested in obtaining samples from such patients under an Institutional Review Board-approved investigational protocol.

In 2001, one patient with evidence of *B. lonestari* infection, and who had been exposed to ticks in Maryland and North Carolina, developed a typical Lyme disease rash. DNA analysis revealed *B. lonestari*. Testing for Lyme disease was negative. The patient was treated with an oral antibiotic and recovered.

Lone star ticks can be found from central Texas and Oklahoma eastward across the southern states and along the Atlantic coast as far north as Maine. Although several studies have demonstrated that between 1 percent and 3 percent of these ticks are infected with a spirochete, a thorough assessment of risk of infection has not been conducted.

Treatment Options and Outlook

As with Lyme disease, prompt treatment with antibiotics cures the infection.

Risk Factors and Preventive Measures

Reducing exposure to ticks lessens the chance of disease. Prevention measures similar to those for Lyme disease will reduce the exposure to infected ticks.

Spanish flu See INFLUENZA.

spinal meningitis See MENINGITIS, MENINGOCOCCAL.

spinal tap The common name for a lumbar puncture, a procedure in which cerebrospinal fluid is removed by using a hollow needle inserted into the lower back, usually between the third and fourth lumbar vertebrae. In infectious diseases, the main use of the spinal tap is to examine the fluid to diagnose infections of the brain and spinal cord, such as MENINGITIS.

The fluid is checked for appearance, white blood cells, sugar, and protein. Examined on a slide in the lab, the fluid is also sent for a special test to help determine what sort of germ is causing symptoms. After the tap is done, the needle is removed, the puncture site is covered with a sterile tape, and the patient must lie flat for at least an hour to prevent a headache. The procedure itself, however, usually takes less than 20 minutes.

While some people worry that a spinal tap will be painful, in fact the procedure is only mildly uncomfortable.

Spirillum minus A species of bacteria in the *Spirillum* genus that causes RAT-BITE FEVER.

spirochetes Slender, coiled bacterial organisms that lack a rigid cell wall and move by flexing their coils. Spirochetes used to be considered protozoa, but they are now classified as bacteria of the Spirochaetales. They include the species *Borrelia, Leptospira,* and *Treponema.*

spoilage bacteria Microorganisms too small to be seen without a microscope that cause food to deteriorate and develop unpleasant odors, tastes, and textures. These one-celled microorganisms can cause fruits and vegetables to get mushy or slimy, or meat to develop a bad odor. Although most people would instinctively avoid spoiled food, ingesting this food would probably not cause illness.

On the other hand, pathogenic bacteria can cause illness. These bacteria grow rapidly in the "Danger Zone"—the temperatures between 40 and 140°F—and do not generally affect the taste, smell, or appearance of food. Food that is left too long at unsafe temperatures could be dangerous to eat, but smell and look just fine. *ESCHERICHIA COLI* O157:H7, *CAMPYLOBACTER,* and *SALMONELLA* are examples of pathogenic bacteria.

There are different types of spoilage bacteria, each of which reproduces at specific temperatures. Some can grow in the low temperatures found in a refrigerator or freezer, whereas others grow well at room temperature.

Bacteria will grow anywhere they have access to nutrients and water. Under the correct conditions, spoilage bacteria reproduce rapidly and the populations can grow very large—sometimes doubling in as little as 30 minutes. It is this large number of microorganisms and their waste products that cause the objectionable changes in odor, taste, and texture.

The spoilage bacteria include

- Mesophiles (found at moderate temperatures ranging from 41 to 50°F)

- Psychrotrophs (can grow at 32°F, but grow best at moderate temperatures)

- Psychrophiles (prefer low temperatures below 32°F, but they can also thrive at moderate temperatures of 59 to 68°F)

- Thermophiles (prefer a warmer temperature between 131 and 149°F; some can grow in temperatures as low as 95°F or as high as 167 to 194°F)

sporotrichosis A chronic fungal infection of the skin that often follows trauma, characterized by painful ABSCESSES and ulcers. The fungus affects both men and women who come in contact with the fungus through soil, vegetation, plants, or decaying vegetables.

Sporotrichosis is caused by the fungus *Sporothrix schenckii.* Outbreaks are common among those who handle sphagnum moss, baled hay, or thorny plants. A number of recent cases have occurred among nursery workers (especially those who handle sphagnum moss topiaries). The fungus enters the skin through a small cut or puncture from thorns, barbs, pine needles, or wires; it can't be spread from one person to another.

Symptoms and Diagnostic Path
There are several forms of the disorder; most patients develop an acute skin condition beginning with a small, painless bump that looks something like an insect bite. It may be red, purple, or pink and usually appears on the finger, hand, or arm at the site where the fungus first entered the skin. The first bump may be followed by one or more bumps, which may resemble boils. The infection can spread to other parts of the body.

While it is possible for the infection to spread to joints, lungs, and central nervous system, this is very rare. Such systemic infections can be fatal. Usually, this occurs only with those who have a disorder of the immune system.

Symptoms may appear any time from one to 12 weeks after exposure; usually, however, the bumps appear within three weeks from the time the fungus enters the skin.

Sporotrichosis is confirmed by culturing the fungus from a swab of the pus or biopsy of a freshly opened skin bump that has been cultured in a lab.

Treatment Options and Outlook
Droplets of potassium iodide for six weeks is the usual method of treatment. The drug itraconazole (Sporanox) may be prescribed, but experience with

this drug is still limited. Amphotericin B and flucytosine also have been used to treat the disease.

Risk Factors and Preventive Measures

Wearing gloves and long sleeves when handling wires, rose bushes, hay bales, pine seedlings, or other materials may help, since it protects against minor skin breaks. Gardeners should avoid skin contact with sphagnum moss, since moss has been implicated as a source of the fungus in a number of outbreaks.

Stachybotrys chartarum mold A potentially fatal green-black mold that may cause health effects ranging from cold- and allergy-like symptoms to skin rashes, respiratory inflammation, bloody noses, fever, headaches, neurological problems, and a suppressed immune system. *Stachybotrys* has been found across the country on school campuses, in courthouses and fire stations, in day-care centers, and in homes.

Molds of any type thrive in damp areas, and on products such as wood or paper. Once building materials get wet, whether from a flood, leaky roof, high water table, or high humidity, the mold can grow. When wet, the mold looks black and slimy, sometimes with white edges; when dry it looks less shiny. It is not the only or the most common black mold to be found in damp conditions, however. Although this dangerous type of black mold is not rare, the U.S. CENTERS FOR DISEASE CONTROL AND PREVENTION (CDC) has no accurate information on how often it is found in buildings.

Some private environmental consulting firms have the ability to conduct home assessments and sample for mold identification. Consulting firms should be familiar with the American Industrial Hygiene Association document entitled "Field Guide for the Determination of Biological Contaminants in Environmental Samples."

To rid a home of black mold, the source of moisture must be eliminated. Then the mold must be removed with a bleachlike solution. All damaged materials, including walls and rugs, must be torn out and replaced. If the wood framing is affected, it must be cleaned and treated with a sealant. Homeowners with a large area of mold growth (more than two square feet) should seek professional help in the cleanup. It is possible to get quite sick during cleanup by inhaling the fungal dust, or by contacting the fungus on the skin.

staphylococcal infections A group of infections caused by staphylococci bacteria and characterized by the formation of abscesses in the skin or other organs. Staphylococci, which grow in grapelike clusters, are a common cause of skin infections—but they also can cause serious internal disorders.

Staphylococcal bacteria are normally found on the skin of most people, but if the bacteria get trapped within the skin by blocked sweat or sebaceous glands, they can cause a wide variety of skin infections including pustules, BOILS, STYES, or CARBUNCLES. The bacteria can cause a severe blistering rash in newborn babies called STAPHYLOCOCCAL SCALDED SKIN SYNDROME.

This type of bacteria also is found in the throats and nose in most people; when mucus is not cleared from the lungs (such as after a viral infection), organisms can build up in the lungs and cause PNEUMONIA.

Staphylococcal infections are among the most common infections in surgical patients, according to the CENTERS FOR DISEASE CONTROL AND PREVENTION. More troubling still, the percentage of hospital-acquired staph infections that are resistant to antibiotics has risen from under 5 percent in 1982 to more than 25 percent in 1992.

BACTEREMIA (bacteria in the blood) caused by a staph infection is common and may lead to endocarditis (a type of heart disease), MENINGITIS, or bone infection (OSTEOMYELITIS). Untreated, multiplying bacteria in the blood (SEPTICEMIA) can lead to fatal cases of SEPTIC SHOCK. Staphylococcal pneumonia may follow a viral disease (such as INFLUENZA). Acute GASTROENTERITIS (food poisoning) may be caused by a toxin produced by certain species of staphylococci in contaminated food.

Among menstruating women (especially those who use highly absorbent tampons), toxin-producing staphylococci may multiply in the mucous membranes lining the vagina, causing TOXIC SHOCK SYNDROME. A separate type of staphlococcal infection can cause URINARY TRACT INFECTIONS.

Treatment for these types of bacterial infections usually includes bed rest, painkillers, and an antimicrobial drug that is resistant to penicillinase (an enzyme secreted by many species of *Staphylococcus*). Surgical drainage of deep abscesses may be necessary.

See also HOSPITAL-ACQUIRED INFECTIONS; VANCOMYCIN-RESISTANT ENTEROCOCI (VRE); METHICILLIN-RESISTANT STAPHYLOCOCCUS.

staphylococcal scalded skin syndrome (SSSS) A blistering skin rash in newborns caused by toxins on the skin released by staphylococcal bacteria. The disorder primarily affects infants between one to three months of age, and occasionally older children and adults.

First recognized as a distinct condition in the mid-1800s, this disease has been incorrectly called by many different names, including Ritter's disease, toxic epidermal necrolysis, and pemphigus neonatorum. The cause of this condition is a toxin-producing strain of *STAPHYLOCOCCUS AUREUS*. Infants with poor immunity or kidney problems are more vulnerable to this infection.

The fatality rate is less than 4 percent. EPIDEMICS have occurred in contaminated nurseries, and the bacteria may be transmitted by a carrier who has no symptoms. The condition has also been reported among adults.

Symptoms and Diagnostic Path

The skin rash strongly resembles a burn, with blistering and peeling skin giving a scalded appearance. Indeed, some parents have been wrongly accused of child abuse as a result of the symptoms of this disease.

First symptoms usually include evidence of a primary staphlococcal infection, including IMPETIGO, eye infection, EAR INFECTION, or SORE THROAT with fever, malaise, or irritability. The skin of the face becomes tender, and the skin around the mouth becomes reddened, weeping, and crusting in a way that resembles potato chips. The trunk also may become involved.

In some patients the rash stabilizes, whereas in other cases flaccid blisters begin to develop all over the skin within 24 to 48 hours. Large areas of skin slough off, and hair or nails may be lost.

Treatment Options and Outlook

The condition should be treated with prompt administration of antistaphylococcal antibiotics. Patients often appear very ill; are dehydrated and they also are at risk of secondary infection. The skin should be covered with wet dressings and antibiotic ointments. Patients usually heal without scarring within a week.

It is important to maintain correct body temperature; infants must be kept warm; any sudden rise in body temperature could indicate blood infection and the immediate need for more aggressive treatment. The skin should be loosely clothed and covered so as to reduce friction. Cotton should be inserted between affected fingers and toes to prevent scarring. Warm baths and soaks help healing and gentle removal of peeling skin will help. Scars from this condition rarely occur.

Staphylococcus aureus A species of *Staphylococcus* that is responsible for a number of infections such as a BOIL, CARBUNCLE, ABSCESS, CELLULITIS, SEPSIS, and OSTEOMYELITIS.

STD See SEXUALLY TRANSMITTED DISEASE.

sterilization The complete elimination or destruction of all forms of microbial life. In hospitals, equipment is sterilized with steam, dry heat, gas, or liquid chemicals. Such sterilization is rarely needed at home. For most in-home needs, such as sterilizing bottles and nipples for babies and heating by boiling (DISINFECTION) is sufficient.

steroids See CORTICOSTEROID DRUGS.

stomach and intestinal infections A number of infections target the stomach and intestines, including APPENDICITIS, *CAMPYLOBACTER*, GIARDIASIS, *HELI-*

COBACTER PYLORI, PINWORMS, ROTAVIRUS, *Salmonella*, *Shigella*, and YERSINIOSIS.

strep throat   A bacterial throat infection caused by *group A beta-hemolytic Streptococcus,* a circular bacterium also known as *Streptococcus pyogenes.* Only group-A strep causes the infection known as strep throat; most kinds of sore throats are *not* strep.

Strep throat occurs all over the world, usually affecting school-age children in winter and spring in the temperate zones of North America. Some people seem to have a tendency toward multiple strep throat infections, while others rarely come down with the disease. It is rare in youngsters under age three.

Because there are many types of group-A strep bacteria, one bout of strep throat does not confer long-term immunity; patients can therefore come down with repeated episodes. Adults may be immune to some types of group-A strep and therefore have fewer infections.

Some people carry group A strep in their throats and nasal passages, although they remain healthy; however, they can spread the infection to others, as can those who are actively ill. However, a person cannot catch strep throat from touching the clothing of an infected person. A sneeze or a cough can project the organisms up to two feet, so it spreads easily in schools and group living situations.

Some EPIDEMICS have been traced to infected health-care workers in operating rooms and to infected food handlers; other outbreaks have occurred by eating contaminated food.

Patients are most infectious in the beginning of the illness; untreated, a patient is infectious for 10 days to three weeks. Carriers are infectious for two to three weeks, although the bacteria may be carried in nose and throat for weeks to several months. Those who receive PENICILLIN are no longer infectious after 24 hours. This means that children with strep can go back to school or child care one to two days after receiving penicillin, if they feel well and have no fever.

Symptoms and Diagnostic Path
Up to half of all children with strep throat have no symptoms, but are considered healthy carriers. In those who do have symptoms, they will appear within one to three days after infection. Young children often have high fevers and red, swollen throats, but their throats are actually less painful than those of adults with the same infection. A few children (one in 10) become quite ill, with extremely high fever, nausea, and vomiting. Such a severe reaction is rare, however. Most people have a sore throat, fever, and pain in swallowing.

A strep throat is different from a run-of-the-mill sore throat that comes with a cold or the flu. With strep throat, there is no runny nose or cough, and symptoms appear abruptly with a fever as high as 104°F, headache, stomach ache, and a red, swollen throat. By the second day, the throat and tonsils may be covered with white or yellow patches that spread together to cover the entire throat. However, it is possible to have a strep throat *without* these telltale white patches, or even without a fever.

Most people also have swollen lymph glands in the front of the neck, just below the point where the ear and jawbone meet. These glands may remain swollen for up to a month after recovery from the infection.

Because almost all of the symptoms of strep throat also can occur with viral infections, lab tests are needed to confirm the diagnosis. Anyone who suspects strep throat should see a doctor for a throat culture or rapid test. A throat culture is the best, most accurate test, but rapid strep tests are also widely used, and can give results within three minutes.

Treatment Options and Outlook
A positive strep test requires antibiotic treatment to prevent complications. Penicillin given seven to nine days after the illness starts will prevent RHEUMATIC FEVER. Benzathine penicillin G is usually injected, since this type of penicillin stays in the body for 10 days. Oral penicillin V must be taken four times a day for 10 days; some studies suggest that oral penicillin may lead to more relapses. Those who are allergic to penicillin may take erythromycin. Oral cephalexin and other new drugs are also effective but are more expensive.

These bacteria are often resistant to tetracycline or sulfonamide.

High fevers may be treated with acetaminophen. Easy-to-swallow foods or cold food (ice cream, frozen juice bars, warm soup, mashed bananas, puddings, gelatins, noodles, soft drinks) are good choices.

Gargling with warm salt water and warm tea with honey and lemon are effective pain reducers. It is not important if the patient does not want to eat, but fluids are critical.

The risk of severe complications is the primary concern with strep throat, and the reason why it is so important to be properly diagnosed and treated. One of the most serious complications is rheumatic fever, a disease that affects up to 3 percent of those with untreated strep infection. Rheumatic fever can lead to rheumatic heart disease.

Kidney inflammation (acute glomerulonephritis) is another possible complication of strep throat, which can appear from 10 days to six weeks after the throat infection. The bacteria do not directly infect the kidneys; instead, the body's immune system response can damage the kidney's filtering mechanism. Warning signs of impending kidney problems include swelling of hands, face, and feet; dark or bloody urine; headaches; vision problems; and decreased urinary output. Children usually recover, albeit slowly, but adults may suffer permanent kidney damage.

EAR INFECTIONS are another possible complication of untreated strep throat.

**WARNING SIGNS OF
COMPLICATIONS IN STREP THROAT**

A doctor should be notified immediately if any of the following symptoms occur:

- breathing problems
- dark, murky urine
- drooling in older child
- extreme problems in swallowing
- fever that goes away and then returns
- headache
- high fever above 105°F
- joint pain
- less urine than normal
- no improvement in two days
- rash
- seal-bark cough
- vision changes

SCARLET FEVER (scarlatina) is an uncommon strep infection that may follow untreated strep throat within two days, producing a fever and a fine red rash over the upper body. With antibiotics, recovery is complete within two weeks, although skin may peel on fingers and toes afterward. A severe form of scarlet fever can cause serious illness, including high fever, convulsions, and death.

Risk Factors and Preventive Measures
People should avoid anyone with strep throat who has not received antibiotics. Children with strep should not be sent to school until they have taken antibiotics for 24 hours, or if there is still a fever and sore throat.

Streptobacillus moniliformis A species of necklace-shaped bacteria that cause RAT-BITE FEVER in humans.

streptococcal infections A group of infections caused by bacteria of the *STREPTOCOCCUS* family, among the most common bacteria in humans. These infections are responsible for a wide range of health problems, including such skin conditions as ERYSIPELAS, SCARLET FEVER, or wound infections.

The name *streptococcus* was first used in 1874, meaning "twisted chain of berries," and refers to the fact that the bacteria grow in long linked chains like strung beads.

Some types of strep bacteria exist harmlessly in the throat; if the bacteria gets in the bloodstream, they are usually destroyed—unless the patient has a heart condition. In this case, a strep infection may lead to bacterial endocarditis. Other types of strep bacteria can cause to sore throats, TONSILLITIS, EAR INFECTIONS, STREP THROAT, or PNEUMONIA. This same bacteria may lead to the serious complications of RHEUMATIC FEVER. Another type of harmless strep is found in the intestines, but if the bacteria gain access to the urinary system, they can cause a URINARY TRACT INFECTION.

Common throughout the world in school-age youngsters, incidence of infections have decreased since the beginning of this century. The danger of resistance to antibiotics were of little concern with these infections until the 1970s, when PENICILLIN-resistant strains of strep bacteria began to appear. As strep A infections became less worrisome, strep-B infections became more virulent; then in the 1980s, strep A became more dangerous again; a much stronger *S. pneumoniae* is part of this resurging tide of infection.

streptococcal pharyngitis See STREP THROAT.

streptococcal toxic shock syndrome (STSS) An uncommon severe condition characterized by very low blood pressure and a rash; it is linked to TOXIC SHOCK SYNDROME caused by staphlococcal infection. STSS can occur after a streptococcus infection of the skin or a wound. It almost never follows a simple streptococcus throat infection (strep throat).

Symptoms and Diagnostic Path

Within 48 hours of infection, the person's blood pressure plummets and other symptoms begin, including fever, dizziness, confusion, difficulty breathing, and a weak and rapid pulse. The skin may be pale, cool, and moist, and there may be a blotchy rash that sometimes peels. The area around an infected wound can become swollen, red, and seriously damaged. The liver and kidneys may begin to fail, and bleeding problems may develop.

STSS can be identified from a physical exam and blood tests that assess liver and kidney function. Doctors may want to rule out conditions such as MEASLES or ROCKY MOUNTAIN SPOTTED FEVER, which can produce similar symptoms. A doctor may also take samples of fluid from an ABSCESS, BOIL, or infected wound to look for a possible source of staphylococcus or streptococcus infection.

Treatment Options and Outlook

STSS is treated with antibiotics, intravenous fluids, and medications to maintain normal blood pressure. Surgery is sometimes necessary to remove areas of dead skin and muscle around an infected wound.

Risk Factors and Preventive Measures

STSS can be prevented by cleaning and bandaging all skin wounds as quickly as possible and by consulting a doctor whenever a wound becomes red, swollen, or tender or if a fever begins. Although STSS almost never follows strep throat, it is wise to check with a doctor whenever a child has a sore throat with fever, particularly if the child's condition is worsening despite treatment.

Streptococcus A genus of gram-positive bacteria classified by letters from A to T. The various species occur in pairs, short chains, and chains. Many of the species can cause disease in humans.

See also STREPTOCOCCAL INFECTIONS; STREP THROAT.

streptococcus, group-A (GAS) Bacteria that are responsible for most cases of strep illness, also known as *Streptococcus pyogenes* ("pus-producing"). Many people carry the bacteria in the throat or skin and have no symptoms at all. When symptoms do occur, they cause relatively mild illnesses. Other strep serogroups (B, C, D, and G) also cause infection.

Diseases caused by group-A strep include STREP THROAT (SCARLET FEVER and RHEUMATIC FEVER are rare complications, usually preceded by a sore throat); skin infections (ERYSIPELAS/CELLULITIS and IMPETIGO), and PNEUMONIA.

Invasive group A strep can cause a severe, sometimes life-threatening infection in which the bacteria spread to other parts of the body, such as the blood, muscle, and fat tissue or the lungs. This includes NECROTIZING FASCIITIS (FLESH-EATING BACTERIA), BACTEREMIA and STREPTOCOCCAL TOXIC SHOCK SYNDROME (STSS).

Early signs and symptoms of necrotizing fasciitis include fever, severe pain and swelling, redness at wound site. Early signs of STSS include fever, dizziness, confusion, rash, and abdominal pain.

In 2001, scientists cracked the genetic code of the bacteria, which may lead to better treatments for the illnesses it causes. Now that the bacteria's complete DNA sequence has been determined, scientists hope they can develop other antibiotics or even vaccinations. During the mapping study, scientists discovered six toxins caused by the strep bacteria that had been previously unknown.

About 10,000 to 15,000 cases of invasive GAS occur in the United States each year, causing more than 2,000 deaths. The CENTERS FOR DISEASE CONTROL AND PREVENTION estimates between 500 and 1,500 cases of necrotizing fasciitis and 2,000 to 3,000 cases of STSS each year in the United States; on the other hand, there are several million cases of strep throat and IMPETIGO each year.

Invasive GAS disease occurs when the bacteria get past the body's immune defenses. The germs are spread by direct contact with nose and throat discharge, or by touching infected skin lesions. The seriousness of the infection is greatest when the person is ill or has an infected wound. Health conditions that impair the immune system make infection with GAS more likely. In addition, there are some strains of GAS that are more likely to cause serious disease.

Most of the people who come in contact with a virulent strain of GAS still will not develop invasive disease; most will have a simple throat or skin infection. Some may not have any symptoms at all. While it is possible for a healthy person to contract invasive GAS, it is people with chronic conditions such as cancer, diabetes, or kidney dialysis, or who use steroid medications, who are at highest risk.

There have been no reports of casual contacts (such as coworkers or classmates) of infected patients developing invasive GAS disease after contact with a patient. However, occasionally close family contacts *have* developed severe disease. There are no current recommendations regarding whether close family contacts should be tested and treated for disease if a family member becomes ill.

Treatment Options and Outlook

Group-A strep bacteria can be treated with common antibiotics; PENICILLIN is the drug of choice for both mild and severe disease. Erythromycin is prescribed for those allergic to penicillin. In addition to antibiotics, supportive care is required. In severe tissue infections, surgery may be needed to remove dead skin. Early treatment can reduce the threat of death, although even the best therapy may not prevent death in every case.

About 20 percent of patients with necrotizing fasciitis and 60 percent of those with STSS will die; only 10 to 15 percent of those with other forms of invasive group-A strep die.

Risk Factors and Preventive Measures

There are no proven vaccines to prevent strep infections. Hand washing may help stop the spread of all types of group-A strep infections, especially after coughing or sneezing, and before preparing food. Those with a strep throat should stay home from work, school, or day care until 24 hours after taking an antibiotic. Wounds should be cleansed and watched for signs of possible infection.

streptococcus, group-B (GBS) A type of bacteria that causes illness in pregnant women, newborns, the elderly, and those with impaired immune systems. It is also the most common cause of life-threatening infections in newborns.

GBS is the most common cause of blood infection (septicemia) and MENINGITIS (infection of the fluid and lining of the brain) in newborns and is a frequent cause of newborn PNEUMONIA. About 8,000 infants in the United States are infected each year, and up to 15 percent of these infants die. Those who survive (especially those who had meningitis) may have complications, including hearing or vision loss or learning disabilities.

In pregnant women, GBS can cause URINARY TRACT INFECTIONS, endometritis, and stillbirth. Other common diseases caused by GBS include skin or soft tissue infections.

While many people carry GBS in their bodies (in bowel, genitals, urinary tract, throat, or lungs), most do not get sick. Between 15 and 40 percent of all pregnant women have GBS in the rectum or vagina.

Symptoms and Diagnostic Path

About 2 percent of infants infected with GBS develop symptoms, which usually appear during the first week of life—usually within a few hours after birth. It is also possible for infants to contract GBS several months after birth; meningitis is more common with this type of later-onset disease.

GBS can be diagnosed by growing bacteria from spinal fluid or blood cultures.

Treatment Options and Outlook

Antibiotics (PENICILLIN or ampicillin) are the treatment of choice. About 20 percent of men and non-pregnant women with GBS infections will die.

Risk Factors and Preventive Measures

Most GBS among newborns can be prevented by giving certain pregnant women antibiotics intravenously during labor. Any pregnant woman who has had a baby with GBS disease or who has a urinary tract infection caused by GBS should receive antibiotics during labor. Women who have been diagnosed with GBS infection at labor are at higher risk if they have fever during labor, rupture of membranes 18 hours or more before delivery, and labor or rupture of membranes before 37 weeks. Women who have GBS but do not have these risk factors have a relatively low chance of delivering a baby with GBS disease.

Unfortunately, some babies still get GBS in spite of testing and antibiotics. Vaccines to prevent GBS disease are being developed.

Streptococcus pneumoniae Any of 70 different types of pneumococci that can cause PNEUMONIA and other diseases in humans. This type of bacteria is one of the most common and clinically important bacterial germs. More and more strains of this bacteria are appearing to be moderately to highly resistant to PENICILLIN.

The most common infections caused by *S. pneumoniae* include SINUSITIS, BRONCHITIS, and pneumonia, followed by BACTEREMIA and MENINGITIS. Other, more unusual infections include soft tissue infection. Pneumococci may also rarely cause pericarditis or endocarditis.

Streptococcus pyogenes See STREPTOCOCCUS, GROUP-A (GAS).

streptogramins A new class of antibiotics with a broad spectrum of activity against gram-positive, gram-negative and intracellular bacteria. They are also effective against many bacteria that are resistant to other drugs, such as quinolones and glycopeptides. The streptogramins work by interfering with protein synthesis.

The first streptogramins in clinical use were a combination of quinupristin/dalfopristin (Syner-cid). This combination is effective against VANCOMYCIN-RESISTANT ENTEROCOCCUS (VRE).

strongyloidiasis An intestinal infestation of tiny parasitic ROUNDWORMS that cause itching and raised red patches where the worms enter the skin. The disease, caused by a type of roundworm known as *Strongyloides stercoralis*, is found throughout the tropics, especially in the Far East. The worms are picked up by walking barefoot on soil contaminated with feces; the larvae enter the skin of the feet and migrate to the small intestines, where they develop into adulthood, burrowing into the intestinal walls and producing larvae.

Symptoms and Diagnostic Path

After infestation, the worms cause redness, swelling, itching, or hives, that fade within two days. If the larvae penetrate the perianal area, skin lesions begin to radiate from the anus down the thigh or across the buttocks or abdomen as itchy bands. While the individual lesions may fade away within a few days, an infestation may continue in the host for many years and cause recurrent problems.

Treatment Options and Outlook

Thiabendazole is the drug of choice. Rarely, death may occur from blood poisoning or MENINGITIS many years after the worms enter the body. PNEUMONIA may occur because of immune system damage.

stye (sty) A small pus-filled ABSCESS (also called a hordeolum) near the eyelashes, caused by a staphylococcal bacterial infection.

Symptoms and Diagnostic Path

A stye begins as a pus-filled swollen bump near the eyelashes that can be reddened and painful.

Treatment Options and Outlook

If the style is painful, warm compresses may help eliminate the pain. Antibiotic ointment designed for the eyes can help prevent a recurrence.

subacute sclerosing panencephalitis (SSPE) A chronic persistent infection of the central nervous system caused by an altered form of the MEASLES virus that affects children and young adults, causing a progressive brain deterioration due to inflammation and nerve cell death. The disease is typically progressive, ending in death within a few years in most patients. There is only a slight (5 percent) chance of spontaneous remission.

SSPE can occur at any time from two to 10 years after the original measles infection. Since the widespread use of the measles vaccine, SSPE has become very rare, although it is far more common in the Middle East and India.

Symptoms and Diagnostic Path

Initial symptoms usually begin with abnormal behavior, irritability, intellectual deterioration, and memory loss. This may be followed by involuntary movements and seizures, followed by further mental deterioration, inability to walk, speech impairment with poor comprehension, swallowing problems, and sometimes blindness. In the final stages, the patient may remain mute or comatose.

Electroencephalograms (EEG) show slow progressive changes in the electrical activity of the brain, as the central nervous system slowly deteriorates. As a result, several staging scales have been used to categorize patients with SSPE according to their symptoms. More recently, a different staging system was developed based on brain scans.

Treatment Options and Outlook

There is no cure. Anticonvulsant therapy and treatment of symptoms may make the patient more comfortable. Some research suggests that treatment with inosine pranobex (oral Isoprinosine) combined with interferon alpha can lead to remission or improvement in half the cases.

When not treated with interferon and antiviral drugs, SSPE is almost always a fatal disease, usually between one and three years after symptoms begin. However, some spontaneous remissions have been reported.

sulfonamides (sulfa drugs) A large group of synthetic drugs used to treat bacterial infections, which are derived from a red dye (sulfanilamide). Drugs in this class prevent the growth of bacteria, they do not kill bacteria. Used in combination with other drugs, they are used to treat a wide variety of conditions such as URINARY TRACT INFECTIONS, BRONCHITIS, PNEUMONIA, skin infections, and EAR INFECTIONS. Most sulfa drugs (including sulfamethoxazole and sulfaphenazole) are quickly absorbed from the stomach and small intestine and should be taken at regular intervals. Others are long-acting (such as sulfadoxine, used to treat LEPROSY and MALARIA) and only need to be taken once a day.

Side Effects

Side effects may include anemia or jaundice, especially if taken for longer than 10 days. More severe side effects include blood disorders, skin rashes, and fever. These drugs are not given during the last trimester of pregnancy or to young babies because of the risk of mental retardation. The drugs are prescribed with caution to patients with kidney or liver problems. In general, patients using these drugs should avoid exposure to direct sunlight, which could provoke a rash.

sushi See ANISAKIASIS.

sweating sickness (English) A contagious disease that appeared in the 15th century that struck and killed victims quickly and violently. It is believed to have been introduced into England by French soldiers recruited by King Henry VII for his army in 1485. Subsequent outbreaks occurred in 1507, 1516, 1529, and 1551. Unlike most other EPIDEMICS of infectious diseases, its appearance was relatively brief, and it permanently disappeared in 1551.

Unlike other infectious epidemics of the 14th and 15th centuries, which tended to strike the poor, the English sweating sickness struck the wealthy with equal vengeance. The most famous victim of "the sweat" was Cardinal Thomas Wolsey of England, who came down with the disease three times in 1517, but survived each time. Also infected were the aldermen and two lord mayors of London, both of whom died within a week during the epidemic of 1485. During this first epidemic, the royal court issued a decree forbidding anyone from appearing at court except on official business.

While it is difficult to tell for sure how many people died from this epidemic, it is believed that the sweats of 1485 and 1507 each killed 10,000 people throughout England. The sweat of 1551 was particularly severe in Devon and Essex.

Although sweating sickness resembled INFLUENZA, SCARLET FEVER, and the PLAGUE, medical historians have never been able to identify it. Although some experts believe it was a milder form of plague, it remains an unsolved medical puzzle.

Striking with fearsome rapidity, the disease lasted only about 24 hours and produced a profuse and drenching sweat from head to foot, together with pains in the back, shoulder, arms, legs, and head, as well as intestinal problems and "passion" in the heart. Reportedly, the disease could kill in as little as two hours.

While primarily affecting people in England, it also occurred in Germany, Scandinavia, Poland, Lithuania, Russia, and the Netherlands. Angry German Catholics swore the disease was God's retribution for Martin Luther's Protestant heresies. The disease never spread into Spain or Italy.

swimmer's ear   See OTITIS EXTERNA.

swimmer's itch   The common name for cutaneous SCHISTOSOMIASIS (or cercarial dermatitis), this is an itchy skin inflammation caused by bites from flatworms. It is characterized by a distinctive patchy, red pinpoint skin rash after swimming in or having contact with freshwater populated by ducks and snails. On the saltwater tributaries of Long Island Sound it is called "clamdigger's itch"; it is known as "duck-feces dermatitis" or "sawah itch" among rice paddy workers of China or Malaysia.

This type of dermatitis is a potential risk whenever people frequent an aquatic area also used by animals and mollusks infested with the flatworms. In the United States, the worst outbreaks occur in the lake regions of Michigan, Wisconsin, and Minnesota, although it also may occur in saltwater areas.

The flatworm parasites are found in migrating birds and mammals; the animal or bird defecates the worm into the water. Snails then ingest the worm; when the larval parasites are released from infected snails, they migrate through water, where they can infect swimmers. Children are most often infected due to their swimming habits. If the victim swims or wades in infested water and then allows water to evaporate off the skin instead of regularly drying off with a towel, the parasites can then burrow under the skin. The problem occurs in summer when the water temperature is warm enough for snails to reproduce and grow rapidly. At the same time, migrating birds infected with the parasite return from their winter habitats, and swimmers enter the water.

Symptoms and Diagnostic Path

After exposure to water affected by the schistosomes, a prickling or itchy feeling begins that can last up to an hour while the flukes enter the skin. Small red macules form, but there may be swelling or wheals among sensitive people. As these lesions begin to disappear, they are replaced after 10 or 15 hours by discrete, very itchy papules surrounded by a red area. Vesicles and pustules form one or two days later; the lesions fade away within a week, leaving small pigmented spots. Different symptoms depend on how sensitive the patient is to the schistosome; each reexposure causes a more severe reaction.

Diagnosis is difficult; skin biopsies are not helpful. There is no widely available blood test that can reveal the worms. Diseases that have been confused with swimmer's itch include IMPETIGO, CHICKEN POX, poison ivy, or HERPES.

Treament Options and Outlook

Treatment may not be needed if there are only a few itchy spots. Calamine lotion or oral antihistamines may help control the itch until the lesions begin to disappear on their own. If symptoms persist for more than three days, a doctor should be consulted.

Risk Factors and Preventive Measures

The best way to alleviate the problem is to destroy the snails by treating the water with copper sulfate and carbonate or with sodium pentachlorophenate. A thick coating of grease or tightly woven clothes can protect against infestation; bathing with a hexachlorophene soap before swimming may help to some degree. Briskly rubbing the skin with a towel after swimming may help remove some organisms.

syphilis A sexually transmitted infection that causes (among other symptoms) a skin sore and rash. Syphilis was first recorded as a major epidemic in Europe during the 15th century, after Columbus returned from his trip to America. Today, the infection is transmitted almost exclusively by sexual contact. Although primary and secondary syphilis in the United States dropped by almost 90 percent from 1990 to 2000, the number of cases has been rising since, from 5,979 in 2000 to 7,352 in 2004. In addition, there was a dramatic increase in cases in men from 2000 to 2002 that reflects syphilis in men who have sex with men. Moreover, HIV infection and syphilis are linked; syphilis increases the risk of both transmitting and getting infected with HIV (the virus that causes AIDS).

Although there are big differences in the reported rates among racial and ethnic groups, these differences have been declining over the past five years. For example, the syphilis rate reported for 2000 among African Americans was 21 times the rate reported among whites, reflecting a substantial decline from 1996, when the rate among African Americans was 50 times greater than that among whites.

Syphilis is caused by a spirochete *Treponema pallidum* that enters broken skin or mucous membranes during sexual intercourse, by kissing, or by intimate bodily contact with an open syphilitic sore. The rate of infection during a single contact with an infected person is about 30 percent. The infection also may be passed to a fetus from an infected mother.

Symptoms and Diagnostic Path

During the first (or *primary*) stage, a sore (chancre) appears between three to four weeks after contact; the sore has a hard, wet, painless base that heals in about a month. In males, the sore appears on the shaft of the penis. In women it can be found on the labia, although it is often hidden so well that the

diagnosis is missed. In both sexes, the sore may be seen on the lips or tongue.

Six to 12 weeks after infection, the patient enters the *secondary* stage, which features a skin rash that may last for months. The rash has crops of pink or pale red round spots, but in black patients the rash is pigmented and appears darker than normal skin. In addition, the lymph nodes may be enlarged, and there may be backache, headache, bone pain, appetite loss, fever, fatigue, and sometimes MENINGITIS. The hair may fall out and the skin may exhibit gray or pink patches that are highly infectious. The secondary stage may last up to a year.

The *latent* stage may last for a few years or until the end of a person's life. During this time, the infected person appears normal; about 30 percent of these patients will develop tertiary syphilis.

Tertiary syphilis (end stage) usually begins about 10 years after the initial infection, although it may appear after only about three years or as late as 25 years later. The person's tissues may begin to deteriorate (a process called gumma formation), involving the bones, palate, nasal septum, tongue, skin, or any organ of the body. The most serious complications in this stage include heart problems, brain damage (neurosyphilis) leading to insanity, and paralysis.

Treatment Options and Outlook

PENICILLIN is the drug of choice for all forms of the disease; early syphilis can often be cured by a single large injection; later forms of the disease require multiple doses of penicillin over time. More than half of syphilis patients treated with penicillin develop a severe reaction within six to 12 hours caused by the body's response to the sudden killing of large numbers of spirochetes.

Risk Factors and Preventive Measures

Infection can be avoided by maintaining monogamous relationships; condoms offer some protection, but they are not absolutely safe. People with syphilis are infectious during the primary and secondary stages, but not in the latter stages of the latent and tertiary stages. The United States is continuing its efforts to eradicate syphilis completely.

taeniasis See TAPEWORM.

tapeworm A parasitic intestinal worm that belongs to the class Cestoda. There are three major species of tapeworms, and all are acquired by humans by eating raw, undercooked, or smoked contaminated meat or fish.

In most tapeworm infestations, the animal or fish has ingested eggs, which develop into larvae, invading the animal's muscles and organs. A human acquires the infection by eating the infected meat.

Beef tapeworm (Taenia saginata) The beef tapeworm is commonly found in undercooked beef in Mexico, South America, Eastern Europe, the Middle East, and Africa. Symptoms may include stomach pain, diarrhea, and weight loss, although it does not usually cause any symptoms. Detached white segments of the worm can emerge spontaneously from the rectum, which is the sign of infestation. Medications are available to treat beef tapeworm.

Pork tapeworm (Taenia solium) The pork tapeworm is commonly found in South America, Eastern Europe, Russia, and Asia. Humans can acquire the tapeworm by eating undercooked pork or raw pork sausage. There are not usually any symptoms other than vague abdominal complaints. Diagnosis is made from white translucent segments of the tapeworm in feces.

Pork tapeworm can lead to a serious complication called cystocercosis, a sometimes-fatal disease. In this illness, a person ingests the eggs, and the larvae then penetrate the stomach wall, invading the tissues (especially the skeletal muscle and the brain) where they form cystlike masses. After several years, the cysts begin to degenerate and produce an inflammatory reaction. At this stage the person may experience epileptic seizures or visual or mental disturbances. Treatment includes drug therapy as well as surgical removal of the cysts.

For this reason, it is important never to eat raw or undercooked pork.

Fish tapeworm infection (diphyllobothriasis) Fish tapeworm occurs after ingesting raw freshwater fish and is found throughout the world. It is particularly common in Scandinavia and the Far East, where consumption of raw fish is high. The infection usually produces a single worm and does not usually cause symptoms other than a vague intestinal discomfort. Pernicious anemia may develop as a result of the worm impairing absorption of vitamin B_{12}. Drug therapy is available.

TB See TUBERCULOSIS.

T cell A type of white blood cell (lymphocyte) involved in the cellular immune response. *Helper T cells* participate in the activation of other T cells; they are targets of the HIV virus, the agent of AIDS. *Suppressor T cells* inhibit the responses of other T cells to antigens. *Cytotoxic T cells* are the cells of the cellular immune system; they recognize and eliminate virus-infected cells.

tetanus An acute, often-fatal bacterial disease commonly known as "lockjaw" because the infection triggers jaw spasms so intense that the patient cannot open the mouth to swallow. The disease affects the nervous system when tetanus bacteria enters the body through a cut or wound. The bacteria can get in through even a tiny pinprick or scratch, but deep puncture wounds or cuts like those made by nails or knives are especially susceptible to infection with tetanus. Tetanus bacteria are present worldwide and are commonly found in soil, dust, and manure. Tetanus is not transmitted from person to person.

About 11 percent of reported cases of tetanus are fatal. Fewer than 50 cases of tetanus occur each year in the United States; deaths are more likely to occur in patients 60 years of age and older. The tetanus vaccine has been available since the 1940s, but anyone who has not been vaccinated as a child or who has not received a booster every 10 years since then is at risk.

A previous infection does not confer immunity; it is possible to get tetanus more than once if the patient was not properly immunized. Experts suggest repeat vaccination every 10 years.

The disease is caused by a bacterium belonging to the Clostridium family, which thrives in the absence of oxygen and is found almost everywhere in the environment—most commonly in soil, dust, manure, and in the digestive tract of humans and animals. The bacteria form spores, which are thick-walled reproductive cells that are hard to kill and that are highly resistant to heat and many antiseptics.

Tetanus cannot be transmitted from person to person but enters the body via a wound—even as small as a pinprick or tiny scratch. Usually, however, a wound that leads to tetanus is a deep puncture or laceration caused by a nail or a knife; because these wounds are hard to clean, bacteria remains deep within the wound. In the presence of dead tissue, tetanus spores can grow and produce the deadly exotoxin that causes symptoms. While tetanus bacteria are found almost everywhere, natural immunity is rare, which is why immunization is so important.

Although most cases are caused by puncture wounds, it is also possible to contract tetanus from animal scratches and bites, in wounds where the flesh is torn or burned, in crushing wounds, and in frostbite. It may even follow minor wounds such as splinters, and can develop after surgery, dental infections, or abortion.

EAR INFECTIONS can lead to a rare form of tetanus called cephalic tetanus, wherein tetanus bacteria are found in the inner ear. Occasionally, tetanus is also found in those with no known injury, wound, or medical condition.

Symptoms and Diagnostic Path

Tetanus affects the central nervous system, producing both stiffness or muscular rigidity and convulsive muscle spasms. While symptoms usually appear within three days to three weeks after infection, the incubation period can be as long as 50 days. The shorter the incubation period, the greater the risk of death. The first symptoms include headache, irritability, and muscular stiffness in the jaw and neck. As more toxin is produced, the jaw, neck, and limbs become locked in spasms, the abdominal muscles become rigid, and the patient may be racked with painful convulsions. The most common symptom is the telltale stiff jaw, caused by spasm of the muscle that closes the mouth.

The affected patient may have other symptoms: difficulty swallowing, restlessness and irritability, fever, headache, and sore throat. As the disease continues, the patient may develop a fixed smile and raised eyebrows because of muscle spasms in the face. Spasms of the diaphragm and the muscles between the ribs may interfere with breathing so that mechanical ventilation may be necessary.

In severe cases, patients become so sensitive to stimulation of any kind (such as a draft or a noise) that their bodies become racked with painful spasms and profuse sweating. These convulsions can be strong enough to break bones.

In addition, overstimulation of the involuntary nervous system may boost blood pressure to dangerous levels or cause irregular heartbeats. Coma may follow repeated convulsions.

Tetanus can be localized so that there are muscle contractions just in the part of the body where the infection began. It also can affect the entire body; about 80 percent of cases are generalized in this latter way.

Treatment Options and Outlook

Powerful tranquilizers and antispasmodic drugs can control symptoms, which last for several weeks and require intensive hospital care. Tetanus immune globulin can confer passive immunization for a few months. Tetanus victims also are given PENICILLIN IV for two weeks and tetanus toxoid vaccine.

Dead skin from the wound must be removed and pus drained.

Tetanus complications may include PNEUMONIA, which occurs in 50 to 70 percent of fatal cases. Other complications may include bone fractures or simple exhaustion due to the muscle spasms. As the disease worsens, patients cannot open their mouth. Constipation and urinary difficulty may occur.

In 1947, 91 percent of the 560 people who got tetanus died. In the period from 1998 to 2000, U.S. doctors reported 43 tetanus cases; 25 patients (all over the age of 40) died. Today, the mortality rate in the United States is about 25 percent and 50 percent worldwide.

Risk Factors and Preventive Measures

Tetanus is totally preventable by routine immunization, which makes the body respond to an inactivated form of the toxin, producing antitoxin that neutralizes the toxins. A booster is needed every 10 years. The only side effect of vaccination is a sore arm for a few days.

Primary immunizations are given in combination with diphtheria and pertussis (DTaP) at two, four, six, and 15 months of age. A booster is given when a child enters school sometime between age four to six years. Every 10 years after, another booster is needed.

There are few side effects with the vaccine, which is virtually 100 percent effective in preventing tetanus. The DTaP shot in children may produce redness or formation of a small hard lump at the site. Some children may have allergic reactions; rarely, serious adverse reactions include rare anaphylaxis (difficulty in breathing or swallowing) and possibly Guillain-Barre syndrome. People who have had a severe reaction should not have any more doses.

Since adults aged 50 or older are responsible for more than 70 percent of tetanus infections, adults must be sure to receive boosters every 10 years.

tetanus immune globulin An injectable solution prepared from the globulin of an immune human that is effective and much safer than administering tetanus antitoxin. It is administered for short-term immunization against tetanus after possible exposure to tetanus.

It should not be substituted for tetanus toxoid (the vaccine that can prevent tetanus). The most serious side effect of immune globulin is an allergic reaction (anaphylaxis). There may also be fever and pain at the injection site.

Thirty Years' War epidemics A wide variety of infectious diseases plagued the soldiers of the Thirty Years' War (1618–48), including TYPHOID FEVER, bubonic PLAGUE, and DYSENTERY. The constant troop movements across Germany led to repeated outbreaks of disease, although a number of local epidemics were unrelated to the war.

Still, many features of the drawn-out conflict boosted the transmission of infectious disease, including the neverending shift of the fronts, the constant troop movements, influx of fresh soldiers from foreign countries, displacement of the German population, and cities swollen with refugees. In this particular war, the extensive contact between soldier and civilian served only to worsen the spread of infectious disease. It has been reported that up to half of the German population died from infections during this war.

throat culture A test to determine the type of organism causing infection in the throat. For this test, a health care worker obtains a specimen from the throat with a long-handled sterile swab. The specimen is placed on a culture plate and read at 24 and 48 hours.

Rapid strep tests are now widely used. These tests react with certain proteins in the bacteria, giving results in just three minutes. They are about 90 percent accurate. Many health care workers do both the rapid test and a backup throat culture to make sure all cases of STREP THROAT are diagnosed.

thrush A yeast infection of the mouth, found often in infants and young children and in those with an impaired immune system.

A yeast infection is a fungal infection, but not all fungi are yeasts. In the case of thrush, the yeast that causes the infection is *CANDIDA ALBICANS*. While there are many different kinds of *Candida* species, albicans causes most human infections and almost all cases of thrush.

An infant may be infected during delivery if the mother has a vaginal yeast infection at birth; infants also may contract thrush from infections on a caregiver's hands or from bottle nipples. Babies born to diabetic mothers are more susceptible to thrush, as are those born with birth defects of the palate or lip. A person is infectious as long as there are lesions in the mouth.

Symptoms and Diagnostic Path

Pain in the mouth, together with raised patches in the mouth, on cheek, tongue, and roof of the mouth, that look like milk curds.

Tests are not needed; the disease can be identified by inspecting the mouth. However, the patches may be swabbed and examined for yeast cells under a microscope; alternatively, the fungus can be cultured.

Treatment Options and Outlook

This condition is treated by painting the mouth with nystatin suspension. Rinsing the mouth often can discourage the spread of thrush.

Risk Factors and Preventive Measures

Mothers with the symptoms of yeast infection should be treated in the last three months of pregnancy. No one should put fingers in a new baby's mouth. If an infant is bottle fed, nipples and bottles should be boiled and hands washed before feeding.

Adults with impaired immune systems, including those with AIDS or patients taking corticosteroid drugs, should be careful to brush the mouth and tongue regularly and rinse the mouth often.

ticks and disease   The tiny bloodsucking pests that commonly plague American dogs and cats, and that can also transmit disease to pet owners. These diseases include BABESIOSIS, EHRLICHIOSIS, and LYME DISEASE, now epidemic in the Northeast. Ticks also can transmit a type of "tick paralysis" in dogs. There are about 200 species of ticks in the United States, found in woods, beach grass, lawns, forests, and cities.

Unlike fleas, ticks are not insects but are arachnids, as are mites, spiders, and scorpions. They have a four-stage life cycle, beginning with eggs, followed by larvae, nymph, and adult. Adult females of some species lay about 100 eggs at a time; her more prolific cousins can lay between 3,000 and 6,000 eggs. Six-legged larvae hatch from these eggs, and after at least one blood meal, the larvae molt into six-legged nymphs (in some species, this happens more than once). Finally nymphs molt into adult males or females with eight legs.

Depending on its species, a tick may take less than a year or up to several years to travel through its entire four-stage life cycle. Ticks need a blood meal at each stage after hatching; some species can survive years without eating anything.

A vaccine to prevent Lyme disease in dogs was licensed in June 1992 and is recommended for dogs at risk for ticks, not those who live in apartments or who live in regions where Lyme disease is not a problem. In most cases, immunity lasts up to about six months with the vaccine; immunity is about 75 percent.

In addition, the Environmental Protection Agency has licensed a product (Damminix) that consists of tubes stuffed with cotton balls treated with the pesticide permethrin. The theory is that the cotton balls mimic the nesting material for deer mice; when placed outdoors in areas inhabited by mice, the cotton kills and repels ticks on the mice.

See also EHRLICHIA; EHRLICHIA CHAFFEENSIS; EHRLICHIOSIS, CANINE; EHRLICHIOSIS, EQUINE; EHRLICHIOSIS, HUMAN MONOCYTIC; EHRLICHIOSIS, HUMAN GRANULOCYTIC.

tinea   Any of a group of common FUNGAL INFECTIONS of the skin, hair, or nails. Most infections are caused by a group of fungi called DERMATOPHYTES and are often called RINGWORM. These common fungus infections are caused by various species of the fungi *Microsporum, Trichophyton,* and *Epidermophyton.* Tinea is highly contagious and can be spread by direct contact or via infected material; infections may be picked up from other people or animals, soil, or an object (such as a shower stall). The term *tinea* is often followed by the Latin term for the part of the body affected by the fungus, such as *tinea pedis* (ATHLETE'S FOOT).

Symptoms and Diagnostic Path

The symptoms vary according to the part of the body affected by the infection; the most common area is the foot (causing athlete's foot), with cracking, itchy skin between the toes. Tinea cruris (JOCK ITCH) is more common in males and produces a red, itchy area from the genitals outward over the inside of the thighs; tinea corporis (ringworm of the body) is characterized by itchy circular skin patches with a raised edge. Tinea capitis (ringworm of the scalp) causes round, itchy circles of hair loss found most commonly in children in large cities or overcrowded conditions. Tinea unguium (ringworm of the nails, or onychomycosis) is characterized by scaling of soles or palms with thick, white, or yellow nails. Ringworm can also affect the skin under a beard (TINEA BARBAE).

Treatment Options and Outlook

Antifungal drugs (creams, lotions, or ointments) can successfully treat most types of tinea. For widespread infection (or those affecting hair or nails), the drug is given as a tablet (usually griseofulvin). Treatment should continue after symptoms have faded to ensure the fungi have been destroyed. Mild infections on the surface of the skin may be treated for four to six weeks; toenail infections may require treatment for up to two years.

tinea barbae Ringworm infection of the skin under the beard, caused primarily by *Tinea mentagrophytes* or *T. verrucosum.*

See TINEA.

tinea capitis The medical term for RINGWORM of the scalp.

tinea corporis The medical term for RINGWORM of the body.

tinea cruris The medical term for JOCK ITCH.

tinea manuum RINGWORM infection most often caused by *Tinea rubrum,* usually found together with a foot infection.

Symptoms and Diagnostic Path

The condition is characterized by thickened outer skin of palms and fingers, especially in the creases of the skin.

Treatment Options and Outlook

Topical imidazole antifungals are the treatment of choice, but topical agents alone do not usually cure this problem; an oral antifungal drug (such as griseofulvin, terbinafine, or ketoconazole) is usually required for between two to three months.

See also TINEA.

tinea nigrapalmaris A superficial RINGWORM infection of the stratum corneum of the palms, although the soles of the feet may also be affected. While the condition is found throughout the world in both men and women of all ages, it is uncommon in North America. Compared to other types of ringworm infections, the incidence of tinea nigrapalmaris is low, even in South America.

While this condition is not fatal, it may mimic malignant melanoma (a type of skin cancer).

Symptoms and Diagnostic Path

The condition is characterized by a single brown-black macule with sharply defined margins (found on the palm or sole) that tend to spread in a circular pattern.

Treatment Options and Outlook

Most infections respond to imidazole cream together with removal by scraping with an emery pad. Recurrence is rare. Surgery is not effective, and there are no established oral medications.

tinea pedis The medical term for ATHLETE'S FOOT.

tinea versicolor A common fungal skin infection (also known as pityriasis versicolor) characterized by patches of white, brown, or salmon-colored flaky skin on the trunk and neck. It primarily affects young and middle-aged adult men and is not contagious.

A fungus (living as a yeast on most people's skin) called *Malassezia furfur* causes the condition when it colonizes the dead outer layer of skin.

Symptoms and Diagnostic Path

The infection is characterized by pale tan patches on the upper trunk and upper arms that may itch and do not tan. In dark-skinned people the lesions may be depigmented.

The patches will show up as fluorescent patches under a special Wood's light and may be easily identified in skin scrapings.

Treatment Options and Outlook

Thorough application of antifungal cream or lotion from ears to knees at night will eradicate the fungus, provided not one spot is missed. It is also important to wash underwear and night clothes thoroughly. The treatment will cure the condition, but it may take many months for the skin patches to return to a normal color.

toe web infection Disorders of the spaces between the toes are usually called ATHLETE'S FOOT, and most are caused by fungal infections. Although the fungus is the primary cause of tissue destruction, subsequent bacterial infiltration can contribute to the problem and interfere with treatment success.

Symptoms and Diagnostic Path

As the infection progresses, the skin between the toes becomes scaly, and then peels and cracks. Toe web infection usually occurs between the fourth and fifth toes.

Treatment Options and Outlook

Because so many different types of organisms are involved in toe web infections, several different types of treatment must be used in order to be effective. If the lesions are dry and scaly, topical antifungal agents (such as *miconazole*, clotrimazole, or ciclopirox olamine) are effective. For soft, wet lesions, treatment must include removal of excess moisture, daily compresses, broad-spectrum topical antimicrobial agents, long-term use of antifungals, and oral griseofulvin.

tonsillitis Infection or inflammation of a tonsil caused by a virus or bacteria. Acute tonsillitis is often caused by *STREPTOCOCCUS* infection. If tonsillitis caused by a strep infection is untreated, it may lead to RHEUMATIC FEVER or kidney disease. Tonsillitis most often occurs in childhood.

The tonsils are believed to help stop infection and protect the upper respiratory tract. However, it is possible for the tonsils themselves to become infected. This happens most often in youngsters under age nine; occasionally, it occurs in teenagers or young adults. Infectious MONONUCLEOSIS often causes tonsillitis.

Symptoms and Diagnostic Path

Severe sore throat, fever, headache, fatigue, swallowing problems, earache, and enlarged, tender lymph nodes in the neck. Acute cases may also be accompanied by SCARLET FEVER. Once in a while, the illness can cause a temporary deafness or an ABSCESS on the tonsil. If symptoms last for longer than 24 hours or if pus is seen on the tonsils, a physician should be consulted.

Treatment Options and Outlook

Tonsillitis can be treated with systemic antibiotics. While a tonsillectomy is still sometimes performed for recurrent cases, this surgical procedure is done much less often today than it was in earlier decades.

See also STREP THROAT.

tonsils The tonsils—a mass of oval lymphoid tissue on either side of the back of the mouth—are one of the body's ways of dealing with invading infections. The tonsils make up part of the lymphatic system, an important part of the body's defense system against infection. Along with the adenoids at the base of the tongue, and posterior oropharynx, the tonsils protect against upper respiratory tract infections. They gradually get bigger after birth, reaching full size at about age seven; after that, they shrink substantially.

An infection of the tonsils is called TONSILLITIS, a common infectious disease of childhood. Quinsy (ABSCESS on the tonsil) is a rare complication. While removal of the tonsils because of infection was once a common treatment in childhood, it is rarely done today.

toothbrushes and infectious disease Despite reports to the contrary, there is little evidence to support the idea that the toothbrush carries germs for the common cold or repeated STREP THROAT.

Instead, experts believe these infections are more likely related to the anatomy of a person's tonsils, or to reexposure to germs from others in the family.

However, the American Dental Association recommends replacing a toothbrush every three to four months (or sooner if the bristles are frayed). Patients who are recently recovered from an infectious illness may still want to replace the toothbrush anyway, or clean it by running it through the dishwasher cycle with the dishes.

toxic shock syndrome (TSS) An uncommon, severe condition characterized by a distinctive skin rash resembling sunburn on the palms and soles. There are two different types of this condition. Toxic shock syndrome (TSS) caused by *STAPHYLOCOCCUS AUREUS* bacteria, and STREPTOCOCCAL TOXIC SHOCK SYNDROME (STSS), caused by streptococcal bacteria.

TSS has been associated with the use of tampons. Although TSS usually occurs in menstruating women, it can affect anyone who has any type of staphylococcal infection, including PNEUMONIA, ABSCESSES, skin or wound infections, blood poisoning (SEPTICEMIA), or a bone infection (OSTEOMYELITIS).

STSS appears after streptococcus bacteria have invaded a cut or scrape, surgical wound, or blisters. It almost never follows a simple streptococcus throat infection. The U.S. Food and Drug Administration (FDA) estimates that one or two of every 100,000 menstruating women develop TSS each year.

Scientists first described TSS as a distinct disease in 1978; two years later, reports of the problem increased among young women who had become ill during or just after menstruation. Studies showed that the use of the high-absorbency tampons was associated with the problem, but the exact connection remains unclear.

The condition is caused by a toxin produced by *S. aureus*, enterotoxin F. It is most common in menstruating women using high-absorbency tampons but has also been seen in newborns, children, and men. Scientists believe that for TSS to develop, the staph bacteria must release one or more toxins into the bloodstream. While the bacteria normally live in the nose, skin, and vagina and cause no problem,

they can also lead to serious infection after a deep wound or surgery or during tampon use.

Symptoms and Diagnostic Path

Symptoms may not begin until the first few days after a woman's period, and develop appear quickly. In addition to the skin rash, symptoms include sudden high fever, vomiting and diarrhea, headache, muscular aches and pains, dizziness, and disorientation. Blood pressure may drop rapidly, and shock may develop.

The sunburn-like rash may not develop until the patient is very ill or may go completely unnoticed if it appears on a small area. The skin on palms and soles may flake or peel.

Once a person has had TSS, he or she is more likely to get it again.

Treatment Options and Outlook

Antibiotic drugs and IV fluids (to prevent shock), plus treatment for any complications as they occur. Recurrence is common; women who have had toxic shock syndrome should not use tampons, cervical caps, diaphragms, or vaginal contraceptive sponges. Death occurs in about 3 percent of cases, usually due to a prolonged drop in blood pressure or lung problems.

Risk Factors and Preventive Measures

A woman can dramatically reduce the risk of TSS by not using tampons. Because the TSS risk increases with tampon absorbency, it is a good idea to use products with the lowest absorbency possible. To help women compare absorbency from brand to brand, the FDA requires that manufacturers use a standard test to measure absorbency and state the findings on the label. The FDA also requires manufacturers to give information about TSS on the box or in a package insert. This information must include a warning about the association between TSS and high-absorbency tampons.

See also STREPTOCOCCUS, GROUP-A; STREPTOCOCCUS, GROUP-B.

Toxocara canis One of two types of ROUNDWORM; this is the variety found in dogs. *T. canis* causes the infestation known as TOXOCARIASIS.

Toxocara cati One of two types of ROUNDWORM; this is the variety found in cats. *T. cati* causes the infestation known as TOXOCARIASIS.

toxocariasis Infection with the larvae of *Toxocara canis* and *T. cati* (the common ROUNDWORM found in dogs and cats). Children between age one and four who eat dirt are at particular risk for this disease. Older children and adults in households with an infected younger child may show evidence of mild infection. The disease is also known as visceral larva migrans.

Ingesting the eggs in soil leads to the spread of tiny larvae throughout the body. In the United States, dogs are often infected with worms that are passed to them as pups before birth, or while they are nursing. Adult worms pass eggs in dogs' feces, which then may find their way into soil or sandboxes. These eggs can remain viable for many weeks—even months. When a child eats soil or sand containing these eggs, the larvae hatch in the child's small intestine, penetrating the intestinal wall and migrating throughout the body. Eventually, the larvae in the child will die.

It is also possible to be infected by eating unwashed vegetables grown in contaminated soil. However, humans cannot pass the infection from one to another.

Symptoms and Diagnostic Path
Most people have no signs of the infestation, and there is a long incubation period. Children who swallow large numbers of worms may experience breathing problems or develop PNEUMONIA, enlarged liver, fever, anemia, fatigue, skin rash, or eye problems. In rare cases, seizures may develop or the child may become blind if larvae enter the eye and die there.

An abnormal blood count with a high number of a certain type of white blood cells and antibodies suggest a diagnosis. Tests for specific antibodies to the worm can be obtained from the CENTERS FOR DISEASE CONTROL AND PREVENTION. The infestation also may be diagnosed by sputum analysis and by a liver biopsy.

Treatment Options and Outlook
There is no specific drug treatment that will cure the infestation. The disease is usually self-limiting even without treatment. In severe cases, the patient should be hospitalized and given the ANTI-HELMINTIC DRUG thiabendazole to control the infestation. Anticonvulsant drugs also may be administered. Steroids have helped some people with heart or nervous system problems.

If the larvae migrate to the liver, lungs, or abdomen, they can cause an enlarged liver, pneumonia, and stomach pain. If they reach a child's eyes, they can damage the retina.

Symptoms of complications include breathing problems, rash, and fever.

Risk Factors and Preventive Measures
Worming pets can help prevent the spread of this disease. All pets at age three weeks should be dewormed, followed by a deworming every two weeks until the pet has had three treatments. They should be checked for worms regularly.

toxoid A bacterial toxin that has been treated with chemicals or with heat to decrease its toxic effect. Inactivation renders the toxin nonpoisonous but preserves its ability to stimulate antibody production by the immune system. Certain toxoids are used to immunize people against specific diseases, such as DIPHTHERIA or TETANUS.

Toxoplasma A genus of crescent-shaped parasites that live within the cells of various tissues and organs of vertebrate animals (especially birds and mammals). They complete their life cycle in the cat. One strain (*T. gondii*) causes TOXOPLASMOSIS.

toxoplasmosis A disease of birds, and mammals (especially cats) that causes a mild illness except in the case of those with impaired immune systems or pregnant women. Cats get the disease by eating infected mice.

More than 60 million people in the United States have been infected with toxoplasmosis by the age of 50; the vast majority of infections produce no symptoms.

The parasite (*Toxoplasma gondii*) is transmitted to humans via undercooked meat, contaminated soil, or by direct contact. In cats, the parasite excretes eggs into the cat's feces, where it then travels to humans and other animals. The eggs of the *T. gondii* migrate to an animals' muscles, where they remain infectious for a long time. Eating undercooked infected beef, mutton, or lamb can transfer the infection. Humans also can get the disease by drinking unpasteurized goat's milk from infected goats, drinking water contaminated with cat feces, or by handling cat feces or infected soil. In humans, the parasite enters the blood and during pregnancy can infect the fetus.

Symptoms and Diagnostic Path

Symptoms are usually mild, characterized by a slight swelling of lymph nodes at various sites in the body together with a low-grade fever, tiredness, sore throat, or slight body rash. The disease is often misdiagnosed as infectious MONONUCLEOSIS. Symptoms usually appear between five and 20 days after exposure. Humans are not infectious to one another. In patients with an impaired immune system, however, the infection can be quite severe, involving multiple organs in the body.

The infection is most serious during pregnancy. While 90 percent of such infected babies are born without disease, 7 percent have minor abnormalities and 3 percent have severe eye or brain damage. The highest risk occurs if the mother is infected during the first six months of pregnancy. Infant abnormalities include eye problems, water on the brain (or microcephaly), low levels of iron in the blood, jaundice, vomiting, fever, convulsions, or mental retardation. In a newborn, the parasite continues to divide, but symptoms may not appear for several years. Postnatal disease may include fever, headache, facial pain, and lymph node swellings. Severe disease includes heart problems (myocarditis), MENINGOENCEPHALITIS, and PNEUMONIA.

Blood tests can reveal the disease; antibodies will remain for life. If a pregnant woman thinks she may have been exposed or her symptoms resemble the disease, blood tests can detect antibodies; some women with an infection during early pregnancy may choose to end the pregnancy. Unfortunately, there is no test that can show whether or not the fetus has been infected.

Tests of newborns can detect those who may have been infected while in the womb; those babies with possible infection can be treated with antibiotics for one year, which can reduce the risk that the baby will have permanent damage. At present, however, this test is not done routinely in all states.

Treatment Options and Outlook

Severe cases are treated with sulfonamides and pyrimethamine. Healthy nonpregnant adults and children do not need treatment.

Pregnant women cannot take pyrimethamine, which can damage the fetus. Pregnant women with suspected or proven toxoplasmosis need counseling to understand the risks and options. No safe and effective drug exists that can be used during pregnancy.

In Europe, the drug spiramycin is used in these cases, where it has proven to decrease (but not eliminate) the risk of infection to the fetus. This drug is not approved for use in the United States and is available here only as an investigational drug requiring special permission to be dispensed.

Complications of infection during pregnancy in the first trimester can include miscarriage, premature birth, and poor growth in the womb. Infants who appear normal at birth may develop eye problems or mental retardation by age 20.

People with impaired immune systems (such as in AIDS) are at risk for complications, including pneumonia, heart infection, and death. These patients often suffer with infection in the brain, especially if dormant organisms that have remained in the muscle for years reactivate. (This does not happen to people with healthy immune systems.)

Risk Factors and Preventive Measures

Pregnant women and those with impaired immune systems should avoid eating raw or undercooked meat. Pregnant women should not touch cat litter or clean cat litter boxes. Cat boxes should be cleaned daily before the feces dry; the eggs are most infectious from dry feces for at least three days. Hands should be washed after handling cats (especially before eating). Cats should be kept indoors, away from infected mice. Stray cats should not be allowed in the house; raw meat should not be fed to cats.

At-risk individuals should not work in gardens accessible to cats.

trachoma   A chronic infectious disease of the eye caused by the bacterium CHLAMYDIA TRACHOMATIS that is fairly rare in the United States today, although it is still found in the southwest in hot, dry climates. The disease is the chief cause of blindness in Third World countries. About 84 million people are infected, causing more than 8 million cases of blindness.

Morocco is expected to be the first country to eliminate trachoma; since 2000, Morocco has reduced its prevalence of active trachoma by 90 percent among children under age 10. Experts hope for global elimination of blinding trachoma by 2020.

Trachoma is one of the earliest-known human diseases, recorded on papyrus in 1500 B.C.E. It was named in 60 C.E. from the Greek word meaning "rough" (a reference to the pustules on the eyelids). The disease spread from the Holy Land during the Crusades, becoming known as Egyptian or "military" ophthalmia.

It is found most often today among children and women who care for them, especially where there is lack of clean water. The organism is spread by direct contact and possibly by flies.

Symptoms and Diagnostic Path

Tearing, inflammation, and eye pain in the presence of light. If untreated, rough thickened scar tissue forms on the upper eyelids, studded with lumps that get bigger until they affect the cornea, eventually causing blindness. Damage to the mucous-secreting cells of the conjunctiva and the tear-producing glands may cause "dry eye." An abnormal growth of blood vessels can reach down into the upper part of the cornea, causing a loss of transparency and loss of vision. More severe damage to the cornea occurs when scarring of the inside upper lid force lashes to rub against the cornea, causing ulcers and secondary bacterial infection.

Treatment Options and Outlook

In the early stages, doctors try to eradicate the organisms causing trachoma, which are sensitive to antibiotics (tetracycline, erythromycin, and topical sulfonamides) given directly into the eye and also by mouth. Established trachoma with scarring is much more difficult to treat. Surgical treatment of the lid deformities and corneal grafts to restore transparency and vision may be needed.

Risk Factors and Preventive Measures

Education and providing water for washing hands, towels, and handkerchiefs are important in eliminating the disease.

traveler's diarrhea   Up to half of all Americans who visit the tropics pick up traveler's diarrhea (also known as "Montezuma's revenge" or *turista*). Areas of high risk include the developing countries of Africa, the Middle East, and Latin America.

The risk of infection varies depending on where the person eats, from low risk (in private homes) to high risk (food from street vendors). Travelers' diarrhea is more common in young adults than in older people and is usually acquired by ingesting food and water contaminated with feces.

Most traveler's diarrhea is caused by a special strain of the common intestinal bacteria ESCHERICHIA COLI. Other bacteria responsible for SALMONELLOSIS and SHIGELLOSIS can also cause diarrhea, as can the parasitic conditions of GIARDIASIS and AMEBIASIS.

Symptoms and Diagnostic Path

Traveler's diarrhea causes diarrhea, nausea, bloating, and malaise that usually lasts from between three to seven days. Even untreated traveler's diarrhea will go away by itself in most cases. Diarrhea that lasts more than four days or is accompanied by severe cramps, bloody stools, or dehydration should be reported to a physician, however.

Treatment Options and Outlook

Patients should drink plenty of fluids to replace water with oral rehydration packets to replace lost minerals. Several prescription and over-the-counter drugs will relieve symptoms or kill bacteria. One of the best treatments for early diarrhea is the antibiotic combination trimethoprim/sulfamethoxazole, which is 90 percent effective against the organisms that cause traveler's diarrhea. Antibiotics can usually shorten the illness and ease the symptoms.

The most widely used antidiarrheal medications are over-the-counter drugs, Pepto-Bismol (bismuth subsalicylate) and Immodium (loperamide). Both treat the symptoms instead of killing the bacteria. Pepto-Bismol should not be used by pregnant women, people subject to seizures, or those taking aspirin or other blood thinners, according to the U.S. Food and Drug Administration (FDA). Immodium can decrease the number of stools, but it can bring complications for those with serious infections. It should not be used by anyone with a high fever or bloody stools.

Risk Factors and Preventive Measures

Since most diarrhea-causing organisms are found in water, they can be passed on in untreated water or on food handled by people who have not properly washed their hands. In order to prevent this type of diarrhea while traveling, travelers should avoid

- drinking tap water or using it to brush teeth (even in good hotels)
- using ice in sodas or alcoholic drinks
- mixing alcohol with water
- drinking milk or dairy products unless they have been pasteurized

Instead, travelers should

- boil water for tooth brushing for five minutes, or add water purification tablets
- avoid bottled water unless it is carbonated (the carbonation process inhibits bacterial growth)
- drink carbonated beverages, bottled beer, wine, coffee, or tea
- wipe off bottle or can tops before drinking
- avoid eating raw vegetables, fruits, meat, or seafood
- avoid cold buffets left in the sun for several hours
- avoid garden or potato salads or food from street vendors
- eat only hot cooked meals, fruit with peels, and packaged foods

Before leaving for a trip, a physician can provide a prescription for antidiarrheal medicine to take along.

Alternatively, Pepto-Bismol appears to be effective in preventing traveler's diarrhea (two ounces four times a day, or two tablets four times a day), but this is not recommended for more than three weeks at a time. Side effects of this preventive treatment include temporary blackening of the tongue and stools, occasional nausea and constipation, and rarely, ringing in the ears. Pepto-Bismol should be avoided by those allergic to aspirin or who have kidney problems or gout. This preventive treatment should be discussed with a doctor before using it with children, adolescents, and pregnant women.

Scientists at West Virginia University have discovered that wine is capable of killing bacteria that cause diarrhea much faster than Pepto-Bismol, tap water, tequila, or pure alcohol. In the case of *Salmonella*, for example, wine destroyed about 10 million bacteria in just 20 minutes; it took the Pepto-Bismol two hours to reach the same effect.

See also DIARRHEA AND INFECTIOUS DISEASE; ANTIDIARRHEAL DRUGS.

trematodes   See FLUKE.

trench mouth   See VINCENT'S DISEASE.

trench fever   See BARTONELLOSIS.

Treponema   A genus of spirochetes, some of which cause diseases in humans including PINTA, SYPHILIS, and YAWS.

Treponema pallidum   An active spirochete that causes SYPHILIS.

Trichinella spiralis   The intestinal ROUNDWORM that causes TRICHINOSIS, which can be ingested when eating uncooked infected meat (usually pork).

trichinellosis See TRICHINOSIS.

trichinosis A food-borne disease caused by the microscopic intestinal ROUNDWORM *Trichinella spiralis*. Anyone who eats undercooked meat of infected animals can develop trichinosis; pork products are most often responsible, although cases have appeared after eating infected bear and walrus.

The parasite may be found in a wide variety of animals, including pigs, dogs, cats, rats, and many wild animals (such as fox, wolf, and polar bear).

Up to 5 percent of Americans have had an infestation, usually without symptoms. It is almost never a problem in countries such as France, where pigs eat root vegetables, not garbage.

Worm larvae exist as cysts in the muscles of infested animals. Within four to six weeks after eating the undercooked or raw meat of an infested animal, the larvae are released from the cysts and develop into adults in the person's intestines. The adult worms produce fresh larvae, which travel in the blood to tissues and organs including the heart, tongue, eye, and brain and to the muscles, where they form cysts. The disease does not spread by person-to-person contact, but infected animals are infectious for months, and the meat from these infected animals remains contaminated unless properly cooked.

Symptoms and Diagnostic Path
The incubation period varies depending on the number of parasites in the meat and how much was eaten. Infestation with only a few worms causes no symptoms, whereas a heavy infestation may cause diarrhea and vomiting, PNEUMONIA, heart failure, or respiratory failure.

Usually within 10 to 14 days after infection, symptoms of fever, muscle aches, pain, and swelling around the eyes will begin. Thirst, profuse sweating, chills, weakness, and tiredness may develop. If the parasite becomes imbedded in the diaphragm (thin muscle separating lungs from abdominal organs), chest pain may result. When the larvae attach to the lining of the intestines, the intestines become inflamed, causing abdominal pain, diarrhea, and weakness. As the larvae begin to increase in length and form cysts in the muscles, muscle soreness and pain in muscle fibers will begin.

Very rarely, a person becomes seriously ill and dies. Those who survive maintain a partial immunity.

A physician may suspect trichinosis from the symptoms; it is confirmed by blood tests that detect antibodies to the larvae or by a muscle biopsy that reveals the larvae themselves.

Treatment Options and Outlook
Painkillers and thiabendazole and corticosteroids may relieve symptoms. Bed rest is recommended to prevent relapse and possible death. After two or three months, the organisms cause no more symptoms. Once the larvae migrate to muscle, mebendazole is the treatment of choice.

Warning signs of complications include breathing problems, swelling, or shortness of breath. Resulting heart failure may be fatal.

Risk Factors and Preventive Measures
The best way to prevent the disease is to ensure meat—especially pork products or wild game—is properly cooked to at least 150°F for 35 minutes per pound. Freezing infected meat no higher than –13°F for 10 days will destroy the parasite. Pork or pork products should never be eaten raw, and even smoked or salted meat may still harbor organisms. Pork should not be ground in the same grinder as other meats; the grinder should then be cleaned well after grinding pork. Hunters should cook walrus, seal, wild boar, and bear meat well before eating.

Routine inspection of carcasses for *Trichinella* organisms is not performed in the United States because the disease is on the decline. Irradiation of pork carcasses also can eradicate the larvae.

Trichomonas vaginalis A protozoan (single-celled microorganism) that causes infection of the vagina (TRICHOMONIASIS).

trichomoniasis A common infection in men and women that is usually sexually transmitted, although it also may be transmitted from an infected washcloth or towel or to a baby during childbirth. The infection may also occur in men, who have an infected urethra, although this does not usually cause symptoms.

A fairly benign condition, trichomoniasis is believed to infect about 7.4 million people each year in the United States. It is the most common sexually transmitted disease in young, sexually active women.

The protozoa *Trichomonas vaginalis* causes trichomoniasis. The parasite is sexually transmitted during intercourse via penis-to-vagina or vulva-to-vulva contact with an infected partner. Women can get the disease from infected men or women, but men usually contract it only from infected women.

Symptoms and Diagnostic Path

The protozoa may exist in the vagina for years without causing symptoms; if symptoms do occur they include painful inflammation and itching of the vagina and vulva, with a profuse, yellow, frothy, foul-smelling discharge. Sex is usually painful.

While men do not usually have symptoms, they may experience urethral discomfort, inflammation of the head of the penis, and signs of urethritis.

Lab examination of vaginal discharge will reveal the disease. Diagnosis is usually difficult in men.

Treatment Options and Outlook

Metronidazole is the treatment of choice; an infected person's partner should be treated at the same time to prevent reinfection.

Partners who are being treated for trichomoniasis should not have sex until they and their partners complete treatment and no longer have symptoms.

Untreated trichomoniasis can cause genital inflammation that may increase a woman's susceptibility to HIV infection if she is exposed to the virus. Having trichomoniasis also may increase the chance that an HIV-infected woman will pass HIV to her sex partner. Pregnant women with trichomoniasis may have babies who are born early or with low birth weight (less than five pounds).

Trichophyton   A genus of fungus that infects skin, hair, and nails.

trichosporosis   A fungal condition in which the hair shafts are coated with hard masses of white (*Trichosporon cutaneum*) or black (*Piedraia hortaei*) fungus. The best treatment is to remove the affected hairs by clipping or shaving.

tropical diseases   Most diseases found in temperate areas are also widespread in the tropics, but many other infectious diseases are largely confined to tropical areas. This is primarily because the people there live in poverty, not because of temperature, humidity, or disease-carrying insects prevalent in this part of the world. War refugees migrating to other areas carry infections with them, and economic and social crises in these areas stress the respective health systems.

Malnutrition is one of the major factors in the development of infectious diseases in the tropics, weakening the body's ability to fight off infections such as DIPHTHERIA or MEASLES. Overcrowding also causes problems, especially in contagious diseases such as TUBERCULOSIS. A vast number of other infectious diseases are due to low standards of public health, food inspection and handling, and lack of sanitary food and water supplies. Diseases associated with contamination by human excrement include TYPHOID FEVER, SHIGELLOSIS, CHOLERA, AMEBIASIS, and TAPEWORM.

Only a few diseases appear to be related to temperature or soil conditions found only in the tropics, such as HOOKWORM or SCHISTOSOMIASIS.

Organisms that cause tropical diseases include bacteria, viruses, and parasites. In temperate climates, many viral and bacterial diseases are spread directly from person to person, either through the air or by sexual contact. In the Tropics, respiratory diseases such as measles, RESPIRATORY SYNCYTIAL VIRUS, tuberculosis, and SEXUALLY TRANSMITTED DISEASES are common, but there are also many other diseases spread by contaminated water and food sources, since clean water and sanitary conditions are often scarce in developing countries. Some tropical disease agents are transmitted by an intermediate carrier—the insect or other carrier picks up the germ from an infected person or animal and transmits it to others.

Viruses are tiny infectious agents that usually consist only of genetic material covered by a protein

---

PREVENTION OF TROPICAL DISEASES

Personal protection is the first line of defense against these diseases. For travelers heading to the tropics, the national Centers for Disease Control and Prevention advises that travelers observe the following guidelines:

At least six weeks before departure, travelers should

- get current health information from the CDC on regions to be visited (other sources may include local health departments, physicians, or travel agencies).

In the Tropics, travelers should

- Avoid rural areas when possible.
- Wear a hat outdoors, long-sleeved shirt tight at the wrists and tucked in at the waist, long pants tight at the ankle and tucked into socks, and shoes covering the entire foot.
- Use a repellent containing permethrin on clothing, (the Environmental Protection Agency recommends applying this repellent to clothing before wearing, letting clothing dry thoroughly first).
- Use a repellent containing DEET (no higher than a 30 percent concentration) on skin. Instructions should be followed carefully; there have been rare cases of toxicity and death with higher concentrations of DEET.
- Use a bed net sprayed with permethrin repellent that is tucked under the mattress if accommodations are not well screened or air conditioned.
- Use a bed net with 18 or more holes per inch for areas with *Leishmania*-infected sand flies.
- Spray screen with permethrin.
- Use aerosol insecticides to clear rooms of insects, and follow instructions carefully.

shell. They can only replicate within cells, which provide the synthetic machinery necessary to produce new virus particles.

Arboviruses (arthropod-borne viruses) are transmitted by mosquitoes, ticks, and flies. DENGUE FEVER, caused by a mosquito-borne flavivirus, is found in tropical and subtropical regions of the Americas, Africa, Asia, and Australia. Infants and children are prone to dengue hemorrhagic fever, a severe and sometimes fatal variation involving circulatory failure and shock. The incidence of both forms of dengue infection has recently been increasing, as expanding populations enlarge the regions inhabited by the AEDES mosquito carrier. Mosquitoes capable of transmitting this disease are also found within the United States. YELLOW FEVER is another arboviral disease limited to tropical South America and Africa, where it is sometimes epidemic in spite of the existence of a safe and effective vaccine. The potential for increased incidence of yellow fever appears to be growing with the expanding distribution of the aedes mosquitoes.

Rotavirus causes watery diarrhea and vomiting in young children, and are found worldwide. They are spread by contact with infected individuals or feces-contaminated objects. Infant mortality is higher in developing countries and is generally associated with severe dehydration.

EBOLA virus causes fever, severe headache, backache, vomiting, diarrhea, and severe hemorrhaging. Experts are not sure how Ebola is transmitted; there have been recent outbreaks in Zaire, Sudan, and Gabon. When humans acquire the infection, it spreads rapidly to those in contact with body fluids from the patient and the death rate is very high. MARBURG VIRUS is related to Ebola, but usually has a somewhat lower death rate.

LASSA FEVER is another often fatal hemorrhagic fever virus that is transmitted by rodents. Symptoms of Lassa fever include sharp backache and/or headache, sore throat, fever, rashes, dehydration, general swelling, skin hemorrhaging, irregular heart beat, and disorientation. Viruses causing several types of South American hemorrhagic fevers belong to the arenavirus family like Lassa, and are also carried by rodents.

Bacterial Diseases

Bacteria are more complex than viruses, and are capable of producing energy and replicating independently. Some bacteria, however, can only reproduce when growing inside a cell, from which they derive required nutrients.

CHOLERA is a diarrheal disease caused by infection with *Vibrio cholerae*, a bacterium most often found in contaminated water and shellfish, which produces a toxin that upsets the biochemical balance of cells lining the intestine and makes them secrete large amounts of water and electrolytes.

Cholera is endemic in a number of tropical countries, and major epidemics break out periodically.

ESCHERICHIA COLI (*E. coli*) bacteria can produce toxins similar to those of cholera, causing illness ranging from mild to persistent diarrhea. An extremely deadly form of these bacteria causes bloody diarrhea and kidney complications that can be lethal in children and the elderly. This form, sometimes known as O157:H7 is often associated with eating undercooked meat, although it has also been found in other foods, including unpasteurized milk and fruit juices. Tuberculosis is caused primarily by the bacterium *Mycobacterium tuberculosis* and is an infection that can last a lifetime, affecting every organ in the body but especially the lungs. Tuberculosis occurs all over the world, and remains a major problem in the developing world, where conditions of poverty, poor nutrition, and crowding contribute to its prevalence. Pulmonary tuberculosis is the most common manifestation worldwide, and is associated with fatigue, weight loss, coughing, and difficulty in breathing. Several drugs are available, but drawbacks include the need for lengthy treatment and increasing development of drug resistance by the bacteria.

Hansen's disease (LEPROSY), is caused by the bacterium *Mycobacterium leprae,* a distant cousin of the agent that causes tuberculosis. While 3.7 million cases are registered, the actual number of cases is at least two to three times higher. The exact mechanism of transmission from person to person remains unknown, but probably involves contact with infected skin or nasal secretions. In its worst form, bacterial growth is uncontrolled, leading to loss of sensation in the affected area which may predispose to trauma and consequent deformity. Presently, no methods for prevention exist, but antibiotics can treat the disease.

Parasites

Parasites include the microscopic protozoa (single-celled organisms more complex than bacteria) and the helminths (worms), which can grow up to three feet in length. Protozoa may live almost anywhere; some types live in red or white blood cells, or in the cells of the muscles, brain, heart, or liver. Other protozoa may live outside cells, in blood, tissues, or mucosal secretions.

Some worms also live within cells, but usually they are found outside cells in the gut, blood, lymph glands, or tissues of the skin and eyes. Many types of parasites undergo complex developmental transformations during their complicated life cycles, unlike bacteria and viruses.

MALARIA affects more than 300 million people each year, killing between 1 and 3 million. Many of these are children living in sub-Saharan Africa. Almost half of the world's population lives in an area where they are at risk of contracting the disease. Each of the four species of malaria parasite causes a different form of the disease, but malaria caused by *Plasmodium falciparum* is the most dangerous form and causes most of the deaths. The malarial parasites are transmitted to humans by mosquitoes; the parasites develop first in liver cells and then infect red blood cells. In 1955, the World Health Organization began an extensive campaign to eradicate malaria, but they have so far been unsuccessful. Parasites also became resistant to chloroquine and other antimalarial drugs. As a result, areas that have been free of malaria have been experiencing outbreaks, and the number of cases have been rising in the Amazon and southeast Asia. In Africa, malaria has been moving from rural areas to the cities.

LEISHMANIASIS is actually a group of diseases caused by infection with about 20 different species of protozoa that are transmitted to humans by female sand flies. Like malaria, leishmaniasis is found in many tropical and subtropical areas of the world, including portions of southern Europe. There are about 12 million infected individuals and another 300 million at risk in 80 countries. Symptoms may range from self-healing skin ulcers to severe life threatening disease. In some individuals, the disease spreads to the mucous membranes of the nose and mouth, resulting in destruction of facial features. The most dangerous form is visceral leishmaniasis, where parasites invade the internal organs.

The protozoa causing TRYPANOSOMIASIS are closely related to leishmania parasites. In the New World form (Chagas disease or American trypanosomiasis, caused by *Trypanosoma cruzi*) affects about 18 million people in Latin America. The trypanosomes responsible for human disease in Africa causes African trypanosomiasis ("sleeping sickness"), which affects 25,000 people per year. These trypanosomes are transmitted to man by the bite of tsetse flies.

SCHISTOSOMIASIS is caused by several species of flatworms that affects about 200 million people, killing about 200,000 of them each year. Many more suffer chronic damage to vital organs including the liver and kidney. This parasite is not transmitted through the bite of an insect, but develops within freshwater snails, leaving the snails and infecting humans in the water. They penetrate the skin, migrating through the blood vessels until reaching the veins of the intestines or bladder. Eggs that are not excreted become lodged in the body's tissues, leading to scarring and interfering with blood circulation and urinary outflow. This can cause death due to rupture of distended blood vessels. FILARIASIS is an infestation of ROUNDWORMS which is not usually life threatening, but it can be debilitating and disfiguring. These roundworms are related to the dog heartworm. Transmitted to man by the bite of infected mosquitoes, filarial worms cause lymphatic filariasis. About 90 million people have the disease, which causes extensive obstruction and damage to the lymphatic system. This leads to a buildup of lymph fluid in arms, legs, and scrotum, which may cause the swelling known as ELEPHANTIASIS.

Two parasitic infections that cause persistent diarrhea in tropical countries are cryptosporidium and CYCLOSPORA. These protozoan parasites are usually acquired by ingesting contaminated water or food. Another water-borne protozoan, giardia, causes diarrheal disease throughout the world.

The protozoan *Entamoeba histolytica* causes severe dysentery and liver disease, and kills up to 100,000 people each year. This parasite is found throughout the world, especially in underdeveloped tropical and subtropical regions. The main source of transmission is people who carry a chronic infection; feces infected with the cyst form of the parasite may contaminate fresh food or water.

Worms

At least one quarter of the world's population is infected with parasitic worms, especially in tropical regions where famine and malnutrition already create health problems. These parasites rob humans of blood and nutrients, affecting the physical and mental development of children. Hookworm infections occur mostly in tropical and subtropical climates, causing mild diarrhea or cramps, but a severe infection can cause profound anemia, slowing growth and mental development. People generally acquire hookworm infection by direct contact with contaminated soil.

Ascaris worms are found in temperate as well as tropical regions and are the most common parasite in the world. While the mortality rate is relatively low (20,000 per year), ascaris infection can be debilitating, causing abdominal pain, weight loss, and sometimes intestinal obstruction.

Other intestinal roundworms are also prevalent in the developing world. Trichuris worms afflict approximately 750 million people, and can cause severe anemia, abdominal pain, nausea, and weight loss. Strongyloides worms infect about 80 million people, causing abdominal pain, nausea, and diarrhea. The tapeworm Taenia solium also causes serious human disease.

trypanosomiasis   A tropical disease caused by protozoa parasites called trypanosomes. In Africa, trypanosomes spread by the TSETSE FLY cause sleeping sickness; other trypanosomes (spread by beetles) cause CHAGAS DISEASE common in South America. Up to 45,000 cases worldwide are reported, but actual numbers are believed to be higher.

African trypanosomiasis is an infection transmitted to man through the bite of the tsetse fly; the protozoa enter the skin through the saliva of the insect.

Symptoms and Diagnostic Path

Symptoms of Rhodesian trypanosomiasis begin two weeks after the bite of the fly, with an inflammation of the skin at the bite site. Fever develops followed by skin rashes; scattered areas of puffy, painful skin; enlarged and painful lymph nodes; and anemia. Later, the person becomes depressed, with tremors, lack of appetite, disturbed speech, and fatigue. The fatigue becomes more pronounced until the person spends almost all his time sleeping; death eventually occurs.

Gambian trypanosomiasis starts six months to several years after the bite of the fly and develops very slowly.

Treatment Options and Outlook

If untreated, most cases are fatal; drugs to treat the disease are very toxic and must be used with great caution. However, if treatment is begun early, the prognosis is good. If not treated soon enough, irreversible brain damage or death is common.

Risk Factors and Preventive Measures

It is important to take precautions against the tsetse fly. Some drugs are available for use in preventing the infection, but these are potentially toxic and should be used only for people at high risk.

tsetse flies Any of several bloodsucking African flies of the genus Glossina, and in the same family as the housefly, that uses its proboscis to inflict a painful bite. Tsetse flies spread the parasitic disease known as SLEEPING SICKNESS (TRYPANOSOMIASIS). A number of the 21 species can transmit the trypanosomes that cause the Gambian and Rhodesian forms of African sleeping sickness. Clearing the brush that the flies inhabit helps to get rid of them; DDT has also been used to exterminate them.

TSS See TOXIC SHOCK SYNDROME.

tsutsugamushi disease Another name for scrub typhus.
See also TYPHUS, SCRUB.

tuberculin test A skin test (tine test) used to determine whether or not a person has been infected with tuberculosis; the test is used to diagnose suspected cases of TUBERCULOSIS and prior to vaccination against the disease.

During the test, the skin is first disinfected and a small dose of tuberculin (a protein extract of the tuberculosis bacilli) is introduced into the skin. The preferred method is the Mantoux test, where the extract is injected between skin layers with a needle.

After a few days, the skin is inspected at the site; if the skin is unchanged, the reaction is negative, indicating the person has never been exposed to tuberculosis and has no immunity. Skin that becomes hard and raised after the injection indicates that the person has been exposed to tuberculosis, either through vaccination or infection.

tuberculosis, skin This condition is caused by direct inoculation of MYCOBACTERIUM TUBERCULOSIS into a wound in people not previously exposed. It is rare in developed countries.

Symptoms and Diagnostic Path

In the localized form of the disease, an inflammatory nodule called the tuberculous chancre is accompanied by inflammation of the lymph nodes and vessels. In immune (or partly immune) patients skin lesions are characterized by patchy lesions with small yellowish nodules on the face. In scrofuloderma, tuberculosis of lymph nodes or bone spreads to the skin, causing ulcers and fistulas underneath ridges of blue skin.

In the disseminated form of the disease, bacteria cause "miliary tuberculosis" in the skin, causing necrotic papules on the face and extremities, with a small dead core that forms chicken pox-like scars.

Treatment Options and Outlook

Administration of standard antituberculosis drugs for six to 12 months is effective.
See also TUBERCULIN TEST.

tuberculosis (TB) A respiratory disease spread from person to person through the air (once known as "consumption," "scrofula," "phthisis," or "wasting"), infecting half the world's population. TB usually affects the lungs, although it can also target other parts of the body, such as the brain, kidneys, or spine. It was once the leading cause of death in the United States. While developed countries such as the United States have had declining numbers of TB cases since the 1990s, 23 countries account for 80 percent of all new TB cases, with more than half concentrated in Bangladesh, China, India, Indonesia, and Nigeria. Most new cases in the United States, and probably a substantial proportion of new cases in other developed countries, occur among individuals born in other countries. Today, it causes more deaths worldwide than any other infectious disease.

People with TB infection but not the disease have the bacteria that cause the infection within their bodies, but the germs are inactive. They cannot spread the bacteria to others, but they may develop TB later on. Because of this, they are often treated to prevent them from developing the disease.

In 1993 the World Health Organization (WHO) declared a "global TB emergency" because of the massive TB epidemic that is spreading around the world. The WHO concluded that worldwide, the disease is the leading killer of women and HIV-positive patients. Among those with hiv, one in 10 per year will develop active TB.

TB kills more adults than all other infectious diseases combined and leaves more orphaned children than any other infectious disease. TB kills more people than AIDS, MALARIA, and TROPICAL DISEASES combined.

About 8 million new cases of TB occur each year; the number of cases reported in the United States increased each year from 1985 to 1992, but the numbers have steadily declined since then with increased vigilance and funding. In the United States, TB has reemerged as a serious public health problem. In 2003, 14,000 active TB cases were reported to the CENTERS FOR DISEASE CONTROL AND PREVENTION (CDC).

Of most concern is that cases of TB resistant to more than one drug have been reported in 17 states in the United States since 1989. More than 50 million people around the world may already be infected with multidrug-resistant TB (MDR-TB). From 1993 to 1997, 43 states reported cases of multidrug-resistant TB. In addition, CDC received numerous reports of outbreaks of MDR-TB in hospitals and prisons. During these outbreaks, MDR-TB has sometimes spread to hospital patients, health care workers, prisoners, and prison guards. Because of this, it is essential to treat TB patients with a recommended four-drug regimen of isoniazid, rifampin, pyrazinamide, and ethambutol or streptomycin, since it is less likely that bacteria can become quickly resistant to multiple drugs at the same time.

Tuberculosis has been the scourge of the world since the dawn of time—evidence of the TB bacteria has been found in neolithic skeletons from 4500 B.C.E. and was described in the Hammurabi Code, circa 2000 B.C.E. Hippocrates described "consump-

tion" (or *phthisis,* in Greek) as the most widespread disease of his time, noting that it was almost always fatal and warning other doctors that if they visited patients in the last stages of the disease, the inevitable deaths might ruin their reputations.

Historians think that TB evolved in the Middle East some 8,000 years ago, from cattle to humans, and could have entered the Americas by human migration from Asia across the Bering Sea.

By the 17th century, doctors were closing in on this dread disease. Sylvius identified actual tubercles in his 1679 *Opera Medica,* noting the consistent change in the lungs of consumptive patients and the inevitable progression to lung ABSCESS. Other 17th-century physicians described the infectious nature of the disease; the Republic of Lucca in Italy required disinfection be carried out after the death of a consumptive.

Up until the 18th century, English citizens thought that the "king's evil" could be cured by the King's touch. But it became a serious problem in England during the Industrial Revolution, when it killed one out of every five London natives. The astonishing idea that TB could be caused by "minute living creatures" was discovered by the 18th-century English physician Benjamin Marten, who decided that it was possible to catch the disease by sharing the same bed, eating utensils, or breathing the same air. However, he wrote in his publication *A New Theory of Consumption* that he did not think simply talking to a person with consumption on a casual basis was enough to transmit the disease.

Not until scientists introduced the idea of putting patients in a sanatorium was there much of a breakthrough in the treatment of TB. Botany student Hermann Brehmer went to the Himalayas to pursue his botany studies while trying to cure his disease; when he did actually succeed in curing himself, he returned home to study medicine in 1854. He built an institution in Gorbersdorf, where patients could breathe clean air and eat healthy food; his hospital became the touchstone for future sanatoriums. The sanatoriums also were a means of isolating the sick from the healthy.

By 1865, French physician Jean-Antoine Villemin discovered that TB could be passed from humans to cattle and on to rabbits, which proved there was a specific microorganism; 20 years later, the great German bacteriologist Robert Koch developed a staining technique that allowed him to actually see and identify the *Mycobacterium tuberculosis.* The word *tubercule* means "a small nodule or growth." But it was not until World War II that drugs that could cure the disease were developed.

Actually, sulfonamide and PENICILLINS were not very effective against TB; in 1940, scientists isolated an effective anti-TB antibiotic—actinomycin—but it was too toxic for humans or animals. Three years later, scientists discovered that streptomycin could control the disease without causing serious side effects. On November 20, 1944, the antibiotic was administered for the first time to a critically ill patient. Almost at once, the disease was stopped, the bacteria disappeared, and the patient rapidly recovered. While the new drug had side effects (especially in the inner ear) it was the first drug that really had an effect on TB.

Over the following years, scientists continued to develop better anti-TB drugs, important, because within a few months TB germs resistant to streptomycin began to appear.

TB is caused by three species of mycobacteria: *Mycobacterium tuberculosis, M. bovis,* and *M. africanum.* When a person breathes in the bacteria, they can settle in the lungs and grow; from here, they can travel through the blood to other parts of the body (such as the kidney, spine, or brain). TB in the lungs or throat is mildly infectious, but the bacteria in other parts of the body are not usually contagious.

TB bacteria are sprayed into the air when a person with the disease of the lungs or throat coughs or sneezes. When another person inhales air that contains TB germs, the person may become infected. People with active TB are most likely to spread it to those they spend time with every day (such as family members or coworkers). The degree of contagiousness is directly related to the number of bacilli expelled into the air. Patients are more likely to be infectious if they have TB in the lungs or larynx, have a cavity in the lung, and cough a lot. Contagion potential is also related to patient behavior, such as failing to cover the mouth when coughing.

Although TB is infectious, it is not highly infectious and is not nearly as contagious as MEASLES or WHOOPING COUGH. Letting fresh air blow through a room will eradicate most of the infectious germs exhaled by a sick patient every day. The bacteria are also sensitive to ultraviolet rays, which means that infection rarely occurs outside in daylight. Indeed, only half of the people who live with an infected patient will contract the disease themselves.

People with TB are most likely to transmit the disease before it has been diagnosed and treated, and at least 12 weeks must pass before a person who has been exposed to the disease will test positive. The infectious state seems to decrease quickly once treatment begins; those who have been treated for two to three weeks, whose symptoms have improved, and who have three consecutive negative sputum tests can be considered non-infectious.

Most people who breathe in the bacteria and become infected are able to fight off the disease; the bacteria become inactive, but they remain alive in the body and can become active later. This is called TB *infection.* People with TB infection have no symptoms, do not feel sick, and cannot spread the disease. However, they usually have a positive skin test for TB, and they can develop the disease later in life if they do not receive preventive treatment. Many people who have the infection never develop the disease, however. In these people, the bacteria remain inactive for a lifetime.

Scientists have recently discovered how TB microbes manage to remain dormant in the lungs for so long before developing into active disease. It appears that TB bacteria contain a gene that regulates dormancy. When the bacterium is under stress (as it is in the lungs), the gene becomes dormant in order to protect itself. If this is true, scientists could then manipulate the bacterium so as to trigger a dormant state in drug-resistant microbes.

Because infants and young children do not have very strong immune systems, they are susceptible to TB, as are those with impaired immune systems. This includes patients with HIV infection; substance abusers; diabetics; those with cancer of head and neck, leukemia, severe kidney disease, or low body weight; and people undergoing medical therapies such as corticosteroid treatment or organ transplant.

Symptoms and Diagnostic Path

The illness does not cause symptoms at first. TB growing in the lungs may cause chest pain or a bad cough that lasts longer than two weeks. The patient may cough up blood or phlegm from the lungs. Other symptoms include fatigue or weakness, weight loss, appetite loss, chills, and fever.

The disease is diagnosed with a tuberculin skin test to determine if a person has the TB organism. It cannot separate those who have active disease from those who do not. For this skin test, a small amount of fluid (tuberculin) is injected within the skin in the lower part of the arm. Two or three days later a health care worker looks for a reaction on the arm.

A positive reaction usually means that the person has been infected with the TB germ, but not necessarily that they have an active infection. Other tests (chest X-ray and sample of phlegm) are necessary to identify active disease.

People should be tested for TB if they have spent time with someone with infectious TB, have HIV, come from a country where TB is common (most countries in Latin America, the Caribbean, Africa, and Asia except for Japan). Others at high risk are those who inject drugs or who live in places in the United States where TB is common (homeless shelters, migrant farm camps, prisons, and some nursing homes) or who are health-care workers.

Because it may take several weeks after infection for the immune system to react to the TB skin test, it may be necessary to be retested 10 to 12 weeks after the last exposure to TB. If the reaction to the second test is negative, there is probably no TB infection present.

The skin test is mandatory in some states and countries for immigrants and students from Africa, Asia, and Latin America, as well as for personnel in schools, hospitals, prisons, food handlers, group homes, child-care centers, and substance abuse centers. Skin tests are also recommended for elderly people. At the moment, screening of children entering kindergarten or day care centers is not required in all school districts, but the CENTERS FOR DISEASE CONTROL AND PREVENTION (CDC) recommends that schoolchildren be tested for TB to ensure that all U.S. citizens are tested at least once in their lives.

A new test can now identify the TB organism much more quickly than in the past. The new test uses nucleic acid amplification to speed the diagnosis of TB from four weeks to two days. Another test in development uses luminescent chemicals from the firefly that can determine, within 24 to 48 hours, which drugs can kill the TB strain a patient carries.

Treatment Options and Outlook

Up to the 1700s it was thought that the touch of a king or queen would cure TB; today, scientists know that TB is cured by taking several drugs for up to nine months long. If patients stop taking the drugs too soon, or if they do not take the drugs correctly, the TB organisms may become resistant. TB that is resistant to drugs is harder to treat.

Patients who have signs of TB should be isolated and tested promptly. After the development of streptomycin, other drugs became available: isoniazid (1952), pyrazinamide (1954), cycloserine (1955), ethambutol (1962), and rifampin (rifampicin 1963). Aminoglycosides (capreomycin, viomycin, kanamycin, and amikacin) and the newer quinolones (ofloxacin and ciprofloxacin) are used in drug-resistant situations. Treatment for 18 months to two years may be necessary, and patients should be given at least three drugs to which the germ is susceptible.

Within a month after treatment begins, the patient should feel well, regain weight, and have no fever. Coughing should have slowed down, and there should be improvements on X-rays. If the disease is severe, however, complete end of treatment may not occur for a year.

If there is no improvement within three months, a change in therapy may be needed. Relapses usually occur within six months after treatment ends and are usually due to patients who do not follow correct drug procedures.

When TB becomes active again in a patient who had been treated before, there is a very good chance that these bacteria will be drug resistant. If the microorganism is resistant to standard drugs, it may be necessary to use more toxic drugs, such as ethionamide, protionamide, pyrazinamide, cycloserine, capreomycin, or viomycin.

Death rates for untreated TB is between 40 and 60 percent. With treatment patients with non-drug resistant TB can be cured more than 90 percent of the time.

Risk Factors and Preventive Measures

Some people who have the TB germ but not active disease are more likely than others to develop an active case. These high-risk individuals include those with HIV infection, those who were recently exposed to someone with TB disease and those with certain medical conditions.

For patients who have TB germs but not the active disease, the Centers for Disease Control recommend taking isoniazid for up to 12 months. Isoniazid may cause liver problems in certain people (especially the elderly and those with liver disease), so patients taking this drug are carefully monitored.

Some people are given preventive therapy if their skin test is negative; this is often done with infants, children, and HIV-infected people who have recently spent time with someone with infectious disease.

Side effects to isoniazid include appetite loss, nausea and vomiting, yellow skin or eyes, fever for more than three days, stomach pain, and tingling in fingers and toes. *Drinking alcoholic beverages while taking isoniazid is dangerous.*

There is a vaccine for TB disease that is used in many countries outside the United States. This vaccine does not completely prevent people from getting TB.

While there is some question as to how effective the BCG vaccine really is against adults, the World Health Organization recommends its use in newborns in developing countries, because it appears to offer some protection in children.

A new TB vaccine from "naked" DNA might work better with less risk of infection than the current BCG vaccine. The traditional BCG vaccine is made from an altered, weakened form of the disease that infects cows. But researchers in 1996 reported that they had made a new vaccine out of a gene taken from the human version of TB. The use of one gene (known as "naked DNA") instead of the many genes contained in TB DNA, appears to be as effective as the earlier cow vaccine. However, trials in humans are still a long way off.

Unlike traditional vaccines, which stimulate the human body to produce disease-fighting antibodies, naked DNA vaccines are incorporated by the cells and the immune response begins there. There is also a lower risk of infection with this new vaccine. While this did not occur often with the old vaccine, it did happen in certain rare cases.

It is also possible to transmit TB on an airplane. In the spring of 1994, a woman on an 8 1/2-hour

United Airlines flight from Chicago to Honolulu infected four passengers sitting near her; all tested positive for the disease, but none have yet become ill. A few days later, the woman died from TB. Because this showed transmission is possible on airlines, the CDC recommended that when airlines learn that a passenger or crew member has traveled with the disease (especially on long flights) they should contact passengers and crew members and inform them. The CDC pointed out that only those passengers sitting near the woman were infected; others sitting farther away breathed air that passed through the plane's filtration system.

Health-care workers who treat TB patients should wear a HEPA filter respirator, collect specimens in a well-ventilated area (if possible, outdoors), and participate in a TB screening and prevention program.

tularemia An infectious disease of wild animals occasionally transmitted to humans, characterized by a red spot at the skin site of infection, eventually forming an ulcer.

Hunters or others who spend a great deal of time outdoors are at greater risk for exposure, since humans may contract the disease through tick bites or by direct contact with an infected animal (such as rabbits, squirrels, or muskrats).

The disease is found only in North America, some parts of Europe, and Asia. There are about 300 cases a year in the United States, primarily in Arkansas, Missouri, and Oklahoma. Eleven people in Oklahoma got sick and two died during a tularemia outbreak in 2000, after being exposed to ticks or dead rabbits. In 2001, scientists traced an outbreak in Martha's Vineyard that sickened 11 and killed one.

The bacteria *Francisella (Pasteurella) tularensis* enters the body through a cut or scratch in the skin, or a bite from a tick, flea, fly, louse, or (rarely) by eating infected rabbit meat. Less common means of spreading tularemia include drinking contaminated water, inhaling dust from contaminated soil, or handling contaminated pelts or paws of animals.

The fact that *Francisella* can spread so readily makes it a possible weapon for bioterrorism, according to some experts, who estimate that a terrorist bomb containing *Francisella* exploded in a city could make tens of thousands of people seriously ill. A widespread infection would make a lot of people very sick for a long time. During the cold war, both the United States and the former USSR stockpiled highly infectious strains of *Francisella*.

Symptoms and Diagnostic Path

Between two and 10 days after contact, symptoms suddenly appear. In addition to the skin lesion, symptoms include enlarged lymph nodes, high fever, swollen glands, throat infection, diarrhea, vomiting, and large, red, skin ulcers, headache. Sometimes the eyes and lungs are affected.

Treatment Options and Outlook

Antibiotics (such as streptomycin or tetracycline) treat the disease with a less than 1 percent fatality rate; untreated, it can be fatal in 5 percent of cases. The disease confers immunity, although occasional reinfection has been reported.

Risk Factors and Preventive Measures

A vaccine is available for those at high risk, such as hunters, trappers, game wardens, or lab workers. Rubber gloves should be worn when skinning or handling animals (especially rabbits). Wild rabbit and rodent meat should be cooked thoroughly before eating.

tumbu fly bites   These fly bites cause myiasis (skin infestation with fly larvae) in South Africa.

See MYIASIS, CUTANEOUS.

tungiasis   A skin infection caused by a burrowing flea found in Africa, the West Indies, and South America.

The female flea burrows under the skin, sucks the victim's blood, swells, and then ejects her eggs.

Symptoms and Diagnostic Path

A localized skin rash appears with lesions containing the live fleas after infestation.

Treatment Options and Outlook

Ethyl chloride spray will kill the fleas when applied to the lesion where they are located. To remove live fleas, tweezers should be used after applying alco-hol. Corticosteroid and antibiotic creams are effective. Exercise or excess warmth should be avoided. Complications may be fatal, and include skin ulcers, GANGRENE, and blood poisoning (SEPTICEMIA).

Risk Factors and Preventive Measures

Avoid contaminated areas and disinfect clothing, bedclothes, and furniture if necessary.

typhoid fever   A serious bacterial infection of the intestinal tract and sometimes the bloodstream, also known as enteric fever. It is caused by eating food or drinking water contaminated with *Salmonella typhi*. An almost-identical disease called PARA-TYPHOID FEVER is caused by a related bacterium.

Typhoid fever today is an uncommon disease in the United States. In 1942 there were 4,000 reported cases, but since 1964 fewer than 400 cases have occurred each year, mostly imported from Mexico or India. Typhoid fever is common in most parts of the world except in industrialized regions such as the United States, Canada, western Europe, Australia, and Japan. Visitors to the developing world should consider taking precautions, especially when visiting Asia, Africa, and Latin America.

An estimated 16 million cases of typhoid fever and 600,000 related deaths occur worldwide.

Before the advent of antibiotics, 12 percent of patients died. Today, fewer than 10 percent of cases are fatal; deaths most often occur in malnourished people, infants, and the elderly.

About 3 percent of those who recover from a mild illness become chronic carriers. There are about 2,000 of these carriers in the United States, almost all of them elderly women with gallbladder disease. Carriers are infectious for years unless the gallbladder is removed or they are treated with antibiotics.

Thomas Willis first described typhoid fever in 1643; typhoid fever was often confused with "typhus" fever until the two were distinguished in 1837, and the name *typhoid* fever—meaning "typhus-like" was coined.

The most famous typhoid patient of all was Typhoid Mary, a cook in New York City who was the first known typhoid carrier in the United States. Although she was healthy, she was infected with typhoid bacteria, which she shed in feces. Her improper hand washing allowed the bacteria to contaminate the food she prepared for others. Between 1900 and 1915, she passed the disease to at least 53 people, three of whom died. Because she refused to stop working as a cook, she was forcibly confined to a hospital by public health authorities. She lived in that hospital for more than 20 years, until she died.

Typhoid fever is caused by the bacterium *Salmonella typhi,* a species of SALMONELLA. While the common *Salmonella* species in the United States live in animals and infect humans via contaminated food (chicken, eggs, etc.), *S. typhi* lives in the intestinal tract of humans. Once ingested, the bacteria lodge in the lower small intestine, where they multiply and invade the bloodstream.

The disease is transmitted via food or water that has been contaminated by the feces of patients or carriers, or from intimate contact with an infected person. It occurs in developing countries by eating shellfish taken from contaminated beds, eating raw fruits, or drinking tainted water supplies. It can also be contracted from food left outdoors accessible to flies. Anyone can get typhoid fever, but the greatest risk is to travelers visiting countries where the disease is common.

People are infectious as long as the bacteria are being shed in feces (usually three to four weeks), but some may remain infectious up to three months. To be considered a noncarrier, a patient must have stool cultures every week until there are three negative cultures in a row.

The most important modern source of the typhoid bacillus (found throughout the world) is the typhoid carrier; these carriers at times contaminate water, milk, or food and set off typhoid epidemics.

Symptoms and Diagnostic Path

Between eight and 14 days after ingesting bacteria, symptoms of fever, headache, joint pains, sore throat, and constipation begin. There may be appetite loss and abdominal pain. Most people have a mild illness and recover without antibiotics. Untreated, the fever will continue to rise for two or three days, remain high for up to two weeks (103 to 104°F) and then fall. Nosebleed and bronchitis are often present. At the height of the fever, the patient appears extremely ill and can be delirious.

Relapses occur in 10 percent of untreated patients, and 20 percent of treated patients about two weeks after the fever abates. If the fever returns, antibiotics must be restarted. Some patients notice rose spots on chest and abdomen during the second week.

Infection confers some immunity, but not enough to protect a patient if there are large numbers of bacteria ingested a second time.

The diagnosis is confirmed by obtaining a culture of typhoid bacteria from a sample of blood during the first week; feces and urine tests reveal the bacillus during the second.

Treatment Options and Outlook

Antibiotics can shorten the disease and reduce chances of complications and death. Otherwise, it can take months to recover. Doctors may prescribe chloramphenicol, ciprofloxacin, ceftriaxone, or cefoperazone. In addition, patients need bed rest and good nutrition. Aspirin, enemas, or laxatives should not be given.

Gloves should be worn when nursing a typhoid patient, and rigorous hand washing is critical. Because the germ is passed in the feces of infected patients, only those with active diarrhea who cannot toilet themselves (infants and some handicapped people) should be isolated.

With early diagnosis and proper treatment, the outlook is usually excellent. Permanent immunity usually follows an attack of typhoid, although relapses are common if the disease is not fully eradicated by thorough antibiotic treatment.

Patients with serious cases can go on to experience frothy, bloody diarrhea in later stages and become apathetic. It can inflame the intestines and in severe cases, intestinal ulcers can perforate, causing severe infections. This can also lead to severe intestinal bleeding, which kill 25 percent of untreated victims.

Risk Factors and Preventive Measures

Typhoid fever is a reportable disease. Typhoid vaccination is not required for international travel, but it is recommended for travel to high-risk areas, including the Indian subcontinent and other developing countries in Asia, Africa, and Central and South America. Vaccination is particularly recommended for those who will be traveling in smaller cities, villages, and rural areas. However, typhoid vaccination is not completely effective and is not a substitute for careful selection of food and drink.

Two typhoid vaccines are currently available for use in the United States—an oral, live-attenuated vaccine (Vivotif Berna vaccine), and a capsular polysaccharide vaccine for injection (Typhim Vi). Both vaccines have been shown to protect 50 percent to 80 percent of recipients.

The time required for primary vaccination differs for each of the two vaccines, and each has a different lower age limit for use among children. Primary vaccination with the oral vaccine consists of a total of four capsules, one taken every other day. The capsules should be kept refrigerated (not frozen), and all four doses must be taken to achieve maximum efficacy. Each capsule should be taken with cool liquid no warmer than 98.6°F, about one hour before a meal. The vaccine manufacturer recommends that Ty21a not be administered to infants or children younger than six years of age, or to immunocompromised travelers, including those infected with human immunodeficiency virus (HIV).

Primary vaccination with the injectable vaccine is given in one dose administered intramuscularly. The manufacturer does not recommend the vaccine for infants younger than two years of age. The injectable vaccine presents theoretically safer alternatives for people with compromised immune systems. The only contraindication to this vaccine is a history of severe local or systemic reactions following a previous dose.

Neither of the available vaccines should be given to travelers with a fever.

Further preventive measures for travelers include drinking only pasteurized milk products, boiled or bottled water or carbonated beverages, eating only cooked food or fruit that is peeled by the diner, eating shellfish boiled or steamed at least 10 minutes, and controlling flies with screens and sprays.

Most infected people may return to work or school when they have recovered, as long as they wash their hands after toilet visits. Children in day care must obtain the approval of the local or state health department before returning to school. Food handlers may not return to work until three consecutive negative stool cultures are confirmed.

See also DIARRHEA AND INFECTIOUS DISEASE.

typhus Any of a group of infectious diseases with similar symptoms, caused by rickettsiae (microorganisms similar to bacteria) that are spread by insects.

In the past, epidemic typhus was the most significant type of this disease, which was spread by body lice. EPIDEMICS of this type of typhus swept across the country, killing hundreds of thousands of people during war, famine, and natural disaster. It is rare today, except in some areas of Africa and South America.

Typhus is caused by rickettsiae; in epidemic typhus, they are ingested by lice from the blood of infected patients. The lice deposit feces containing the rickettsiae on other people's skin; when the person scratches the skin, the microorganisms enter the bloodstream.

Endemic (or murine) typhus is found in rats; about 50 cases occur in the United States each year, spread to humans through the bite of fleas. Scrub typhus is spread by mites in India and Southeast Asia. ROCKY MOUNTAIN SPOTTED FEVER is another disease similar to typhus.

Symptoms and Diagnostic Path

Epidemic typhus is characterized by a measles-like rash, severe headache, back and limb pain, high fever, confusion, prostration, weak heartbeat, and delirium. Untreated, the patient may die from blood poisoning, heart or kidney failure, or pneumonia. Other types of typhus have similar symptoms and complications.

Particular types of typhus are diagnosed by tests that detect certain blood products produced in reaction to the rickettsial organisms.

Treatment Options and Outlook

Antibiotic drugs treat typhus fever; other treatment is aimed at relieving the rest of symptoms. It may take a long time to recover from the disease, especially among the elderly.

Risk Factors and Preventive Measures

Epidemic typhus may be prevented by vaccination and control of infestations via insecticides. Other types of typhus may be prevented by wearing protective clothes to prevent tick, mite, and flea bites.

See also RICKETTSIAL INFECTIONS.

typhus, endemic flea-borne   A mild type of TYPHUS that is less severe than louse-borne typhus and occurs around the world, usually in places where people and mice live in the same buildings. It is found in the United States along the southern Atlantic and Gulf coasts.

Endemic flea typhus is transmitted to humans through the bite of an infected rat flea (*Xenopsylla cheopis* in the order Siphonaptera), which leaves feces while sucking blood. It is also possible to inhale infected flea feces.

Symptoms and Diagnostic Path

Between one and two weeks after a flea bite, symptoms of fever and rash on the trunk appear, lasting up to about two weeks.

Treatment Options and Outlook

Antibiotics treat this disease, which is rarely fatal.

Risk Factors and Preventive Measures

The disease can be prevented by controlling rats and the fleas they carry.

See also TYPHUS, EPIDEMIC LOUSE-BORNE.

typhus, epidemic louse-borne   An infectious form of TYPHUS caused by a parasite of the body louse (*Pediculus humanus*), found in mountainous regions of Mexico, Central and South America, the Balkans and eastern Europe, Africa, and many parts of Asia.

The more crowded the conditions, the more likely the disease will be transmitted from person to person because of a heavy infestation with lice. When a louse sucks the blood of someone infected with the parasite, the parasite enters the louse and grows. When the infected louse then bites another person, the infected louse feces is rubbed into a wound or the eye of the human host.

Symptoms and Diagnostic Path

Within 10 to 14 days after infection, symptoms appear suddenly, including headache, aches, pains, and chills. A fever follows these signs, and a rash appears over the body except for the face, palms of the hands, and feet. The flu-like symptoms can worsen into delirium and stupor that can lead to coma and death if untreated.

Treatment Options and Outlook

Drug therapy can effectively cure typhus. The fever can be reduced with tepid baths or cool temperatures. Isolation is required until all lice have been removed from the patient.

Risk Factors and Preventive Measures

Anyone who has had contact with the patient must be quarantined for 15 days. Immunization, louse control, and good personal hygiene are effective ways of protecting against typhus. No typhus cases are known to have occurred in an American traveler since 1950, and no typhus vaccine is available in the United States. The risk to a U.S. traveler of contracting typhus is very small.

See also TYPHUS, SCRUB; TYPHUS, ENDEMIC FLEA-BORNE.

typhus, scrub   A mite-borne disease also known as tsutsugamushi disease, tropical TYPHUS, or mite-borne typhus, found in southeast Asia, the western Pacific, and Australia. It is most often found in scrubby land, forest clearings, or other mite-infested areas.

The infected parasites of rodents are transmitted by mites that spend most of their life on vegetation, where they can bite humans and transmit the infection.

Symptoms and Diagnostic Path

One to three weeks after the mite bite, the patient feels tired and chilled, with a severe headache and backache. At the mite-bite site, a small swelling is followed by blisters and then by a black flat scab. Fever gradually rises over one week, followed by a rash over the trunk. If untreated, other symptoms including heart problems and delirium may follow, and the disease may be fatal.

Treatment Options and Outlook

With appropriate treatment, recovery is quick and complete.

Risk Factors and Preventive Measures

Avoiding mites or applying a miticide in outdoor and indoor living areas can prevent the disease. Insect repellent on clothing and skin can provide some protection.

U

ulcers and infectious disease See *HELICOBACTER PYLORI.*

universal blood and bodily fluids precautions See UNIVERSAL PRECAUTIONS.

universal precautions An approach to hospital infection control designed to prevent transmission of blood-borne infections such as AIDS and HEPATITIS B in health care settings.

The precautions were first developed in 1987 by the U.S. CENTERS FOR DISEASE CONTROL AND PREVENTION. The guidelines include specific recommendations for use of gloves and masks and protective eyewear when there is the risk of contact with blood or body secretions containing infected blood.

See also HOSPITAL-ACQUIRED INFECTIONS.

upper respiratory infections See RESPIRATORY TRACT INFECTIONS.

urethritis Inflammation of the urethra usually caused by one of a variety of infectious organisms, the best known of which is the bacterium that causes GONORRHEA.

Nonspecific urethritis may be caused by one of a number of different types of microorganisms, including BACTERIA, YEASTS, or CHLAMYDIAL INFECTIONS. Bacteria may spread to the urethra from the skin or rectum.

Symptoms and Diagnostic Path
A burning sensation and pain when urinating that can be severe. The urine may be stained with blood; if gonorrhea is the underlying cause, there may be a yellow pus-filled discharge. The infection may be followed by scarring that narrows the urethra, which can make urinating more difficult.

Treatment Options and Outlook
Treating the underlying infection will cure the urethritis. Gonorrhea is usually cured by PENICILLIN or other antibiotic. Treatment of nonspecific urethritis depends on what organism is causing the infection. If the urethra is scarred (urethral stricture), a physician may try to stretch and widen the tube under anesthesia.

urinary tract infection (UTI) This condition, also known as a bladder infection, is the most common bacterial infection in adult women and the most common medical problem of pregnancy, resulting in 8.3 million doctor visits each year. Most of the time, the problem is caused by fecal bacteria in the bladder, usually *ESCHERICHIA COLI. Gardnerella* (which causes VAGINITIS in women) also may infect the urinary tract.

Women most likely to get UTIs are older or who are sexually active. A woman with a UTI is not infectious to others. UTIs in men are uncommon and may indicate that there is an abnormality in the urinary tract.

The bacteria that cause UTI usually originate in the rectum or vagina, and then move up into the bladder. Because the urethra in women is so close to other body openings, bacteria can more easily contaminate the urinary tract. This happens most often during sexual intercourse; one study found that 75 percent of women with UTIs reported having sex within 24 hours before the start of the infection. The bacteria do not come from a woman's partner, however, but originate within the woman's own body.

UTIs are 14 times more likely to occur in women because of their shorter urethra, their failure to empty their bladders as fully as men, and because the opening of the urethra in women is always contaminated by germs from the vagina and anus.

While most women have a natural defense mechanism in the walls of the bladder that interferes with bacterial growth, some women appear to lack this mechanism. In addition, as women age and their estrogen levels fall, they are more prone to thinning of mucous membranes and more frequent UTIs. UTIs in men are often caused by an obstruction, such as a urinary stone or an enlarged prostate, or as the result of having a catheter.

Symptoms and Diagnostic Path

Burning and pain during urination plus the frequent urge to urinate even when the bladder is empty. It is also possible to have a UTI with no symptoms. Untreated, a UTI could lead to a serious kidney infection. It usually takes 24 hours for the bacteria to reach the bladder before symptoms appear.

While some physicians may start treatment without testing for bacteria, a urinalysis—and usually a urine culture—should always be performed. Culture results take between 24 to 48 hours. It is possible to have a high levels of bacteria in the urine without having any pain or symptoms.

Treatment Options and Outlook

There are many different antibacterials available to treat UTIs. Plenty of fluids will help to flush the bladder and dilute the urine; water, fruit juice, or caffeine-free soft drinks are best choices.

For those women with recurrent UTIs, an antibiotic will be prescribed for up to 10 days together with a pain reliever.

Kidney infections are treated with a variety of antibiotics over a longer period of time. A relapse within 10 days could indicate the presence of kidney stones or kidney disease. Those with a severe kidney infection, or pregnant women, are usually hospitalized and given intravenous drugs.

The first step in treating a UTI in men is to identify the infecting organism and the drugs to which it is sensitive. Usually, doctors recommend longer treatment for men, partly as a way of preventing prostate infections. Prostate infections (called chronic bacterial prostatitis) are more difficult to cure because antibiotics cannot penetrate infected prostate tissue very well. As a result, men with prostatitis often need long-term antibiotic treatment. UTIs in older men are often associated with acute bacterial prostatitis, which can have serious consequences if not treated right away.

Untreated UTIs can lead to kidney infection (especially in pregnant women), with high fever, chills, severe flank pain, and painful urination. There also may be nausea and vomiting.

Risk Factors and Preventive Measures

There is no sure way to prevent UTIs, but there are ways to reduce the risk. Women should completely empty the bladder as often as possible (at least once every three hours) and after sex, and wipe from front to back after a bowel movement to avoid contaminating the urethra. It may help to cut down on caffeinated drinks (cola, coffee, or tea), which can irritate the bladder.

While many women can successfully prevent infections by drinking cranberry juice, which increases the acidity of the urine and interferes with bacterial growth, cranberry tablets are now available for the same purpose.

In the future, a new vaccine may help women ward off recurring UTIs in those plagued by several episodes a year. Children and women who get recurrent UTIs often lack proteins, called immunoglobulins, that fight infection. Children and women who do not get UTIs are more likely to have normal levels of immunoglobulins in their genital and urinary tracts. Research suggests that a vaccine helps patients build up their own natural ability to fight infection. The experimental vaccine prompts the body to produce antibodies that can later fight against UTI bacteria. Researchers are testing injected, oral, and vaginal suppository vaccines to see which works best.

Reducing recurrent urinary infections without the use of antibiotics would be helpful, since antibiotics can cause allergic reactions and women who take them continuously risk developing resistant strains that cannot be killed by any medicine.

V

vaccine A tiny dose of a specific protein of the organism that causes disease, given to prevent that disease. When a person is vaccinated, the vaccine helps build protective substances in the body to fight off any invasion by the disease-causing organism.

At present, there are vaccines for ANTHRAX, some types of PNEUMONIA, CHICKEN POX, DIPHTHERIA, GERMAN MEASLES, MEASLES, HEPATITIS A, HEPATITIS B, HIB, INFLUENZA, LYME DISEASE (for dogs), MALARIA, MUMPS, WHOOPING COUGH, PLAGUE, POLIOMYELITIS, Q FEVER, RABIES, ROTAVIRUS, SMALLPOX, TETANUS, TUBERCULOSIS, TYPHOID, and YELLOW FEVER.

Despite the fact that immunization is required by the time a child reaches school age, far too many U.S. children are still not vaccinated. From time to time, there are EPIDEMICS among those who are not, such as the 1990–91 epidemic of measles that swept through the Philadelphia area. Measles infected almost 56,000 Americans between 1989 and 1991, killing 166 of them. Most were babies, young children, and teens. Today, more and more vaccines are required for children. Yet the concept of vaccination is not without some controversy. Some parents worry that side effects of vaccines can harm their children.

Experts reply that most vaccine adverse events are minor and temporary, causing only a sore arm or mild fever, which can often be controlled by taking acetaminophen before or after vaccination. More serious adverse events occur rarely (about one per thousands to one per millions of doses), and some are so rare that risk cannot be accurately assessed.

Fatal reactions to vaccines are so rare that it is hard to assess the risk statistically. Of all deaths reported between 1990 and 1992, only one is believed to be even possibly associated with a vaccine. Each reported death is thoroughly examined to ensure that it is not related to a new vaccine-related problem, but little or no evidence suggests that vaccines have contributed to any of the reported deaths. The Institute of Medicine in its 1990–2001 report states that the risk of death from vaccines is "extraordinarily low." The death rate ranged from 1.4 percent to 2.3 percent of all adverse reports.

Moreover, the experience in several developed countries who let their immunization levels drop as a result of vaccine fears show what can happen when children are not vaccinated. Great Britain, Sweden, and Japan cut back the use of pertussis vaccine because of fear about the vaccine. In Great Britain, a drop in pertussis vaccination in 1974 was followed by an epidemic of more than 100,000 cases of pertussis and 36 deaths by 1978. In Japan at about the same time, a drop in vaccination rates from 70 percent to 20–40 percent led to a jump in pertussis from 393 cases and no deaths in 1974 to 13,000 cases and 41 deaths in 1979. In Sweden, the annual incidence rate of pertussis per 100,000 children up to six years of age increased from 700 cases in 1981 to 3,200 in 1985. Government experts believe that these experiences show that the end of vaccinations would bring these diseases back.

Experts believe as many people as possible should be vaccinated. Even if the chances of getting an infectious disease is small, the diseases still exist

---

WHO SHOULD NOT BE VACCINATED

- anyone who has had a serious allergic reaction to a previous shot
- anyone with a severe allergy to eggs should not receive MMR, flu, or yellow fever vaccines, except under special medical situations
- anyone with a high fever or serious illness

(except for smallpox) and can still infect anyone who is not protected. And because there are a few people who cannot be vaccinated because of severe allergies to vaccine components, and a small percentage of people do not respond to vaccines, their only hope of protection is that people around them are immune and cannot pass disease along. A successful vaccination program depends on the cooperation of every individual to ensure the good of all.

Those who believe they were injured by a vaccine may have compensation through the VACCINE INJURY COMPENSATION PROGRAM passed by Congress in 1986.

The doctor must keep a record of what vaccines were given, together with the date, manufacturer, lot number, and signature of person giving the vaccine. Patients will be given an information booklet, and parents must sign a consent form before the child is vaccinated. Most doctors offer immunization record forms for parents to keep track of all shots. School and day care programs require proper, up-to-date vaccinations.

RECOMMENDED IMMUNIZATION SCHEDULE FOR ADULTS BY AGE, HEALTH, JOB

All ages

- Td (tetanus, diphtheria) every 10 years
- Anyone born after 1957 should have two doses of measles vaccine given at least one month apart. Most high schools and colleges now require this.

Adults over age 65

- Td every 10 years
- Influenza vaccine every fall
- One dose pneumococcal pneumonia vaccine (with booster every six years for transplant patients or those with chronic kidney failure or no spleen)

Health-care/public-safety workers

- Hepatitis B vaccine (three-dose series)
- Influenza vaccine every fall
- MMR (unless proof of immunity) or birthdate before 1957

Medical or research lab workers

- Inactivated polio vaccine for those who have not received three doses of OPV
- Plague vaccine for anyone working with plague (three-dose series; booster every one to two years)
- Anthrax vaccine for anyone working with anthrax bacteria
- Rabies vaccine for anyone testing or isolating rabies virus

Veterinarians or small animal handlers

- Rabies vaccine and blood test every two years, with booster if needed

- Plague vaccine for those in western states (three-dose primary series; boosters every one to two years)

Field personnel

- Plague vaccine (three-dose primary series; boosters every one to two years)
- Rabies vaccine and blood tests every two years, with booster if needed
- Anthrax vaccine for those in contact with imported animal hides, furs, bonemeal, wool, animal hair (especially goat), and bristles

Homosexually active males or anyone with multiple partners

- Hepatitis B vaccine (three-dose series)
- Influenza

Injection drug users

- Hepatitis B vaccine (three-dose series)
- Td vaccine

Developmentally disabled residents of institutions

- Hepatitis B vaccine (three-dose series)
- Influenza vaccine every fall

Household contacts of hepatitis B carriers

- Hepatitis B vaccine (three-dose series)

Pregnant women

- Booster of Td if more than 10 years have elapsed
- Hepatitis B if woman is at risk of exposure because of lifestyle or household contact with carrier
- Influenza vaccine if there are medical conditions that increase risk of flu

(Table continues)

RECOMMENDED IMMUNIZATION SCHEDULE FOR ADULTS BY AGE, HEALTH, JOB *(continued)*

- Yellow fever and polio vaccines should be given only if she is traveling to areas where there is high risk of exposure and travel cannot be postponed until after delivery.
- Pregnant women who are not immune to measles, mumps, or rubella should receive these live virus vaccines immediately after delivery.

People with weakened immune systems

- Influenza vaccine every fall
- Pneumococcal vaccine; one dose (booster in six years)

HIV-infected patients

- Influenza vaccine every fall
- Pneumococcal vaccine; one dose (booster in six years)
- MMR vaccine (two doses)
- Hib (primary series)
- eIPV (inactivated polio vaccine) if not immune

Hemodialysis and kidney transplant patients

- Influenza vaccine every fall

- Pneumococcal vaccine; one dose (booster in six years)
- Hepatitis B vaccine (three-dose series)

Those with abnormal or absent spleens

- Pneumococcal vaccine
- Meningococcal vaccine

Clotting disorder patients who receive factor VIII or IX

- Hepatitis B vaccine (three-dose series)

Alcoholics

- Pneumococcal vaccine
- Influenza
- Ta

Patients with chronic lung, heart or kidney disease; diabetes; sickle-cell anemia

- Influenza vaccine every fall
- Pneumococcal vaccine

All adults over 65

- Pneumococcal vaccine

VACCINE TIME LINE

Pre–1950s Vaccines		***1970s***	
1798	Smallpox	**1970**	Anthrax vaccine manufactured by the Michigan Department of Public Health.
1885	Rabies		
1897	Plague	**1971**	Routine smallpox vaccination ceases in
1917	Cholera; typhoid (parenteral)		the United States. Measles/mumps/rubella
1923	Diphtheria		(MMR)
1926	Pertussis	**1976**	Swine flu: Largest public vaccination pro-
1927	Tuberculosis (BCG); tetanus		gram in the United States halted by link
1935	Yellow fever		with Guillain-Barré syndrome.
1940s	DTP (three-disease vaccine—diphtheria, tetanus, pertussis)	**1977**	Last indigenous case of smallpox (Somalia)
		1978	Fluzone flu vaccine by Aventis Pasteur
1945	Influenza	**1979**	Last case of polio (caused by wild virus) acquired in the United States
1950s–1960s			
1955	Inactivated polio vaccine (IPV); tetanus and diphtheria toxoids adsorbed (Td for adults)	***1980s***	
		1980	Smallpox declared eradicated from the world.
1959	Initial call for global smallpox eradication		
1961	Monovalent oral polio vaccine	**1981**	Meningococcal polysaccharide, groups A,
1963	Trivalent oral polio vaccine (OPV); measles		C, Y, W135 combined (Menomune)
1967	Mumps vaccine	**1982**	Hepatitis B
1969	Rubella (57,600 rubella cases reported this year)	**1983**	Pneumococcal vaccine, 23 valent
		1986	The National Childhood Vaccine Injury Act

establishes a no-fault compensation system for those injured by vaccines and requires adverse health events following specific vaccinations be reported and those injured by vaccines be compensated.

1988 Worldwide Polio Eradication Initiative launched; supported by WHO, UNICEF, Rotary International, CDC.

1989– 1991 Major resurgence of measles in the United States; two-dose measles vaccine (MMR) recommended

1990s

1990 The Vaccine Adverse Reporting System (VAERS), a national program monitoring the safety of vaccines established. *Haemophilus influenzae* type B (Hib) polysaccharide conjugate vaccine licensed for infants. Typhoid vaccine (oral)

1991 Hepatitis B vaccine recommended for all infants; acellular pertussis vaccine (DTaP) licensed for use in older children aged 15 months to six years.

1993 Japanese encephalitis

1994 Polio elimination certified in the Americas. Vaccines for Children (VFC) program established to provide access to free vaccines for eligible children at the site of their usual source of care.

1995 Chicken pox; hepatitis A vaccine licensed.

1996 Acellular pertussis vaccine (DTaP) licensed for use in young infants.

1998 First rotavirus vaccine licensed.

1999 First rotavirus vaccine withdrawn from the market as a result of adverse events; Lyme disease vaccine approved, FDA recommends removing mercury from all products, including vaccines; efforts begun to remove thimerosal, a mercury-based additive, from vaccines.

2000s

2000 Worldwide measles initiative launched; measles declared no longer endemic in the United States. Pneumococcal conjugate vaccine (Prevnar) recommended for all young children.

2001 September 11 results in increased concern of bioterrorism. The United States establishes a plan to reintroduce smallpox vaccine if necessary, a vaccine thought never to be needed again.

2002 Lyme disease vaccine withdrawn from the market by the manufacturer because of lawsuits and lack of demand for the vaccine.

2003 Measles declared no longer endemic in the Americas. First live attenuated influenza vaccine licensed (FluMist) for five- to 49-year-olds; first adult immunization schedule introduced.

2004 Inactivated influenza vaccine recommended for all children six to 23 months.

2005 Rubella declared no longer endemic in the United States; Boostrix (booster against diphtheria, whooping cough, and tetanus) approved for ages 10 to 18, replacing Td booster (against just tetanus and diphtheria) new single-shot vaccine (Proquad) that protects children against measles, mumps, rubella, and chicken pox

2006 A combination booster vaccine (Adacel) that confers protection against tetanus, diphtheria, and pertussis in both adults and adolescents aged 11 to 64. New rotavirus vaccine approved. New vaccine (Gardasil) against certain papillomaviruses, designed to prevent cervical cancer.

Vaccine Adverse Event Reporting System A cooperative reporting program for vaccine safety that tracks any unusual event that occurs after a vaccination was given. Since 1990, VAERS has received more than 123,000 reports, most of which describe mild side effects such as fever. Very rarely, people experience serious side effects after immunization. By monitoring such events, VAERS helps to identify any important new safety concerns.

VAERS is a post-marketing safety surveillance program, collecting information about side effects that occur after the administration of U.S. licensed vaccines. Reports to the VAERS program are welcome from all patients, parents, health-care providers, pharmacists, and vaccine manufacturers. Most reports are sent in by vaccine manufacturers (42 percent) and health-care providers (30 percent). The rest are obtained from state immunization programs (12 percent), vaccine recipients or their parents (7 percent), and other sources (9 percent). The Center for Biologics Evaluation and Research and the Centers for Disease Control and Prevention (CDC) jointly manage the Vaccine Adverse Event Reporting System.

In order to collect all information that may be of value, there is no restriction on the time lapse between the vaccination and the start of the event, or between the event and the time the report is made.

The toll-free VAERS information line is (800) 822-7967. It is also possible to submit a report on the Internet, by visiting the VAERS Web site at http://secure.vaers.org/VaersDataEntryintro.htm. Consumers are encouraged to get help from their family doctor in reporting the event.

In addition to any reports by consumers, the NATIONAL CHILDHOOD VACCINE INJURY ACT of 1986 requires health care providers to report any event listed by the vaccine manufacturer as a contraindication to subsequent doses of the vaccine, and any event listed in the Reportable Events Table that occurs within the specified time period after vaccination.

Vaccine Injury Compensation Program   A special program established in 1988 that provides compensation for children who experience adverse effects after receiving vaccines. All claims are reviewed by medical staff, and awards are decided by a group of attorneys of the U.S. Claims Court. The program, which is paid for by a surtax on all vaccines, applies to DPT, MMR, OPV, and Td vaccines. The VICP is administered jointly by the U.S. Department of Health and Human Services (HHS), the U.S. Court of Federal Claims (the court), and the U.S. Department of Justice (DOJ).

To report an adverse event after a vaccine, a parent should call the doctor where the child received the shot to report any reactions. Complete information should be given about what happened and when it occurred. The doctor should report any unusual or serious reactions to the VACCINE ADVERSE EVENT REPORTING SYSTEM at (800) 822-7967 or at the VAERS Web site.

vaccinia   A viral cattle disease ("cowpox") inoculated in humans to produce an antibody against SMALLPOX. Vaccinia is the source of the word *vaccine*.

vaginal infections   Any infection of the vagina caused by bacteria or yeast. Together with a physical exam and history, lab tests are needed to examine vaginal fluid microscopically. Some vaginal infections cause VAGINITIS, an inflammation of the vagina that may include discharge, irritation, and itching.

Some of the most common vaginal infections are bacterial VAGINITIS, TRICHOMONIASIS, and VAGINAL YEAST INFECTION.

vaginal warts   See WARTS.

vaginal yeast infection   A type of infection (also known as CANDIDIASIS) that infects the vagina, caused by yeast, which lives normally in the vagina. However, when certain conditions upset the delicate balance, a vaginal yeast infection also can occur. These conditions include

- diabetes (the high sugar content in urine helps yeast grow)
- obesity (thick folds of fat favor yeast, which grow in warm moist environments)
- pregnancy (hormone balance changes that are favorable to yeast)
- antibiotics (kill off bacteria, allowing yeast to grow)
- steroids (disturb immune system)

Yeast infections commonly occur after a woman has been taking antibiotics for a different infection. PENICILLINS, tetracyclines, and cephalosporins are particularly associated with this problem.

There is conflicting evidence as to whether birth control pills are associated with infections.

It is not clear whether a woman can give yeast infections to her sexual partner; some studies suggest male partners of women with infections have positive cultures for yeast, but do not have symptoms. It is possible to pass the infection to a newborn during delivery, causing thrush in the baby in the first few weeks of life.

Symptoms and Diagnostic Path

White, thick, cheesy discharge that can cause severe itchiness and discomfort; the vulva or vagina may be red and swollen. Some infections are mild, with only slight itchiness and redness. The outer lips of the vulva may feel dry or scaly.

A vaginal culture is the most accurate test.

Treatment Options and Outlook

Creams and suppositories are available over the counter to cure yeast infections. They are inserted into the vagina for two to seven nights, depending on the brand. If there is no improvement in three days, a doctor visit is recommended, since the condition could be caused by something other than a yeast infection. Pregnant women should wait until they have passed 14 weeks of pregnancy before inserting vaginal antifungal yeast infection medicine.

If one course of medicine does not work, the doctor may try a different drug; if this fails, ketoconazole pills may be prescribed, which will eradicate yeast in most women with a chronic problem.

Because yeast grows best in dark, moist places, the area should be kept open to air as much as possible. This means avoiding underwear, and wearing a loose dress or nightgown. When underwear must be worn, it should be white 100 percent cotton; no panty hose or tight-fitting pants should be worn.

vaginitis (vaginosis) Any mild infection or inflammation of the vagina. It may be called bacterial vaginosis or nonspecific vaginitis when a specific organism (such as TRICHOMONAS) is not identified.

The bacterium *Gardnerella vaginalis* has been associated with vaginosis, although studies suggest a mixture of bacteria may be associated with the infection. Most of these bacteria are normally found in the vagina, but when they multiply excessively they can cause symptoms.

It is not clear how women get vaginitis, although women who are sexually active and those who have more than one sexual partner have higher rates of disease. Women in their teens and twenties have more infections than older women. While vaginitis may be related to sexual activity, it is not passed directly from one person to another.

Symptoms and Diagnostic Path

Symptoms include gray or frothy vaginal discharge with a foul or fish-smelling odor. It rarely causes itch, burning, or irritation.

Inspection of vaginal discharge or microscope investigation will diagnose the infection.

Treatment Options and Outlook

Vaginosis is easily treated with the antibiotic metronidazole (Flagyl), which is also used to treat TRICHOMONIASIS. A woman should not take metronidazole during the first 14 weeks of pregnancy.

Sexual intercourse should be avoided during treatment because it may worsen symptoms. Douching is not recommended, since it upsets normal flora in the vagina and will make symptoms worse. Patients should bathe or shower daily with plain soap and water. Bubble baths and bath salts or oils should be avoided until the infection clears.

Pregnant women with vaginosis are 40 percent more likely to give birth to premature, low-birth-weight babies than are uninfected pregnant women. Scientists recommend that pregnant women mention any symptoms of vaginal infection to their doctors and get treatment if they have bacterial vaginosis.

vaginosis See VAGINITIS.

valley fever The common name for COCCIDIOIDOMYCOSIS (or "cocci" for short).

vancomycin-resistant enterococcus (VRE) A common bacteria that can infect patients in intensive-care units, and that is resistant to vancomycin, the antibiotic of last resort. Vancomycin-resistant enterococcus (VRE) infections are especially aggressive and have been associated with mortality rates of 60 to 70 percent. They are now the second-leading cause of hospital-acquired infections in the United States, and their prevalence is increasing. Enterococci normally exist in the stomach and intestines and on the skin; generally, they do not cause disease, but they can cause infections (especially in patients weakened by another illness). There are many types of this bacteria, most of which rarely cause disease. Many people carry the bacteria without symptoms.

What makes this particular bacteria so dangerous is that many strains are now able to resist antibiotics, including PENICILLINS, cephalosporins, and aminoglycosides. As a result, for many years doctors relied on the antibiotic vancomycin to treat serious enterococcal infections. In the late 1980s, however, strains of enterococci began to appear that resisted even this drug. VRE infection was first documented in Europe in the 1980s and is now emerging as a new threat to patients in the United States.

The most common types of infections attributed to VRE are URINARY TRACT INFECTIONS, ENDOCARDITIS, MENINGITIS, BACTEREMIA, and abdominal infections. Bloodstream infections are linked to use of catheters or indwelling devices, and intra-abdominal infections are usually associated with ABSCESSES or surgery.

In the United States, VRE are most commonly found in teaching hospitals and hospitals with more than 500 beds. Reports also suggest that it is rare for a patient who has not been in a hospital to have VRE. However, in Europe, VRE can be found in waste waters and in the feces of both nonhospitalized patients and healthy volunteers.

VRE are spread by direct or indirect contact with an infected person; they are not spread through the air.

There is no proven treatment for VRE; chlorhexidine (but not regular soap) kills the bacteria.

Guidelines published by the CENTERS FOR DISEASE CONTROL AND PREVENTION suggest hospital labs periodically test patients for VRE and isolate those patients who are infected. Health-care workers who treat these patients should wear protective clothing. Because VRE can live on dirty telephones, walls, and patient charts, hospitals should improve simple housekeeping, according to the CDC.

varicella   See CHICKEN POX.

varicella-zoster immune globulin (VZIG)   An immune globulin obtained from the blood of healthy people with high levels of varicella-zoster antibodies. The immune globulin can be administered to anyone exposed to CHICKEN POX to prevent or modify symptoms of the infection.

varicella-zoster virus (VZV)   A member of the family of herpes viruses, (HSV) which causes the diseases varicella (CHICKEN POX), and herpes zoster (SHINGLES). When the virus enters the upper respiratory tract of a nonimmune host, it produces skin lesions of chicken pox. The virus then passes from skin to sensory ganglia, where it establishes a latent infection. When the patient's immunity to HSV fades away, the virus replicates within the ganglia and results in shingles.

The virus is highly contagious and may be spread by direct contact or droplets. Dried crusts of skin lesions do not contain the virus.

variola   Another name for SMALLPOX.

venereal disease   Another name for SEXUALLY TRANSMITTED DISEASE. Its name is a reference to Venus, goddess of love.

venereal warts   See WARTS, GENITAL.

Vessel Sanitation Program   A program aimed at keeping cruise ships free from disease, established by the U.S. CENTERS FOR DISEASE CONTROL AND PREVENTION (CDC) in the early 1970s. The program was developed after several major infectious diseases broke out on board cruise ships.

The program helps cruise ships develop and implement comprehensive sanitation programs in order to minimize the risk for gastrointestinal diseases. Every ship traveling abroad that carries 13 or more passengers and calls on a U.S. port is subject to unannounced twice-yearly inspections (and when necessary, to reinspection). The ship owner pays a fee for all inspections.

Currently more than 140 cruise ships participate in the program, which gives each ship a score based on a 100-point scale. To pass the inspection, a ship must score 86 or above. If the ship fails an inspection, it will be reinspected within 30 to 45 days.

Depending on the size of the ship, an inspection may take from five to eight hours to complete. The inspection focuses on

- how safely water is stored, distributed, protected, and disinfected
- filtration and disinfection of spas and pools
- safe food storage, preparation, and service
- potential for contamination of food and water
- employee practices and personal hygiene
- ship's cleanliness and condition
- training programs in general environmental and public health practices

Inspection scores and reports are published on the VSP website (http://www2.cdc.gov/nceh/vsp/default.htm). In addition, scores are published every month in the Summary of Sanitation Inspections of International Cruise Ships (the "green sheet"). This sheet is distributed to more than 3,000 travel-related services around the world. In general, the lower the score the lower the level of sanitation, but a low score does not necessarily imply immediate health risks.

Since the program began, the number of disease outbreaks on ships has declined despite significant growth in the number of ships sailing and the number of passengers carried.

The VSP staff continually monitors reports of diarrheal illness on each ship, and each vessel is required to maintain a list of gastrointestinal illnesses for each cruise. The list contains information on passengers and crew members who had reported diarrhea, including the number of cases of gastrointestinal illnesses by dates of onset and the total numbers of passengers and crew members. If at least 3 percent of the ship's passengers and crew have gastrointestinal illness, the VSP may conduct

an investigation to determine if an outbreak of gastrointestinal illnesses occurred. If an unusual gastrointestinal illness pattern or characteristic is found even when the illness rate is less than 3 percent, an investigation may also take place.

In the 1970s and early 1980s, 12 to 15 outbreaks of diarrheal illness occurred each year on cruise ships. In 2002, a rash of diarrheal illnesses on several cruise lines were linked to a Norwalk-like virus.

vibrio   Any bacterium that is curved and capable of unconscious movement, with a tail that makes them good swimmers. Vibrio includes bacteria that belong to the genus *Vibrio*. These include *V. cholerae* (the cause of CHOLERA), *VIBRIO PARAHAEMOLYTICUS* (the cause of a type of seafood poisoning); *V. alginolyticus* and *V. vulnificus* can infect wounds received in warm salt water; *V. vulnificus* can cause blood poisoning if swallowed, especially in people with impaired immune systems or liver problems; *V. vulnificus* has been identified in raw Gulf Coast oysters and has been responsible for at least 13 fatalities since 1992.

Several other marine vibrios have been implicated in human disease. Some may cause wound or ear infections and others cause gastroenteritis. These include *V. alginolyticus, V. carchariae, V. cincinnatiensis, V. damsela, V. fluvialis, V. furnissii, V. hollisae, V. metschnikovii,* and *V. mimicus.*

See also DIARRHEA AND INFECTIOUS DISEASE; TRAVELER'S DIARRHEA; *VIBRIO PARAHAEMOLYTICUS* GASTROENTERITIS.

Vibrio cholerae   A species of comma-shaped bacillus that causes CHOLERA.

See also VIBRIO.

Vibrio parahaemolyticus   A type of bacterium often isolated from ocean fish and shellfish that can cause a type of food poisoning.

See also VIBRIO; *VIBRIO PARAHAEMOLYTICUS* GASTROENTERITIS.

Vibrio parahaemolyticus gastroenteritis   A type of food poisoning caused by eating fish or shellfish contaminated with the bacteria *V. parahaemolyticus.* Sporadic outbreaks of this type of gastroenteritis have occurred in the United States. It is also very common in Japan, where large outbreaks regularly occur.

The disease occurs when the bacterium attaches itself to a person's small intestine and secretes an as-yet-unidentified toxin. Infections with this organism have been associated with eating raw, improperly cooked contaminated fish and shellfish, especially during the warmer months. Improper refrigeration of contaminated seafood allows the bacteria to flourish, increasing the chance of infection.

Symptoms and Diagnostic Path

Between four and 96 hours after ingestion, the victim may experience diarrhea, abdominal cramps, nausea and vomiting, headache, fever, and chills. The illness is usually mild, although some cases require hospitalization.

The organism can be cultured from stool.

Treatment Options and Outlook

Symptomatic, including plenty of clear fluids. In most cases, the infection will clear up of itself.

See also ANTIDIARRHEAL DRUGS; DIARRHEA AND INFECTIOUS DISEASE; SHELLFISH POISONING, DIARRHEIC; TRAVELER'S DIARRHEA.

Vincent's disease Also known as trench mouth, this is a painful bacterial infection and ulceration of the gums, known medically as acute necrotizing ulcerative gingivitis. The condition is relatively rare.

Vincent's disease is caused by abnormal growth of microorganisms that are usually harmlessly found in pockets in the gums. Predisposing factors include poor dental hygiene, smoking, throat infections, emotional stress, and impaired immune system. It is usually preceded either by gingivitis or periodontitis (gum infections).

Symptoms and Diagnostic Path

Over several days, the gums become sore and inflamed, bleeding at the slightest pressure. Ulcers which bleed spontaneously develop on the gums between the teeth. This is accompanied by bad breath, foul taste, and sometimes swollen glands.

As the disease worsens, the ulcers spread along the gum margins and into deeper tissues. Sometimes, the infection spreads to the lips and the lining of the cheeks, causing tissue destruction.

Treatment Options and Outlook

Mouthwash containing hydrogen peroxide may help relieve pain and inflammation. After a few days, when the gums are less painful they can be scaled to remove hardened mineral deposits and plaque from the teeth. In severe cases, antibacterial drugs may be prescribed to treat the infection.

viral infection An infectious disease that are caused by a virus, the smallest known kind of infectious agent. About half to a hundredth the size of the smallest BACTERIA, viruses also have a much simpler structure and method of multiplication.

Scientists debate whether viruses are really living organisms or just collections of large molecules capable of self-replication under favorable conditions. They take over cells of other organisms, where they proceed to make copies of themselves. Outside living cells, viruses are inert and not capable of metabolism or other activities typically found in living organisms.

It is believed that there are more viruses than any other type of organism, and they parasitize all recognized life-forms (mammals, birds, reptiles, insects, plants, algae, and even bacteria).

Viral infections may be mild (such as WARTS or the common cold) or they can be extremely serious, including RABIES, AIDS, SMALLPOX, and POLIOMYELITIS. There are no specific cures for most viral diseases, although it is possible to treat their symptoms.

However, it is possible to prevent some of the viral diseases through vaccination, including smallpox, measles, and polio.

virucide Any agent that can destroy a VIRUS.

virus The smallest known type of infectious agent. These tiny parasitic microorganisms are much smaller than bacteria, and they do not have any independent metabolic activity. Viruses are about half to a hundredth the size of the smallest bacteria, and they lack bacteria's complex structure.

A virus includes a core of nucleic acid (genetic material RNA or DNA), surrounded by a layer of protein—really just a movable bit of genetic information. Viruses lack the ability to independently reproduce unless they enter a living cell and take over that cell's reproductive apparatus, directing the cell to manufacture viral components instead of its normal ones. The damage that results from this takeover produces the symptoms of viral disease. Scientists believe viruses began as bits of genetic material that escaped from cells, eventually acquiring the ability to move from one organism to the next.

More than 200 viruses have so far been identified as causing human disease, divided into at least 20 types, including ADENOVIRUS, ARENAVIRUS, CORONAVIRUS, ENTEROVIRUS, HERPESVIRUS, POXVIRUS, PICORNAVIRUS, RHINOVIRUS, and RETROVIRUS. They are responsible for an astonishingly wide variety of diseases, ranging from the mild common cold to WARTS, AIDS, and RABIES. The number of viruses

VIRUS TYPES	
Family	Examples of Diseases
Adenoviruses	Respiratory and eye infections
Arenaviruses	Lassa fever
Coronaviruses	Common cold
Enteroviruses	Viral meningitis
Herpesviruses	Cold sores, genital herpes, chicken pox, shingles, glandular fever, congenital abnormalities
Orthomyxoviruses	Influenza
Papovaviruses	Warts
Paramyxoviruses	Mumps, measles, rubella
Picornaviruses	Polio, viral hepatitis types A and B, respiratory infections, myocarditis
Poxviruses	Cowpox, smallpox, molluscum contagiosum
Retroviruses	AIDS, degenerative brain disease, possibly cancer
Rhabdoviruses	Rabies
Togaviruses	Yellow fever, dengue, encephalitis

probably exceeds the number of types of all other organisms, and they invade all other types of life-forms—mammals, birds, reptiles, insects, plants, algae—even bacteria. While not all viruses cause disease, many do.

They enter the human body by a variety of ways: They are swallowed, inhaled, or taken into the skin via a puncture (such as an insect bite). They may enter directly via the mucous membranes of the genitals during sexual intercourse and by the conjunctiva of the eye during accidental contamination. Once inside the body, some viruses enter the lymph nodes near where they invaded the body. Many pass into the blood, spreading throughout the body within a few minutes. From there, they may invade the skin, brain, lungs, or liver.

When they invade cells, they may disrupt or destroy cellular activities; this can cause serious disease if vital organs are involved. The body's immune system rallies to fight off the viral attack, leading to symptoms of fever and fatigue.

The healthy immune system is often able to fight off a viral attack fairly quickly, within a few days to weeks. Typically, the immune system is so sensitized by this attack that a second illness from the same virus is rare (such as in MEASLES). However, some viruses attack so fiercely and fast that serious damage or death may occur before the immune system can muster its defenses (as in the case with polio or rabies). Other times, a virus can hide from the immune system, leading to a chronic infection. This is what happens with many herpes infections, such as genital herpes and SHINGLES. In the case of the AIDS virus, the weakened immune system opens the door to many OPPORTUNISTIC INFECTIONS.

The name *virus* comes from the Latin word for "poison," first used during the late 19th century for any infectious microbe that caused a disease. It was not until 1892 that Russian bacteriologist Dmitri Ivanovski discovered the sap of a tobacco plant with tobacco mosaic disease could be filtered through a bacteria-trapping filter and still produce the disease. After several other scientists discovered other filter-passing agents, Dutch botanist Martinus Beijerinck named this organism that was able to pass through bacteria filters a *filterable virus.* The two-word term was used for many years, eventually shortened to *virus.* The first human virus was identified by name in 1901 by U.S. army surgeon Walter Reed, who showed that YELLOW FEVER was caused by a filterable virus. Still, it was not until 1927 that its viral heritage was fully understood.

Unlike bacteria, which are easily killed by antibiotics, it is not easy to design a drug that will kill a virus without killing its host cell. Still, scientists have made progress, such as with the antiviral drugs used to treat herpes infections.

INTERFERONS are a group of natural substances produced by infected cells that protect uninfected cells from viral attack. Some interferons are now produced artificially and are being studied against a wide variety of viral infections.

Far easier than curing a viral infection once it occurs is vaccination—protecting against infection before it occurs. Highly effective vaccines are available to prevent a wide variety of viral infections, including polio, measles, MUMPS, RUBELLA, HEPATITIS B, yellow fever, and rabies. The SMALLPOX vaccine has resulted in the total eradication of that disease from the face of the earth.

vulvovaginitis Inflammation of the vulva and vagina usually caused by bacteria, yeast, viruses, parasites, SEXUALLY TRANSMITTED DISEASES, or chemicals.

Symptoms and Diagnostic Path
Symptoms include profuse vaginal discharge, irritation, itching, odor, and discomfort during urination.

Treatment Options and Outlook
Antifungal or antibiotic drugs, cortisone creams, or antihistamines are effective in treating the disease.

walking pneumonia See PNEUMONIA, MYCOPLASMA.

warts Generally harmless small, rough, hard, round raised bumps, which usually appear on hands and fingers, around the knees, or on the genitals.

Warts are caused by one of the more than 58 types of HUMAN PAPILLOMAVIRUS (HPV). A person gets a wart by touching someone else's wart, touching something a wart-infected person has touched, or by self-inoculation. People who bite on their own warts can spread them to other areas of their own bodies.

The incubation period between first infection and the appearance of the wart averages between two to three months, but it may be as long as 20 months. The person is infectious as long as the wart exists.

Symptoms and Diagnostic Path

Common warts appear on backs of hands, fingers, and knees, and are usually about a quarter inch in size. Sometimes a few of these bumps blend together, but they usually appear separately. Tiny black specks in the wart are caused by small clots of blood.

Digitate warts are dark-colored growths with fingerlike projections.

Filiform warts look like long, slender growths that occur on the eyelids, armpits, or neck they are usually found in overweight middle-aged people.

Flat warts are small (about 1/16 inch) tan, flat, round, and are grouped together on the face, wrists, backs of hands, and shins. They may itch.

Plantar warts are flat, rough warts that appear on the soles of the feet. They occur alone or in groups; they are flat because of the pressure of the rest of the body.

Most warts are diagnosed by appearance; rarely, a doctor may biopsy a piece of wart to make a diagnosis.

Treatment Options and Outlook

More than 65 percent of warts disappear on their own within two years. There is no specific medication that kills the virus, although different treatments can eradicate the wart itself. Over-the-counter removal preparations include topical medications containing salicylic acid, which peels off the affected skin. The virus is killed as well, since it is inside the tissue. The skin should be softened first before applying the medicine; a few times a week, the dead skin should be removed with an emery board.

If the warts do not disappear with this treatment, a dermatologist may apply liquid nitrogen to freeze the wart solid; as it thaws, it forms a blister that lifts off the wart. This takes four to six weeks. Sometimes a blister-producing liquid (cantharidin) or a corroding acid may be used. Some doctors may use heated electrical needles. Since wart treatment can cause scars, it is best to wait for the warts to disappear on their own.

warts, genital Soft warts that grow in and around the entrance of the vagina, the anus, and the penis. Genital warts are the most common viral SEXUALLY TRANSMITTED DISEASE in the United States, outranking even genital HERPES.

Almost 5.5 million Americans are treated for new cases of genital warts each year, and most cases are diagnosed in women between the ages of 15 and 24. About 20 million Americans are already infected. Older people may have the virus, but their immune systems control the outbreaks. Those who are most at risk are people with more than one sex partner and those who do not use condoms.

Eight different types of HUMAN PAPILLOMAVIRUS (HPV) are associated with genital warts. There are high-risk and low-risk types of HPV. High-risk HPV may cause abnormal Pap smear results and can lead to cancers of the cervix, vulva, vagina, anus, or penis. Low-risk HPV also may cause abnormal Pap results or genital warts. HPV types 16 and 18 are associated with cervical cancer, and these are not usually visible. The different types of virus can only be distinguished in a research lab. The virus is transmitted during unprotected sex with an infected partner. A person is infectious when visible warts are present in the genital area; however, even if the warts have disappeared, the virus may still be present in the body.

Genital warts are very contagious and are spread via skin-to-skin contact during vaginal, anal, or rarely oral sex with an infected partner. About two-thirds of people who have sexual contact with an infected partner also will develop warts, usually within three months of contact.

Some doctors inject the antiviral drug alpha interferon directly into stubborn warts that have returned after removal by traditional means. The drug is expensive, however, and does not stop genital warts from returning again.

Symptoms and Diagnostic Path

Genital warts are pink to gray, soft, raised, or flat, and may cause itching, burning, or bleeding around the genital area. They may appear alone or in clusters, ranging in size from pinpoint to a small mass. Men usually notice the warts on the penis, although they can also appear in the anus or the urethra. Men may completely miss small warts.

Women may find warts on the vulva, vagina, or anus; occasionally they may occur on the cervix. Incubation period is unknown. The warts will not be painful, but they can grow and block the openings of the vagina, anus, urethra, or throat.

A doctor can diagnose the condition from the wart's appearance; a magnifying glass may be needed to find small warts. Odd-looking warts may require a biopsy. A Pap smear will identify warts on the cervix or those deep inside the vagina.

Treatment Options and Outlook

In 2006, the first vaccine to prevent cervical cancer caused by the papillomavirus was approved. The vaccine, Gardasil, prevents four types of wart virus, which are responsible for 70 percent of cervical cancers and 90 percent of genital warts. It may be used for girls and women aged nine to 26 years.

There is no way to remove all traces of the HP virus from the body. Instead, treatment aims at removing or shrinking the warts, whether by freezing, using a topical solution or laser, or with conventional surgery. Unfortunately, warts often reappear after treatment.

Podophyllin topical solution is applied by a doctor to external warts only (it should not be used in the cervix, rectum, or while pregnant). The solution must not touch the surrounding skin, as it can be irritating. If there are no results after four weeks, another treatment method should be used. Podofilox 0.05 percent is a prescription topical solution that can be applied by the woman for external warts. It works by killing wart tissue.

Cryotherapy freezes the wart off; it is sometimes used for cervical or rectal warts. Laser therapy is performed in a doctor's office and is sometimes used for cervical warts.

Electrosurgery is also performed in a doctor's office for rectal warts.

As a last resort, a doctor may turn to surgical removal if the warts are very large or causing problems. Still, 20 percent of the time warts grow back after this treatment.

Pregnant women with genital warts may have problems during delivery because hormonal changes can cause the warts to grow in size and number. Occasionally, babies exposed to warts in the birth canal develop warts in the throat and a few develop warts on the genitals or eyes. Warts also may multiply and grow larger among those with weakened immune systems or diabetes.

Two or more strains of the HPV strain have been associated with a higher risk of cervical cancer, especially among women with persistent warts and many sex partners.

Risk Factors and Preventive Measures

Infected partners should avoid sex when the warts are large, bleeding, or painful. Anyone who has genital warts or who has been diagnosed in the past should always use a condom during sexual intercourse. A doctor should be consulted if warts block rectal openings or if there is trouble urinating.

All women with anogenital warts need a Pap test every six to 12 months to detect early signs of cervical cancer. Young girls with cervical HPV should have regular Pap tests to treat any changes in the cervix. Most cervical problems take care of themselves, but those with a positive Pap test should seek medical help regularly to monitor the changes.

The best way to prevent the disease is by not having sex. Condoms may reduce the risk of HPV, but research has not proven they can completely prevent infection.

water, contaminated   Water can be a source of infection if it contains infective or parasitic organisms and is drunk, swum in, or comes into contact with food. Throughout the world, tainted water is a major source of the spread of infectious disease, including viral HEPATITIS A, DIARRHEA, TYPHOID FEVER, CHOLERA, AMEBIASIS, and some types of worm infestation. Water can become contaminated by feces (either human or animal) that contain infective material in rivers, lakes, reservoirs, or wells. Contamination can also occur via untreated sewage or leakage between sewage and water supplies.

The risk of water-borne infection in the United States is far less than in the Third World because of adequate sanitary facilities, sewage treatment and disposal, and the sterilization and testing of municipal water supplies. This does not mean that all U.S. drinking water is safe, however. The CRYPTOSPORIDIOSIS parasite is believed to infect millions of Americans each year through tainted tap water.

In 1993, more than 400,000 Milwaukee residents became ill after drinking contaminated tap water. Those infected reported nausea, severe abdominal cramps, diarrhea, and low-grade fever. Some deaths were reported. The parasite, which is not killed by chlorination, can also be found in pools, lakes, rivers, hot tubs, ice cubes, and on fruits and vegetables. Symptoms usually strike two to 10 days after exposure. Similarly, the microorganism *Cyclospora* can cause many of the same symptoms in those who drink tainted water or food.

To avoid infection outside the United States, travelers should use bottled or canned water and drinks of well-known brand names. Ice should not be put into drinks. Rainwater is usually free from infective organisms if it not allowed to stand for a long period before drinking.

Water that may be tainted should be boiled before drinking for five minutes, since this will kill any infective organisms. Alternatively, the water can be filtered and then sterilized chemically. Various filters can remove bacteria and other infective organisms as well as inanimate particles. Chemical sterilization methods use pills containing chlorine or iodine; water should be left for 20 to 30 minutes after chemical treatment before being used.

Swimming in polluted water may lead to an EAR INFECTION. Swimmers who inadvertently swallow water may contract a disease transmitted in polluted drinking water. This is why swimmers should avoid swimming in polluted rivers or in the ocean near large coastal resorts. In tropical countries, swimming in rivers, lakes, or ponds is not recommended because of the risk of SCHISTOSOMIASIS, a serious disease caused by a river fluke that can burrow through the swimmer's skin. SWIMMER'S ITCH is caused by a similar type of fluke. Outbreaks of swimmer's itch have occurred in the United States.

Finally, fish and shellfish that live in polluted water may accumulate infective organisms in their own bodies and, if improperly cooked, can pass on infections to consumers.

Although the responsibility for ensuring a safe water supply lies with local government, consumers can reduce their risk from waterborne disease by:

- washing raw or unpeeled fruits and vegetables
- complying with any emergency water advisory issued by local or state authorities
- having private wells tested by a state or U.S.-certified laboratory
- boiling contaminated water for one minute to kill harmful microorganisms; a home filter must be used to remove cryptosporidium or giardia. Reverse osmosis filters are effective against viruses and bacteria, as well as these protozoa, and must be changed regularly

- never drinking water directly from lakes, streams, reservoirs, or rivers without boiling it first
- not swallowing water when swimming, especially in lakes, ponds, and rivers that are open to contamination by human and animal wastes. Local swimming pools and those at recreational water parks can also become contaminated by fecal accidents and can cause illness in those who accidentally swallow pool water.

Waterhouse-Friderichsen syndrome   A very rare, serious condition caused by an overwhelming infection of the bloodstream. The condition is almost always fatal unless it is immediately intensively treated in a hospital.

Bacteria of the meningococcus group cause this disease; therefore, MENINGITIS is often associated with this syndrome.

Symptoms and Diagnostic Path

The onset of symptoms is abrupt; within hours, the patient sinks into a coma as blood pours into the adrenal glands, leading to acute adrenal failure and shock. Rapidly enlarging purple spots appear on the skin.

Treatment Options and Outlook

Emergency treatment includes administration of vasopressor drugs, intravenous fluids, plasma, and oxygen. No sedatives or narcotics should be given. Specific treatment for BACTEREMIA is intensive antibiotic therapy until symptoms subside.

Weil's syndrome   A severe form of LEPTOSPIROSIS, this infectious disease is caused by organisms of the genus *Leptospira*. Weil's syndrome was named after German physician Adolph Weil, who identified this syndrome as a type of "infectious jaundice" in 1886.

The organisms are transmitted to human beings via the urine of a wide variety of wild and domestic animals, including rats, mice, deer, dogs, bats, foxes, rabbits, pigs, goats, birds, frogs, snakes, fish, raccoons, and so on. The germs attack humans by entering the skin.

Symptoms and Diagnostic Path

Weil's syndrome can lead to liver and kidney problems, vomiting, and MENINGITIS.

Treatment Options and Outlook

It can be treated with antibiotics.

West Nile fever   A mild illness caused by infection with the WEST NILE VIRUS that does not affect the brain as do more serious infections with this virus. Although doctors are required to report cases of West Nile fever, the number of cases reported may be limited by whether patients go to the doctor for care, whether lab tests are ordered, and whether the doctor actually does report the case. About one in 150 people infected with the virus develop a more severe form of disease resulting in ENCEPHALITIS, MENINGITIS, or MENINGOENCEPHALITIS, requiring hospitalization. There are no apparent long-term effects from this infection.

Symptoms and Diagnostic Path

West Nile fever causes mild flu-like symptoms of fever, headache, and body aches; a skin rash on the body, and swollen lymph glands that last only a few days. However, about 80 percent of patients infected with the virus never have any symptoms at all.

Treatment Options and Outlook

No treatment is necessary for West Nile fever, other than treating symptoms to make the patient more comfortable.

Risk Factors and Preventive Measures

The risk for severe complications from West Nile virus infection increases with age, chronic illness, impaired immunity, and poor health. Infection can be prevented only by avoiding mosquitoes; there is no vaccine.

See also ENCEPHALITIS, WEST NILE; MENINGITIS, WEST NILE.

West Nile virus   A virus that can cause a fatal ENCEPHALITIS, commonly found in humans and birds in Africa, Eastern Europe, West Asia, and the Middle East.

Until 1999, the virus had not been documented in the Western Hemisphere. That year, 62 cases of severe disease, including seven deaths, occurred in New York, followed by 21 more cases the next year, including two deaths. Nearly 3,000 cases of the virus were recorded throughout the country in 2005, with the highest concentration in California, where 928 residents contracted the illness and 18 died. This was fewer than the worst outbreak years in 2002 and 2003, when 14,000 Americans were stricken and 548 died in two seasons. But as the virus settles in among wild birds and mosquitoes in nearly all the nation's most populated regions, experts warn that the potential for future outbreaks has never been greater. No reliable estimates are available for the number of cases of WEST NILE VIRUS ENCEPHALITIS or WEST NILE VIRUS POLIOMYELITIS that occur worldwide.

The virus is transmitted to humans via the bite of infected mosquitoes, which become infected when they feed on infected birds. The virus is located in the mosquito's salivary glands. During blood feeding, the virus may be injected into the animal or human, where it may multiply, possibly causing illness. Following transmission, West Nile virus multiplies in a person's blood and crosses the blood-brain barrier to reach the brain, where it inflames brain tissue and interferes with central nervous system function. Among those with severe illness due to West Nile virus, the fatality rates range from 3 percent to 15 percent.

However, even in areas where mosquitoes do carry the virus, very few mosquitoes (fewer than 1 percent) are infected. If the mosquito is infected, less than 1 percent of people who get bitten and become infected will be severely ill. The chances that any one person will become severely ill from a single mosquito bite are extremely small. The virus is not spread by touching or kissing a person who has the disease, or from a health-care worker who has treated someone with the disease. Although ticks infected with West Nile virus have been found in Asia and Africa, their role in the transmitting the virus is uncertain. There is no information to suggest that ticks played any role in the cases identified in the United States.

While experts do not know from where the U.S. virus originated, it is most closely related genetically to strains found in the Middle East. West Nile virus was first isolated from a feverish woman in the West Nile district of Uganda in 1937. A more virulent form appeared in eastern Europe in the 1990s. As the virus moved across the United States by the end of that decade, it killed 782 Americans and inflicted more than 8,000 with neurological problems ranging from persistent headache to a form of paralysis similar to POLIOMYELITIS.

The virus is now considered to be endemic in the United States, like its cousin St. Louis encephalitis, which has periodically affected parts of the country for 80 years. West Nile virus and St. Louis encephalitis occur primarily in birds and are spread by the same families of mosquitoes. However, St. Louis encephalitis has been unpredictable and sometimes explosive, with a huge national outbreak in 1975. West Nile virus also could become unpredictable, with far more serious consequences, because West Nile virus is a much more lethal germ than its St. Louis cousin. Birds infected with West Nile have hundreds of more viruses in their bloodstream.

Mosquitoes become infected when they feed on infected birds; they then spread WNV to humans and other animals when they bite. WNV is not spread through casual contact such as touching or kissing a person with the virus. In a very small number of cases, WNV also has been spread through blood transfusions, organ transplants, breast-feeding, and occasionally during pregnancy from mother to baby.

Symptoms and Diagnostic Path

Within three to 14 days of being bitten, about 80 percent of people infected with WNV have no symptoms at all. Most of the rest who become infected experience fever, headache, body aches, nausea, vomiting, and sometimes swollen lymph glands or a skin rash on the chest, stomach, and back. Symptoms can last for as short as a few days, though even healthy people have become sick for several weeks.

About one in 150 people infected with WNV will develop severe illness, with high fever, headache, stiff neck, stupor, disorientation, coma, tremors, convulsions, muscle weakness, vision loss, numbness, and paralysis. These symptoms may last several weeks, and neurological effects may be permanent. Some research suggests people with diabetes may be at higher risk for developing more serious symptoms.

Treatment Options and Outlook

There is no specific treatment for WNV infection. People with milder symptoms such as fever and aches will get better on their own, although even healthy people have become sick for several weeks. In more severe cases, people usually need to go to the hospital, where they can receive supportive treatment including intravenous fluids, help with breathing, and nursing care.

Risk Factors and Preventive Measures

People over age 50 are more likely to develop serious symptoms of WNV if they do get sick and should take special care to avoid mosquito bites. The more time people spend outdoors, the more likely they could be bitten by an infected mosquito.

All donated blood is checked for WNV before being used, and the risk of getting WNV through blood transfusions and organ transplants is very small.

To prevent being bitten by infected mosquitoes, people should:

- stay indoors at dawn, dusk, and in the early evening
- wear long-sleeved shirts and long pants outdoors
- spray clothing with repellents containing permethrin or DEET
- apply insect repellent sparingly to exposed skin. An effective repellent contains 35 percent DEET (higher concentrations provides no additional protection)

Although the vast majority of infections have been identified in birds, the virus can infect horses, cats, bats, chipmunks, skunks, squirrels, and domestic rabbits. While there is no evidence that a person can get the virus from handling live or dead infected birds, people should avoid bare-handed contact when handling any dead animals and use gloves or double plastic bags to place the carcass in a garbage can. Normal veterinary infection control precautions should be followed when caring for a horse suspected to have this or any viral infection.

Dead birds have proven to be a remarkably effective predictor of human outbreaks. Using a computer program originally developed in New York and Chicago, public-health experts can track West Nile with remarkable accuracy.

West Nile virus encephalitis Normally seen in the Middle East and some parts of Europe and Asia, the WEST NILE VIRUS can cause ENCEPHALITIS in some people.

The first outbreak of West Nile Virus encephalitis occurred in 1999 in the Western hemisphere, with 62 cases of human encephalitis or MENINGITIS and seven fatalities in New York City and adjacent Long Island and Westchester County. In addition, mosquitoes and more than 20 bird species were found to be infected with West Nile virus in New Jersey, Connecticut, New York State, and Maryland. In the hardest hit section of Queens, 2.5 percent of humans tested were found to have been infected with West Nile virus. Fatal infection was also seen in horses on Long Island.

The future impact of West Nile virus is uncertain. States on the eastern bird flyway have received federal funding to conduct monitoring activities and perform diagnostic assays. This effort will be expanded nationwide.

While all residents of areas where virus activity has been identified are at risk of getting West Nile encephalitis, people over age 50 are at highest risk of severe disease.

The virus, which normally circulates in birds and mosquitoes, crosses to humans who are bitten by an infected mosquito. The virus then multiplies in the person's blood and eventually crosses the blood-brain barrier to reach the brain. At this point, the virus interferes with normal central nervous system functioning and inflames brain tissue.

Symptoms and Diagnostic Path

Symptoms of West Nile encephalitis typically appear between five and 15 days after a mosquito bite and include headache, high fever, neck stiffness, muscle weakness. More severe infections may include disorientation, confusion, stupor, tremors, convulsions, paralysis, and coma. This infection is rarely fatal. Symptoms are most severe in the very young and the very old. The death rate is between 3 and 15 percent.

A sample of blood confirms the diagnosis.

Treatment Options and Outlook

Treatment is supportive and includes hospitalization, fluids, and breathing support. Severely ill patients may need to be hospitalized.

West Nile virus poliomyelitis An inflammation of the spinal cord that causes a syndrome similar to POLIOMYELITIS. This is a complication of infection with WEST NILE VIRUS. WNP causes a sudden onset of weakness in the limbs or breathing muscles, also called "acute flaccid paralysis."

West Nile poliomyelitis was first widely recognized in the United States in 2002, but experts do not know for sure how often West Nile poliomyelitis occurs, although it is clear that it occurs less often than MENINGITIS or ENCEPHALITIS.

Although most people with West Nile virus who have "acute flaccid paralysis" suffer from West Nile poliomyelitis, which is an inflammation of the spinal cord, some patients with the infection may instead develop an illness similar to Guillain-Barré syndrome, which is a disease of the peripheral nerves and not the spinal cord.

Symptoms and Diagnostic Path

Patients with West Nile poliomyelitis may develop sudden or rapidly progressing weakness affecting one side of the body more than the other, or sometimes involving only one limb. The weakness is generally not associated with any numbness or loss of sensation but may occur together with severe pain. In very severe cases, the virus affects nerves to the muscles that control breathing, which can cause a rapid respiratory failure. This weakness may occur without any sign of meningitis, encephalitis, fever, or even a headache, so that it may be hard to recognize that the weakness is due to WNV infection.

Weakness of the facial muscles may also develop in patients with WNV infection, but while many people with WNV infection experience fatigue and feel weak all over, this is not the same as acute flaccid paralysis.

Treatment Options and Outlook

Although there is no treatment for WNV infection itself, the person with severe disease often needs to be hospitalized. Care may involve IV fluids, respiratory support, and preventing secondary infections.

Some people recover completely, others recover partially, and there are still others who have not shown significant recovery after a year.

Risk Factors and Preventive Measures

People of any age can be affected by West Nile poliomyelitis, but those over age 65 are at highest risk for all forms of WNV neurological complications, including poliomyelitis. However younger people also can develop West Nile poliomyelitis. In fact, West Nile poliomyelitis may affect people who are otherwise healthy and without prior medical conditions.

Whipple's disease A rare intestinal disorder found most often among middle-aged men. People with the disease become severely malnourished. The cause is unknown, but is probably due to an unidentified bacterial infection.

Symptoms and Diagnostic Path

Onset of symptoms is slow, and include malabsorption, diarrhea, abdominal pain, progressive weight loss, joint pain, swollen lymph nodes, anemia, and fever, grey-brown skin, and memory loss.

The disease can be diagnosed with small bowel biopsy.

Treatment Options and Outlook

Antibiotics (PENICILLIN and tetracycline) should be given for at least one year, together with dietary supplements.

whipworm infestation (trichuriasis) Whipworms are parasitic roundworms of the species *Trichuris trichiura* that infect the intestinal tract. Adults worms are 30 to 50 mm long and look somewhat like a whip. The eggs are remarkably hardy and may resist freezing; they can remain alive in the environment for years. Infestation is not common in the United States but occurs in 700 to 800 million people in other parts of the world.

Whipworm infection occurs when a person comes in contact with and ingests whipworm eggs in fecal-contaminated soil. Whipworms are small worms about one or two inches long that can live in the intestines for up to 20 years. The eggs hatch, and the whipworm embeds itself into the mucous membrane. While the worms live in the large intestine (predominantly in the cecum) and appendix, they may infest the colon as well.

Symptoms and Diagnostic Path

Light infestation causes few symptoms, but a heavier worm load may cause bloody diarrhea that appears to contain mucus.

Examination of stool can reveal the presence of whipworm eggs.

Treatment Options and Outlook

Mebendazole can kill the worms, although a serious case may require more than one treatment.

In very severe cases, dehydration and anemia can occur as a result of the bloody diarrhea. Rarely, rectal prolapse can occur.

Risk Factors and Preventive Measures

Good public health practices, including covered sewers and safe garbage disposal, can reduce the incidence of whipworms.

Whitmore's disease The common name for melioidosis, an uncommon bacterial infection of rodents. It is caused by *Pseudomonas pseudomallei,* which is endemic in southeast Asia and Australia.

The disease is also found in pigs, cattle, sheep, and horses. The exact mode of transmission in unknown, but it is thought to be acquired by humans through breathing in the bacteria or through contact with broken skin. The bacteria are also found in soil and water (especially rice paddies).

Symptoms and Diagnostic Path

The exact incubation period is not known; it may be months or years. There may be no symptoms at all. If there are, in humans, the disease takes three forms—an acute septicemic (blood poisoning) with diarrhea; a typhoidal form with local ABSCESS formation and severe hives; and a chronic form.

Treatment Options and Outlook

Abscesses must be surgically drained; antibiotics are administered (tetracycline with chloramphenicol, piperacillin, gentamicin, or doxycycline).

whooping cough The common name for "pertussis," an acute infection of the upper respiratory tract featuring violent, loud bouts of coughing that end in a whoop. Vomiting usually occurs at the end of the coughing spell. Most serious in young children, whooping cough is highly contagious and will infect virtually all susceptible people who come in contact with the bacterium. It can lead to seizures, PNEUMONIA, brain damage, and death.

Before the vaccine was available in the 1940s, about 200,000 children were sickened each year, and about 8,000 died. Because the disease can be deadly in infants, babies should be isolated from anyone with whooping cough.

Although the number of cases has declined since the introduction of the vaccine, the disease is far from eradicated. In 2002, there were nearly 10,000 cases and 18 deaths, up from 1,900 cases of whooping cough, in 2000 with 16 deaths.

Often considered to be a childhood disease, 28 percent of whooping cough cases in the United States occur in adults. Although most Americans were vaccinated against whooping cough as children, the older vaccine only gives protection for less than 10 years. A new safe and effective whooping cough vaccine is now available to prevent adults from contracting this disease.

New guidelines released in January 2006 by the American College of Chest Physicians strongly recommend that adults up to age 65 receive a new adult vaccine for whooping cough. Because antibiotics are only effective early on in the infection, preventing whooping cough with a vaccine is the only way to eventually eliminate the disease.

Whooping cough affects people of all ages all over the world, and is a common cause of death in the developing countries. The disease is most serious in babies, who may often develop pneumonia; babies younger than three months of age get the worst cases. Seventy percent of deaths occur in young babies (about one in 200 infected babies will die).

Doctors must report any suspected or confirmed cases of whooping cough to the health department. If the child attends school or child care, the parent must notify the principal so staff and other children can be given preventive medicine.

The disease is caused by a rodshaped bacterium called *BORDETELLA PERTUSSIS*, which produces a toxin that invades the lining of the throat, windpipe, and bronchial tubes. The tissue damage causes very thick mucus production that is irritating, leading to severe coughing spells as the victim tries to expel the mucus. The thick mucus often leads to pneumonia. A similar but less common bacterium called *B. parapertussis* may cause a milder form of the disease.

The disease is spread during coughing, which spews the bacteria outward for several feet. These bacteria can survive on tissue or bed covers for a short time; the disease can also be passed on when another person touches these items. Whooping cough is infectious enough so that it will be spread to everyone in the household from one infected patient.

Symptoms and Diagnostic Path

The most infectious time is at the beginning of the illness. Whooping cough occurs in three stages in children; the first stage starts slowly with coldlike symptoms (sneezing, red or sore eyes, and a low-grade fever) and an irritating dry cough for one or two weeks. This is the period when the patient is most infectious.

These initial symptoms are followed by intense, violent spasms of repeated coughing with no time to breathe between spasms. There is a repetitive series of eight or 10 rapid coughs on one breath that often end in gagging or vomiting. The coughs may end in a characteristic "whoop" as the patient tries to take a breath. (Babies under six months of age will choke but will not make the whooping sound; these youngest patients can become very sick.) The infected person may appear blue, with bulging eyes and a dazed, apathetic expression. Infants may experience temporary apnea (cessation of breathing) after a coughing spasm. The periods between coughing are comfortable; there is little fever. This stage may last about two weeks.

The final stage dwindles down into a chronic cough for three to four weeks; some children experience a cough of more than two months.

Adults can get whooping cough, although there is not usually a whoop and the cough is milder. Public health experts suggest that whooping cough should be suspected in anyone who has a cough lasting more than seven days. Some adults may be infected without symptoms; these adults are capable of spreading the disease to children.

The disease is diagnosed by identifying the bacterium in a culture grown from a nasal swab taken in the early stages of the illness. There are two tests, neither of which is 100 percent accurate, and there are many false negatives. The rapid test gives results in a few minutes; a blood test done in mid-disease may identify the bacterium or detect antibodies.

Treatment Options and Outlook

If the illness is recognized early enough, antibiotics such as erythromycin or clarithromycin are often given; they may shorten the duration of illness and the period of contagiousness, although they are not particularly helpful once the severe coughing stage of the illness has begun.

Patients should be kept warm, given small, frequent meals and plenty to drink and protected from things that produce coughing (such as drafts or smoke). An infant or child who becomes blue or keeps vomiting after coughing needs to be admitted to the hospital.

Once whooping cough takes hold, the coughing patient is at risk of serious complications from coughing, such as vomiting, breaking ribs, passing out, and passing the infection on to others. Children with the infection can develop ear infections or pneumonia. One in 500 infants under age six months may experience seizures, brain damage, and coma.

Risk Factors and Preventive Measures

In the past, the pertussis vaccine was usually given as part of the DTP (diphtheria-tetanus-pertussis) vaccine in infancy and childhood to prevent the disease for children at two, four, and six months of age in the United States. A booster dose was given at age five.

This pertussis vaccine was made from killed whole pertussis cells or a whole bacterium. While some babies had no side effects after whole cell pertussis immunization, about half suffered from swelling and pain in the arm, fever, crankiness, drowsiness, or poor appetite for a day or two after the shot.

The pertussis part of the DTP vaccine was controversial because some parents and scientists believed a few children developed more serious side effects, including seizures, brain damage, or death. Very rarely (about one in every 100,000) a baby had a severe reaction with high-pitched screaming or seizures. About one in 300,000 suffered permanent brain damage.

An improved vaccine called DTaP was introduced in 1997. This vaccine uses only the parts of the bacteria that help children develop immunity, and leaves behind the parts that may have been responsible for the harmful side effects of the old DTP vaccine. (The "a" in DTaP stands for "acellular," which means there are no whole bacteria in the vaccine.) The DTaP is about 10 times less likely to cause adverse reactions such as fever, vomiting, and mild seizures. The DTaP has dramatically reduced the rate of high fever (one or two in 35,000) and seizure (0 percent).

Further improvements were introduced on March 7, 2001, when the U.S. Food and Drug Administration (FDA) approved a new version of the DTaP vaccine—this one without preservatives and with only a trace amount of thimerosal. This approval is significant because now all routinely recommended pediatric vaccines are available as either completely thimerosal-free or without any significant amounts of thimerosal, a preservative that contains mercury. Although thimerosal is a very effective preservative, the Public Health Service recommended that thimerosal should be reduced or eliminated from vaccines as soon as possible to minimize the exposure of infants and young children to mercury.

The new vaccine now contains less than 0.5 micrograms of mercury per dose—more than a 95 percent reduction in the amount of thimerosal per dose compared to the original version. The pediatric vaccines that are recommended for routine use are: DTaP, hepatitis B, Haemophilus conjugate (Hib), pneumococcal conjugate, inactivated poliovirus, varicella, measles, mumps, and rubella. Since 1999, pediatric formulations of hepatitis B vaccines that either contain no thimerosal (Recombivax HB) or trace amounts (EngerixB) have been approved.

Mercury is found in the environment, in food, and in household products. Although no harmful effects have been reported from thimerosal at doses that were used in vaccines, the government, the American Academy of Pediatrics, and vaccine manufacturers agreed that thimerosal should be reduced or eliminated in vaccines to make already safe vaccines even safer.

The DTaP shots are given at a baby's two-, four-, six-, and 12- or 18-month checkups, and then again when the child is four to six years old. At 11 or 12 years of age and every 10 years after that, a child should get a booster shot to prevent diphtheria and tetanus.

If a child has had a severe reaction to either the DTP or the DTaP, including difficulty breathing, hives, fainting, high fever, or seizure, the child should not receive another dose of the DTaP vaccine. Children also should avoid the DTaP if they have had any swelling of the brain within seven days of any vaccination not known to be due to another cause.

Children who are moderately to severely ill at the time the vaccine is scheduled should probably wait until they recover before getting the shot.

Boostrix is a new whooping cough vaccine that also protects against tetanus and diphtheria for teens between 10 and 18. Boostrix, or Tdap, includes the tetanus toxoid (T), reduced diphtheria toxoid (d), and acellular pertussis (ap) vaccine in a single shot. The Boostrix replaces the tetanus booster (Td).

Other patients who should not be given further doses of the vaccine include those who, after initial vaccination have had persistent uncontrollable crying for more than three hours, a fever higher than 105°F not caused by another illness, or collapse *unless* there is a serious outbreak in the patient's area.

If the percentage of vaccinated children drops significantly (as it did in the United Kingdom in the 1970s), the number of children who contract the disease skyrockets. Because the illness is potentially deadly, it is important that all infants suitable for vaccination be treated. The risks of vaccination are far less than the dangers of having whooping cough.

worms   See HELMINTH.

wound care   For skin to heal best, it is essential to keep the wound clean and protected. As many as 72 percent of Americans care for wounds and scrapes incorrectly. Contrary to popular belief, wounds to not need to "air out" and form a scab in order to heal. Patients should clean the cut, and protect it with a simple bandage.

yaws One of the world's most prevalent infections, this childhood skin disease is found throughout the poorer subtropical and tropical areas of the world. Also known as frambesia, pian, or bouba, yaws is not a SEXUALLY TRANSMITTED DISEASE. It occurs between the tropics of Cancer and Capricorn, where more than 50 million people have been treated with PENICILLIN in an effort to eradicate the disease. As a result, the incidence of the disease has dropped in many areas, although it still occurs in many communities.

The disease is not believed to have been known in the ancient world. It was first noted in the West Indies after the discovery of America; it is believed that was brought from Africa to America by the slave trade. It is very rare in India, and it is almost unknown in Europe, Japan, New Zealand, and Tasmania.

Yaws is caused by the spirochete *Treponema pertenue*, a close cousin of *T. pallidum*, the spirochete that causes SYPHILIS. The relationship between the two diseases is not clear. However, unlike syphilis, yaws appears to be acquired by direct contact with an infected person, not by sexual intercourse.

Symptoms and Diagnostic Path

While not a fatal disease, yaws is very disfiguring and often disabling. About a month after infection, symptoms of malaise, low fever, and headache appear. In the primary stage, a highly contagious, itchy red raspberry-like growth appears on the site of the infection. In places where people regularly go barelegged and barefoot, these growths usually appear on the soles of the feet and the lower legs. Scratching spreads the infection, leading to development of more growths on other parts of the skin.

During the next few weeks, the growths develop into blisters, which begin to ooze and then form a crust. Sores then develop. The nearby lymph glands may become swollen, and the joints and bones may ache. There may be an irregular fever. The initial sores may disappear with no other problems except for scarring. More typically, they last for several months.

The secondary stage is the most infectious, usually developing three months after onset of the disease. At this point, areas of rash and sores appear all over the body; as some sores disappear (leaving discolored patches), others enlarge and develop into nodules. These lesions are usually painless (except on the soles of the feet), but they may be very itchy. This stage lasts for three to six months in children, and from six months to a year in adults.

The tertiary stage—characterized by the destruction of large areas of the bones, nose, and joints by the ulcers—may last for years, but it does not always occur.

Treatment Options and Outlook

A single dose of penicillin will cure this disease. Without treatment, growths heal slowly over about six months, but recurrence is common. About 10 percent of untreated patients experience the tertiary stage.

Risk Factors and Preventive Measures

There is no way to prevent yaws, but in places where the disease is widespread, proper care of injuries or wounds will lessen the chance of contracting the disease.

yeast infection A skin infection caused by types of FUNGI, the most important of which is *CANDIDA ALBICANS*, which causes CANDIDIASIS. *Candida* can normally be found in the mouth, vagina, and large intestine, but for unknown reasons it can sometimes turn against its host—most commonly in those who take antibiotics, oral steroids, and birth control pills, and in diabetics and the overweight. This type of yeast causes THRUSH (white patches on the inside of the cheeks), cheesy vaginal discharge, or monilial intertrigo (damp red eruptions under the breasts, the foreskin, and under body folds in the obese). It also causes *Candida* paronychia (redness and swelling around the nails).

Candidal infections usually respond to topical broad-spectrum antibiotics or specific preparations designed to fight yeasts (nystatin).

See also VAGINAL YEAST INFECTIONS.

yellow fever A short-acting infectious viral disease that gets its name from its symptom of yellowed skin. The three varieties of yellow fever include urban, jungle, and sylvan, and can range from mild to fatal. In general, the disease is a risk only for those who travel to sub-Saharan Africa or tropical South America. Eradication of the mosquito from populated areas has greatly reduced the incidence of the disease. It is fatal only about 5 percent of the time.

Still, EPIDEMICS of yellow fever can occur when large numbers of susceptible humans and infected mosquitoes coexist. The disease has been known since the time of the first explorations of Africa; every few years since, many thousands of Africans have gotten yellow fever, and as many as half of those infected will die. Nigerian epidemics between 1986 and 1988 killed 10,000 people.

Epidemics of yellow fever end when the dry season comes and the mosquitoes who carry the virus become less abundant. Epidemics have also ended when the surviving human population becomes immune, either through infection or mass vaccination.

The disease was considered to be the American PLAGUE, profoundly affecting the development of the New World in the wake of Columbus's arrival. After his visit, the yellow fever virus helped to exterminate entire civilizations on the new continent. Dreadful epidemics in coastal cities such as Philadelphia, New Orleans, and Charleston were devastating to the new settlers as well as the native American populations. In 1793, Philadelphia was struck by a severe yellow fever outbreak that was to kill 4,000 of its citizens (15 percent of the total population of the city) in three months. The outbreak, which was blamed on German and Haitian immigrants, virtually brought the city to a standstill and was one reason why the former great seaport dropped behind New York City in maritime importance.

In the late 19th century, the origin of the disease was discovered to be the AEDES mosquito, which explained why it was not contagious and why it occurred only during the summer months. The fact that port cities faced the most severe epidemics helps support the theory that ships transported the mosquitoes to the United States. Moreover, the mosquitoes' inability to fly over great distances limited the spread of the disease.

The virus was identified by Adrian Stokes in 1927 at the Rockefeller Foundation's Yellow Fever Research Institute in Lagos, Nigeria. Dr. Stokes was one of four Foundation scientists who died of laboratory infections with yellow fever virus while working at the institute (two others died in labs in Mexico and Brazil).

The yellow fever virus is included in a group of viruses called flavivirus (from the Latin word *flavus*, meaning "yellow"). This is the same group of viruses that contains St. Louis and Japanese ENCEPHALITIS. There is no difference in the way the three types of yellow fever (urban, jungle, and sylvan) affect victims; the three types differ only in their natural cycles.

Yellow fever virus mostly infects monkeys and mosquitoes, although it sometimes is transmitted via monkeys, who pass it on to humans. In cities ("urban yellow fever"), the disease is transmitted between humans by *Aedes aegypti* mosquitoes. This mosquito is found in the southeastern United States, but no disease has been reported since 1905 in New Orleans. However, the potential for the disease to spread in this country remains.

Most yellow fever is of the *jungle* type, which is transmitted to monkeys in Africa by forest mosquitoes. Countries reporting cases in 1995 include Angola, Cameroon, Gabon, Gambia, Ghana, Guinea, Mali, Nigeria, Sudan, Zaire, Bolivia, Brazil, Colombia, Ecuador, and Peru and West Africa.

Sylvan yellow fever is transmitted to forest monkeys in South America by treetop-living species of mosquitoes (not *Aedes*) that only bite humans when giant trees, are cut down, bringing the mosquitoes down to ground level.

While people cannot directly transmit the disease to other humans, mosquitoes can be infected from just before symptoms appear to about five days into the illness. The infected mosquitoes remain infectious for their entire life span. For these reasons, patients should be isolated and standard blood and body fluid precautions should be taken by caregivers.

Major epidemics can reappear in towns and cities that do not control the mosquitoes. In the forests, the virus cycle is carried by forest mosquitoes to monkeys. When monkey populations increase, there are more nonimmune monkeys, and the virus spreads among them. In addition, as the monkey populations increase, more of them venture into farmers' fields, where other mosquitoes become infected and they in turn infect farmers.

Symptoms and Diagnostic Path

Many people have no symptoms; some have a mild illness, and a few (about 5 percent of those infected) become very sick and die. In those who have symptoms, between three and six days after infection there is a sudden fever and headache, backache, nausea, and vomiting. Characteristic signs are slow pulse as temperature rises and albumin in the urine; in those with serious disease, those signs progress to nosebleeds, bleeding from the mouth, dark vomit due to blood in the stomach, and black stool due to digested blood.

In most people, these symptoms pass in about three days; others experience neck, back, and leg pain; fever; chills; weakness; restlessness; and irritability.

Most people recover because their immune systems are able to fight off the disease and develop antibodies that destroy the virus. Recovery in these cases is slow but complete, without permanent damage. One episode of yellow fever provides lifetime immunity. Yellow fever is diagnosed by high levels of albumin in urine; low levels of white blood cells; antibodies to the virus in blood samples is conclusive.

Treatment Options and Outlook

No drug is effective against the yellow fever virus, so treatment is aimed at lowering fever, maintaining blood volume via transfusion of fluids and avoiding liver damage. In mild or moderate cases the prognosis is excellent: up to 95 percent of patients will survive.

Some patients begin to feel better but then, after three to nine days progress to the second stage of yellow fever, including liver and kidney damage, jaundice and kidney failure, and agitation. The gums bleed, vomit contains blood, stools turn black, and skin and eyes become yellow tinged. Some cases proceed to delirium, coma, and death.

Risk Factors and Preventive Measures

Vaccination confers long-lasting immunity and should always be obtained before traveling through affected areas. Although the vaccination is effective for life, international regulations require revaccinations every 10 years. The vaccine is effective beginning 10 days after the first dose. The yellow fever vaccine is given only at approved yellow fever vaccination centers.

Reactions to the vaccine are usually mild. Between two and five percent of vaccinated patients have mild headaches, low-grade fevers, or other minor symptoms between five and 10 days later. Immediate hypersensitivity reactions (including rash, hives, or asthma) are extremely uncommon (less than one in a million). They occur primarily in those with egg allergies.

However, scientists are questioning the safety of the 60-year-old vaccine after six suspicious deaths have been linked to the shot. The deaths of three Americans, two Brazilians, and an Australian after vaccination are the first deaths that may have been linked to the vaccine virus. Still, experts strongly recommend travelers to South America and Africa should continue to get the shots.

The vaccine, which has been given to about 400 million people, has always been considered one of the safest. Now researchers suspect that other deaths over the years may have gone unnoticed. Still, severe reactions are very rare, and yellow fever causes about a thousand times more illness and death than does EBOLA virus.

The vaccine uses an altered, but still live virus, which gives people a mild form of the disease. If vaccinated people are later exposed to the virus, the immune system recognizes it and attacks. It now appears that a few people can get very sick from the vaccine itself, which may be linked to a genetic weakness.

The symptoms in people having a severe reaction are typical of yellow fever, including vomiting, fever, muscle pain, jaundice, and kidney failure.

A yellow fever vaccination certificate is required to enter to many countries. Travel plans that include visits to any country in Africa or South America require a yellow fever vaccination and certificate before leaving the United States.

Countries where yellow fever is reported are listed every two weeks in the Summary of Health Information for International Travel ("the blue sheet"), available 24 hours a day from the Centers for Disease Control (CDC) Fax Information Service for International Travelers or by calling the CDC international travelers' hot line at (404) 332-4559. The blue sheet is also available from state or local health departments. In Canada, information can be found at the Tropical Health and Quarantine Division at the Laboratory Center for Disease Control at (613) 957-8739 or fax (613) 998-6413.

All those who cannot be vaccinated for medical reasons must obtain a medical waiver instead of the yellow fever certificate. This will include a doctor's letter stating the reasons against the vaccine; the waiver is obtained from the consular or embassy officials of the country to be visited before leaving the United States. Those medical reasons include infants under six months of age, pregnant women, people hypersensitive to eggs, or patients with an immunosuppressed condition associated with AIDS or HIV infection, or those whose immune system has been altered by either diseases such as leukemia and lymphoma or through drugs and radiation. People with HIV infection but who do not have symptoms may be vaccinated if exposure to yellow fever cannot be avoided.

The World Health Organization must be notified within 24 hours about new cases of yellow fever in areas previously free of the disease, including cases in monkeys.

Yersinia enterocolitica   A member of the *Yersinia* genus of small bacteria that cause enterocolitis and other diseases.

See also YERSINIOSIS.

Yersinia (Pasteurella) pestis   A small gram-negative bacterium that causes PLAGUE, transmitted from rodents to humans usually via the flea *Y. pestis* can live for a long period of time in infected carcasses, soil, or sputum. It is also known as *Pasteurella pestis.* It is named for the 19th-century French bacteriologist Alexandre E. J. Yersin.

See also YERSINIOSIS.

Yersinia pseudotuberculosis   A member of the *Yersinia* genus of bacteria that causes pseudotuberculosis.

yersiniosis   A common but underreported foodborne illness caused by the *Yersinia* bacteria that was first recognized in the United States in 1976, where it was traced to tainted chocolate milk. Infants and children are the most common victims; children with abnormally high iron levels in their blood are particularly susceptible.

While it can occur at any time, most cases appear during the winter in North America.

The disease is caused by eating tainted food or touching sick pets or contaminated people. The illness is caused by two species of rod-shaped bacteria, *YERSINIA ENTEROCOLITICA* and *YERSINIA PSEUDOTUBERCULOSIS* both of which are related to *YERSINIA PESTIS* (the bacterium that causes human PLAGUE). All three belong to the family Enterobacteriacae (which also includes *SALMONELLA*). The bacteria are found in swine and swine waste, cows, dogs, cats (especially those from animal shelters), poultry, shellfish, ice cream, fruit, and vegetables, but most outbreaks are traced to chocolate milk, milk, mussels, oysters, tofu, pork, and contaminated water.

Because the bacteria can grow even when refrigerated, high-risk foods include undercooked pork, beef that has been vacuum packed or fresh packed, unpasteurized milk, and cheese.

Outbreaks are fairly common among day-care centers. Infected pups and kittens can infect small children. The water from untreated wells, lakes, rivers, and streams may also be a source for the disease.

Symptoms and Diagnostic Path

Symptoms include high fever (up to 104°F), nausea and vomiting, bloody or mucousy diarrhea, abdominal pain (similar to appendicitis pain). Yersiniosis is often misdiagnosed as appendicitis. Children may be quite ill and may also suffer headache, sore throat, and loss of appetite. Symptoms usually last up to 10 days, although some children may be ill for a month. It is almost never fatal, however.

Some women experience a painful skin rash on the front of the legs. The bacteria may remain in the stool for up to three months afterward.

Stool culture is the best test, although yersiniosis is not easy to diagnose. Blood tests may detect antibodies a few weeks after the illness appears.

Treatment Options and Outlook

Antibiotics are effective and should be taken up to seven days; serious illness may require hospitalization and administration of intravenous medication. Analysis of stool samples can determine which antibiotic to use.

Bone or bloodstream infection, or MENINGITIS, may follow yersinosis, but these are rare except in the very old or those with weakened immune systems.

Risk Factors and Preventive Measures

If yersiniosis is suspected, the health department should be contacted. Any cases with these symptoms at a child-care center should prompt an investigation to determine if others have a similar illness.

APPENDIXES

APPENDIX I
DRUGS USED TO TREAT INFECTIOUS DISEASES

acetaminophen (Trade names: Tylenol, Datril, Temora, Volatile) Over-the-counter painkiller and fever reducer used in many nonprescription pain relievers. Often prescribed for mild to moderate pain or fever, it is not effective in treating inflammation.

Side Effects
Overdose can cause fatal liver problems.

acyclovir (Trade name: Zovirax) An antiviral drug prescribed for the treatment of herpes simplex, shingles, and chicken pox that is available in oral or topical form. Acyclovir works by inhibiting the synthesis of DNA in cells infected by herpes viruses. The drug also has been helpful to patients receiving bone marrow transplants to prevent the subsequent development of herpes simplex infection.

Acyclovir is effective in managing both initial and recurrent infections of herpes and localized shingles. It can prevent subsequent herpes attacks if taken continuously soon after infection. However, in cases of recurrent genital herpes, acyclovir therapy does not make the lesions heal quicker or ease symptoms.

The topical form does not prevent new herpes lesions from forming during the course of the disease. When applied to an existing blister, however, it may relieve symptoms, speed healing, and shorten the duration of the infection and the contagious period.

Side Effects
Adverse effects are rare. The ointment may cause skin irritation or rash. Taken by mouth, the drug may cause headache, dizziness, nausea/vomiting. Rarely, acyclovir injections may lead to kidney damage.

adenosine monophosphate (AMP) A compound containing adenine, ribose, and one phosphate group (AMP), this metabolism byproduct seems to help ease the pain of shingles. The treatment has no side effects and works best within the first few months of pain, when the nerve endings have experienced minimal damage.

amantadine hydrochloride (Trade names: Symmetrel, Symadine) An antiviral drug that is prescribed to prevent and (in the early stages) to treat type-A influenza virus. It is believed to act by preventing a virus from penetrating into the host's cells.

Side Effects
Among the most serious adverse effects are central nervous system effects; nervousness, blurred vision, and slurred speech also may occur. The drug should be used with caution in patients with congestive heart failure or during pregnancy and breast-feeding.

amikacin Antibiotic used to treat serious infections, including bacterial septicemia; burns; and infections of the respiratory tract, bone and joints, central nervous system, skin, soft tissue, urinary tract, and abdomen.

Side Effects
This drug may cause kidney failure that is usually reversible. There may occasionally be damage to hearing.

amoxicillin (Trade names: Amoxil, Moxilin, Wymox) A semisynthetic oral penicillin antibiotic, similar to ampicillin. This broad-spectrum antibiotic is prescribed in the treatment of infections caused by gram-positive and gram-negative bacteria, including bronchitis, cystitis, gonorrhea, and ear and skin infections.

Side Effects

Side effects include nausea and diarrhea; allergic reactions include rash, fever, swelling of the mouth, itching, and breathing problems.

amphotericin B (Trade name: Fungizone)   An antibiotic drug used to treat deep fungal infections of the skin, available as drops, lotion, or cream. It is inactive against both bacteria and viruses. While it can be given by mouth, it is given by intravenous injection to treat serious systemic infections such as cryptococcosis and histoplasmosis. This drug is usually administered in a hospital setting.

Side Effects

Adverse effects are likely only when given as injection; these side effects may include muscle pains, vomiting, fever, headache, or (rarely) seizures. There is also a risk of kidney damage.

ampicillin (Trade names: Amcill, Omnipen, Polycillin, Principen)   A penicillin-type semisynthetic antibiotic used to treat conditions caused by a broad spectrum of gram-negative and gram-positive organisms in the urinary, respiratory, biliary, and intestinal tracts. Some of these conditions include cystitis, bronchitis, gonorrhea, typhoid fever, and ear and eye infections. It is inactivated by penicillinase, and therefore cannot be used against organisms that produce this enzyme.

Side Effects

Symptoms include nausea, vomiting, fever, or diarrhea. Allergic reactions may include symptoms of rash, diarrhea, and (rarely) fever; swelling of the mouth and tongue; itching; and breathing problems.

azidothymidine (AZT)   See ZIDOVUDINE.

azithromycin (Trade name: Zithromax)   Antibiotic used to treat exacerbations of chronic obstructive pulmonary disease; tonsillitis or sore throat; infections of the skin, urethra, and cervix; community-acquired pneumonia; acute middle ear infection, bronchitis; Legionnaires' disease; and acute sinusitis.

Side Effects

There may be stomach upset, diarrhea, nausea, abdominal pain, vaginitis, and reversible hearing loss.

AZT   See ZIDOVUDINE.

bacitracin (Trade name: Bacitracin, Bactine Triple Antibiotic)   An antibiotic contained in many over-the-counter antibiotics that is used to treat minor cuts, scrapes, and burns. It is often used for topical treatment of wounds, although most experts are unconvinced that topical antibiotics can promote wound healing, prevent infection, or treat infection effectively.

Side Effects

Allergic reactions may occur with use of this medication.

benethamine penicillin   An antibiotic that is effective against most gram-positive bacteria, such as streptococci, staphylococci, and pneumococci. This drug is a derivative of benzylpenicillin and can be administered by mouth, although it is usually given as an intramuscular injection.

Side Effects

As with all penicillins, allergic reactions are common.

benzathine penicillin G (Trade names: Bicillin, Permapen)   Long-acting antibiotic given by mouth or injection that is slowly absorbed and effective against most gram-positive bacteria, including streptococci, staphylococci, and pneumococci.
    See also PENICILLIN.

Side Effects

As with all penicillins, allergic reactions are fairly common.

benzoyl peroxide   An antibacterial agent that is extremely effective in suppressing the bacterium *Propionibacterium acnes,* associated with acne. Probably the most popular of the over-the-counter products, it draws the peroxide into the pore where it releases oxygen, killing the bacteria that can aggravate acne. Benzoyl also suppresses fatty acid cells that irritate pores. It is most effective for patients with inflammatory acne; by inhibiting bacteria, it decreases the inflammatory components in the skin. Benzoyl peroxide is sold in strengths ranging between 5 to 10 percent, but the lower concentration is just as effective and less likely to cause irritation. Most over-the-counter products contain benzoyl peroxide in a lotion base; prescription products contain the chemical in a gel base. A fairly new preparation combining 3 percent erythromycin with 5 percent benzoyl peroxide in a gel base may be more effective than either component by itself.

Side Effects

Some irritation may follow use with benzoyl peroxide, and allergic sensitization has occasionally occurred. *Benzoyl peroxide is closely related to products containing vitamin A (such as Retin-A and Accutane) and they should not be used together.*

bleomycin (Trade name: Blenoxane)   An antibiotic obtained from a soil fungus, bleomycin is effective in treating warts that have not responded to other treatment. It is administered by injection.

Side Effects

Bleomycin can cause toxic side effects in skin and lungs and should not be used with patients who have problems with kidney function or lung disease. Other side effects include localized swelling and the development of pneumonitis or rash.

butoconazole nitrate (Trade name: Femstat)   An antifungal drug derived from imidazole, used to treat vaginal mycotic infections caused by *Candida* species. Pregnant women should use the drug only in the second and third trimesters.

Side Effects

Rarely, side effects include burning or itching.

capsaicin (Trade name: Zostrix)   An ointment used to ease the pain of shingles. Its active ingredient is capsaicin, a red pepper derivative used to make chili powder. *Zostrix should be used only after all blisters have disappeared.* Capsaicin blocks the production of a chemical necessary for pain impulse transmission between nerve cells. It also has been tested as a treatment for psoriasis; however, it has been approved so far by the Food and Drug Administration only for use with shingles.

Side Effects

As a counter-irritant, Zostrix should be used only on patients with unbroken skin still experiencing pain from shingles, not for those with open, oozing infections. Zostrix does burn, and it will not be effective unless used often and continuously for three weeks. However, the burning lessens or vanishes if treatments are continued.

caspofungin acetate (Cancidas)   The first in a family of antifungal medications called echinocandins that work by attacking fungal cell walls. Cancidas has been approved to treat aspergillosis infections in seriously ill immune-compromised patients for whom other treatments have failed. Cancidas is not a first-line treatment for newly-diagnosed patients, nor should it be used together with cyclosporin, a common drug given to transplant recipients.

Side Effects

The most common side effects were fever, infused vein complications, nausea, flushing, and vomiting.

cefaclor (Trade name: Ceclor)   A common cephalosporin-type antibiotic used to treat ear infections, upper and lower respiratory-tract infections, urinary tract infections, skin infections, pharyngitis (sore throat), and tonsillitis. Given by mouth, the drug should be used with caution in patients who are allergic to penicillin.

Side Effects

Severe diarrhea, nausea and vomiting, or skin eruptions.

cefadroxil monohydrate (Trade names: Duricef, Ultracef)   A cephalosporin antibiotic used to treat certain bacterial infections, including urinary tract infections, skin infections, sore throat, and tonsillitis. Given by mouth, it is administered with caution to patients who have a history of allergy to penicillin.

Side Effects

Symptoms include allergic reactions, generalized itching, severe diarrhea, and nausea and vomiting.

cefazolin sodium (Trade name: Ancef; Kefzol)   A cephalosporin antibiotic used to treat certain bacterial infections, including respiratory, urinary tract, skin, biliary, bone, joint, and genital infections, and septicemia ("blood poisoning"). It is administered with caution to patients with a history of allergy to penicillin.

Side Effects

Side effects include severe diarrhea, nausea, and vomiting.

cefepime (Trade name: Maxipime)   A cephalosporin antibiotic used to treat pneumonia, cellulitis, bronchitis, and infections of the abdomen, skin, and urinary tract.

Side Effects

This drug may cause phlebitis at the infusion site, diarrhea, and, rarely, fever and encephalopathy.

cefotaxime sodium (Trade name: Claforan)   A cephalosporin antibiotic used to treat lower respiratory tract, genitourinary, gynecologic, intra-abdominal, skin, bone, and joint infections and septicemia. Intravenous route only.

Side Effects

Itching, colitis, and fungal infections.

cefixime (Trade name: Suprax)   A cephalosporin antibiotic is used to treat gonococcal infection, middle ear infection, and infections of the respiratory tract and urinary tract.

Side Effects

This drug may cause diarrhea and nausea, and occasionally lead to allergic reactions and colitis.

cefoxitin sodium (Trade name: Mefoxin)   A cephalosporin antibiotic used to treat certain bacterial infections. It should be administered with caution to patients allergic to penicillin or other cephalosporins. Intravenous route only.

Side Effects

Allergic reactions, phlebitis, and pain at the injection site.

ceftazidime (Trade names: Ceptaz, Fortaz, Pentacef, Tazicef, Tazidime)   A cephalosporin-type of antibiotic used to treat infections of the lower respiratory tract, urinary tract, skin, abdomen, blood, bones and joints, and the central nervous system. It should not be used for anyone allergic to cephalosporin antibiotics, and should be used with caution in those allergic to penicillin.

Side Effects

Side effects include itching, fever, skin rash, diarrhea, or phlebitis.

ceftriaxone (Trade name: Rocephin)   A cephalosporin-type broad-spectrum antibiotic prescribed for infections of the lower respiratory tract, urinary tract, skin, abdomen, bones, joints, and the central nervous system. It is used to treat gonorrhea, septicemia, and meningitis, and is administered as an IV or intramuscular injection.

Side Effects

This drug is usually well tolerated. Occasionally, side effects may include local pain at the injection site, allergic reaction (rash, itching, fever, or chills), blood problems, gastrointestinal problems, headache, or dizziness.

cephalexin (Trade names: Keflex, Biocef, Cephalexin)   A cephalosporin antibacterial prescribed orally to treat certain infections, including respiratory tract, skin, bone, and ear infections.

Side Effects

Side effects include nausea, diarrhea, and allergic reactions.

chloramphenicol (Trade names: Chloromycetin, Chloroptic)   An antibiotic and antirickettsial drug derived from the bacterium *Streptomyces venezuelae* (and that is also produced synthetically). It is effective against a wide variety of microorganisms. Because of its severe side effects, it is usually reserved for serious infections (such as typhoid fever), when less toxic drugs are not effective. It should not be given to pregnant or breastfeeding women or to anyone with only a mild infection.

Side Effects

The most serious side effect of this medication is the potential damage to bone marrow.

chlorhexidine (Trade name: Hibiclens)   An antimicrobial agent used as a surgical scrub, hand rinse, and topical antiseptic. It is used in solution, creams, gels, and lozenges and in some preparations combined with cetrimide. In very dilute solutions, it can be used as a mouthwash to control mouth infections.

Side Effects

Rarely, a skin sensitivity to this product can develop.

chloroquine (Trade name: Aralen)   An antimalarial drug prescribed to treat malaria and amebiasis

and certain skin conditions (such as lupus erythematosus). It is administered by mouth or injection.

Side Effects

Side effects include gastrointestinal problems, headache, visual disturbances, and itching. Those with retina or visual problems or porphyria should not use this drug. Long-term use can lead to eye damage.

chlorproguanil   A drug administered by mouth to prevent or treat malaria.

Side Effects

Rarely, large doses may cause stomach discomfort and vomiting.

ciclopirox olamine (Trade name: Loprox)   A broad-spectrum, topical agent used to treat fungus infections such as ringworm by inhibiting the growth of dermatophytes and *Candida albicans.*

Side Effects

The incidence of adverse reactions with this medication is low. A few patients may notice itching at the application site.

cimetidine (Trade name: Tagamet)   An antihistamine and antiulcer drug that may be a possible drug treatment for chronic hives and for multiple warts in children.

Side Effects

Side effects include diarrhea, dizziness, and rash.

ciprofloxacin (Trade name: Cipro)   An antimicrobial used to treat lower respiratory and urinary tract infection, infections of skin, bone and joints, and gastrointestinal disease. It is administered by mouth or IV.

Side Effects

Side effects include nausea and vomiting, diarrhea, abdominal pain, and headache.

clarithromycin (Trade name: Biaxin) This macrolide antibiotic is used to treat tonsillitis and sore throat, sinusitis, chronic bronchitis, community-acquired pneumonia, middle ear infection, *Mycobacterium avium* infections, duodenal ulcer, and infections of the skin.

Side Effects

This drug occasionally causes stomach upset, diarrhea, and a metallic taste. Rarely, it may cause headache, colitis, and a reversible hearing loss.

clavulanate potassium (Trade name: Augmentin) An oral antibacterial combination of the antibiotic amoxicillin and clavulanate potassium (a potassium salt of clavulanic acid, which is produced by the fermentation of *Streptomyces clavuligerus*). It is used to treat infections caused by susceptible strains of a variety of organisms that may be resistant to other antibiotics. Some of the conditions it may be used to treat include lower respiratory tract infections, ear infections, sinusitis, skin infections, urinary tract infections, and bite wounds.

Side Effects

This drug is usually well tolerated; most side effects (when they occur) are mild and may include diarrhea, skin rash and itching, vomiting, and vaginitis.

clindamycin (Trade name: Cleocin) An antibacterial drug used to treat acne and serious anaerobic infections that have not responded, or are resistant, to other antibiotics. Clindamycin is especially effective against most anaerobic bacteria, including *Propionibacterium acnes*. It is also an excellent agent against *Staphylococcus aureus* and streptococcal species.

Side Effects

Side effects include colitis and severe gastrointestinal problems.

clofazimine (Trade name: Lamprene) A dye used primarily in the treatment of leprosy. This drug has a remarkable lack of toxicity, and although there is no evidence of birth defects, it does cross the placenta and cause pigmentation changes in offspring. Administered by mouth, it should be taken with meals or milk. For most skin conditions, the drug needs to be taken for at least two months before benefit is seen. The drug should not be taken by women during the first three months of pregnancy, by patients prone to diarrhea or recurrent abdominal pain, or by those with kidney or liver disease.

Side Effects

The most obvious side effect is a pink, red, or brownish-black discoloration of the skin, especially in areas exposed to sunlight. Hair, sweat, sputum, urine, and feces also may be discolored. These pigmentation side effects are related to dosage, however, and begin to fade when therapy is stopped. Other side effects, include itching, sensitivity to sunlight, and acne-like skin eruptions. There also may be nausea and vomiting, abdominal pain, and diarrhea.

clotrimazole (Trade names: Gyne-Lotrimin, Lotrimin, Mycelex) A broad-spectrum drug used in topical applications to treat fungal and yeast infections including ringworm and infections of the genital organs. It is applied as a cream or solution or as vaginal pessaries. Contact with eyes should be avoided.

Side Effects

Severe skin allergic reactions may occur, as can mild burning or irritation.

cloxacillin (Trade names: Cloxapen, Tegopen) A penicillin-type antibiotic used to treat staphylococcal infections that are resistant to penicillin. Administered by mouth or injection, it should not be taken with acidic fruits or juices or aged cheese. Taken with alcohol, this drug could cause stomach irritation. Use with birth control pills may impair the efficacy of the contraceptive.

Side Effects

Side effects include stomach discomfort and rash, diarrhea, or allergic reactions in those sensitive to penicillin.

dapsone (4,4'-diaminodiphenyl-sulfone) An antibacterial drug and a derivative of sulfone used to treat leprosy and dermatitis herpetiformis. Results with this drug (the most often-used of the sulfones) have been variable, but in some cases there have been excellent results. Its mechanism of action is unknown.

The introduction of the sulfones in the 1950s had a dramatic impact on the treatment of leprosy, since dapsone was the first safe and effective drug available that stopped the disease and eliminated the need for patient isolation.

Although bacterial resistance to dapsone is becoming widespread, it remains the drug of choice in the treatment of leprosy in conjunction with other medication. According to reports, millions of patients have been successfully treated with dapsone for years with a relatively low rate of toxic side effects. Pregnant women should not use dapsone.

Side Effects
The adverse effects of this drug tend to be dose related and are uncommon in low doses. Concerns over the safety may have been exaggerated by the high doses used in some early studies. Severe allergic reactions may occur. Other side effects may include nausea, vomiting, and, rarely, damage to the liver, red blood cells, and nerves. During long-term treatment, blood tests are conducted to monitor liver function and the red blood cell level. Neurological symptoms (such as psychosis) are believed to be dose related; those with a history of psychiatric problems may be more likely to develop mental problems with this drug.

dideoxyinosine An antiretroviral drug used to treat HIV infections, restricting the viral replication activity.

doxycycline (Trade names: Vibramycin, Adoxa Doryx, Monodox) A tetracycline drug used to treat a variety of infections caused by bacteria and other microorganisms, including anthrax due to *Bacillus anthracis*, including inhalation anthrax (post-exposure), Q fever, rickettsial pox, Rocky Mountain spotted fever, typhus infections, urethritis, and yaws.

Side Effects
Side effects are the same as other tetracyclines: Gastrointestinal disturbances, phototoxicity, and discoloration of teeth of children under age eight or in utero. It should not be used in patients with kidney or liver problems or to sensitivity to other tetracyclines, nor should it be prescribed for pregnant women or children under age eight.

econazole (Trade name: Spectrazole) An antifungal drug used to treat ringworm of the scalp, athlete's foot, jock itch, "sun fungus," nail fungus, and candidiasis. Available in powder, cream, lotion, ointment, or vaginal tablet, the medication acts quickly (often within two days), killing fungi by damaging the fungal cell wall. The drug may take up to eight weeks to completely cure the infection.

Side Effects
Rarely, the drug may cause skin irritation.

erythromycin (Trade names: E-mycin, Erythro, Erythrocin, Robimycin, Ery-Tab, Erycette) A drug used to treat many bacterial and mycoplasmic infections, especially those that cannot be treated with penicillin. In children under age eight, it is the alternative to tetracycline (an antibiotic that can permanently stain developing teeth). Because erythromycin is destroyed by acid in the stomach, the drug should be taken in coated forms or as a compound. Patients with liver disease should not use this drug.

Side Effects
Possible side effects include nausea and vomiting, abdominal pain, diarrhea, and an itchy rash. Certain brands of erythromycin may be taken with food to reduce the chance of irritating the stomach.

ethambutol (Trade name: Myambutol) An antibiotic drug used to treat pulmonary tuberculosis in conjunction with other drugs. It is not recommended for small children or for those with optic neuritis.

Side Effects

Side effects include diminished visual acuity and allergic reactions (such as rashes). It may sometimes cause visual problems that ease when the drug is withdrawn.

ethionamide (Trade name: Trecator-SC) An antibacterial drug used to treat tuberculosis, usually in conjunction with other drugs. It is administered by mouth or as a suppository. Patients with liver damage should not use this drug.

Side Effects

Loss of appetite, nausea, and vomiting are common. Other side effects include skin rash, jaundice, mental depression, or gastrointestinal problems.

famciclovir (Trade name: Famvir) An antiviral drug active against the herpes viruses, including herpes simplex 1 and 2 (cold sores and genital herpes) and varicella-zoster (shingles and chicken pox). It interferes with the replication of viral DNA necessary for viruses to reproduce themselves. Famciclovir does not directly attack viruses but is converted to penciclovir in the body; it is the penciclovir that attacks the viruses. Because famciclovir has a longer duration of action, it can be taken fewer times each day.

foscarnet (phosphonoformic acid, trisodium salt) An antiviral that acts directly on the viral DNA of herpes simplex viruses and cytomegalovirus, and on retroviruses. The major use of foscarnet has been to treat severe infections caused by acyclovir-resistant herpes simplex viruses.

furazolidone (Trade name: Furoxone) A drug prescribed for certain bacterial or protozoal infections of the gastrointestinal tract. This drug is not prescribed for infants under age one.

Side Effects

Among the more serious reactions are fever and hemolytic anemia (destruction of red blood cells).

Skin rash and stomach pain may occur. This drug should not be taken with monoamine oxidase (MAO) inhibitors (a class of drugs used primarily to treat depression).

gamma benzene hexachloride (lindane) (Trade name: Scabene) A medication used to treat lice that is no longer recommended by the National Pediculosis Association because of its potential toxicity. Other products, according to the association, work equally well with less risk. It is not usually given to infants or pregnant women and should not be applied to the face.

Side Effects

Among the most serious reactions are neurologic damage and aplastic anemia (a deficiency of the elements of the blood). Eyes or skin may be irritated by topical use. Lindane also may irritate the skin and scalp, or cause itching.

ganciclovir sodium (Trade name: Cytovene) A drug related to acyclovir used to prevent cytomegalovirus infection after bone marrow transplantation and in AIDS patients. It is administered intravenously, orally, and via ocular implants.

Side Effects

During clinical trails, this drug was withdrawn in about 32 percent of patients because of adverse reactions, including most frequently liver and kidney problems and fever, rash, and malaise. Other side effects include headache, confusion, blood infection, swelling, high or low blood pressure, disturbing and intrusive thoughts and dreams, nausea and vomiting, loss of appetite, diarrhea, and abdominal pain.

gentamicin (Trade names: Gentacidin, Bristagen, Garamycin, Genoptic Liquifilm) An aminoglycoside antibiotic prescribed to ease the effects of a wide variety of severe bacterial infections. It can be administered by injection or applied as a cream, or as drops to the ears and eyes. It should not be used together with other drugs that may be potentially harmful to the kidneys or hearing. It should be used cautiously with patients who have kidney problems. Blood tests may be given during treatment to monitor kidney function.

Side Effects

The more serious adverse reactions (especially at high doses) include kidney, hearing, or balance problems and problems along the pathways between brain and muscles.

griseofulvin (Trade names: Griseofulvin, Fulvicin, Grisactin)

One of the oldest antifungal drugs available in America, it is used to treat infections of the skin, nails, or hair. It is particularly effective against superficial dermatophytes infections of the scalp, beard, palms, soles, and nails, including ringworm of the scalp (tinea capitis), ringworm of the body (tinea corporis), and athlete's foot. It is not effective against bacteria, deep fungi, or *Candida albicans*. Even with prolonged treatment, many nail infections do not respond completely or else they recur. Resistance may develop to this drug. When griseofulvin is taken with a high-fat meal, it is better absorbed and tolerated. Griseofulvin should not be taken by patients suffering with acute intermittent porphyria, since it may cause an acute abdominal attack. The drug may also interact with birth control pills, producing breakthrough bleeding or pregnancy.

Side Effects

The most common side effects are headache and gastrointestinal problems; others include loss of taste, rashes, and increased sun sensitivity. Long-term treatment may cause liver or bone marrow damage. The most serious problems include abnormal blood conditions.

hydrogen peroxide

A colorless topical antiseptic used to treat skin infections, to cleanse open wounds, or as a deodorant mouthwash. The solution combines with catalase (an enzyme present in the skin) to release oxygen, which kills bacteria and cleanses the infected areas.

Side Effects

Strong solutions sometimes irritate the skin.

idoxuridine (IDU)

An antiviral drug that acts by being incorporated into newly synthesized DNA; this drug is highly toxic to host cells. Thus, clinical use has been limited to topical therapy of herpes simplex infections of the eye because of its high systemic toxicity.

Side Effects

When used in the eye, it may cause irritation, pain, itching, and inflammation or swelling of the eyelids; rare allergic reactions and light sensitivity have been reported.

interferons

Natural cellular products released from infected host cells in response to viral (or other foreign) nucleic acids. While scientists do not fully understand how they act, they know that interferon selectively blocks translation and transcription of viral RNA, stopping viral replication without interfering with normal host cell functions. Interferon may be active against many viruses, but it can only be used in the same species that initially produced it.

Interferon-alpha is approved for use in some patients with hairy cell leukemia, Kaposi's sarcoma, or condylomata acuminata. Studies have shown that interferon-alpha2 nasal spray can prevent upper respiratory infections caused by rhinoviruses. Interferon is also effective against shingles in patients with impaired immune systems.

Combining interferon with either acyclovir or vidarabine is useful in treating various versions of hepatitis. Thanks to recombinant DNA technology, interferon is now available in large enough quantities from bacterial cells and many studies around the country are currently under way.

isoniazid (isonicotinic acid hydrazide, INH) (Trade names: Cotinazin, INH, Nydrazid)

An antibacterial used to prevent and treat tuberculosis, usually given by mouth. Isoniazid may be given to close contacts of patients who have TB to prevent the spread of the disease. Because TB bacteria soon become resistant to isoniazid, it is usually given in combination with streptomycin or other antibacterial drugs. Since the drug may hasten the depletion of pyridoxine (vitamin B_6) in the body, B_6 supplements are usually given to prevent nerve damage.

Side Effects

Because long-term treatment may be associated with liver problems, isoniazid should not be used by patients with liver disease. High doses or prolonged treatment has been associated with problems with the peripheral nervous system (the motor and sensory nerves outside the brain and spinal cord). Other side effects that commonly occur are rash and fever; occasionally, patients may experience dry mouth and digestive problems.

kanamycin (Trade names: Kantrex, Kantrim, Klebcil) An aminoglycoside antibiotic used to treat certain severe bacterial infections, especially those resistant to other antibiotics. It should not be used at the same time as other ototoxic drugs (medicines potentially harmful to hearing). It is given mainly by injection, but it is administered by mouth for infections of the intestines, and by inhalation for respiratory infections.

Side Effects

Mild side effects occasionally occur, including skin rash, fever, headache, nausea and vomiting, and tingling sensations. Other more serious side effects include renal failure and deafness.

ketoconazole (Trade name: Nizoral) A drug prescribed to treat fungal diseases, including tinea versicolor, candidiasis, coccidiomycosis, and histoplasmosis when other antifungal preparations have not been effective. It should not be used to treat fungal meningitis.

Side Effects

The most serious—but rare—adverse reactions are liver disorders. Ketoconazole may also cause nausea, but this may be avoided by taking the drug with food; it should not be taken at the same time as antacids. Other side effects include itching, headache, dizziness, abdominal pain, constipation, diarrhea, nervousness, or rash. Occasionally, patients may experience hives and allergic reactions with the first dose. Drug interactions with ketoconazole can be serious; this drug should not be taken with rifampin, isoniazid, warfarin, cyclosporine, or phenytoin.

lindane See GAMMA BENZENE HEXACHLORIDE.

linezolid (Zyvox) The first in a new class of antibacterial drugs designed to treat serious infections resistant to other antibiotics, such as vancomycin-resistant Enterococcus faecium. It also was approved to treat hospital-acquired pneumonia and severe skin infections.

Zyvox is the first in a new class of synthetic drugs (the oxazolidinone class) approved for use in the United States. It is the first drug in more than 50 years to be introduced for the treatment of methicillin-resistant Staphylococcus aureus.

Side Effects

The most reported side effect are headache, nausea, diarrhea, and vomiting, together with a decrease in platelet count. Zyvox may interact with other drugs such as over-the-counter pain medications that contain pseudoephedrine or phenylpropanolamine, leading to a rise in blood pressure.

mebendazole (Trade name: Vermox) A drug used to treat infestations of pinworms, whipworms, roundworms, and hookworms. Pregnant women should not use this drug.

Side Effects

Abdominal pain and diarrhea are among the most serious side effects.

mefloquine (Trade name: Lariam) An antimalarial drug that is effective in preventing and treating chloroquine-resistant falciparum and vivax malaria.

Side Effects

Vomiting, dizziness, nausea and fever, chills, diarrhea, or fatigue.

metronidazole (Trade names: Flagyl, Metro I.V., Metryl, Protostat, Satric) An antibiotic particularly useful in fighting infections caused by anaerobic bacteria infecting the genital, urinary, and digestive systems, such as amebiasis, trichomonas, and giardiasis. It is administered by mouth or in suppositories. It should not be used by pregnant women in the first trimester or by patients with organic disease, central nervous system disorders, or blood conditions.

Side Effects

Possible side effects include severe nausea and vomiting, appetite loss, abdominal pain, dark-colored urine, dizziness, neurological disturbances, or decrease in certain white blood cells (neutropenia). Many patients report that this drug creates a metallic taste in the mouth. Drinking alcohol during treatment with this drug can trigger particularly unpleasant reactions such as nausea, vomiting, hot flashes, and headache.

miconazole (Trade names: Micatin, Monistat) An antifungal medicine used on the skin to treat certain fungal infections of the skin and vagina, such as ringworm of the scalp, body, and feet, fungal meningitis, coccidioidomycosis, and candidiasis. It is given intravenously or by injection to treat systemic fungal infections, as well as topically or intravaginally.

Side Effects

Among the more serious reactions following application to the skin are irritation and burning. When used systemically, the drug may trigger nausea, itching, phlebitis, and anemia.

minocycline (Trade names: Minocin, Myrac, Dynacin) A tetracycline antibiotic used to treat acne, granuloma inguinale, lymphogranuloma venereum caused by chlamydia, psittacosis, Q fever, rickettsial pox, Rocky Mountain spotted fever, typhus, urethritis, and yaws.

Side Effects

Common side effects include vertigo, nausea and vomiting, and stomach problems. This drug will stain the teeth of children under eight years of age. Occasionally, it may cause liver toxicity, diarrhea, candidiasis, phlebitis, and sensitivity to the sun.

mupirocin (Trade name: Bactroban) This topical antibiotic is used to treat methicillin-resistant *S. aureus* infections and *Streptococcus pyogenes*.

Side Effects

Occasionally, this drug causes stinging or irritation of mucous membranes, pain, itching, and rash.

neomycin (Trade names: Mycifradin, Myciguent, Neobiotic) An aminoglycoside antibiotic used to treat infections of the intestine, eyes, and (topically) of the skin caused by a wide range of bacteria. It is usually applied in creams or drops with other antibiotics, but it can also be given by mouth. Neomycin should not be used by anyone with kidney problems or an intestinal obstruction.

Side Effects

Possible adverse effects include nausea and vomiting, rash, itching, diarrhea, hearing loss, dizziness, and tinnitus (ringing in the ears). Application of this medication to the skin may lead to allergic reactions.

niclosamide (Trade name: Niclocide) An anthelminthic prescribed to treat beef or fish tape-worm infestation. Its safety for small children, pregnant women, or nursing mothers has not been established.

Side Effects

Side effects include rectal bleeding, palpitations, hearing loss, swelling, nausea, and vomiting.

norfloxacin (Trade names: Chibroxin, Noroxin) An oral antibacterial drug prescribed for the treatment of urinary tract infections. It is not recommended for children or pregnant women. Nitrofurantoin drugs should not be used together with this medicine.

Side Effects

Nausea, dizziness, and headache have been reported.

nystatin (Trade names: Mycostatin, Nilstat, Nystex, O-U Statin) An antibiotic prescribed for the treatment of fungal infections of the gastrointestinal tract, vagina, and skin. It is applied as a cream for skin infections, by mouth for oral and intestinal infections, as pessaries or suppositories for vaginal and anal infections, or as eye drops for eye infections.

Side Effects

There are no known serious side effects; some patients may experience mild gastrointestinal irritation or mild skin reactions.

ofloxacin (Trade name: Floxin) A broad-spectrum injectable and oral antimicrobial used to treat adults with mild to moderate infections caused by susceptible strains of certain microorganisms in a variety of infections involving the lower respiratory tract, skin, urinary tract, and prostate. It is also used to treat a variety of sexually transmitted diseases. It should not be given to anyone allergic to drugs in the quinolone group.

Side Effects

Nausea, insomnia, headache, dizziness, diarrhea, vomiting, rash, itching, vaginitis, tendonitis, and tendon rupture.

oseltamivir (Trade name: Tamiflu) An antiviral drug used to treat influenza A and B infection and H5N1 (bird flu) in adults within the first two days after symptoms have appeared. Tamiflu also can be used to prevent the flu during an outbreak or epidemic. More expensive than rimantidine or amantadine, it is also more effective than those two drugs against influenza B and bird flu.

Side Effects

This drug may cause nausea, vomiting, or diarrhea.

oxytetracycline (Trade name: Terramycin) One of the tetracyclines, this antibiotic is used to treat a wide variety of bacterial and rickettsial infections, including chlamydia, syphilis, Rocky Mountain spotted fever, and cholera. It is administered by mouth or injection, or applied to the skin as a cream. Oxytetracycline should be used with caution in patients with kidney or liver problems.

Side Effects

Possible side effects include rash, increased skin sensitivity to the sun, nausea, and vomiting. Because it may discolor developing teeth, it is not prescribed for pregnant women or children under age eight.

para-aminosalicylic acid (PAS) A drug chemically related to aspirin that is used (together with isoniazid or streptomycin) to treat various types of tuberculosis. It is administered by mouth.

Side Effects

Side effects include nausea and vomiting, diarrhea and abdominal pain, fever, rash, goiter, hypokalemia (loss of potassium in the blood), and acid-base imbalance.

penciclovir (Trade name: Denavir) An antiviral cream used to treat the symptoms of cold sores around the mouth. Although topical penciclovir will not cure cold sores, it may help relieve the pain and discomfort and may help the sores heal faster.

penicillin (penicillin G [benzylpenicillin]) (Trade names: Bicillin, Cilloral, Crystapen, Falapen, Liquapen, Pentids, Permapen, Pfizerpen) An antibiotic derived from cultures of species of the mold *Penicillium notatum* used to treat a wide variety of bacterial infections, such as meningococcal, pneumococcal, and streptococcal infections, syphilis and many other diseases. It is rapidly absorbed when injected, but it is inactivated by stomach acid. It is often not effective against staphylococcus aureus. There are several similar drugs prepared from *P. notatum* (benethamine penicillin and benzathine penicillin) and a group of antibiotics derived from the penicillins, known as semisynthetic penicillins (including ampicillin and cloxacillin).

Side Effects

Allergic reactions are common, and include skin rash, hives, and anaphylaxis. Any patient who has had an allergic reaction to one type of penicillin should not be given any other. Other side effects include vomiting and diarrhea.

penicillin V (phenethicillin)   An antibiotic similar to penicillin that is active against gram-positive bacteria (except certain strains of staphylococci). It can be administered by mouth.

Side Effects
Diarrhea and allergic reactions.

permethrin (Trade names: Elimite, Rid)   A drug used on the skin to treat head lice and their nits. It should not be used by anyone allergic to pyrethrine, pyrethroids, or chrysanthemum flowers.

Side Effects
Reported reactions include itching, mild burning or stinging, numbness, discomfort, mild redness, or scalp rash.

piperazine (Trade names: Antepar, Bryrel)   A drug used to treat infestations by roundworms and thread worms. It is administered by mouth.

Side Effects
Rarely, side effects (nausea and vomiting, headache, tingling, and rashes) may follow high doses.

podofilox (Trade name: Condylox)   An antimitotic drug synthesized from plants used to treat external genital warts (condyloma acuminatum). It is not used to treat perianal or mucous membrane warts. Correct diagnosis of the lesions is essential.

Side Effects
There is a likelihood of side effects, including burning, pain, inflammation, erosion, and itching; burning and itching occur more often among women. Other, more rare side effects include pain with intercourse, insomnia, tingling, bleeding, tenderness, chafing, bad odor, dizziness, scarring, blisters, crusting, and swelling.

polymyxin B (Trade name: Aerosporin)   An antibiotic prescribed for infections caused by *Pseudomonas,* such as urinary tract infections, septicemia (blood poisoning), and eye infections.

Side Effects
This drug it should be used with extreme caution in patients with kidney problems. Drug fever, kidney, and liver problems may be caused by this drug. Mild dizziness also may occur.

polymyxins   A group of antibiotics derived from the bacterium *Bacillus polymyxa* used to treat gram-negative bacterial infections that cause a variety of conditions such as meningitis, corneal ulcers, and ear infections. The polymyxins include colistin and polymyxin B.

Side Effects
Taken orally, colistin is associated with pseudomembranous enterocolitis—a severe, life-threatening type of diarrhea sometimes caused by antibiotics. It also may cause liver problems and various neurologic changes when taken internally. When applied on the skin, irritation and allergic reactions may occur.

praziquantel (Trade name: Biltricide)   A drug used to treat schistosome infections and infections of liver flukes.

Side Effects
Praziquantel is usually well tolerated; side effects are usually mild and do not last long. They include headache, dizziness, abdominal discomfort, fever, or hives.

pyrantel pamoate   A drug used to treat infestation of roundworms or pinworms. It should be used with caution in patients with anemia or severe malnutrition.

Side Effects
Side effects include nausea, abdominal cramps, diarrhea, dizziness, and skin rash.

pyrazinamide   An antimycobacterial drug prescribed in combination drug therapy to treat hospitalized patients with tuberculosis who do not respond to other drugs. Patients with severe liver damage should not use this drug.

Side Effects

Side effects include joint pain, fever, and rash. At high doses, the drug may cause toxic effects on the liver.

pyrethrin (Trade name: A-200 shampoo) Used together with piperonyl butoxide, this is a fixed-combination medication used to treat head, body, and pubic lice, and scabies. Patients with a sensitivity to ragweed should not use this medication.

Side Effects

Side effects include irritation of skin and mucous membranes.

pyrimethamine (Trade names: Daraprim, Fansidar) A drug prescribed in the treatment of malaria and toxoplasmosis. It should not be used to treat chloroguanide-resistant malaria, and it should be prescribed cautiously in patients with toxoplasmosis because the dosage needed may be near toxic levels. It also may be used together with sulfadozine to treat malaria. This combination should not be used to treat pregnant women at term or while nursing, infants under age two months, or patients with the blood disorder megaloblastic anemia.

Side Effects

Adverse reactions occur especially at large doses, and may include blood disorders, very sore tongue (atrophic glossitis), low levels of some types of white blood cells (leukopenia), and convulsions. Side effects to the pyrimethamine and sulfadoxine combination may include pancreatitis, depression, convulsions, hallucinations, and several types of blood disorders.

quinacrine (Trade name: Atabrine) A drug used since World War II to suppress malaria; it is now used to treat intestinal infections, giardiasis, or cestodiasis. It should not be used during pregnancy or together with the drug primaquine, and it should

be administered with caution to patients over age 60 or to anyone with a history of psychosis.

Side Effects

Possible adverse effects include nausea and vomiting, and yellow discoloration of the skin and urine. Prolonged use can cause blood disorders or psychological problems. Other side effects include severe psoriasis, aplastic anemia, acute kidney problems.

quinine (Trade names: Quinamm, Quinine) The oldest drug treatment for malaria. Quinine had been abandoned and replaced by more effective, less toxic drugs, but in the wake of resistant forms of malaria it is being reintroduced as a potential malaria treatment. Today, it is used mainly to treat strains of the disease that are resistant to other antimalarial drugs (especially in malaria caused by *Plasmodium falciparum*). Patients with certain types of heart problems should not use this drug.

Side Effects

Large doses of this drug are needed, and therefore there is a high risk of adverse effects: headache, fever, nausea and vomiting, confusion, hearing loss, ringing in the ears, and blurred vision.

quinupristin/dalfopristin (Synercid) The first streptogramin (a new antibiotic class) available in the United States approved for treatment of patients with serious or life-threatening infections associated with vancomycin-resistant Enterococcus faecium (VREF) bacteremia. Synercid is also approved for complicated skin and skin structure infections caused by *Staphylococcus aureus* (methicillin susceptible) or *Streptococcus pyogenes* (Group A strep).

The most common adverse drug reactions are inflammation and pain at the infusion site, muscle and joint pain, and nausea. Drugs including cyclosporin A, midazolam, nifedipine, and terfenadine should be used with caution and monitored when coadministered with Synercid, because when used together they may lead to temporary heart rhythm problems.

ribavirin (Trade names: Virazole, Copegus, Rebetol, Rebetron, Ribasphere)   An aerosol drug prescribed to treat respiratory syncytial virus (RSV) infections of the lower respiratory tract, and other RNA and DNA viruses in infants and small children. It is not recommended for infants who need help in breathing, and its role in healthy children remains to be defined. It also appears to have some effectiveness against influenza A and B, but its role in treating these diseases is not defined. It has also been used successfully against lassa fever.

Side Effects

Reported side effects include bacterial pneumonia, pneumothorax, breathing cessation (apnea), low blood pressure, and cardiac arrest (these reported conditions could have been caused by the underlying disease and not the medication). Other side effects may include eye infection, impaired breathing function, and an increase in immature red blood cells (reticulocytosis).

rifampin (Trade names: Rifadin, Rimactane)   A drug prescribed to treat various infections, particularly tuberculosis. It is also used to prevent meningococcal meningitis in people who are exposed to someone with the disease. It is usually prescribed with other antibacterials because some strains of bacteria quickly develop resistance to rifampin alone. The drug should not be used by pregnant women or anyone with liver problems.

Side Effects

Liver toxicity and a syndrome that resembles influenza. Other side effects include a harmless, orange-red discoloration of urine, saliva, and other body secretions; gastrointestinal distress; aches and cramps; jaundice; rash; or itching.

rimantadine (Trade name: Flumadine)   An analog of amantadine used to treat flu that has the same effectiveness.

Side Effects

Side effects include light-headedness, insomnia, and nervousness.

saquinavir (Trade names: Invirase, Fortovase)   An antiretroviral drug used to treat HIV infection in combination with other antiretrovirals.

Side Effects

This drug may cause nausea, diarrhea, abdominal pain, high blood sugar, and high cholesterol.

silver sulfadiazine (Trade name: Silvadene)   A topical antibacterial cream used to prevent infections in skin grafts or second- and third-degree burns. It is especially helpful in keeping burn sites sterile, reducing the chance of secondary infection.

Side Effects

Possible side effects include allergic reactions (with rash, itching, or burning). Rarely, long-term use may rarely produce serious blood disorders or kidney damage. It is not recommended for patients who are sensitive to sulfonamide drugs, nor should it be used for newborns or premature infants.

streptomycin   An aminoglycoside antibiotic derived from *Streptomyces griseus* that is used to treat a wide variety of bacterial infections, including tularemia, plague, brucellosis, and glanders. It is administered by injection and is sometimes given together with a penicillin drug to treat endocarditis (inflammation of the lining of the heart and its valves). Streptomycin was once used to treat a variety of other infections, but it has now been surpassed by newer, more effective drugs with less serious side effects. When it was discovered, it was the first effective drug treatment for tuberculosis; it is still sometimes used (together with isoniazid) to treat a resistant strain of TB bacteria. Streptomycin should be used with caution by the elderly and those with kidney problems.

Side Effects

Its most serious adverse affect is the possibility of damage to the inner ear, disturbing balance and causing dizziness, ringing in the ears, and deafness. For this reason, patients with labyrinthine disease should not take this drug. It also must be used with caution in patients with kidney problems and the elderly. Other possible problems include facial numbness, tingling in the hands, headache, malaise, nausea, and vomiting.

sulfacetamide (Trade names: Bleph-10, Cetamide, Sebizon, Sulamyd, Sulf-10, Sulfacet-R) A topical sulfonamide-type of antibacterial drug used to treat pinkeye (conjunctivitis) and sometimes given to treat inflammation of the eyelids blepharitis. It also may be used to prevent infection after an eye injury or the removal of a foreign object. Those with impaired kidney function should not use this drug.

Side Effects
Side effects include stinging and possible allergic reactions such as itching, redness, and swelling of the eyelids.

Sulfacet-R Brand name drug for a topical combination medicine containing a scabicide (sulfur), an antibacterial (sulfacetamide sodium), and an antiseptic and astringent (zinc oxide).

sulfachlorpyridazine A sulfonamide-type of antibacterial drug used to treat infection (especially of the urinary tract). It should not be used if the urinary tract is blocked.

Side Effects
Among the more serious reactions are photosensitivity and severe allergic reactions.

sulfacytine A sulfonamide antibacterial used to treat infection, especially pyelonephritis and cystitis. It should not be used in patients who have porphyria or an obstructed urinary tract.

Side Effects
Side effects include photosensitivity, severe allergic reactions, a variety of blood conditions, or crystals in the urine (crystalluria).

sulfadiazine Sulfonamide antibacterial prescribed to treat infection (especially of the urinary tract)

and to prevent the development of rheumatic fever. This drug should not be used with patients who have porphyria or an obstructed urinary tract.

Side Effects
Side effects include photosensitivity, severe allergic reactions, a variety of blood conditions, or crystals in the urine (crystalluria).

sulfamethoxazole (Trade name: Gantanol) A sulfonamide-type antibacterial used to treat ear infection (otitis media), pinkeye, skin infections, or certain urinary tract infections. When combined with the antibacterial drug trimethoprim (as Bactrim or Septra), the two are given to treat a variety of respiratory tract infections, including pneumocystic pneumonia. It should not be given during the last trimester of pregnancy, during breast-feeding, or to children under age two months.

Side Effects
Side effects include rash, fever, nausea, vomiting, diarrhea, headache, dizziness, muscle or joint pain, or crystals in the urine.

sulfonamides (sulfa drugs) A large group of synthetic antibacterial agents effective in treating infections caused by many gram-negative and gram-positive microorganisms responsible for urinary tract infections, some types of pneumonia, and middle-ear infections, among other diseases. The sulfonamides are derived from a red dye known as sulfanilamide. Before the development of penicillin drugs, the sulfonamides were widely used to treat infections. Most sulfonamides are given by mouth and are available in a range of effectiveness from short- to long-acting, depending on the speed with which they are excreted from the patient's body. Most (including sulfamethoxazole and sulfaphenazole) are quickly absorbed from the stomach and small intestine and should be taken at frequent intervals. Some (such as sulfadoxine) are used for leprosy and malaria; sulfalene is a long-acting drug that need only be taken once a day. Others (such as sulfaguanidine) are poorly absorbed and are used to treat infections of the gastrointestinal tract, such as bacillary dysentery and gastroenteritis.

Side Effects

Side effects include hemolytic anemia, agranulocytosis, thrombocytopenia or aplastic anemia, drug fever, or jaundice, or allergic reactions. Adverse effects are more common with the long-acting sulfonamides that are given for more than 10 days. Sulfonamides also are given cautiously to people with impaired liver or kidney function. They are not given in the last three months of pregnancy or to infants, because of the risk of mental retardation. In general, patients should avoid exposure to direct sunlight when taking these drugs. Prolonged use of these drugs leads to the development of resistant strains of microorganisms in the gut.

sulfones One of a group of drugs closely related to the sulfa drugs in their structure and the way they act. Sulfones are powerful agents in the fight against the bacteria that cause leprosy and tuberculosis. Patients who take these drugs require frequent evaluation, including complete blood counts, a chemistry profile (including liver and kidney tests), and urine tests.

sulfisoxazole (Trade name: Gantrisin) A sulfonamide-type of antibacterial drug used to treat urinary tract infections (including vaginitis, cystitis, and pycloncphritis) and eye infections (pinkeye).

Side Effects

Side effects include nausea, vomiting, appetite loss, diarrhea, headache, dizziness, or rash. There may be a severe hypersensitivity reaction. The drug is not given during the last trimester of pregnancy, or to children under age two months.

tetracycline (Trade names: Achromycin, Cyclopar, Panmycin, Polycycline, Sumycin, Tetracyn, Tetrex, Topicycline) Any one of a group of broad-spectrum antibiotics derived from cultures of *Streptomyces* bacteria (chlortetracycline, doxycycline, oxytetracycline, and tetracycline). They are prescribed for the treatment of many bacterial and rickettsial infections, including respiratory-tract

infections, syphilis, and acne. Because tetracycline may cause permanent discoloration of the teeth, it is not used during the last half of pregnancy or during a child's first eight years of life. Patients with significant liver or kidney problems should not use this drug.

Side Effects

Nausea and vomiting and diarrhea are fairly common side effects. Others include more severe gastrointestinal disturbances, kidney and liver damage, inflammatory lesions in the anal-genital area, hemolytic anemia, and rash. Patients may also be susceptible to infection with tetracycline-resistant organisms.

thiabendazole (Trade name: Mintezol) An anthelmintic used to treat a variety of worm infestations, including roundworms, pinworms, and hookworms. People with erythema multiforme (an allergic syndrome associated with some drugs) or Stevens-Johnson syndrome (a severe form of erythema multiforme) should not use this medication.

Side Effects

Side effects include loss of appetite, central nervous system effects, severe gastrointestinal problems, dizziness, and low blood pressure.

tobramycin (Trade name: Tobi) An aminoglycoside antibiotic used to treat septicemia, lower respiratory tract infections, central nervous system infections, abdominal infections (including peritonitis), and infections of the skin, bone, urinary tract, and eyes. It is also used to manage cystic fibrosis.

Side Effects

This drug may cause kidney failure that is usually reversible, and irreversible vestibular or hearing problems.

tolnaftate (Trade names: Aftate, Tinactin) An antifungal drug used to treat superficial fungus infections of the skin, including some types of ringworm (including athlete's foot, ringworm of the body, and tinea versicolor). It is available without a prescription as a cream, powder, or aerosol. Tolnaftate is not effective in candidiasis.

Side Effects
In rare cases, it may cause skin irritation or rash.

trifluridine (trifluorothymidine) This antiviral drug interferes with DNA synthesis and is effective in treating eye infections caused by herpes simplex 1 and 2.

Side Effects
Side effects include burning or stinging in the eye.

trimethoprim (Trade names: Proloprim, Trimpex) An antibacterial drug used to treat various infections such as malaria, chronic infections of the urinary tract, and infections of the middle ear and bronchi. It should not be used to treat streptococcal pharyngitis (strep throat). It is often administered by mouth in a combined preparation with sulfamethoxazole (Bactrim, Septra).

Side Effects
Side effects include a range of blood abnormalities, allergies, gastrointestinal problems, and central nervous system problems. Long-term treatment may impair bone marrow production.

trimethoprim and sulfamethoxazole (Trade names: Bactrim, Septra) A combination antibacterial drug used to treat urinary tract infections, ear infections, and shigellosis. It is not recommended for use in infants under age two months, or in the last three months of pregnancy. It should be used with caution by patients with kidney or liver problems, or who have a possible folate deficiency.

Side Effects
Side effects include crystals in the urine, rash, fever, and allergic reactions.

undecylenic acid (Trade names: Breezee Mist Foot Powder; Fungi-Nail Solution, Gordochom solution) An antifungal agent used to treat athlete's foot and ringworm. It is applied to the skin as a powder, ointment, lotion, or aerosol spray, but should not be used in the eyes or on mucous membranes. Diabetic patients should use this drug with caution.

Side Effects
Side effects include skin irritation and allergic reactions.

valacyclovir (Trade name: Valtrex) An antiviral drug active against the herpes viruses. It is also effective against shingles and genital herpes, and works by interfering with the replication of viral DNA necessary for viruses to reproduce themselves. Valacyclovir is converted to acyclovir in the body, and it is the acyclovir that is active against the viruses. (Acyclovir itself is available as a topical, oral, and intravenous medication.) However, valacyclovir stays in the body longer than does acyclovir, so it does not have to be taken as often.

vancomycin (Trade names: Vancocin) Antibiotic used to treat bone and joint infections, pneumonia, septicemia, endocarditis, colitis, and enterocolitis.

Side effects
Phlebitis is most common. Occasionally, there may be flushing, low blood pressure, or itching. Rarely, there may be lowered white blood count, fever, or allergic reactions.

vidarabine An antiviral that interferes with viral DNA synthesis. It is used to treat herpes simplex infections and appears to be less susceptible to development of drug-resistant viral strains than idoxuridine (used to treat herpes simplex infections of the eye).

When used against herpes simplex encephalitis, it has cut mortality from 70 percent to 28 percent; therapy is most effective when started early, and is least effective when begun once the patient is comatose. It is also effective in treating shingles infections in those with an impaired immune system, shortening the period of viral shedding and lessening the incidence of postherpetic neuralgia.

While vidarabine is effective, however, studies have shown that acyclovir is more effective than vidarabine against both shingles and herpes simplex encephalitis.

Side Effects

Possible side effects of eye treatment include tearing, irritation, pain, and sensitivity to light. Systemic use may cause nausea, vomiting, tremor, and phlebitis at the infusion site. This drug may be toxic to bone marrow and liver when given in high doses.

Zostrix   See CAPSAICIN.

zalcitabine (Trade name: Hivid)   An anti-retroviral drug used in combination with AZT (zidovudine) to treat adult patients with advanced HIV infection whose condition is deteriorating.

Side Effects

Side effects that have been reported include oral ulcers, nausea, loss of appetite, abdominal pain, vomiting, rash and itching, dizziness, headache, fatigue, and sore throat.

zidovudine (Trade name: Retrovir)   An antiviral drug formerly known as azidothymidine (AZT) that is used in the treatment of AIDS and severe AIDS-related complex. The drug slows the growth of HIV infection in the body but cannot cure the infection; it works by interfering with DNA synthesis. It is used in conjunction with other drugs that help eradicate HIV.

Side Effects

Side effects include nausea, headache, and insomnia.

APPENDIX II
HOME DISINFECTION

Most of the items needed to keep infections from spreading at home are readily available:

- sanitary running (hot and cold) water
- separate eating, bathing, and sleeping areas
- towels
- soap
- paper towels
- washing machine/dryers.

"Disinfection" means the elimination of most germs on household surfaces. The following products are used to disinfect:

Antiseptic: a germicide used for human skin (not inanimate objects), such as

- alcohol
- iodine
- povidone-iodine (Betadine)
- hydrogen peroxide
- chlorhexidine

Disinfectant: A chemical germicide used to disinfect surfaces; most must not be used on human skin. All common disinfectants if used properly kill HIV, other viruses, and bacteria. Any household product called a "disinfectant" contains either ethyl alcohol (ethanol), isopropyl alcohol (isopropanol), a chlorine compound, ammonia, phosphoric acid, or pine oil.

- alcohol (also an antiseptic); can be used to wipe off thermometers

- ammonium (quaternary ammonium compounds) are used in hospitals to wipe down floors, walls, and furniture
- chlorine (household bleach) usually found in a liquid called sodium hypochlorite; can be used to wipe down bathroom, diaper changing table and pail, toys, and cutting boards. To use, 1/4 cup bleach is mixed in one gallon of cool water or one tbs. bleach in one quart of water in a spray bottle; a fresh mixture should be made every few days.

BATHROOM CLEANING

Viral, bacterial, and yeast infections can be spread from contaminated surfaces and cloth towels. To limit infection, any household disinfectant can be used to

- wipe bathroom faucets, toilets, and light switches regularly when family members are sick
- wash hands after using the toilet
- wash hands after changing a baby's diaper

KITCHEN CLEANING

To eliminte germs, consumers should

- wipe countertops with hot soapy water and let dry thoroughly
- wipe cutting boards with hot soapy water; clean in dishwasher if possible
- thoroughly wash hands before preparing food and after handling raw meat

APPENDIX III
ORGANIZATIONS

AIDS

AIDS Education Office of the American Red Cross
2025 East Street NW
Washington, DC 20006
(202) 303-4498
http://www.redcross.org/services/hss/resources/
refcent.html

CDC National AIDS Information Hotline
(800) 232-4636 (24 hours); (888) 232-6348
(Spanish and TDD)

CDC Clinical Trials Information Service
(800) 874-2572 (English and Spanish);
(888) 480-3739 (TDD)

CDC National Prevention Information Network
(800) 458-5231 (English and Spanish);
(800) 243-7012 (TDD)
http://www.cdcnpin.org/scripts/index.asp

Center for AIDS Prevention Studies
AIDS Research Institute
UCSF
50 Beale Street
Suite 1300
San Francisco, CA 94105
(415) 597-9100
http://www.epibiostat.ucsf.edu/capsweb

Elizabeth Glaser Pediatric AIDS foundation
2950 31st Street, #125
Santa Monica, CA 90405
(310) 314-1459; (888) 499-HOPE (4673)
http://www.pedaids.org

Gay Men's Health Crisis
The Tisch Building
119 West 24th Street

New York, NY 10011
(212) 367-1000
http://www.gmhc.org

Immune Deficiency Foundation
40 West Chesapeake Avenue
Suite 308
Towson, MD 21204
(301) 461-3127; (800) 296-4433
http://www.primaryimmune.org

National Association of People With Aids
1413 K Street NW
Suite 700
Washington, DC 20005
(202) 898-0414
http://www.napa.org

National Center for HIV, STD and TB Prevention
1108 Corporate Square
Atlanta, GA 30329
(404) 639-8040
http://www.cdc.gov/nchstp/od/nchstp.html

National Indian AIDS Hotline
(800) 283-2437

Red Ribbon Foundation
1155 Camino del Mar, Suite 521
Del Mar, CA 92014
(888) 649-6905
http://www.redribbon.net

Creutzfeldt-Jakob Disease (CJD) Foundation Inc.
P.O. Box 5312
Akron, OH 44334
(800) 659-1991
http://www.cjdfoundation.org

CJD Aware!
2527 South Carrollton Avenue
New Orleans, LA 70118
(504) 861-4627
http://www.cjdaware.com

FOOD SAFETY

Food Safety and Inspection Service
Room 1175-South Building
1400 Independence Avenue SW
Washington, DC 20250
(202) 720-7943
http://www.fsis.usda.gov

USDA Meat and Poultry Hotline
(888) 674-6854 (202) 720-3333 (TTY)
(Washington, D.C., area); 800-256-7072 (TDD/TTY)

For help with restaurant food problems
Call the local Health Department

For help with non-meat or poultry food products (such as cereal)
Call or write to the Food and Drug Administration (FDA)

Turkey hotline
(800) 535-4555 (10 A.M.–4 P.M.)

GOVERNMENT ORGANIZATIONS

Centers for Disease Control and Prevention
1600 Clifton Road
Atlanta, GA 30333
(404) 639-3311; (800) 311-3435
http://www.CDC.gov

National Institute of Allergy and Infectious Diseases
6610 Rockledge Drive
MSC 6612
Bethesda, MD 20892
(301) 496-5717
http://www3.NIAID.NIH

Food and Drug Administration
5600 Fishers Lane
Rockville, MD 20857
(301) 472-4750; (888) 463-6332
http://www.FDA.gov

GROUP B STREP

Group B Strep Association
P.O. Box 16515

Chapel Hill, NC 27516
http://www.groupbstrep.org

HELICOBACTER PYLORI

Helicobacter Foundation, The
P.O. Box 7965
Charlottesville, VA 22906-7965
http://www.helico.com

HEPATITIS

The American Liver Foundation
75 Maiden Lane, Suite 603
New York, NY 10038
(800) 465-4837; (212) 668-1000
http://www.liverfoundation.org

Hepatitis Information Network
http://www.hepnet.com

Hepatitis Foundation International
504 Blick Drive
Silver Spring, MD 20904
(301) 622-4200 or (800) 891-0707
http://www.hepfi.org

Hepatitis B Foundation
700 East Butler Avenue
Doylestown, PA 18901
(215) 489-4900
http://www.hepb.org

Hepatitis C Information Center
http://www.hepatitis-central.com

HERPES

(See also SEXUALLY TRANSMITTED DISEASES)

American Herpes Foundation
433 Hackensack Avenue
Hackensack, NJ 07601
(201) 342-4441
http://www.herpes-foundation.org

Herpes Information
http://www.herpeshelp.com

Herpes Resource Center
American Social Health Association
P.O. Box 13827
Research Triangle Park, NC 27709
(800) 230-6039
National Herpes Hotline: (919) 361-8488
http://www.ashastd.org/herpes-overview.cfm

INFECTIOUS DISEASES

Infectious Diseases Society of America
66 Canal Center Plaza
Suite 600
Alexandria, VA 22314
(703) 299-0200
http://www.idsociety.org

International Society for Infectious Diseases
1330 Beacon Street
Suite 228
Brookline, MA 02446
(617) 277-0551
http://www.isid.org

National Foundation for Infectious Diseases
4733 Bethesda Avenue, Suite 750
Bethesda, MD 20814
(301) 656-0003
http://www.nfid.org

Pediatric Infectious Diseases Society
66 Canal Center Plaza
Suite 600
Alexandria, VA 22314
(703) 299-6764
http://www.pids.org

National Center for Infectious Diseases
Division of Bacterial and Mycotic Diseases
1600 Clifton Road NE, MS-D63
Atlanta, GA 30033
(800) 311-3435
http://www.cdc.gov/ncidod

INTERNATIONAL TRAVEL

National Center for Infectious Diseases Traveller's Health
CDC
1600 Clifton Road
Atlanta, GA 30333
(404) 639-3311
http://www.cdc.gov/travel/index.htm

International Association for Medical Assistance to Travelers
1623 Military Road #279
Niagara Falls, NY 14304
(716) 754-4883
http://www.iamat.org

Vessel Sanitation Program
National Center for Environmental Health
Centers for Disease Control and Prevention (CDC)
4770 Buford Highway NE
Building 101, MS-F23
Atlanta, GA 30341-3724
(770) 488-7070; (800) 323-2132
http://www.cdc.gov/nceh/vsp

KIDNEY INFECTIONS

National Kidney and Urologic Diseases Information Clearinghouse
3 Information Way
Bethesda, MD 20892
(800) 891-5390
http://kidney.niddk.nih.gov

National Kidney Foundation
30 East 33rd Street
New York, NY 10016
(800) 622-9010
http://www.kidney.org

LEPROSY

American Leprosy Missions
1 ALM Way
Greenville, SC 29601
(800) 543-3135 or (864) 271-7040
http://www.leprosy.org

LYME DISEASE

American Lyme Disease Foundation
P.O. Box 684
Somers, NY 10589
(914) 277-6970
http://www.aldf.com

Lyme Disease Association, Inc.
P.O. Box 1438
Jackson, NJ 08527
(888) 366-6611
http://www.lymediseaseassociation.org

Lyme Disease Network
43 Winton Road
East Brunswick, NJ 08816
http://www.lymenet.org

NECROTIZING FASCIITIS

National Necrotizing Fasciitis Foundation
http://www.nnff.org

PROFESSIONAL GROUPS

American Society for Rickettsiology
http://www.cas.umt.edu/rickettsiology

American Society for Virology
http://www.mcw.edu/asv

Association for Professionals in Infection Control and Epidemiology
1275 K Street NW
Suite 1000
Washington, DC 20005
(202) 789-1890
http://www.apic.org/AM/Template.
   cfm?Section=Home

Association for Tropical Biology and Conservation
http://atbio.org

Society of Infectious Diseases Pharmacists
823 Congress Avenue
Suite 230
Austin, TX 78701
(512) 479-0425
http://www.sidp.org

Society of Nematologists
P.O. Box 311
Marceline, MO 64658
(660) 256-3331
http://www.nematologists.org

Surgical Infection Society
http://www.sisna.org

World Health Organization
Avenue Appia 20
1211 Geneva 27
Switzerland
(+ 41 22) 791 21 11
http://www.who.int/en

RABIES

CDC Division of Viral and Rickettsial Diseases
(404) 639-1075
http://www.cdc.gov/ncidod/dvrd

RESPIRATORY DISEASES

American Lung Association
61 Broadway, Sixth Floor
New York, NY 10006
http://www.lungusa.org

SEXUALLY TRANSMITTED DISEASES

(See also HERPES)

American Social Health Association
P.O. Box 13827
Research Triangle Park, NC 27709
(919) 361-8400
http://www.ashastd.org

Herpes Resource Center
P.O. Box 13827
Research Triangle Park, NC 27709
(919) 361-8488
http://www.ashastd.org/herpes/herpes_overview.
   cfm

TROPICAL DISEASES

American Society of Tropical Medicine and Hygiene
60 Revere Drive
Suite 500
Northbrook, IL 60062
(847) 480-9592
http://www.astmh.org

TUBERCULOSIS

CDC Division of TB Elimination
CDC
1600 Clifton Road NE
MS E-10
Atlanta, GA 30333
(404) 639-8135
http://www.cdc.gov/nchstp/tb/default.htm

International Association for Paratuberculosis
2015 Linden Drive
Madison, WI 53706-1102
(608) 262-8457
http://www.paratuberculosis.org

National Center for HIV, STD and TB Prevention
1108 Corporate Square
Atlanta, GA 30329
(404) 639-8040
http://www.cdc.gov/nchstp/od/nchstp.html

VACCINE INJURY

National Vaccine Compensation Program
Parklawn Building, Room 11C-26
5600 Fishers Lane
Rockville, MD 20857
(800) 338-2382
http://www.HRSA.gov/vaccinecompensation/
   default.htm

National Vaccine Information Center
204 Mill Street
Suite B1
Vienna, VA 22180
(703) 938-DPT3; (800) 909-SHOT
http://www.909shot.com

GLOSSARY

abscess   A clearly defined walled-off inflammatory area (usually caused by infection) that contains pus.

acute condition   A condition that appears suddenly.

adjuvant   A substance used in a vaccine to improve the immune response so that less vaccine is needed to stimulate an immune response.

anaphylaxis   An immediate and severe allergic response that can cause sudden severe breathing problems, severe drop in blood pressure, and loss of consciousness. Anaphylactic shock can be fatal if not treated promptly.

antibiotic   A drug that kills or slows the growth of bacteria. Antibiotics are used to fight bacterial infections; they have no effect on viruses.

antibiotic resistance   The ability of a bacterium to change its characteristics so that it is no longer sensitive to a particular antibiotic.

antibody   A protein that is manufactured by white blood cells to identify, neutralize, or destroy bacteria, viruses, and other harmful microorganisms.

antigen   A substance that can trigger an immune response, causing the production of an antibody as part of the body's defense against infection. Many antigens are not found naturally in the body; they include microorganisms, toxins, and tissues from another used in an organ transplant.

ARC   Abbreviation for "AIDS related complex," a collection of signs and symptoms that often appear as HIV infections progress from a no-symptom state to full-blown AIDS.

arthropod   Insects and ticks capable of transmitting bacteria or viruses that cause infectious disease in humans.

attenuated   A medical term meaning "weakened." An attenuated vaccine is one that has been weakened by chemicals or other processes so that it will produce an adequate immune response without causing the serious effects of an infection.

biopsy   Removal and examination of a small piece of tissue.

bone marrow   Tissue contained within the internal cavities of the bones.

bubo   Enlarged, inflamed lymph node (especially under the arm or in the groin) caused by infections such as plague, tuberculosis, or syphilis.

canker sore   A small, painful ulcer, usually found on the mouth or lips.

carbuncle   A staphylococcal infection of skin and skin tissue made up of a cluster of furuncles.

carrier   A person who harbors the microorganisms that cause a particular disease without experiencing symptoms of infection, but who can transmit the disease to others.

chancre   An ulcer at the site of a skin infection caused by disease, such as syphilis or tuberculosis.

congenital   Present at birth.

contagious   Capable of being transmitted to others.

contagious disease   Originally, a disease that was transmitted only by physical contact. Today, the term is usually used to mean "communicable disease."

corticosteroid   A group of drugs based on the structure of cortisone (a hormone produced by the adrenal glands), which has antiinflammatory properties.

culture   Growth of microorganisms on artificial media; cultures are used to diagnose a particular bacterium or virus.

curettage   The removal of skin tissue with a curet (sharp blade).

disinfection   Eliminating most germs on surfaces.

ecthyma   A shallow bacterial infection that often causes scarring.

endemic Occurring frequently in a particular region or population.

enteric Pertaining to the intestines.

epidemic A sudden outbreak of infectious disease that spreads rapidly through the population, affecting a large number of people. Narrowly defined, *epidemic* refers to outbreaks in human populations and *epizootic* to outbreaks in animal groups.

exposure The condition of being subject to an infectious disease as a result of contact with an infected person or contaminated environment.

fungus Simple parasitic life-forms that make up a plant phylum (including yeasts, rusts, molds, smuts, mushrooms, mildews, and so on).

gram-negative bacteria A type of bacteria that resists the chemical stain used in "Gram's method" of identifying microorganisms for characterization purposes. Some of the most common gram-negative bacteria include *Bacteroides fragilis, Brucella abortus, Escherichia coli, Haemophilus influenzae, Klebsiella pneumoniae, Neisseria gonorrhoeae, Proteus vulgaris, Pseudomonas aeruginosa, Salmonella typhi, Shigella dysenteriae,* and *Yersinia pestis.*

gram-positive bacteria A type of bacteria that retains the violet color of the stain used in "Gram's method" of staining microorganisms. Some of the most common kinds of gram-positive bacteria are *Bacillus anthracis, Clostridium, Mycobacterium leprae, M. tuberculosis, Staphylococcus aureus, Streptococcus pneumoniae,* and *S. pyogens.*

Gram's stain A laboratory staining test used to identify bacteria. A bacterium will either retain or resist a chemical stain depending on what type of cell wall it has. Bacteria that accept stain are "gram-positive," those that do not are "gram-negative."

host The insect, animal, or human on which a microorganism is able to live and reproduce.

immune disorder Any temporary or permanent condition that weakens the immune system.

immune globulin Human blood plasma from many sources that contain protective antibodies to a particular disease.

immune system The network of cells and proteins that is designed to fight infection in the human body.

The system includes the spleen, lymph glands, white blood cells, and antibodies.

immunity A state of protection against a disease through the activities of the immune system. Natural immunity is present from birth and is the first line of defense against most infectious agents. Acquired immunity is the second line of defense, that develops either through exposure to microorganisms or as a result of immunization.

immunization The injection of weakened or killed microorganism to trigger the production of antibodies to provide protection against a particular disease (active immunization). Passive immunization is the injection of antibodies against a specific microbe from donated blood plasma from a person already exposed, to give protection against a disease for up to about three months.

immunocompromised A condition in which a person's immune system can't respond adequately to an invading organism. Such an impaired immune system makes a patient vulnerable to infection.

immunoglobulins A specific protein substance, produced by plasma cells to help fight infection.

immunosuppression Impairment of a person's immune system by using certain drugs, in order to treat cancer or stop the rejection of transplanted organs.

incubation period The time between exposure to an infection and the first appearance of symptoms.

infection The establishment of a colony of disease-causing microorganisms such as bacteria, viruses, or fungi in the body. The organisms reproduce rapidly and cause disease by damaging cells or producing damaging toxins. Infection usually triggers a response from the immune system, which causes many of the symptoms commonly seen in diseases.

infestation Colonization by parasites such as mites, ticks, or lice in the skin or by worms (such as tapeworms) in the body.

latency A quiescent period during which a pathogen either does not reproduce or reproduces very slowly. During this time, symptoms of the disease may not appear.

lymphocyte A category of white blood cells with specialized functions in the immune system. B lymphocytes create antibody-producing cells; T lymphocytes activate other white blood cells (such as B lymphocytes) or kill infected cells directly.

mutation A change in the genetic material within a living cell (the DNA).

pandemic A disease that occurs over a large geographical area that affects a high proportion of the population.

parasite Any organism living in or on any other living creature, deriving advantages from doing so, while causing disadvantage to the host.

pathogen Bacteria, viruses, parasites, or fungi that can cause disease in humans.

plasmid A loop of DNA that occurs in bacteria that contain genes coding for toxin production, antibiotic resistance, and ability to invade host cells. Plasmids can be transferred between bacteria.

Plasmodium A genus of protozoans (single-celled organisms) that live as parasites within the red blood cells and liver cells of man. The parasite completes the sexual phase of its development in the stomach and digestive glands of a bloodsucking *Anopheles* mosquito; four species cause malaria in man (*P. vivax, P. ovale, P. falciparum, P. malariae*).

pus A liquid caused by inflammation. It consists of leukocytes, dead tissue, and fluid.

pyoderma A condition of the skin involving pus-filled lesions.

retrovirus A member of a family of viruses that use RNA as genetic information and transcribes this information into DNA. The family Retroviridae includes HIV and HTLV (human T-cell lymphotropic virus, human T-cell leukemia virus, or human T-cell leukemia/lymphoma virus).

spleen An organ that removes and destroys worn-out red blood cells and helps fight infection. It fights infection by producing some of the antibodies, phagocytes, and lymphocytes that destroy invading microorganisms. If it is removed, its duties can be taken over by other parts of the lymphatic system, although this makes the patient more susceptible to infection.

T cells One of the two main classes of a type of white blood cell. T cells play an important part in the body's immune system defenses against infection.

thymus A gland that makes up part of the immune system, by making lymphocytes become T cells. These T cells play an important part in the body's defense against viruses and other infections.

toxin A poisonous protein produced by disease-causing bacteria such as *Clostridium tetani* (which causes tetanus). Bacterial toxins are sometimes subdivided into endotoxins (released from inside dead bacteria), exotoxins (released from the surface of live bacteria), and enterotoxins (which inflame the intestine).

trematodes Parasitic flatworms in the class Trematoda, commonly called "flukes."

trypanosomes Single-celled parasites that cause diseases such as sleeping sickness.

vector Any animal that transmits a particular infectious disease. A vector picks up an organism from a source of infection, carries them within the body, and later deposits them where they infect a new host. Mosquitoes, fleas, lice, ticks, and flies are the most important vectors of disease to humans.

virus The smallest known type of infectious agent, causing diseases that range from mild (warts and the common cold) to extremely serious (rabies, AIDS, and probably some types of cancer).

white blood cells Also known as leukocytes, their principal role is to protect the body against infection. There are three main types of white blood cells: granulocytes, monocytes, and lymphocytes. These cells circulate in blood, lymph, and body tissues and either directly or indirectly destroy invading organisms and infected or damaged cells.

zoonosis Any infectious or parasitic disease of animals that can be transmitted to humans. Many disease organisms can infect only humans or particular animals, but zoonotic organisms are more flexible. They can adapt themselves to many different species. Zoonoses are usually caught from animals closely associated with humans (dogs, cats, parrots, pigs, cattle, rats). Examples include cat-scratch disease, fungal infections, psittacosis, brucellosis, trichinosis, leptospirosis.

BIBLIOGRAPHY

Acheson, D. W. "Food safety: Bovine spongiform encephalopathy (mad cow disease)," *Nutrition Today.* 37, no. 1 (January–February 2002): 19–25.

Adler, Stuart. "Risk of Human Parvovirus B19 Infections," *Journal of Infectious Diseases* 168 (1993): 361–368.

Adler, Tina. "Mauling mosquitoes naturally: New ways to silence the buzz," *Science News* 149 (April 27, 1996): 270–271.

Akue, J. P., T. G. Egwant, and E. Devaney. "High levels of parasite-specific IgG4 in the absence of microfilaremia in Loa loa infection," *Tropical Medical Parasitology* 45 (1994): 246–248.

Alexander, D. J. "Should we change the definition of avian influenza for eradication purposes?" *Avian Disease* 47, no. 3 (2003): 976–981.

Alibek, K. *Biohazard.* New York: Random House, 1999.

Almond, J. W., et al. "Will bovine spongiform encephalopathy transmit to humans?" *British Medical Journal* 311 (November 25, 1995): 1,415–1,121.

American Lyme Disease Foundation. Available at: http://www.aldf.com. Updated 2005.

Anasari, A., et al. "Comparison of Cloth, Paper and Warm Air Drying in Eliminating Viruses and Bacteria from Washed Hands," *American Journal of Infection Control* 19, no. 5 (1991): 243–249.

Anderson, Kenneth N., ed. *Mosby's Medical, Nursing and Allied Health Dictionary.* 4th ed. Boston: Mosby, 1994.

Barbour, Alan G., and Durland Fish. "The biological and social phenomenon of Lyme disease," *Science* 260 (June 11, 1993): 1,610–1,616.

Barreto, M. L., M. G. Teixeira, and E. H. Carmo. "Infectious diseases epidemiology," *Journal of Epidemiology and Community Health* 60, no. 3 (March 2006): 192–195.

Barthold, S. W. "Antigenic stability of borrelia burgdorferi during chronic infections of immunocompetent mice," *Infection and Immunity* 61, no. 12 (December 1993): 4,955–4,961.

Bausch, D. G., and T. G. Ksiazek. "Viral hemorrhagic fevers including hantavirus pulmonary syndrome in the Americas," *Clinical Laboratory Medicine* 22 (2002): 981–1,020.

Bausch, D. G., M. Borchert, T. Grein, et al. "Risk factors for Marburg hemorrhagic fever, Democratic Republic of the Congo," *Emerging Infectious Diseases* 912 (2003): 1,531–1,557.

Bausch, D. G., A. H. Demby, M. Coulibaly, et al. "Lassa fever in Guinea: I. Epidemiology of human disease and clinical observations," *Vector Borne Zoonotic Diseases* 14 (2001): 269–281.

Beardsley, Tim. "Trends in preventive medicine: Better than a cure," *Scientific American* 272 (January 1995): 88–95.

Beeler, J., F. Varricchio, and R. Wise. "Thrombocytopenia after immunization with measles vaccines: Review of the Vaccine Adverse Events Reporting System (1990 to 1994)," *Pediatric Infectious Disease Journal* 15 (1996): 88–90.

Berenbaum, May R. *Bugs in the System: Insects and Their Impact on Human Affairs.* Boston: Addison-Wesley, 1995.

Berenguer, J., M. Santiago, and F. Laguna. "Tuberculous meningitis in patients infected with the HIV virus," *New England Journal of Medicine* 326 (1992): 668–672.

Biddle, Wayne. *A Field Guide to Germs.* New York: Doubleday, 1995.

Bishop, Jerry. "Study suggests cause and cure for ulcers," *Wall Street Journal,* May 1, 1992, B-1.

Blake, P. A. "Epidemiology of Cholera in the Americas," *Gastroenterology Clinics of North America* 22 (1993): 639–660.

Blumenthal, Susan. "Another ear infection?" *Ladies' Home Journal* 112 (June 1995): 118.

Bocchino, M., S. Greco, Y. Rosati, G. Mattioli, et al. "Cost determinants of tuberculosis management in a low-prevalence country," *International Journal of Tuberculosis and Lung Disease* 10, no. 2 (February 2006): 146–152.

Bower, Bruce. "Virus may trigger some mood disorders," *Science News* 147 (June 17, 1995): 132.

Breiman, R., et al. "Emergence of Drug-Resistant Pneumococcal Infections in the United States," *JAMA* 271, no. 23 (1994): 1,831–1,835.

Breman, J. G., and D. A. Henderson. "Poxvirus dilemmas: Monkeypox, smallpox and biological terrorism," *New England Journal of Medicine* 339 (1998): 556–559.

Bren, L. "FDA continues work to help prevent mad cow disease," *FDA Consumer* 36, no. 3 (May–June 2002): 31–32.

Briesel, T., et al., "Identification of a Kunjin/West Nile-like favivirus in brains of New York encephalitis patients," *Lancet* 354 (1999): 1,261–1,262.

Briseno-Garcia, B., H. Gomez-Dantes, E. Argott-Ramirez. "Potential risk for dengue hemorrhagic fever. The isolation of serotype dengue-3 in Mexico," *Emerging Infectious Diseases* 2, no. 2 (1996): 841–844.

Brown, E. E., D. A. Peura. "Diagnosis of *Helicobacter pylori* infection," *Gastroenterology Clinics of North America* 22, no. 1 (March 1993): 105.

Brown, Kathryn Sergeant. "Skip the flu: It can be done," *Woman's Day*, October 10, 1995, 100.

Bryce, J. "New Estimates for the Causes of Child Deaths Worldwide," *Lancet* 365, no. 9465 (March 26, 2005): 1,147–1,152.

Bulbin, A., and M. S. Simberkoff. "Prevention of pneumonia in the elderly," *Infections in Medicine* 12, no. 8: 385, 389–394, 1995.

Bull, J. J. "Virulence," *Evolution* 48 (1994): 1,423–1,437.

Burkot, T. R., G. R. Mullen, R. Anderson, et al. "*Borrelia lonestari* DNA in adult *Amblyomma americanum* ticks," *Emerging Infectious Diseases* 7, no. 3 (May–June 2001): 471–473.

Butler, D. "Alarms rising over bird flu mutations," *Nature* 439, no. 7074 (January 2006): 19,248–19,249.

Call, S. A., M. A. Vollenweider, C. A. Hornung, et al. "Does this patient have influenza?" *Journal of the American Medical Association* 293, no. 8 (February 23, 2005): 987–997.

Capua, I., and D. J. Alexander. "Avian influenza: Recent developments," *Avian Pathology* 33, no. 4 (August 2004): 393–404.

Carey, R. F., W. A. Herman, et al. "Effectiveness of latex condoms as a barrier to human immunodeficiency virus-sized particles under conditions of simulated use," *Sexually Transmitted Diseases* 19 (1992): 230–234.

Carruthers, J., and A. Carruthers. "Mad cows, prions, and wrinkles," *Archives of Dermatology* 138, no. 5 (May 2002): 667–670. Review.

Centers for Disease Control and Prevention. "Condoms for prevention of sexually transmitted diseases," *Morbidity and Mortality Weekly Report* 37 (1988): 133–137.

———. "Screening for tuberculosis and tuberculosis infection in high-risk populations," *Morbidity and Mortality Weekly Report* 39 (1990): 1–7.

———. "Summary of Notifiable Diseases, United States," *Morbidity and Mortality Weekly Report*. Atlanta: Centers for Disease Control and Prevention, 1992.

———. "The Management of Acute Diarrhea in Children: Oral Rehydration, Maintenance and Nutritional Therapy," *Morbidity and Mortality Weekly Report* 41 (1992): RR–16.

———. "E. Coli O157:H7 Information Package," March 1993. *Morbidity and Mortality Weekly Report* 42 (1993): RR–1.

———. "Initial therapy for tuberculosis in the era of multi-drug resistance: Recommendations of the Advisory Council for the elimination of tuberculosis," *Morbidity and Mortality Weekly Report* 42 (1993): 1–8.

———. "Summary of Notifiable Diseases, United States," *Morbidity and Mortality Weekly Report*. Atlanta: Centers for Disease Control and Prevention, 1993.

———. "Outbreak of Powassan Encephalitis—Maine and Vermont, 1999–2001," *Morbidity and Mortality Weekly Report* 50, no. 35 (September 7, 2001): 761–764.

———. "Bovine spongiform encephalopathy in a dairy cow—Washington state," *Morbidity and Mortality Weekly Report* 52 (2003): 1,280–1,285.

———. "Outbreaks of avian influenza A (H5N1) in Asia and interim recommendations for evaluation and reporting of suspected cases: United States, 2004," *Morbidity and Mortality Weekly Report* 53, no. 5 (February 13, 2004): 97–100.

———. "Preventing Tetanus, Diphtheria, and Pertussis among Adolescents: Use of Tetanus Toxoid, Reduced Diphtheria Toxoid and Acellular Pertussis Vaccines: Recommendations of the Advisory Committee on Immunization Practices (ACIP)," *Morbidity and Mortality Weekly Report* 55 (February 23, 2006): 1–34.

———. "Influenza vaccination of health-care personnel: Recommendations of the Healthcare Infection Control Practices Advisory Committee (HICPAC) and the Advisory Committee on Immunization Practices (ACIP)," *Morbidity and Mortality Weekly Report* 55, RR–2 (February 24, 2006): 1–16.

———. Mumps outbreak at a summer camp: New York, 2005," *Morbidity and Mortality Weekly Report* 55, no. 7 (February 24, 2006): 175–177.

———. "Update: Influenza activity—United States, February 5–11, 2006," *Morbidity and Mortality Weekly Report* 55, no. 7 (February 24, 2006): 183–184.

———. "Bacteria take new role as cancer vaccine," *Science News* 148 (November 25, 1995): 357.

———. "New drug sweeps clean in HIV model," *Science News* 148 (November 18, 1995): 324.

———. "Basic information about SARS." Available at: http://www.cdc.gov/ncidod/sars/factsheet.htm. Updated 2005.

———. "Epidemic/epizootic West Nile virus in the United States: Guidelines for surveillance, prevention and control," March 2000, available at: http://www.cdc.gov/ncidod/dvbid/arbovirus_pubs.htm.

———. "Hendra virus and Nipah virus." Available at: http://www.cdc.gov/ncidod/dvrd/spb/mnpages/dispages/nipah.htm. Updated August 2004.

————. "Lyme Disease." Available at: http://www.cdc.gov/ncidod/dvbid/lyme. Updated September 29, 2005.

————. "Noroviruses." Available at: http://www.cdc.gov/ncidod/dvrd/revb/gastro/norovirus.htm. Updated April 22, 2005.

————. "SARS: Information for patients and close contacts." Available at: http://www.cdc.gov/ncidod/sars/closecontacts.htm. Updated May 3, 2005.

Centers for Disease Control Yellow Book. "Marburg hemorrhagic fever." Available at: http://www2.ncid.cdc.gov/travel/yb/utils/ybGet.asp?section=dis&obj=viral_hemorrhagic.htm&cssNav=browseoyb. Updated 2006.

Centofanti, Marjorie. "Just lookin' for a home: Many bacteria sneak into cells via entry routes already in place," *Science News* 149 (January 6, 1996): 12–13.

Chan, M. C. W., C. Y. Cheung, W. H. Chui, et al. "Proinflammatory cytokine responses induced by influenza A (H5N1) viruses in primary human alveolar and bronchial epithelial cells," *Respiratory Research* 6, no. 1 (November 11, 2005).

Chapnick, Edward K., John Protic, et al. "Congratulations: It's a worm!" *Infections in Medicine* 13, no. 8 (1996): 653–654.

Check, E. "US urged to provide smallpox vaccines for emergency crews," *Nature* 417, no. 6891 (June 20, 2002): 775–776.

Chen, H., G. J. Smith, S. Y. Zhang, et al. "Avian flu: H5N1 virus outbreak in migratory waterfowl," *Nature* 436, no. 7048 (July 14, 2005): 191–192.

Child Health Alert. "Hepatitis B vaccine encouraged for all newborn infants. . . and do multiple vaccines overwhelm a child's immune system?" *Child Health Alert* 20 (February 2002): 1.

Clancy, Cornelius J., et al. "Fungemia caused by *Candida lusitaniae*," *Infections in Medicine* 13, no. 11 (1996): 940, 948–951.

Clemens, J. D., D. A. Sack, and J. R. Harris. "Field trial of oral cholera vaccines in Bangladesh: Results from three-year followup," *Lancet* 335 (1990): 270–273.

Coffin, S. E. "Rotavirus vaccines: Current controversies and future directions," *Current Infectious Disease Reports* 2, no. 1 (February 2000): 68–72.

Corbett, E. L., R. W. Steketee, F. O. ter Kuile, A. S. Latif, A. Kamali, and R. J. Hayes. "HIV-1/AIDS and the control of other infectious diseases in Africa," *Lancet* 359, no. 9324 (June 22, 2002): 2,177–2,187.

Cordell, R. L. "A public health perspective on infectious disease aspects of the revised standards for health and safety in out-of-home child care," *Pediatric Annals* 31, no. 5 (May 2002): 307–312.

Cortes, L. M., S. W. Hargarten, and H. M. Hennes. "Recommendations for water safety and drowning prevention for travelers," *Journal of Travel Medicine* 13, no. 1 (January–February 2006): 21–34.

Covacci, A., S. Censini, M. Bugnoli, et al. "Molecular characterization of the 128-kDa immunodominant antigen of Helicobacter pylori associated with cytotoxicity and duodenal ulcer," *Proceeds of the National Academy of Science* 90 (1993): 5,791–5,795.

Cover, T. L., M. J. Blaser. "Helicobacter pylori: A bacterial cause of gastritis, peptic ulcer disease and gastric cancer," *American Society of Microbiology Newsletter* 61 (1995): 21–26.

Crabtree, J. E., et al. "Expression of 120 kilodalton protein and cytotoxicity in Helicobacter pylori," *Journal of Clinical Pathology* 45 (1992): 733–734.

Crawford, P. C., E. J. Dubovi, W. L. Castleman, et al. "Transmission of equine influenza virus to dogs," *Science* 310, no. 5747 (October 21, 2005): 482–485.

Crosby, Alfred W. *America's Forgotten Pandemic: The Influenza of 1918*. New York: Cambridge University Press, 1990.

Crowcroft, N. S., and J. Britto. "Whooping Cough—A continuing problem," *British Medical Journal* 324, no. 7353 (June 29, 2002): 1,537–1,538.

Custer, Joseph. "Croup and Related Disorders," *Pediatrics in Review* 14, no. 1 (1993): 17–28.

Das, P. "Infectious disease surveillance update," *Lancet Infectious Disease* 2, no. 5 (May 2002): 267.

Dealler, S. F., and R. W. Lacey. "Transmissible spongiform encephalopathies: The threat of BSE to man," *Food Microbiology* 7 (1990): 253–279.

De Jong, M. D., T. T. Thanh, T. H. Khanh, et al. "Oseltamivir resistance during treatment of influenza A (H5N1) infection," *New England Journal of Medicine* 353, no. 25 (December 22, 2005): 2,667–2,672.

De Manzione, N., R. A. Salas, H. Pardes, et al. "Venezuelan hemorrhagic fever: Clinical and epidemiological studies of 165 cases," *Clinical Infectious Disease* 26, no. 2 (1998): 308–313.

Digre, K. B. "Infectious Disease," *Journal of Neurophthalmology* 22, no. 2 (June 2002): 141–142.

Do, A. N., S. K. Fridkin, A. Yechouron, et al. "Risk factors for early recurrent Clostridium difficile-associated diarrhea," *Clinical Infectious Diseases* 26 (1998): 954–959.

Dobkin, Jay F. "Influenza and HIV in '97: The big one?" *Infections in Medicine* 14, no. 1 (1997): 10.

Ebert, D. "Virulence and local adaptation of a horizontally transmitted parasite," *Science* 265 (1994): 1,084–1,086.

Enserink, M. "Fort Detrick. On biowarfare's frontline," *Science* 296, no. 5575 (June 14, 2002): 1,954–1,956.

———. "Bioterrorism. In search of a kinder, gentler vaccine," *Science* 296, no. 5573 (May 31, 2002): 1,594.

———. "Bioterrorism. How devastating would a smallpox attack really be?" *Science* 296, no. 573 (May 31, 2002): 1,592–1,595.

Epstein, P. R. "Climate change and infectious disease: stormy weather ahead?" *Epidemiology* 13, no. 4 (July 2002): 373–375.

Esposito, S., G. Faldella, A. Giammanco, S. Bosis, O. Friscia, M. Clerici, and N. Principi. "Long-term pertussis-specific immune responses to a combined diphtheria, tetanus, tricomponent acellular pertussis and hepatitis B vaccine in pre-term infants," *Vaccine* 20, no. 23–24 (July 26, 2002): 2,928–2,932.

Ewald, P. W. *The Evolution of Infectious Disease.* Oxford: Oxford University Press, 1994.

———. "Guarding against the most dangerous emerging pathogens: insights from evolutionary biology," *Emerging Infectious Diseases* 2, no. 4 (1996): 245–257.

———. "The hepatitis G enigma: researchers corner new viruses associated with hepatitis," *Science News* 149 (April 13, 1996): 238–239.

Farci, P. "Lack of protective immunity against reinfection with hepatitis C virus," *Science* 258 (October 2, 1992): 135–140.

Farley, Dixie. "On the teen scene: TSS—reducing the risk," *FDA Consumer* (October 1991): 24.

———. "Help for cuts, scrapes and burns: OTC options," *FDA Consumer* (May 1996): 13–15.

———. "Fighting Fleas and Ticks," *FDA Consumer* (July–August 1996): 23–29.

———. "Treating Tropical diseases," *FDA Consumer* (January–February 1997): 26–30.

Farrington, P., et al. "A new method for active surveillance of adverse events from DTP and MMR vaccines," *Lancet* 345 (1995): 567–569.

———. "Multifactorial nature of human immunodeficiency virus disease: implications for therapy," *Science* 262 (1993): 1,008–1,011.

———. "Pandemic influenza threat and preparedness," *Emerging Infectious Diseases* 12, no. 1 (January 2006): 73–76.

FDA Consumer. "Penicillins," *FDA Consumer* (July–August 1990): 29–30.

———. "Report on rotavirus vaccine," *FDA Consumer* (July–August 1995): 3.

———. "HIV-Related use of antibiotic," *FDA Consumer* (November 1996): 3.

———. "First drug for rare parasitic diseases," *FDA Consumer* (September 1996): 4.

———. "New pertussis vaccine safer for infants," *FDA Consumer* (October 1996): 2.

———. "New drug for AIDS-related eye infection," *FDA Consumer* (October 1996): 4.

———. "First urine test for HIV," *FDA Consumer* (October 1996): 5.

———. "AIDs drug approved in 119 days," *FDA Consumer* (October 1996): 5.

———. "Drug for testing HIV wasting gets early approval," *FDA Consumer* (November 1996): 2.

———. "FDA Warning concerning certain Italian cheese," *FDA Consumer* (November 1996): 3–4.

———. "Breath Test for Ulcer Bacterium," *FDA Consumer* 31, no. 1 (January–February 1997): 3.

———. "Certain antimicrobial drugs related to tendon problems," *FDA Consumer* 31, no. 1 (January–February 1997): 4.

Felz, M. W., F. W. Chandler, Jr., J. H. Oliver, Jr., D. W. Rahn, and M. E. Schriefer. "Solitary erythema migrans in Georgia and South Carolina," *Archives of Dermatology* 135, no. 11 (November 1999): 1,317–1,326.

Feng, P. "Escherichia coli Serotype O157:H7: Novel vehicles of infection and emergence of phenotypic variants," *Emerging Infectious Diseases* 1, no. 2 (1995): 47–52.

Fikrig, E. Barthold, et al. "Protection of mice against the Lyme disease agent by immunizing with recombinant OSPA," *Science* 250 (October 26, 1990): 553–556.

Finch, R. "Antibiotic resistance—From pathogen to disease surveillance," *Clinical Microbiology and Infection* 8, no. 6 (June 2002): 317–320.

Francesconi, P., Z. Yoti, S. Declich, et al. "Ebola hemorrhagic fever transmission and risk factors of contacts, Uganda," *Emerging Infectious Diseases* 9, no. 11 (2003): 1,430–1,437.

Franco, Eduardo. "Human Papillomavirus and the National History of Cervical Cancer," *Infections in Medicine* (January 1993): 57–64.

Furley, Dixie. "Treating tropical diseases," *FDA Consumer* 31, no. 1 (January–February 1997): 26–30.

Gale, J. L., et al. "Risk of serious acute neurological illness after immunization with diphtheria-tetanus-pertussis vaccine," *JAMA* 271 (1994): 37–41.

Gantz, Nelson, et al., eds. *Manual of Clinical Problems in Infectious Disease.* Boston: Little, Brown, 1994.

Garraud, O., et al. "Identification of recombinant filarial proteins capable of inducing polyclonal and antigen-specific IgE and IgG4 antibodies," *Journal of Immunology* 155, no. 1316–25: 1995.

Garrett, Laurie. *The Coming Plague.* New York: Farrar, Straus and Giroux, 1994.

Georgia Department of Human Resources, Division of Public Health, Epidemiology Branch. "Tick Bites and Erythema Migrans in Georgia: It Might NOT be Lyme

Disease!" *Georgia Epidemiology Report* 17 (August 2001): 1–3.

Girgis, N., et al. "Dexamethasone adjunctive treatment for TB meningitis," *Journal of Pediatric Infectious Disease* 10 (1991): 179–183.

GlaxoSmithKline. "Boostrix." Available at: http://www. boostrix.com. Updated 2006.

Goddard, Jerome. "Viruses transmitted by mosquitoes: dengue fever," *Infections in Medicine* 13, no. 11 (1996): 933–934.

Goldfarb, L. G. "Genetics and infectious disease: convergence at the prion." *Epidemiology* 13, no. 4 (July 2002): 379–381.

Gottfried, Robert S. *The Black Death.* New York: Free Press, 1983.

Granoff, D. M. "Assessing efficacy of Haemophilus influenzae type b combination vaccines," *Clinical Infectious Disease* 33, suppl. 4 (December 15, 2001): S278–S287.

Gray, G. C., K. B. Chesbrough, M. A. Ryan, et al. "The millennium Cohort Study: A 21-year prospective cohort study of 140,000 military personnel," *Military Medicine* 167, no. 6 (June 2002): 483–488.

Griffin, M. R. et al. "Risk of seizures and encephalopathy after immunization with the DTP vaccine," *Journal of the American Medical Association* 263 (1990): 1,641–1,645.

Gubler, D. J., and G. G. Clark. "Dengue/dengue hemorrhagic fever: The emergence of a global health problem," *Emerging Infectious Diseases* 1, no. 2 (1995): 55–57.

Guinee, Vincent F. "Epidemic," *Colliers Encyclopedia.* CD-ROM. Released February 28, 1996.

Gutman, L. T., J. Moye, and B. Zimmer. "Tuberculosis in HIV-exposed or infected U.S. children," *Journal of Pediatric Infectious Disease* 13 (1994): 963–968.

Harden, Virginia. *Rocky Mountain Spotted Fever.* Baltimore: Johns Hopkins University Press, 1990.

Harvard Women's Health Watch, "New clue to CFS," *Harvard Women's Health Watch,* November 1995: 6.

Haslam, R. H. "Role of computed tomography in the early management of bacterial meningitis," *Journal of Pediatrics* 119 (1991): 152–159.

Hayden, F. C., R. L. Atmar, and M. Schilling, et al. "Use of the selective oral neuraminidase inhibitor oseltamivir to prevent influenza," *New England Journal of Medicine* 341 (1999): 1,336–1,343.

Henretig, F. M., T. J. Cieslak, M. G. Kortepeter, and G. R. Fleisher. "Medical management of the suspected victim of bioterrorism: An algorithmic approach to the undifferentiated patient," *Emergency Medical Clinics of North America* 20, no. 2 (May 2002): 351–364.

Hill, A. V. S., et al. "Common West African HLA antigens are associated with protection from severe malaria," *Nature* 252 (1991): 595–600.

Hingley, Audrey. "Rabies on the Rise," *FDA Consumer* (November 1996): 25–29.

Hitt, E. "Poor sales trigger vaccine withdrawal," *Natural Medicine* 8, no. 4 (April 2002): 311–312.

Hobby, Gladys. *Penicillin: Meeting the Challenge.* New Haven, Conn.: Yale University Press, 1985.

Hoeprich, Paul D., et al., eds. *Infectious Diseases,* 5th ed. Philadelphia: Lippincott, 1994.

Hoke, C. H., et al. "Protection against Japanese encephalitis by inactivated vaccines," *New England Journal of Medicine* 319 (1988): 608–614.

Holman, R. C., et al. "Epidemiology of Creutzfeldt-Jakob disease in the United States 1979–1990," *Neuroepidemiology* 14 (1995): 174–181.

Horgan, John. "The no-name virus: Questions linger after the four corners outbreak," *Scientific American* 271, no. 6 (December 1994): 34.

Hotez, Peter J., and David I. Pritchard. "Hookworm Infection," *Scientific American* 272, no. 6 (June 1995): 68–74.

Hughes, J. M., and F. C. Tenover. "Infectious disease challenges of the 1990s," *Infections in Medicine* 13, no. 9 (1996): 788, 798–799.

Inglesby, T. V., D. A. Henderson, J. G. Bartlett, et al. "Anthrax as a biological weapon: medical and public health management," *Journal of the American Medical Association* 281 (1999): 1,735–1,745.

Institute of Medicine. *Adverse effects of pertussis and rubella vaccines.* Washington, D.C.: National Academy Press, 1991.

———. *Emerging Infections: Microbial Threats to Health in the United States.* Washington, D.C.: National Academy Press, 1992.

———. *Vaccines against Malaria: Hope in a Gathering Storm.* Washington, D.C.: IOM Board on International Health, 1996.

———. *Assessment of Future Scientific Need for Live Variola Virus.* Washington, D.C.: National Academy Press, 1999.

James, A. M., D. Liveris, G. P. Wormser, et al. "Borrelia lonestari infection after a bite by an Amblyomma americanum tick," *Journal of Infectious Diseases* 183, no. 12 (June 15, 2001): 1,810–1,814.

Johnson, Hillary. *Osler's Web: Inside the Labyrinth of the Chronic Fatigue Syndrome Epidemic.* New York: Crown, 1996.

Johnson, Howard, et al. "How interferons fight disease," *Scientific American* 270, no. 5 (May 1994): 68–75.

Kammer, A. R., and H. C. Errl. "Rabies vaccines: From the past to the 21st Century," *Hybrid Hybridomics* 21, no. 2 (April 2002): 123–127.

Kantor, Fred S. "Disarming Lyme disease," *Scientific American* 271, no. 3 (September 1994): 34–39.

Kayhty, Helena, and Juhani Eskola. "New vaccines for the prevention of pneumococcal infections," *Emerging Infectious Diseases* 2, no. 4 (1996): 289–298.

Kelly, D. J., A. L. Richards, J. Temenak, D. Strickman, and G. A. Dasch. "The past and present threat of rickettsial diseases to military medicine and international public health," *Clinical Infectious Diseases* 34, suppl. 4 (June 15, 2002): 5,145–5,169.

Keusch, G. T., J. Wilentz, and A. Kleinman. "Stigma and global health: Developing a research agenda," *Lancet* 367, no. 9509 (February 11, 2006): 525–527.

Khouri, Y., et al. "Mycobacterium TB in children with human HIV type 1 infection," *Journal of Pediatric Infectious Disease* 11 (1992): 950–955.

King, Linda. "The facts on feline AIDS," *McCall's,* October 1996: 166.

Kiple, Kenneth, ed. *The Cambridge World History of Human Disease.* Cambridge: Cambridge University Press, 1993.

Kirkland, K. B., T. B. Klimko, R. A. Meriwether, et al. "Erythema migrans-like rash illness at a camp in North Carolina: A new tick-borne disease?" *Archives of Internal Medicine* 157, no. 22 (December 8–22, 1997): 2,635–2,641.

Kirsche, M. L. "FDA panel requests more safety data, surveillance for LYMErix," *Infectious Disease News* 14 (2001): 36–37.

Klion, A. D., et al. "Loiasis in endemic and nonendemic populations: Immunologically mediated differences in clinical presentation," *Journal of Infectious Diseases* 163 (1991): 1,318–1,325.

Knight-Ridder Newspapers. "Public at risk from old, new diseases," January 17, 1996.

Kolasa, M. S., T. J. Petersen, E. W. Brink, I. D. Bulim, J. M. Stevenson, and L. E. Rodewald. "Impact of multiple injections on immunization rates among vulnerable children," *American Journal of Preventive Medicine* 21, no. 4 (November 2001): 261–266.

Kolata, G. "A Litigation Nightmare." In *FLU: The story of the great influenza pandemic of 1918 and the search for the virus that caused it.* New York: Farrar, Straus and Giroux, 1999.

Koopmans, M., B. Wilbrink, M. Conyn, et al. "Transmission of H7N7 avian influenza A virus to human beings during a large outbreak in commercial poultry farms in the Netherlands," *Lancet* 363, no. 9409 (February 21, 2004): 587–593.

Kraut, Alan M. *Silent Travelers.* New York: Basic Books, 1994.

Krieg, Joann P. *Epidemics in the Modern World.* New York: Macmillan/Twayne, 1992.

Kubic, Mike. "New Ways to prevent and treat AIDS," *FDA Consumer* 31, no. 1 (January–February 1997): 7–11.

Kuiken, T., G. Rimmelzwaan, D. van Riel, et al. "Avian H5N1 influenza in cats," *Science* 306, no. 5694 (October 8, 2004): 241.

Lacey, R. W. "Bovine spongiform encephalopathy is being maintained by vertical and horizontal transmission," *British Medical Journal* 312 (January 20, 1996): 180–181.

Lang, M. M. "Antimicrobial resistance in pediatric upper respiratory infection: a prescription for change," *Pediatric Nursing* 25, no. 6 (November–December 1999): 607–616.

Lederberg, Joshua, et al., eds. *Emerging Infections.* Washington, D.C.: National Academy Press, 1992.

LeDuc, J. W., and J. Becher. "Current status of smallpox vaccine," *Emerging Infectious Diseases* 5 (1999): 593–594.

Leigh Brown, A. J., and E. C. Holmes. "Evolutionary biology of the human immunodeficiency virus," *Annual Review of Ecology and Systematics* 25 (1994): 127–162.

Lemonick, Michael. "Germ Warfare: Infectious diseases can strike anywhere, anytime," *Time,* September 13, 1996: 59–62.

Levin, Bruce R. "The evolution and maintenance of virulence in microparasites," *Emerging Infectious Diseases* 2, no. 2 (1996): 93–102.

Levin, B. R., and J. J. Bull. "Short-sighted evolution and the virulence of pathogenic microorganisms," *Trends in Microbiology* 2 (1994): 76–81.

Levine, Arnold J. *Viruses.* New York: Scientific American Library, 1992.

Levy, S. B. *Antibiotic Paradox: How Miracle Drugs Are Destroying the Miracle.* New York: Plenum Press, 1992.

Llewelyn, C. A., P. E. Hewitt, R. S. G. Knight, et al. "Possible transmission of variant Creutzfeldt-Jakob disease by blood transfusion," *Lancet* 363, no. 9407 (February 2004): 417–421.

Lin, J. S., et al. "Underdiagnosis of Chlamydia trachomatis infection: Diagnostic limitations in patients with low-level infection," *Sexually Transmitted Diseases* 19 (1992): 259–65.

Lipkin, R. "New 'design rule' yield novel drugs," *Science News* 147 (June 17, 1995): 374.

Lipotov, A. S., R. J. Webby, E. A. Govorkova, et al. "Efficacy of H5 influenza vaccines produced by reverse genetics in a lethal mouse model," *Journal of Infectious Diseases* 191 (April 15, 2005): 1,216–1,220.

Lippi, D., and A. A. Conti. "Plague, policy, saints and terrorists: A historical survey," *Journal of Infection* 44, no. 4 (May 2002): 226–228.

Lipsitch, M., and M. L. Nowak. "The evolution of virulence in sexually transmitted HIV/AIDS," *Journal of Theoretical Biology* 174 (1995): 427–440.

Long, C. O., E. A. Greenberg, and R. L. Ismeurt. "Infectious Disease," *Home Healthcare Nurse* 20, no. 7 (July 2002): 472–473.

Long, Michael. "In the woods, an unspotted fever," *Health* 8 (March 1, 1994): 17.

Los Angeles News Service. "Researchers: Immune system fix possible," January 27, 1997.

Ludlam, C. A., W. G. Powderly, S. Bozzette, M. Diamond, et al. "Clinical perspectives of emerging pathogens in bleeding disorders," *Lancet* 367, no. 9506 (January 21, 2006): 252–261.

Luke, C. J. and K. Subbarao. "Vaccines for pandemic influenza," *Emerging Infectious Diseases* 12, no. 1 (January 2006): 66–72.

Lutwick, L., et al. "There is always something small that's too big for some of us," *Infections in Medicine* 13, no. 9 (1996): 761–762, 767.

Lutwick, L. "Prion's progress: Are you what you eat?" *Infections in Medicine* 13, no. 12 (1996): 1,037, 1,041–1,043.

Lyme Disease Network. Available at: http://www.lymenet.org. Updated March 6, 2006.

Macaluso, A., A. Petrinca, L. Lanni, S. Saccares, et al. "Identification and sequence analysis of hepatitis A virus detected in market and environmental bivalve molluscs," *Journal of Food Protection* 69, no. 2 (February 2006): 449–452.

Marshal, B. J. *"Helicobacter pylori,"* American Journal of Gastroenterology 89, no. 81 (August 1994): S-116.

Marshall, E. "Hantavirus Outbreak Yields to PCR," *Science* 262 (1993): 832–836.

Maupin, R. T. "Obstetric infectious disease emergencies," *Clinical Obstetrics and Gynecology* 45, no. 2 (June 2002): 393–404.

Mayo Foundation. "SARS." Available at: http://www.mayoclinic.com/health/sars/DS00501. Updated October 2004.

McCarthy, S. A., et al. "Toxigenic Vibrio cholerae 01 and Cargo Ships Entering Gulf of Mexico," (letter) *Lancet* 339 (1992): 624–625.

Michels, K. M., K. J. Hofman, G. T. Keusch, and S. H. Hrynkow. "Stigma and global health: Looking forward," *Lancet* 367, no. 9509 (February 11, 2006): 538–539.

Michigan Nurse editors. "Change suggested in hepatitis B vaccinations for infants," *Michigan Nurse* 72, no. 8 (September 1999): 35.

Miller, D. L., et al. "Pertussis immunization and serious acute neurological illnesses in children," *British Medical Journal* 307 (1993): 1,171–1,176.

Miller, E., et al. "Risk of aseptic meningitis after measles, mumps and rubella vaccine in UK children," *Lancet* 341 (1993): 979–995.

Monastersky, Richard. "Health in the hot zone: How would global warming affect humans?" *Science News* 149 (April 6, 1996): 218–219.

Moore, J. E., and B. C. Millar. "Spelling of emerging pathogens," *Emerging Infectious Diseases* 11, no. 11 (November 2005): 1,796–1,797.

Moore, Patrick S., and Claire V. Broome. "Cerebrospinal meningitis epidemics," 271, no. 5 (November 1994): 38–45.

Moore, Patrick S. "Meningococcal meningitis in subsaharan Africa: A model for the epidemic process," *Clinical Infectious Diseases* 14, no. 2 (February 1992): 515–525.

Morbidity and Mortality Weekly Report, "Cholera associated with an international air flight," *MMWR* (1992): 134–135.

———. "Importation of cholera from Peru," *MMWR* 4 (1991): 258–259.

———. "Dengue fever at the U.S.-Mexico border, 1995–1996," *MMWR* 45, no. 39 (1996): 841–844.

———. "World Health Organization consultation on public health issues related to bovine spongiform encephalopathy and the emergence of a new variant of Creutzfeldt-Jakob disease," *MMWR* 45, no. 14 (1996): 295–303.

———. "Surveillance for Creutzfeldt-Jakob disease—United States," *MMWR* 45, no. 31 (1996): 665–669.

———. "Prevention and control of influenza: Recommendations of the Advisory Committee on Immunization Practices," *MMWR* 49, no. RR-3 (2000): 1–38.

———. "Summary of notifiable diseases—United States, 2000," *MMWR* 49, no. 53 (June 14, 2002): i–xxii, 1–100.

———. "Hepatitis B vaccination—United States, 1982–2002," *MMWR* 51, no. 25 (June 28, 2002): 549–552, 563.

Moris, G., and J. C. Garcia-Monco. "The challenge of drug-induced aseptic meningitis," *Archives of Internal Medicine* 59 (1999): 1,185–1,194.

Moro, M. L., D. Resi, B. Lelli, A. Nicoli, et al. "Barriers to effective tuberculosis control: A qualitative study," *International Journal of Tuberculosis and Lung Disease* 9, no. 12 (December 2005): 1,355–1,360.

Morrison, D. C., and J. L. Ryan, eds. *Novel Therapeutic Strategies in the Treatment of Sepsis.* New York: Marcel Dekker, 1996.

Morse, Stephen S., ed. *Emerging Viruses.* New York: Oxford University Press, 1993.

Murdoch, Guy. "Swimmer's ear," *Consumer's Research Magazine* 75 (August 1, 1992): 2.

Musgrove, C., et al. *"Campylobacter pylori:* Clinical, histological and serological studies," *Journal of Clinical Pathology* 41 (1988): 11,316–11,321.

Nair, S., D. Yadav, M. Corpuz, et al. "Clostridium difficile colitis: Factors influencing treatment failure and relapse—a prospective evaluation," *American Journal of Gastroenterology* 93 (1998): 1,873–1,876.

Newell, D. G., et al. "Estimation of prevalence of Helicobacter pylori infection in an asymptomatic elderly population comparing urea breath test and serology," *Journal of Clinical Pathology* 44 (1991): 385–387.

NewScientist.com "Nanobacteria revelations provoke new controversy." Available at: http://www.newscientist.com/article.ns?id=dn5009. Updated: May 2004.

Nguyen, T. M., D. Ilef, S. Jarraud, L. Rouil, et al. "A community-wide outbreak of Legionnaires disease linked to industrial cooling towers—how far can contaminated aerosols spread?" *Journal of Infectious Diseases* 193, no. 1 (January 1, 2006): 102–110.

Nowak, Rachel. "Cause of fatal outbreak in horses and humans traced," *Science* 268 (April 7, 1995): 32.

Nursing. "Lymerix. Lack of demand kills Lyme disease vaccine," *Nursing* 32, no. 5 (May 2002): 18.

Official Mad Cow Disease Home Page. "Bovine CJD: Do you have it?" Available at: http://www.mad-cow.org. April 2001.

Ortolon, K. "Short on shots," *Texas Medicine* 98, no. 5 (May 2002): 30–32.

Palumbo, P., et al. "Population-based study of measles and measles immunization in HIV-infected children," *Pediatric Infectious Disease Journal* 11 (1992): 1,008–1,014.

Pang, T. "The impact of genomics on global health," *American Journal of Public Health* 92, no. 7 (July 2002): 1,077–1,079.

Parashar, U. D., E. G. Hummelmann, J. S. Bresee, M. A. Miller, et al. "Global illness and deaths caused by rotavirus disease in children," *Emerging Infectious Diseases* 9, no. 5 (May 2003): 562–572.

Parsonnet, J., et al. "*Helicobacter pylori* infection and the risk of gastric carcinoma," *New England Journal of Medicine* 325 (1991): 1,127–1,131.

Patchett, S., et al. "*Helicobacter pylori* and duodenal ulcer recurrence," *American Journal of Gastroenterology* 87 (1992): 24–27.

Patlak, Margie. "Book reopened on infectious diseases," *FDA Consumer* 30 (April 1996): 19–23.

Patterson, P. and J. A. Reinarz. "Smallpox: Mass vaccinations or not?" *Texas Medicine* 98, no. 6 (June 2002): 43–44.

Paul, John R. *A History of Poliomyelitis*. New Haven, Conn.: Yale University Press, 1971.

Payer, Lynn. *Disease-Mongers*. New York: John Wiley, 1992.

Peeling, R. W. "Chlamydia trachomatis and *Neisseria gonorrhoeae:* pathogens in retreat?" *Current Opinion in Infectious Diseases* 8 (1995): 26–34.

Peeling, R. W., and Robert C. Brunham. "Chlamydiae as pathogens: New species and new issues," *Emerging Infectious Diseases* 2, no. 4 (October–December 1996): 307–319.

Pennisi, E. "Infectious disease: Cholera strengthened by trip through gut," *Science* 296, no. 5574 (June 7, 2002): 1,783–1,784.

Podolsky, Doug. "Kill the bug and you kill the ulcer," *U.S. News & World Report,* May 13, 1991, 94.

Pounds, J. A., M. R. Bustamante, L. A. Coloma, J. A. Consuegra, et al. "Widespread amphibian extinctions from epidemic disease driven by global warming," *Nature* 439, no. 7073 (January 12, 2006): 161–167.

Prusiner, S. B. "Molecular biology of prion diseases," *Science* 252 (June 14, 1991): 1,515–1,522.

———. "The prion diseases," *Scientific American* 272, no. 1 (January 1995): 48–57.

Prusiner, S. B., ed. *Prion Biology and Diseases.* 2nd ed. Cold Spring Harbor, N.Y.: Cold Spring Harbor Laboratory Press, 2004.

Quetel, Claude. *History of Syphilis.* Baltimore: Johns Hopkins University Press, 1992.

Raloff, Janet. "How climate perturbations can plague us," *Science News* 148 (September 23, 1995): 196–197.

———. "Oldest Lyme-carrying microbes found," *Science News* 148 (December 2, 1995): 373.

———. "Pesticides may challenge human immunity," *Science News* 149 (March 9, 1996): 149.

———. "Stress undercuts flu shots," *Science News* 149 (April 13, 1996): 231.

———. "Antibiotics take a bite out of bad gums," *Science News* 149 (May 18, 1996): 308.

Ramsey, B. W., M. S. Pepe, J. M. Quan, et al. "Intermittent administration of inhaled tobramycin in patients with cystic fibrosis," *New England Journal of Medicine* 340 (1999): 23–30.

Ranger, Terence, and Paul Slack. *Epidemics and Ideas.* Cambridge: Cambridge University Press, 1992.

Rantala, J., et al. "Epidemiology of Guillain-Barre syndrome in children: Relationships of oral polio vaccine administration to occurrence," *Journal of Pediatrics* 124 (1994): 220–223.

Rich, S. M., P. M. Armstrong, R. D. Smith, et al. "Lone star tick-infecting borreliae are most closely related to the agent of bovine borreliosis," *Journal of Clinical Microbiology* 39, no. 2 (February 2001): 494–497.

Rose, C. D., P. T. Fawcett, and K. M. Gibney. "Arthritis following recombinant outer surface protein A vaccination for Lyme disease," *Journal of Rheumatology* 28, no. 11 (November 2001): 2,555–2,557.

Rotavirus Vaccine Program. "Rotavirus." Available at: http://www.rotavirusvaccine.org. Updated 2006.

Sabin, Francene. *Microbes and Bacteria.* Mahwah, N.J.: Troll, 1985.

Saracco, A., et al. "Man-to-woman sexual transmission of HIV: Longitudinal study of 343 steady partners of infected men," *Journal of Acquired Immune Deficiency Syndrome* 6 (1993): 497–502.

Schaechter, M., et al., eds. *Microbial Disease.* Baltimore: Williams & Wilkins, 1993.

Schrag, S., and P. Wiener. "Emerging infectious diseases: What are the relative roles of ecology and evolution?" *Trends in Ecology and Evolution* 10 (1995): 319–323.

Schubert, C. R., K. J. Cruickshanks, T. L. Wiley, R. Klein, B. E. Klein, and T. S. Tweed. "Diphtheria and hearing loss," *Public Health Reports* 116, no. 4 (July–August 2001): 362–368.

Schumm, W. R., E. J. Reppert, A. P. Jurich, et al. "Self-reported changes in subjective health and anthrax vaccination as reported by over 900 Persian Gulf War era veterans," *Psychological Reports* 90, no. 2 (April 2002): 639–653.

Science News. "Turning DNA into an antibiotic," *Science News* 149 (January 20, 1995): 47.

———. "Another round in the prion debate," *Science News* 147 (June 17, 1995): 383.

———. "Tuberculosis gene may explain dormancy," *Science News* 149 (April 20, 1996): 255.

———. "Nitric oxide at war with homocysteine?" *Science News* 149 (April 27, 1996): 269.

———. "Get the infection, not the disease," *Science News* 148 (September 2, 1995): 153.

Seachrist, Lisa. "The once and future scourge: Could common anti-inflammatory drugs allow bacteria to take a deadly turn?" *Science News* 148 (October 7, 1995): 234–235.

———. "Amount of virus sets cancer risk," *Science News* 148 (September 23, 1995): 197.

Shen, Chen-Yang, et al. "Cytomegalovirus Transmission in Special Care Centers for Mentally Retarded Children," *Pediatrics* 91, no. 1 (1993): 517–521.

Shoji, Y., Shimada, J., and Mizushima, Y. "Drug delivery system to control infectious diseases," *Current Pharmaceutical Design* 8, no. 6 (2002): 455–465.

Shulman, Stanford T., et al., eds. *The Biologic and Clinical Basis of Infectious Diseases.* 4th ed. Philadelphia: Saunders, 1992.

Simone, P. M., and M. D. Iseman. "Drug resistant tuberculosis: A deadly and growing danger," *Journal of Respiratory Disease* 13 (1992): 960–971.

Singleton, Paul. *Introduction to Bacteria.* 2nd ed. New York: John Wiley, 1992.

Smeltzer, Suzanne, and Brenda Bare, eds. *Brunner and Suddarth's Textbook of Medical and Surgical Nursing.* 7th ed. New York: Lippincott, 1992.

Smith, A., ed. "Antibiotic Update," *Pediatric Annals* 22, no. 3 (1993).

Smith, J. D. G., et al. "PCR detection of colonization by Helicobacter pylori in conventional euthymic mice based on the 16S ribosomal gene sequence." *Clinical Diagnostic Lab Immunol.* 3 (1996): 66–72.

Squires, Sally. "The most misused medicine in America," *Good Housekeeping,* November 1995, 90–93.

———. "New treatment helps ease pain of shingles," Washington Post News Service, October 24, 1995.

Stanley, S. K., et al. "Effect of immunization with a common recall antigen on viral expression in patients infected with HIV type 1," *New England Journal of Medicine* 334 (1996): 1,222–1,230.

Starke, J. R., R. F. Jacobs, and J. Jereb. "Resurgence of tuberculosis in children," *Journal of Pediatrics* 120 (1992): 839–855.

Steffen, R., and R. H. Behrens. "Travelers' malaria," *Parasitology Today* 8 (1992): 61–66.

Sternberg, Steve. "Human version of mad cow disease?" *Science News* 149 (April 13, 1996): 228.

———. "Chance reveals deadly rotavirus secret," *Science News* 149 (April 6, 1966): 213.

Stoffman, Phyllis. *The Family Guide to Preventing and Treating 100 Infectious Illnesses.* New York: Wiley, 1995.

Stromdahl, E. Y., S. R. Evans, J. J. O'Brien, and A. G. Gutierrez. "Prevalence of infection in ticks submitted to the human tick test kit program of the U.S. Army Center for Health Promotion and Preventive Medicine," *Journal of Medical Entomology* 38, no. 1 (January 2001): 67–74.

Tapper, M. L. "Emerging viral diseases and infectious disease risks," *Haemophilia* 12 (March 2006): 3–7.

Taylor, Jeffrey, et al. "Amebic meningoencephalitis," *Infections in Medicine* 13, no. 12 (1996): 1,017, 1,021, 1,024.

Temte, J. L. "The 2006 Childhood and Adolescent Immunization Schedule: Reflections at the 50th anniversary of the polio vaccine," *American Family Physician* 73, no. 1 (January 1, 2006): 37–40.

Theuretzbacher, U., and J. H. Toney. "Nature's clarion call of antibacterial resistance: Are we listening?" *Current Opinions in Investigational Drugs* 7, no. 2 (February 2006): 158–166.

Tompkins, L. S., and S. Falkow. "The new path to preventing ulcers," *Science* 267 (1995): 1,621–1,622.

Tournier, J. N., A. Jouan, J. Mathieu, and E. Drouet. "Gulf war syndrome: Could it be triggered by biological warfare-vaccines using pertussis as an adjuvant?" *Medical Hypotheses* 58, no. 4 (April 2002): 291–292.

Travis, John. "AIDS update '96: New drugs, new tests, new optimism mark recent AIDS research," *Science News* 149 (March 23, 1996): 184–186.

————. "Body's proteins suppress AIDS virus," *Science News* 148 (December 9, 1995): 388.

————. "Swallowing *Shigella:* Can bacteria that cause food poisoning deliver oral DNA vaccines?" *Science News* 149 (May 11, 1996): 302–303.

————. "Digging into TB's history with genetics," *Science News* 147 (June 3, 1995).

————. "Making big mountains out of tiny bacteria," *Science News* 148 (September 23, 1995): 197.

————. "HIV-2 offers protection against HIV-1," *Science News* 147 (June 17, 1995): 373.

————. "Body's proteins suppress AIDS virus," *Science News* 148 (December 9, 1995): 388.

————. "The worm turns: Into a source of new drugs," *Science News* 149 (March 9, 1996): 148.

U.S. Food and Drug Administration. "Bovine spongiform encephalopathy." Available at http://www.fda.gov/oc/opacom/hottopics/bse.html. June 2005.

Vaz, A., L. Glickstein, J. A. Field, G. McHugh, V. K. Sikand, N. Damle, and A. C. Steere. "Cellular and humoral immune responses to Borrelia burgdorferi antigens in patients with culture-positive early Lyme disease," *Infectious Immunology* 69, no. 12 (December 2001): 7,437–7,444.

Velin, Bob. "FDA takes aim at mad cow disease," *USA Today,* September 12, 1996.

Vento, S., and F. Cainelli. "Childhood infections and autoimmune diseases," *New England Journal of Medicine* 346, no. 22 (May 30, 2002): 1,749–1,750.

Vila, Ileana, et al. "Chronic Q fever in an avian," *Infections in Medicine* 13, no. 11 (1996): 977–988.

Vinetz, J. M., et al. "Sporadic urban leptospirosis," *Annals of Internal Medicine* 125 (1996): 794–798.

Vlacha, V., et al. "Recurrent thrombocytopenic purpura after repeated MMR vaccination," *Pediatrics* 97 (1996): 73–79.

Vogt, Shelly. "Psittacosis," *Veterinary Technician* 15 (September 1, 1994): 483.

Walker, D. H., and J. S. Dumler. "Emergence of the erlichioses as human health problems," *Emerging Infectious Diseases* 2, no. 1 (1996): 18–29.

Wallace, M. R., B. R. Hale, G. C. Utz, P. E. Olson, K. C. Earhart, S. A. Thornton, and K. C. Hyams, "Endemic infectious diseases of Afghanistan," *Clinical Infectious Diseases* 34, suppl. 5 (June 15, 2002): S171–S207.

Walsh, J. H., and W. Peterson. "The treatment of *Helicobacter pylori* infection in the management of peptic ulcer disease," *The New England Journal of Medicine* 333, no. 15 (October 12, 1995): 984.

Watson, D. A., and D. M. Musher. "The pneumococcus: sugar-coated killer," *Infections in Medicine* 13, no. 5, (1996): 373–376, 379–381, 429–432.

Whitley, R. J., and D. T. Durack, eds. *Infections of the Central Nervous System.* New York: River Press, 1991.

Will, R. G., et al. "A new variant of Creutzfeldt-Jakob disease in the UK," *Lancet* 347 (1996): 921–925.

Williams, D., and D. Churchill. "Ulcerative proctitis in men who have sex with men: An emerging outbreak," *British Medical Journal* 332, no. 7533 (January 14, 2006): 99–100.

Williams, Gurney. "8 New Health Threats: How to protect your family," *Family Circle,* October 8, 1996, 66–76.

Williams, J. D., and J. Burnie, eds. *The Epidemiology of Acute Bacterial Meningitis in Tropical Africa.* New York: Academic Press, 1987.

Wilson, Mary E. *A World Guide to Infections.* New York: Oxford University Press, 1991.

Woolhouse, M. E., and S. Gowtage-Sequeria. "Host range and emerging and reemerging pathogens," *Emerging Infectious Diseases* 11, no. 12 (December 2005): 1,842–1,847.

World Health Organization. "Nipah virus." Available at: http://www.who.int/mediacentre/factsheets/fs262/en. Updated September 2001.

Wotherspoon, A. C., et al. "*Helicobacter pylori*–associated gastritis and primary B-cell gastric lymphoma," *Lancet* 338 (1991): 1,175–1,176.

Wynia, M. K., and L. Gostin. "Medicine. The bioterrorist threat and access to health care," *Science* 296: 5573 (May 31, 2002): 1,613.

Yamauchi, T., et al. "Transmission of live, attenuated mumps virus to the human placenta," *New England Journal of Medicine* 290 (1974): 710–712.

Yoshikawa, T. T. "Resistant pathogens: considerations in geriatrics and infectious disease," *Journal of the American Geriatric Society* 50, no. 7 (July 2, 2002): 225.

Young, M. H., N. C. Engleberg, Z. D. Mulla, and D. M. Aronoff. "Therapies for necrotising fasciitis," *Expert Opinions in Biological Therapy* 6, no. 2 (February 2006): 155–165.

Zamula, Evelyn. "Adults need tetanus shots, too," *FDA Consumer* (July–August 1996): 13–18.

Zhang, Y., K. Post-Martens, and S. Denkin. "New drug candidates and therapeutic targets for tuberculosis therapy," *Drug Discoveries Today* 11, no. 1–2 (January 2006): 21–27.

Zimmerman, R. K. "Lowering the age for routine influenza vaccination to 50 years AAFP leads the nation in influenza vaccine policy," *American Family Physician* 60 (1999): 2,061–2,070.

Zitter, J. N., P. D. Mazonson, D. P. Miller, S. B. Hulley, and J. R. Balmes. "Aircraft cabin air recirculation and symptoms of the common cold," *Journal of the American Medical Association* 288, no. 4 (July 2002): 483–486.

Zoloth, L., and S. Zoloth. "Don't be chicken: Bioethics and avian flu," *American Journal of Bioethics* 6, no. 1 (January–February 2006): 5–8.

INDEX

Page numbers in **boldface** indicate major treatment of a topic.

A